*The Columbia University
College of Physicians
and Surgeons*

COMPLETE
GUIDE TO
EARLY
CHILD CARE

The Columbia University College of Physicians and Surgeons

MEDICAL EDITORS

NICHOLAS CUNNINGHAM, M.D., DR. P.H.
*Professor of Clinical Pediatrics and
Director of Pediatric Services
Columbia Presbyterian Medical Center*

DONALD F. TAPLEY, M.D.
*Senior Deputy Vice-President for Health Sciences
Alumni Professor of Medicine*

EDITORIAL DIRECTOR
GENELL J. SUBAK-SHARPE, M.S.

ASSOCIATE EDITOR
DIANE M. GOETZ

COMPLETE GUIDE TO EARLY CHILD CARE

Crown Publishers, Inc.

NEW YORK

Figures 21.2, 21.3, 21.4, and 21.5 from *If Your Child Has a Congenital Heart Defect: A Guide for Parents*,
copyright © 1987, reproduced by permission of the American Heart Association.
Figures 21.6, 23.2, 34.1, 34.2, 34.3, 34.4, and 34.5 from *The Columbia University College of Physicians
and Surgeons Home Medical Guide*, rev. ed., copyright © 1989, reproduced by permission of Crown
Publishers, Inc.

Published by Crown Publishers, Inc., 201 East 50th Street, New York, New York 10022

CROWN is a trademark of Crown Publishers, Inc.

Manufactured in the United States of America

Library of Congress Cataloging-in-Publication Data

The Columbia University College of Physicians and Surgeons complete guide to early child care /
   edited by the College of Physicians and Surgeons at Columbia University.
      p.   cm.
   Bibliography: p.
   Includes index.
      1. Children—Health and hygiene.   2. Children—Diseases.
   3. Pediatrics—Popular works.   I. Columbia University. College of Physicians and Surgeons.
   RJ61.C69 1990
   618.92—dc20   89-15859
                                                                                  CIP

ISBN 0-517-57217-6

10 9 8 7 6 5 4 3 2 1

First Edition

Contents

Acknowledgments

COMPILING A BOOK OF THIS SCOPE and comprehensiveness obviously requires the knowledge, skills, and dedication of scores of people—far too many to list on a single page. While it is impossible to cite every person who has worked on this book, there are some whose efforts certainly must be acknowledged.

Foremost, we are deeply indebted to the scores of dedicated physicians, nurses, and other health professionals at the Columbia University College of Physicians and Surgeons and the Columbia-Presbyterian Medical Center who have worked on this book. It is their special insight gained only through years of patient care, teaching, and research that makes this book truly unique. These busy health professionals have found time in their already overloaded schedules to write chapters, check facts, and provide invaluable guidance. In addition to the contributors of various chapters, a note of appreciation goes to Drs. Lawrence Savetsky and Hugh Moss, who reviewed chapter drafts and added useful suggestions.

A team of medical writers and editors also has been instrumental in creating this book. They include Sue Berkman, Jean Fitzpatrick, Connie Grzelka, Judy Hoffmann, Rebecca Hughes, Susan Ince, Marjorie Joyce, Hedi Levine, Dawn Micklethwaite, Joy Nowlin, Prabhu Ponkshe, George Ryan, Caroline Tapley, Antonia van der Meer, Graham Yost, and Stephanie Young. They have been assisted by Desiree Cooper, Sara Gelbaum, Elena Villegas, Hope Subak-Sharpe, and Sarah Subak-Sharpe.

A team of talented medical artists and illustrators also have worked on this book. The original drawings have been provided by Lauren Keswick and Hilda R. Muiños. Art also has been supplied by Marsha Dohrmann, Neil Hardy, and the American Heart Association.

To our editors at Crown—Betty Prashker, David Groff, and Laurie Stark, as well as Pamela Stinson, producton editor, and Bill Peabody, production supervisor—go our special thanks for their support, patience, and sharp eyes. Copy editor Margaret Wolf and designer Peggy Goddard deserve special mention for their efforts in bringing this manuscript to fruition.

Finally, hats off to the many spouses who have pitched in to do everything from babysitting to proofreading. Their help and understanding have soothed frazzled tempers and calmed jittery nerves—the inevitable occupational hazards in creating any book.

The Editors

DONALD F. TAPLEY, M.D., Alumni Professor of Medicine and Senior Deputy Vice President for the Health Sciences, has spent most of his medical career at the College of Physicians and Surgeons. After completing a fellowship at Oxford University, he joined the P&S faculty as an assistant professor of medicine in 1956, rising to dean in 1974. During his ten-year tenure as dean, Dr. Tapley presided over the tremendous growth of the institution and is widely acknowledged as one of the most notable medical school deans in the nation. His medical specialty is endocrinology, and over the years he has published a number of papers in this field, with special emphasis on the role of the thyroid hormones.

NICHOLAS CUNNINGHAM, M.D., DR. P.H., started at Columbia as a pediatric resident in 1959, with degrees from Harvard and Johns Hopkins. After a neonatal fellowship at Babies Hospital, he was appointed volunteer leader of the first U.S. Peace Corps medical project in Togo. Today he continues his international health interest as a pediatric consultant to the Nigerian government. Returning to Columbia Presbyterian Medical Center in 1977, he was appointed director of the division of general pediatrics. As Professor of Clinical Pediatrics and Public Health at the College of Physicians and Surgeons, he became interested in the epidemiology of child maltreatment. In 1981 Dr. Cunningham cofounded and now directs the Presbyterian Hospital Therapeutic Nursery, which serves as a locus for teaching and research, as well as providing clinical services to troubled families.

GENELL J. SUBAK-SHARPE, M.S., is a medical writer and editor who began her journalism career on the metropolitan staff of the *New York Times*. Since then, she has served as vice president of Biomedical Information Company and as editor of a number of magazines for both physicians and consumers and is the author, coauthor, or editor of more than thirty books in health and medicine. She is now president of her own medical communications company.

DIANE M. GOETZ is a medical writer and editor who specializes in preventive health topics for the general public. She was on the staff of the American Heart Association, New York City Affiliate, for ten years, ultimately serving as vice president for communications. She holds a B.A. in journalism from the University of Wisconsin and an M.B.A. from New York University. She is editor of *Weight Watchers Women's Health* and *Fitness News*, a monthly newsletter.

Contributors

FRED AGRE, M.D.
Clinical Professor of Pediatrics

ELIZABETH ANISFELD, PH.D.
Associate Research Scientist

STEPHEN J. ATWOOD, M.D.
Associate Professor of Clinical Pediatrics

ROSEMARY BARBER-MADDEN, ED.D.
Associate Clinical Professor of Public Health
Director, Maternal and Child Health Program

FRED BOMBACK, M.D.
Associate Clinical Professor of Pediatrics

CAROL ANN BROWN, R.N., M.S.
Associate in Clinical Nursing
Pediatric Nurse Practitioner

PENELOPE BUSCHMAN, R.N., M.S.
Assistant Professor of Clinical Nursing
Research Nurse Clinician

ALLAN S. CUNNINGHAM, M.D.
Associate Clinical Professor of Pediatrics
Attending Pediatrician, The Mary Imogene
Bassett Hospital, Cooperstown, N.Y.

NICHOLAS CUNNINGHAM, M.D., DR. P.H.
Professor of Clinical Pediatrics and Clinical
Public Health

LESLIE DAVIDSON, M.D.
Assistant Professor, Pediatrics and Public Health
(Epidemiology) in the G. H. Sergievsky Center

MARTIN J. DAVIS, D.D.S.
Director, Division of Pediatric Dentistry, and
Chief, Comprehensive Care Section

WILLIAM J. DAVIS, M.D.
Clinical Professor of Pediatrics
Director, Division of Allergy

RICHARD J. DECKELBAUM, M.D.
Associate Professor of Pediatrics
Director, Division of Gastroenterology
and Nutrition

DARRYL DEVIVO, M.D.
Sidney Carter Professor of Neurology
Professor of Pediatrics
Director of Pediatric Neurology

JOHN M. DRISCOLL, JR., M.D.
Professor of Pediatrics

CANDACE ERICKSON, M.D.
Assistant Professor of Clinical Pediatrics
Director of Behavioral and Developmental
Pediatrics

CHARMAINE FITZIG, R.N., DR. P.H.
Associate Director, Nurse Anesthesia Program,
Harlem Hospital
Lecturer, Columbia University School of Public
Health

ANNE A. GERSHON, M.D.
Professor of Pediatrics
Director of Pediatric Infectious Disease

WELTON M. GERSONY, M.D.
Professor of Pediatrics
Director, Division of Pediatric Cardiology

ARTHUR H. GREEN, M.D.
Medical Director, Family Center
Clinical Director, Therapeutic Nursing
Associate Clinical Professor of Psychiatry
Associate Clinical Professor of Psychiatry of
Pediatrics

TERRY W. HENSLE, M.D.
Professor of Clinical Urology
Director of Pediatric Urology

MATILDE IRIGOYEN, M.D.
Associate Clinical Professor of Pediatrics

STANLEY JAMES, M.D.
Professor of Pediatrics and of Obstetrics
and Gynecology

KENNETH KATZ, M.D.
Assistant Professor of Clinical Pediatrics

JOSEPH LEVY, M.D.
Associate Professor of Clinical Pediatrics
Director of Clinical Gastrointestinal Service

HARRIET McGURK, M.D.
Associate Clinical Professor of Pediatrics

ROBERT B. MELLINS, M.D.
Professor of Pediatrics
Director, Pediatrics Pulmonary Division

MARTIN A. NASH, M.D.
Associate Professor of Clinical Pediatrics
Director of Pediatric Nephrology

MICHAEL NOVOGRODER, M.D.
Associate Professor of Pediatrics

SERGIO PIOMELLI, M.D.
Professor of Pediatrics

KENNETH PITUCH, M.D.
Assistant Professor of Clinical Pediatrics

DAVID ROYE, M.D.
Assistant Professor of Orthopedic Surgery

DAVID SHAFFER, M.D.
Irving Philips Professor of Child Psychiatry
Professor of Psychiatry and Pediatrics
Director, Division of Child Psychiatry

MARGARET STILLMAN, M.D.
Assistant Clinical Professor of Pediatrics

PAUL D. TRAUTMAN, M.D.
Assistant Professor of Clinical Psychiatry

GAIL A. WASSERMAN, PH.D.
Associate Professor of Psychiatry

FOREWORD
How to Use This Book

THERE IS LITTLE DOUBT that parenting today is much different from only a generation ago when the norm was that mothers tended home and children, and fathers were the financial providers. Today, more than half of all mothers work outside the home, and fathers are expected to assume a greater role in child rearing.

In the past, there usually were grandparents, aunts, and other relatives—often in the same household or at least nearby—to give advice and lend a hand when needed. Today, generations are likely to be scattered across the country and unavailable to pitch in.

Even when it comes to medical problems, today's parents are expected to assume a greater responsibility than in the past. Thanks to advanced medical knowledge and technology, many diseases that went untreated a few years ago are now highly treatable. Much of this treatment is delivered by parents in the home.

Attitudes toward child rearing also have changed. Parents today are apt to be older and to have fewer children than in past generations. And they are more determined than ever to "do it right." Faced with increased responsibilities and demands but with fewer resources for help, these parents need all the good information they can get. This book is intended to provide that information.

Dozens of leading pediatric specialists at Columbia University's College of Physicians and Surgeons have participated in creating the *Complete Guide to Early Child Care*. It differs from other books for parents in that it combines in one convenient volume in-depth discussions of normal growth and development as well as routine and more serious medical problems. Any parent will find useful the practical issues such as outfitting a nursery, picking a daycare center, and caring and feeding a newborn that are covered. Fortunately most parents are not faced with caring for seriously ill babies, but those who are also can turn to this book.

Obviously, this book is not intended to substitute for your pediatrician or family physician. Your family doctors are the best source of advice regarding your child. But you should use this book as a point of reference, both to better understand a particular problem or issue and to determine whether you should seek advice from a health professional. Many of the routine illnesses of childhood quickly resolve themselves; others require prompt medical attention. This book is designed to help you tell one from the other. With it, you can be a more informed partner in caring for your child's medical needs. And you can turn to it for practical advice and information on dealing with the day-to-day nonmedical aspects of child care.

1 Before the Baby Is Born

Fred Bomback, M.D.

INTRODUCTION

DURING THE LATTER part of pregnancy, many women (and some men) experience an urge to prepare for the baby's arrival that is popularly known as the "nesting instinct." Happily, it tends to inspire parents to do all they can to make life safer and healthier for the baby after birth.

CHOOSING A PEDIATRICIAN

THE MOST SENSIBLE TIME to choose a pediatrician is in advance of delivery. Most parents-to-be schedule a prenatal visit with a pediatrician, or several pediatricians, late in the third trimester of pregnancy. At this interview they may decide which pediatrician they wish to select, or if they have made that decision, ask questions about baby care—thus benefiting from the pediatrician's advice in considerably greater calm than will be possible in later visits.

The relationship parents develop with their child's pediatrician is often unique. Over the years, through checkups and crises, most get to know the pediatrician better than any other physician. Meeting the pediatrician in advance is important. For mothers, it helps provide a smooth transition from the rapport with her obstetrician, with whom she shared her concerns during pregnancy, to that with the pediatrician who will be a partner in her child's health care. For the father, this is an opportunity to begin to share as an equal partner in parenting.

Prenatal visits are recommended for all parents, but especially for those with high-risk pregnancies, complications, multiple gestation (twins, triplets), and those who have previously experienced miscarriage or stillbirth. Usually there is no charge for this visit, although some pediatricians will send a bill if the parents choose not to use them later on.

The pediatrician views the prenatal visit as an opportunity to establish a relationship with the family, to obtain medical information (such as how the pregnancy has been, the parents' medical histories, and the family history), and to stress the importance of safety issues (such as the need for a car seat on the trip home from the hospital).

The parents may wish to discuss preparations for the baby's arrival, issues surrounding the delivery and hospital stay, including childbirth classes, rooming-in, breastfeeding, and circumcision. This is a good time to ask questions about the pediatrician's role at and after delivery, office and telephone procedures, and approach to the type of feeding (breast or bottle) that the parents are considering. (See box atop next page for common questions.) In addition to obtaining specific information, this is a valuable opportunity to gauge the physician's overall atti-

QUESTIONS FOR PARENTS TO ASK THE PEDIATRICIAN

- What are the usual intervals for routine examinations and immunizations?
- What are the pediatrician's office hours? Do the hours accommodate working parents?
- Is the pediatrician willing to attend to a child accompanied by a caretaker other than the parents? If so, is previous authorization required?
- How busy is the pediatrician? How long does it take to get an appointment?
- Does the pediatrician have a telephone calling hour? If not, are there particular hours when he or she prefers to be called?
- With which hospital or hospitals is the pediatrician affiliated?
- What are the usual fees?
- Who is on call when the pediatrician is not available?
- If this is a group practice, may the parents choose which physician to see?
- What is the policy concerning insurance?
- Is the pediatrician willing to participate in early discharge (through early examination of the baby and follow-up exams during the first few days)?
- What is the pediatrician's attitude toward breastfeeding?
- What if the mother can't breastfeed?
- Will there be someone to help the mother with breastfeeding in the hospital?
- If the baby is a boy, should he be circumcised?
- Does the pediatrician recommend any parenting classes in the area?
- Does the pediatrician recommend any books for parents to read or have on hand?
- How does the pediatrician assess appropriate weight gain in infants?
- When does the pediatrician start infants on solid foods?

tude and personality so that the parents can decide whether they feel comfortable with the doctor.

In today's mobile society, new mothers and fathers are often unable to turn to their own parents for advice or support, and they often have had little experience or exposure to children. As a result, pediatricians are often pressed into a role much like that of the old "family doctor." With the increasing awareness among parents of the importance of the child's emotional health, the pediatrician is often turned to for advice in areas that go beyond direct health care questions. (The box below lists

QUESTIONS THE PEDIATRICIAN MAY ASK

These may be asked personally or by means of a questionnaire that the parents fill out in the office before the interview.

- Are there any genetic diseases or birth defects in the parents' families?
- Does either parent have any allergic, metabolic, neurologic, cardiovascular, respiratory, or other serious disease?
- Has this been an "easy" pregnancy or have any problems developed?
- Are the parents married? How long have they been married?
- Is this the couple's first pregnancy?
- What have the parents read about baby care?
- Are the parents attending prenatal classes?
- Is the mother planning to breastfeed?
- Who lives in the parents' household?
- Who will help with the housework and siblings when the baby comes home from the hospital?
- Do the parents smoke?
- Have the parents bought a car seat?
- Are there smoke detectors or fire extinguishers in the home?
- What is the educational background of the parents?
- What do the parents do for a living?
- Are both parents planning to return to work after the birth? If so, how soon afterward?
- Have the parents decided about circumcision if the baby is a boy?
- Was this a convenient time for the parents to have a baby?
- How do the parents think having a baby will change their lives?
- Do the parents plan to bring up the baby as they were raised? What do they intend to do differently?
- Any special worries?

the kinds of questions a pediatrician may ask parents.)

For this reason, the parents should feel that the pediatrician is responsive to their concerns. No parent should feel ill at ease about asking questions. Nor should any parent be made to feel ignorant for his or her queries. Some pediatricians schedule specific telephone hours each morning, others answer questions throughout the day. Many have the office nurse field some of the questions and direct others to the doctors. None should object if the parents call at night with a real problem. There is no need for parents to feel guilty or foolish about their anxieties —pediatricians themselves have plenty of anxiety about their own children. If a child suddenly develops a large bruise, for example, the typical parent might wonder whether the child is being bullied in the playground. The pediatrician, on the other hand, may recognize such a bruise as a possible symptom of a blood disorder.

TOURING THE HOSPITAL

HOSPITALS VARY CONSIDERABLY in their routines, facilities (birthing chair, birthing room), visiting policies (hours for fathers and siblings), and the type of support they offer new families after the birth (newborn care classes, breastfeeding advice, 24-hour "warm line" parents can call after mother and child have returned home for advice). During the third trimester, a visit to the maternity unit where the baby will be born can be a very reassuring experience for both parents and siblings. The opportunity to see the labor, delivery, and birthing rooms, and to talk with the nurses, makes the coming birth more real and the hospital less strange. And looking through the glass, if there is one, at the nursery may reassure parents-to-be, who inevitably worry about the health of their baby: they can see how many healthy babies, in a variety of shapes, sizes, and temperaments, are born every day. If they are considering rooming-in, they can see the arrangement of rooms provided for this purpose.

This visit may be a regular part of the parents' childbirth education classes, or they may prefer to schedule one privately. The accompanying box lists some questions to ask during the hospital tour. It is helpful to obtain specific answers to these questions, but more important is the opportunity to get a sense of the staff's overall attitude and approach to birth and the newborn—whether the hospital is providing care that is sensitive and personal, or highly conservative and routine.

QUESTIONS FOR PARENTS TO ASK OF HOSPITAL STAFF MEMBERS

- What procedures (shaving, enema, IV, fetal monitoring, silver nitrate drops or ointment) are done routinely?
- What is the policy concerning the presence of husbands and others during labor and delivery? Must the father show proof of attendance at a childbirth preparation course? May he attend a cesarean birth?
- What is the hospital's attitude toward prepared childbirth? Are the nurses trained in Lamaze or another prepared childbirth method?
- Does the hospital have a birthing chair?
- Is the hospital willing to cooperate with a Leboyer birth (dimming the lights during delivery, allowing the mother to hold the baby immediately, delaying cutting the cord, allowing the father to give the newborn a warm bath)?
- Is there rooming-in, or modified rooming-in? This enables the mother to keep the baby with her—for nursing, cuddling, bathing, and diaper changing— right from the start. If the hospital does not have this policy, the baby will be brought in on a regular feeding schedule or on demand, but will be cared for primarily in the nursery.
- What are the visiting hours and who can visit? This includes hospital policy on fathers, siblings, and grandparents.
- Are there parenting classes? Many maternity units offer lessons—either to groups of new parents or informally—in how to bathe the baby, or how to breastfeed successfully. They may also hold group discussions where new mothers can share their feelings and anxieties about the birth and the new baby.
- Is the staff supportive of breastfeeding? If the mother is planning to nurse her baby, it is important that the maternity unit nurses be attuned to her wishes: whether she wants to be awakened for night feedings, does not want the baby fed sugar water, needs help with positioning during the first few feedings, or seeks advice about breast care.

THE PEDIATRICIAN AT THE BIRTH

THE PEDIATRICIAN'S ROLE at the time of the birth depends primarily on the procedure followed by the hospital and the obstetrician. The obstetrician will inform the pediatrician of any condition that may call for his or her attendance at the birth. These may include maternal disease (such as toxemia) or chronic medical conditions (hypertension, pulmonary disease, or diabetes); fetal prematurity, or birth before 37 weeks of gestation, or postmaturity, after 42 weeks; conditions that may require a cesarean section; an abnormal fetal heart rate; meconium-stained amniotic fluid; multiple births; an abnormal pattern or length of labor; or unusual presentation (such as a breech birth).

Virtually all tertiary-care facilities require a pediatrician to be in attendance in the case of a cesarean section. But in a smaller community hospital, pediatricians may not be as readily available, and the obstetrician and anesthesiologist are invariably experienced in newborn resuscitation. The fact that a pediatrician is called in to attend a birth should be no cause for alarm—nine out of ten times this is nothing more than a precautionary measure.

The baby will be examined extensively by the pediatrician within 24 hours of delivery. (The pediatrician may see the baby sooner, but if the birth occurs right after pediatric rounds, the baby will be seen on the next rounds.) But parents can rest assured that the baby will be examined at least twice during the first 24 hours—for color, activity, and cry —by the nursing staff and the obstetrician or midwife. From then on, the pediatrician will examine the baby at least every other day until the time of discharge, assuming the baby is his only patient in the hospital nursery. If he has others there, he will often see each one daily.

If the baby is a boy, a circumcision may be performed in the hospital after he has had some time to recover from the trauma of birth. Before the due date, parents should discuss with the pediatrician whether or not they wish to have a boy circumcised. (See box.)

Circumcisions are usually performed by the obstetrician, but the pediatrician should provide parents with enough information to enable them to make a rational decision. Also, the parents can ask about what type of anesthesia is available for the procedure.

CIRCUMCISION CONSIDERATIONS

Circumcision is the surgical removal of the sleeve of skin (the prepuce or foreskin) that covers the head of the penis. Although circumcision is the most commonly performed operation in the United States (it is estimated that two-thirds of American males have been circumcised), it is beginning to decline in popularity. Outside of English-speaking countries, the operation has never been routinely done except for religious reasons, and it is gradually being abandoned everywhere. In England, for example, less than one percent of newborn males are now circumcised.

In addition to the reason of religious practice, circumcision continues to be popular in the United States because many parents believe that it is medically indicated or because they believe there will be a psychological impact on their son if he does not look like his circumcised father or other boys.

Parents considering circumcision for other than religious reasons should be aware that there is no evidence that the procedure protects against disease, with the possible exception of urinary tract infection. In fact, both the American Academy of Pediatrics and the American College of Obstetrics and Gynecology have taken a position against routine circumcision of infants. Most physicians believe that parents can adequately reassure their son about a difference in the appearance of his penis, just as they would other differences in appearance.

Circumcision is painful, even with local anesthesia, which should be used if not proscribed by religious practice. There may also be side effects, although these are relatively rare. One of the most common is irritation of the meatus—the hole through which the urine is passed.

Although urinary tract infection in boys is rare, it does appear to be more common in uncircumcised baby boys. This may be related to attempts by the parent or caregiver to retract the foreskin during bathing. There is no reason to do so; the foreskin should be gently sponged along with the rest of the penis.

Sometime before the child starts school, usually by age two or three, the uncircumcised foreskin will separate naturally from the glans of the penis. After this happens, the foreskin can be gently pushed back during bathing in order to clean any secretions from the glans.

PLANNING THE BABY'S ROOM

AS PARENTS BEGIN to ready the baby's room or sleeping area, there are many factors to consider. In addition to making the room attractive and providing visual stimulation for the baby, it is important to keep comfort and safety in mind.

For the first few weeks, or until the bassinet has been outgrown, many parents choose to keep the baby in their room. However, it is probably a mistake not to plan for a separate sleeping area in advance. Eventually a separate area will be needed, and planning a nursery before the baby is born is considerably less hectic than doing it afterward. Of course, the baby does not necessarily need a room of his or her own, but a quiet place to sleep and be changed is essential.

Although a newborn can sleep in a crib, a cozier space is preferable. A bassinet, "Moses basket," or even a laundry basket or drawer can be fitted with a small mattress and blanket for the newborn. Some parents may want the baby in bed with them for the first few months. However, after six weeks or two months, depending on the size of the baby, most families find that it is time to move the baby into the crib.

Be sure to select a crib with slats less than 2⅜ inches apart and a snug-fitting mattress (the parent should not be able to fit two fingers between the mattress and the sides of the crib). Do not use a crib with missing slats. Avoid cribs with high corner posts (these can sometimes be unscrewed) or cutouts in the head- or footboards (these have caused strangulation, either by trapping the baby's head or catching onto clothes or pacifiers). The crib should have teething rails; if these are missing, replacements are widely available. (See figure 1.1 for safety features.) Avoid placing the crib near a window. If a used crib is to be repainted, it is important to use nontoxic paint and to paint in a well-ventilated area, especially if the expectant mother does the painting.

To prevent the baby from banging his or her head against the slats, bumper pads are available. The vinyl type are often inexpensive and can be wiped clean, but cloth bumpers are far more comfortable for the baby and are machine-washable. Be sure there are enough ribbons or ties to secure them tightly to the sides of the crib. Cribs usually only have fitted bottom sheets, no top sheets. A soft quilt will suffice to keep the baby warm. Decorative crib pillows are widely sold but they are a hazard to

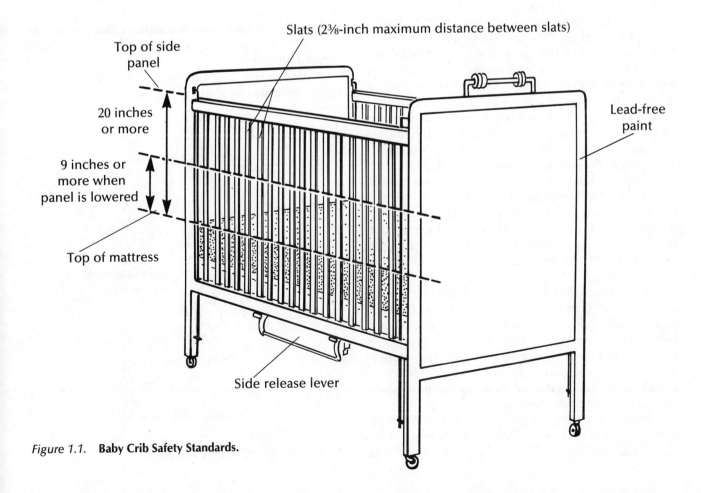

Figure 1.1. **Baby Crib Safety Standards.**

infants, who risk being smothered because they cannot raise their heads.

In selecting window coverings, keep in mind that although the baby's sleep patterns are unlikely to be synchronized with night and day at first, a toddler will fall asleep much more readily in a darkened room. Room-darkening shades, blinds, or draperies are all good choices, but avoid those with hanging cords (children have strangled on them). Tension wheels that attach drapery cords to the wall can be purchased, or the cords can be tied up during the day when the baby is on the floor.

Changing tables designed for the purpose are widely available, as are dressers with changing tops that can be removed when the child is out of diapers. But any sturdy surface about waist height can be used for changing the baby if an inexpensive changing pad is put on top. A pad can also be placed right in the crib at changing time.

If the thermostat is set low in order to save fuel, a space heater in the baby's room may be useful. Kerosene heaters are unsafe, and others can give a crawling baby a bad burn. Many parents prefer small electric blower heaters that can be placed high out of reach, or oil-circulating heaters that can be set low and operate in much the same way as hot-water radiators. Do not place the heater near the crib or beside any flammable material.

Many infants benefit from increased humidity in the room while they are sleeping, especially in cold weather when heating systems make indoor air very dry. Inexpensive cold-water humidifiers are widely available, but also consider an ultrasonic humidifier, which is far less messy to use and will not soak the baby's blankets when placed near the crib. To prevent bacteria from building up inside, the humidifier should be cleaned regularly; solutions are available to prevent the growth of molds.

Until the baby can sit up—at around six months—neither a highchair nor a walker will be needed; the use of either before this age may cause back problems. Many parents put babies three or four months old in a playpen occasionally to get them used to it, but a playpen can be borrowed or purchased later.

A mobile, either purchased or homemade, is an excellent first crib toy. Try to find one that is bright and appealing from the baby's perspective. If parents decide on a "crib gym," it is important to remember that a number of infants have been caught in them and strangled to death. Crib gyms should be removed as soon as the baby can push up on hands or knees, around five months.

Until about eight weeks, a newborn baby cannot hold a toy but will enjoy focusing on things—especially parents' faces. But bright rattles and balls, especially red ones, will attract interest. Rattles small enough to be swallowed should be avoided, as should those that seem likely to break into pieces small enough to pose a choking hazard. Newborn infants cannot grasp things, but there are rattles that can be attached to the baby's wrist.

A windup swing is often a wonderful way to lull an infant to sleep. Some infant swings come with a bassinet attachment suitable for a baby too young to sit up; the child should always be strapped in and never left unattended.

THE MOBILE BABY

THE MOST IMPORTANT piece of equipment parents can buy for today's traveling infant is a car safety seat. By some estimates, car seats can reduce traffic deaths among young children by as much as 80 percent. All states now have child-restraint laws requiring that children under a certain age or weight ride in an approved car seat. In choosing a car seat, be sure to check that the seat will fit in the family car; some rear and bucket seats, and some seatbelts will not hold rear-facing infant seats or large car seats. Practically speaking, the best car seat is one that comes with a clear set of instructions and is simple to use—because it is essential that the car seat be used every single time the child rides in the car. (Figure 1.2 shows a model that includes essential safety features.)

Infant seats are designed to be used in the rear-facing position so that in the event of an accident,

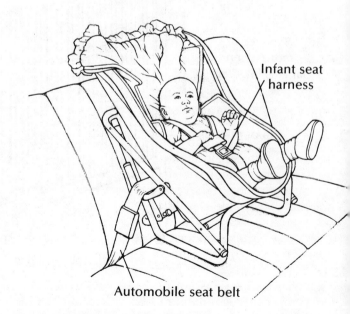

Infant seat harness

Automobile seat belt

Figure 1.2. **Model Infant Car Seat.**

the baby will be pressed down into the car seat, and the back—which is the strongest part of the baby's body—will absorb most of the impact. (At this stage, the head and neck are not strong enough to withstand a crash if the baby is facing forward). The safest place for a baby to ride is in the middle of the back seat. However, some parents feel this presents a driving hazard—it is impossible to keep an eye on the road *and* on the baby—and prefer to put the infant seat (still facing backward) on the front passenger seat. Inexpensive locking clips are available to fit shoulder-harness seatbelts; placed across both the lap and shoulder portion of the belt at the buckle, they keep the belt from sliding through the eye of the buckle and loosening its hold on the infant seat.

Although many seats are designed to be convertible from infant to toddler sizes, they often provide little support for an infant. Parents can buy a car-seat liner or use a rolled-up blanket to support a newborn's head. A cloth cover is more comfortable next to the baby's skin than the seat's vinyl upholstery, and protects against burns when the car has been left out in the hot sun. Cloth upholstery is difficult to clean unless it is designed for easy removal.

If a seat of the older design that requires a tether is bought or borrowed, the tether must be in place —bolted to the cargo floor—or the car seat will not be effective.

It is important to be sure there are no large, loose objects—such as stereo speakers—in the car, because these can hurt a child (even if in a car seat). And adults and other children riding in the car must also be belted in since they might crush a baby in the event of an accident.

A reclining stroller is a better investment than a carriage because the baby can ride in it as an infant, and ride seated in it later. Also, it can be easily folded and put into the car. A model with a reversible handle that allows the parent to walk facing the baby is best. The stroller should have a seatbelt or harness as well as a brake.

Even better than a stroller, for the first few months, is a soft baby carrier. This front carrier pouch, strapped onto the parent's shoulders, provides a convenient way for the parent to hold the baby close and still have two free hands. The carrier should have wide shoulder straps for stability for the parent's comfort, and it should provide ample head and neck support for the baby. The baby should be carried as much as possible, indoors as well as out, and by the father as well as the mother. For times when it is not practical to have the baby in the soft carrier, an infant seat, which can be easily carried from one room to another, is a good investment. It gives the baby a "perch" from which to watch household goings-on. It should have a stable base and a safety belt or harness. Neither a front carrier nor an infant seat is safe to use as a car seat.

For changing and feeding the baby away from home, a diaper bag with space for diapers, wipes, bottles, and other paraphernalia is essential. Do not store milk or formula, except in unopened cans, in the bag—even in a thermal container.

CLOTHING AND ACCESSORIES

IN THE PAST, parents tended to overdress their children—particularly in cold weather. Today most pediatricians recommend that babies be dressed more or less like their parents, with the addition of a cap or hat for warmth in the winter and protection from the sun in the summer. In the winter, babies' feet need to be kept warm. The traditional booties are impractical because they are easily kicked off; fortunately, many infant garments come with attached "feet."

Clothing made of 100 percent cotton is most comfortable against the baby's skin. However, the law requires that sleepwear be made of flame-retardant materials, which usually means synthetic fabrics. Although TRIS, a chemical flame retardant believed to cause skin cancer, has been banned by the Consumer Product Safety Commission, it has not disappeared from the marketplace; check labels carefully, and avoid buying sleepwear without labels. Many fibers lose their flame-resistance when washed with soap or soap flakes; use regular laundry detergent.

No matter how charming a baby's clothing looks, it is unlikely to have lasting appeal for parents unless it can be quickly and easily taken off for frequent diaper changes. Look for snaps under the crotch, zipper and Velcro fasteners, and simple, one-piece styles such as the popular "stretchie." Since babies grow quickly, most parents buy three- or six-month clothing for newborns. Keep in mind that sizes vary considerably from one brand to another, and garments shrink in the wash. Unless the baby is premature, limit purchases of newborn-size clothes to one outfit to be worn home from the hospital.

Even if disposable diapers are going to be used, it is a good idea to have a dozen cloth diapers on hand to protect parents' clothing while feeding or burping the baby. And even though the baby will not be eating solid food for a few months, bibs are useful for keeping the baby's clothes clean.

The best way to prevent diaper rash is to change the baby as necessary, rather than relying on powders, creams, and oils. Oils and lotions may stop the

BABY CHECKLIST

No baby needs every item on the list. Choices and quantities should be based on each family's time, space, and financial resources.

Furniture and Accessories

Soft baby carrier
Bassinet
Crib
Crib sheets
Crib blankets
Waterproof mattress
Waterproof mattress pads
Bumper pads
Mobile
Changing table
Dresser with shelves
Humidifier
Heater

Basic Clothing

Sleep gowns
Receiving blankets
Stretch overalls
T-shirts
Bibs
Snowsuit or bunting
Hat
Cardigan sweaters

Diapers and Accessories

Disposable diapers
Wipes
Zinc oxide cream
Cloth diapers
Diaper bag

Bath Items

Hooded towels
Mild soap
Baby shampoo
Infant bathtub
Blunt nail scissors

Feeding Items

Bottles (regular or disposable)
Nipples and rings
Breast pump
Nursing bras
Nursing pads

Travel Items

Car seat
Reclining stroller
Infant seat

Miscellaneous

Alcohol (to clean end of umbilical cord)
Nasal aspirator
Syrup of ipecac (to induce vomiting in case of poisoning)
Cotton swabs (to apply ointments, never for cleaning ears)
Infant acetaminophen (liquid)
Vitamin drops (as prescribed by the pediatrician)
Oral electrolyte maintenance solution (such as Pedialyte—for diarrhea)
Thermometer (rectal or digital)

---

skin from "breathing" and tend to promote diaper rash rather than prevent it. Baby powder (talcum) should not be used, since it has been demonstrated to be an aspiration hazard and can irritate the skin. Baby cornstarch powder is safe, however. Disposable wipes are useful during diaper changes, although soft paper towels and plain water work just as well. In the event of diaper rash, have some zinc oxide cream on hand.

Surprisingly, diaper pails are a proven safety hazard: babies have been known to drown in them. Be sure to choose a pail with a securely locking cover.

Nursing mothers should buy pads to line their brassieres. Mothers who plan to return to work while nursing, and those who expect to spend time away from their babies on occasion, will need a breast pump to express their milk. The manual cylinder or plunger-type pump, consisting of two cylinders, one inside the other, is the easiest to use. Naturally, parents intending to bottle-feed their babies will need bottles (disposable or regular), nipples, and rings. Today most pediatricians believe sterilization to be unnecessary, but parents may

wish to buy an inexpensive basket to hold nipples and rings in the dishwasher. (The box above lists items parents may wish to buy in advance.)

ENGAGING A NURSE

FOR AT LEAST the first three weeks of a newborn's life, parents are usually exhausted from lack of sleep, the excitement of the birth, and (in the mother's case) labor and delivery. Lacking the traditional support of an extended family, many mothers choose to hire a baby nurse or a housekeeper. A baby nurse, usually found through a nursing agency, cares primarily for the child. Some couples prefer a housekeeper who will take over cooking, cleaning, and other chores so that they themselves can concentrate on caring for the new member of the family. In some areas a *doula*, who cares for the mother after the birth, may be available to prepare meals, do light housekeeping, run errands, and answer parents' questions about feeding, infant care, and maternal postpartum care.

It may be less expensive to be discharged early from the hospital and have a home nurse than to stay in the hospital for the traditional three days. Many health maintenance organizations and health insurers are beginning to reimburse a postpartum health care program that includes visiting nurses and home health aides.

Whether a couple hires help or is assisted by a family member such as a mother or sister, it is important to set up guidelines on the helper's role. Discuss in advance whether the helper is to participate in baby care or whether "parent care" would be most appreciated. It is especially important to clarify the question of feeding—nursing mothers will want to be sure that bottles of formula or water are not being fed to their infants unless they so wish.

OTHER SAFETY CONSIDERATIONS

DURING PREGNANCY, when parents have more leisure time than they will for months after the birth, the home should be prepared for the presence of a curious baby. The thermostat on the hot-water heater should be set to 120 degrees in order to prevent burns. Poisons of all sorts should be placed well out of reach. The list includes detergents, medicines (these should be put in a safe place with child safety caps), nail polish remover, drain cleaners, oven cleaner, furniture polish, soaps, felt-tip markers, alcoholic beverages, poisonous plants, fertilizers, weedkillers, insecticides, gasoline, antifreeze, mothballs, and insect poisons.

THE NEEDS OF SIBLINGS

THERE ARE MANY ways to involve older children in preparing for the advent of the new baby, depending on their ages. One of the best ways is to expose them as often as possible to infants (especially the siblings of their own friends). Parents can point out the mother's expanding belly and discuss the baby inside, including information on conception, pregnancy, and childbirth, if the child is old enough to understand. A three- or four-year-old may be able to understand the physical process of birth, and older children may be ready for more specific details of conception and delivery. Siblings can also play an active role in preparing the baby's room and choosing clothes and toys.

Check with the hospital to find out whether there are tours of the maternity unit and nursery for siblings. Some communities offer sibling preparation classes in hospitals or maternity centers, or childbirth education programs. If parents have arranged for sibling attendance at the birth, classes to prepare the child for this experience may be offered at the hospital or maternity center. Finally, there are many excellent books on the market to help the first child cope with having a new sibling.

During the third trimester, parents need to arrange for someone to care for the older child while the parents are in the hospital. Since grandparents often live too far away to arrive at a moment's notice when the mother goes into labor, other arrangements need to be made. If a babysitter is hired, she should be someone with whom the child is familiar. If possible, try not to take the child to someone else's house at this time, but have the sitter come to your house instead. At some point during the third trimester, be sure to talk to your child about how long you expect to be away at the hospital.

Many mothers are surprised to find how much they miss their first child during the hospital stay. Be sure to telephone the child from the hospital and try to arrange for visits as the hospital permits. (Many maternity units now allow siblings to visit.)

Once the whole family is home, the first child is bound to exhibit some signs of stress in response to the presence of the "usurper." Toddlers may regress in toilet training, and some children behave aggressively toward the infant. A newborn baby should never be left alone with a toddler.

THE MARRIAGE

ONE OF THE MOST difficult things for any couple to prepare for is the enormous change in their relationship a new baby invariably brings. Despite the great joy new parents share, they also share exhaustion, stress, lack of confidence in their abilities to care for the infant, and worries about the state of their sex lives and social lives. There can be added stress if a working woman decides to stay home for an extended period with the new baby—not only lack of money but the need for both spouses to adjust to new roles that may bring to mind stereotypes from past decades. During pregnancy, couples can best prepare for all these changes by taking time to discuss them and plan on how best to cope with them.

If the birth of a baby will mean the loss of one income, the parents can review their financial picture and together find the best ways to manage their available resources. Many couples make the mistake of deciding during pregnancy that they need a much larger house—often far from their present home—to accommodate the new baby. In fact, infants take up little space. Moving at this time not only constitutes an added financial stress, but is a further drain on the parents' physical energy. New families are often better off staying close to friends in a familiar environment at this stage.

It is important for fathers, who often feel left out during the months of pregnancy, to have the opportunity to share as much as possible in the preparations for parenting. After the birth, men sometimes feel that their wives are totally absorbed in the demands of caring for the new baby. Women, on the other hand, may feel overwhelmed by demands from both spouse and child. For most couples, arranging to get babysitting help right from the beginning, even if only to allow themselves to take a nap, go for a walk together, or steal a few moments' quiet rest, can work wonders and ensure a happy start for the new family.

2 Caring for the Newborn

Nicholas Cunningham, M.D., Dr. P.H.

INTRODUCTION

PARENTS-TO-BE RARELY MANAGE to anticipate what it is really going to be like once the baby joins the family. All through a pregnancy, they hear dire warnings—from friends, family, and even perfect strangers—about how profoundly having a baby will change their lives: "What with feedings, colds, and teething, you'd better forget about having a good night's sleep for the rest of your life," they are told. Or, "Good luck keeping the spit-up off your new living-room furniture after the baby comes," and, "Enjoy your honeymoon days now—you won't believe how much time and attention a baby demands!"

But somehow, during the glow of the pregnancy, expectant parents remain confident that these warnings don't really apply to them. Being organized, intelligent people who are used to effective problem-solving in their working lives, they feel certain they will manage to take infant care in stride. Or they just let themselves be carried away by excitement and joyful anticipation.

Unfortunately this means that today's couples often experience a rude awakening when they do bring the baby home. No matter how organized and intelligent parents may be, a newborn invariably succeeds in making them feel bewildered, at times incompetent, and inevitably, exhausted. They may wonder if life will ever get back to normal. The good news is that it will, although "normal" with a baby in the house will be different from "normal" before the arrival. But as parents get to know and understand their infant, the family will gradually settle into a routine. The difficulties of the first few weeks will not last forever.

During these early days, wise parents will not consider it a sign of weakness or inexperience to devote the vast majority of their time and effort to baby care rather than "snapping out of it" and "getting on with real life." Instead, they will understand that offering *contingent responsiveness*, or trying to

11

be as sensitive as possible to all of their newborn's needs, is the best way to help the baby settle down, to gain confidence in their own ability to provide care, and to fully appreciate the incomparable joy a child can bring.

IN THE HOSPITAL

SOON AFTER BIRTH, if there have been no complications, the baby will be placed in the mother's arms. The baby will be examined to be sure that he or she has come through the birth process in a healthy state. Heart rate, breathing, muscle tone, reflexes, and skin color are evaluated at one minute and again at five minutes after birth and an Apgar score is assigned, based on criteria developed by the late Dr. Virginia Apgar of The Columbia Presbyterian Medical Center. A first (one-minute) score of 6 or 7 is considered normal for a healthy baby, and the second score is usually higher. (See table 2.1.) If the score is under 6, the respiratory passages may be at least partially obstructed, and the medical personnel will try to clear them, suctioning off any mucus or *vernix* (a white, cheesy substance that protects the skin while the baby is still in the uterus).

Table 2.1 **APGAR SCORE**

Sign	2 Points	1 Point	0 Points
Heart rate	Over 100 beats per minute	Under 100 beats per minute	Not heard
Respiration (breathing)	Breathing well and/or crying	Irregular, inadequate	None
Muscle tone	Arms and legs well-flexed	Some tone, flexible limbs but little resistance to extension	Limp
Reflexes (when suctioned)	Crying, coughing, sneezing, grasping	Grimace	None
Color	Pink all over	Blue hands and feet	Blue or white

Next the umbilical cord is clamped and cut (either by the obstetrician or the mother's "coach"), and the baby's eyes are usually treated with silver nitrate or erythromycin antibiotic ointment to prevent infection. Usually the newborn is given vitamin K to help blood clotting. Although some hospitals place the baby in an artificial warmer, maternity unit staff are becoming more sensitive to the desire of the mother to hold the baby and aware that the mother's body heat is sufficient to warm the infant. In a normal birth there is no reason for the baby to be taken away for an extended period, and parents who wish to hold their babies at this deeply emotional time should insist on it.

Hospitals are increasingly concerned about neonatal infection, and, in fact, birthing centers and a more natural delivery do provide the advantage of more natural bacterial flora. Once they go home, babies quickly acquire "normal" bacteria, both on their skin and in their gastrointestinal tracts. One of the commonest sites of infection is the eye, although infection should be distinguished from the irritation caused by the medication given at birth. Infection, evident by the presence of redness, pain, and pus, should be treated promptly.

The First Complete Physical

This detailed exam usually takes place within the first 24 hours after the birth. Ideally it occurs in the presence of the parents or at least the mother, affording the opportunity to learn more about the baby and to ask questions.

Skin. Babies of all races are usually pinkish. Some are born covered with vernix, a cheeselike substance that protects the baby's skin from becoming waterlogged in the amniotic fluid. The body may be covered with dark, fine hair known as *lanugo* and the skin may be wrinkled and scaling. Babies of dark-skinned parents often have highly pigmented areas on the lower back that look like bruises. Sometimes called "Mongolian spots," these disappear within the first four years. Fair-skinned babies may have pink or red marks (sometimes called "stork bites") on their faces or necks. These go away within the first year (see chapter 32, Childhood Skin Disorders).

Reflexes. Newborns exhibit several reflexes that disappear over the next few weeks and months. When startled, for example, the baby will fling out the arms and legs as if trying to grasp something. This is known as the *Moro reflex.* The *gag reflex* helps protect the baby against choking. The examiner will test it using a tongue depressor. (See chapter 8, The First Year, for more information.)

Head and Neck. The newborn should be able to move the head from side to side and lift it up when lying on the stomach. There are two soft spots, known as *fontanels*, at the top of and near the back of the head where the bones have not yet joined. (See figure 2.1.) The soft spot allows the baby's head

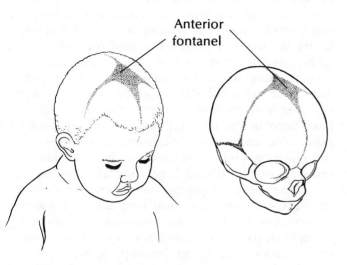

Anterior fontanel

Figure 2.1. **The Baby's "Soft Spot."**

more flexibility during the delivery. It also permits the brain to grow normally, as it would be dangerous for the bones of the skull to join or fuse before the brain finishes its growth. The soft spot near the back of the head closes within a few weeks after birth while the other one shrinks and disappears by around 18 months.

The baby's head may be pointed as a result of "molding" during the trip down the birth canal: the head is wider in circumference than the mother's pelvis, and the bones of the skull overlap in order to allow passage. In addition, the scalp tissue may be swollen because of pressure during the birth. Both the swelling and pointedness should disappear within a day or two. If there is a definite swelling on one side of the head (cephalhematoma), it may take a few months to disappear.

It is not dangerous to stroke or wash the baby's head or touch the fontanel. The soft spot should feel flat, and it may pulse with the heartbeat. If at any time after birth the fontanel feels bulging or sunken, the doctor should be contacted immediately.

Eyes. Contrary to what people once believed, a baby's eyes will follow light, brightly colored objects, and the human face. The eyelids may be puffy, either from the pressure of the birth canal or from the eyedrops given after birth, but this will disappear within a few days. Eye color is not determined until at least three months of age.

Nose. The nose may be flattened after the passage through the birth canal. Babies tend to sneeze to clear mucus out of their nasal passages. There may also be tiny white spots called *milia* under the skin on the nose and chin; they will usually disappear in a few weeks.

Ears. Babies can hear at birth. If the earlobes have been bent during the birth, they should quickly return to their normal shape.

Chest and Abdomen. The examiner will check the chest, breasts, heart, and lungs. A small bulge may appear when the baby breathes; this is only the cartilage at the bottom of the breastbone and should not cause concern. Breast tissue may be swollen, and nipples may secrete fluid, in both boys and girls, as a result of maternal hormones that cross the placental barrier and circulate in the baby's blood before birth. This will subside.

Infants have a rapid heart rate (usually 120 or more beats a minute). A mild heart murmur will usually disappear within a few hours or days. It is normal for breathing to be irregular, varying from deep to shallow, slow to fast. The examiner will also check the umbilicus and the abdomen to feel the internal organs, including the kidneys, which usually can be felt in newborns.

Genitalia. The genitals appear large in both boys and girls. The examiner will check a boy's scrotum to see whether the testes have descended. Often baby girls have a white secretion (sometimes tinged by a small amount of blood) from the vagina during the first two weeks after birth.

Rectum. The examiner may check to see that the anus is open by taking the baby's temperature with a rectal thermometer. Soon after birth, the baby usually passes *meconium* or black, sticky stool.

Legs. Because the baby is in a curled-up position before birth, he or she may be bow-legged and pigeon-toed. While the examiner will check the hips, legs, and feet carefully for abnormalities, most of the positional effects are self-correcting and parents should be assured that legs and feet will straighten out with time.

Blood tests. Sometime during the second day, the newborn is also given a blood test for *phenylketonuria* (PKU), a congenital condition in which an enzyme needed to metabolize certain proteins properly is lacking. Untreated, this condition can lead to brain damage. Because the PKU test is accurate only if the blood is drawn at least 24 hours after birth, mothers who opt for early discharge from the hospital should arrange to have the test done at the pediatrician's office within the first week. The blood that is drawn from the baby's heel for this test will also be used to test for a number of other conditions, including thyroid malfunction, blood type, Rh factor, hemoglobin, and bilirubin level. Bilirubin is a pigment released by the breakdown of excess red blood cells no longer needed after birth. If the amount in the blood is excessive, the condition may be dangerous and the infant will require close monitoring for hours or days. (For additional information see box on Newborn Screening.)

COMING HOME

A GENERATION AGO, new mothers and babies were usually kept in the hospital for a week or more after the birth. Today, with the emphasis on a natural approach to childbirth rather than one that treats both mother and infant as sick patients, hospital stays tend to last three days or less after a low-risk vaginal delivery. This is possible in part because fewer drugs are now used during labor. Breastfeeding may be easier to establish at home than in the hospital, and the reduced stay can cut hospitalization costs and minimize the chance of infection. A quick return home can provide a wonderful opportunity for the new family to spend time alone together, if they have set up a workable support system beforehand. If the mother is able to go home and concentrate on baby care and getting enough rest, her recovery may be more rapid than it would have been in the hospital environment. If, on the other hand, she is immediately catapulted into cooking, cleaning, and caring for older children, she will probably find it difficult to get the rest she needs.

Fortunately for mothers who do not or cannot choose early discharge, most hospitals and maternity centers now offer family-centered care, encouraging both parents to help meet their infant's daily needs (from bathing to feeding), and providing rooming-in or modified rooming-in and sibling visits.

NEWBORN SCREENING

Certain genetic disorders of metabolism make it impossible for an infant to break down and use certain components of food. With an inherited block in metabolism, often due to the lack of a necessary enzyme, nutrition is hampered and levels of intermediary chemicals can build to dangerous levels, causing serious illness or permanent damage to the brain and other organs. Although the inborn error of metabolism cannot yet be corrected or cured, for some disorders damage can be prevented by dietary changes or supplements started early in life. For this reason, states test all newborns for several of these rare disorders so that treatment can be offered.

Each state has its own newborn screening laws, selecting the disorders for screening on the basis of their frequency, cost of the test, and availability of successful early treatment. Usually the law requires that all newborns be screened unless parents request an exemption on religious grounds. Physicians and midwives are responsible for properly obtaining and submitting a small blood sample for the test. If an abnormality is found on a newborn screening test, parents will be asked to bring the infant for more definitive diagnostic testing. In many hospitals, it is standard practice to review the results of newborn screening at the six-week checkup.

The first newborn screening began in the 1950s when a simple test for phenylketonuria (PKU) was developed. Children with PKU are unable to metabolize one of the essential amino acids, phenylalanine. If PKU is undetected, they develop seizures and severe mental retardation. When diagnosed, they are treated with a special low phenylalanine diet for at least the first several years of life.

An inherited lack in thyroid hormone, congenital hypothyroidism, occurs in approximately one in 4,000 births. If untreated, an infant will have irreversible mental damage by three to six months of age. If diagnosed so that thyroid hormone treatment begins promptly, the damage is avoided. It is not unusual for premature infants to have low levels of thyroid hormone on initial screening and to require a second test.

Galactosemia, an inherited inability to metabolize galactose and milk sugar (lactose) which occurs in one in 50,000 infants, can cause jaundice, enlarged liver, mental retardation, cataracts, and failure to gain weight. It is very simply treated by removing sources of galactose and lactose from the diet. This disorder, which can be fatal if not treated, is not the same as the more common lactose intolerance.

A disorder recently included in some newborn screening programs is biotinidase deficiency, an inability to recycle and use vitamin B in the body. If undetected, infants may develop frequent infections, hearing loss, seizures, uncoordinated movements, mental retardation, and sometimes death. When extra biotin is provided to affected children, the damage is avoided.

Two other rare metabolic disorders are included in many state screening programs: maple syrup urine disease (which occurs in one of every 225,000 newborns and is fatal or severely damaging if untreated) and homocystinuria (which can produce mental retardation, skeletal and eye problems).

Newborn screening for sickle-cell anemia is included in a few state programs, often on a voluntary basis.

Setting Up a Support System

Good prenatal planning requires looking beyond the assembling of the layette and setting in place a workable support system. New mothers are physically and psychologically recovering from the birthing experience, and for both parents, caring for a newborn is an astonishingly time-consuming and challenging task. First-time parents are often not sure what is considered normal and what is not. Typically, a pediatrician can expect many calls during the first few months. (See box.) Mothers who

---

WHEN TO CALL THE PEDIATRICIAN

Most parents will have interviewed the pediatrician or nurse-practitioner prior to the birth of the baby, and they should feel comfortable calling for help and advice as early and as often as necessary. Later on, they can learn when to call and when not to call. If the health care practitioner is not in agreement with this approach, parents should find another one. Many parents learn to recognize when the baby "is not right" and good practitioners learn to listen to these feelings.

The parents should call if the infant:

- Does not pass meconium (the first dark greenish-black bowel movement) within 36 hours of birth.
- Appears to be getting jaundiced or yellow (check the whites of the eyes).
- Vomits forcefully or more frequently than usual.
- Refuses feedings for more than 6–8 hours.
- Has a fever of 100.5 degrees F or higher.
- Has a cough that persists.
- Cries much more or less than usual, or very intensely or loudly.
- Begins to sleep markedly more or less.
- Seems unusually cranky or restless, or unusually passive and lethargic.
- Turns very pale or flushed (except when stooling).
- Appears dehydrated—urinates less, lacks saliva, is drowsy, lethargic, feverish, or has a very dry nose, lips, and cheeks.
- Has bad diarrhea (frequent, very watery stools), which can lead to dehydration.
- Has a marked change in the color or consistency of bowel movements. There is great variability in frequency among babies (some stool only at 3–4 day intervals; others every time they feed), but the important thing to watch for is a change in the baby's established pattern.

---

were working before the birth often find the transition to life at home difficult, whether for a few years or for only a few weeks or months. Most of their friends are still at the office, and infant care tends to entail far more minute-by-minute attention—and far less tangible reward—than most paid jobs. New fathers often have trouble coping with their wives' preoccupation with the infant, as well as with the total dependency of the newborn. For these reasons, it is important to find people with whom to talk and share experiences. And it is essential to have help with meals, housework, and baby care.

Traditionally couples have invited one of the new grandmothers to stay with them for a week or two, although some hire baby nurses or housekeepers instead. If a relative offers to come and stay with the family around the time the baby is born, it is important to clarify her role in advance. Most new parents find it better in the long run if they themselves take charge of newborn care, so that they have the opportunity to form an intimate bond with their child from the start, while the helper assists with meals and household tasks. The helper should be sensitive to the parents' need to be alone and alone with the baby.

If a baby nurse is hired, she usually devotes herself to the newborn, and for this reason many parents prefer to hire a housekeeper to assist them with meals and cleanup while they devote themselves to the baby.

When friends and relatives come to admire the baby, new parents need to shake off the urge to offer the customary food and drink and realize that this is a time to rest, not to worry about entertaining. Guests should be encouraged to keep their visits brief. Friends and relatives can be a tremendous help if parents are not too shy to answer yes when asked if they can be of help; visitors are often quite willing to bring over a casserole or stop at the supermarket for a few badly needed items, or even take the other children out for a few hours. Some parents, on the other hand, may find it more restful to restrict all but the closest friends and relatives until they and the baby have settled into their new life together.

Advice and emotional support can come from a variety of sources—family, friends, other new parents (met at childbirth education or parenting classes, for example, or at a prenatal exercise program), and the hospital "warm line" that is often available for round-the-clock advice from the nursery.

Attachment

Although fathers play an important role in parenting, during these early weeks the infant's primary attachment is still to the mother. There is a large body of research that points up the baby's need to form an early one-on-one attachment to one person, by regularly seeing her face and smile, smelling her body, having skin-to-skin contact, and hearing her voice. This does not mean the mother has to be the only person who feeds, diapers, carries, or plays with the baby; such activities can and should be shared with the father and others. This is a critical period for both parents to establish themselves as nurturers, and the longer it lasts, the better.

Some mothers and fathers are dismayed to discover that they lack a feeling of closeness with their newborns at first. But they usually find that as they nurture and care for the baby, feelings of warmth and intimacy develop. Some researchers have observed that working mothers may occasionally fail to attach strongly because they are preoccupied with the thought of returning to work and are perhaps afraid to fall too deeply in love with their babies for fear it will be too difficult to leave. Childbirth work-leaves in the United States are rarely sufficient to provide optimal early infant care and parents should do everything possible to increase this time for both mother and father. Noted child psychologist Selma Fraiberg has called this "every child's birthright." It seems likely that an investment of time early on will pay rich dividends later in terms of a securely attached child with a firm cultural base for later development.

Even if she has only a brief maternity leave, it is important for a mother to give herself totally to the experience during this time. Regardless of how much time the parents are able to devote to the baby later on, it is crucial to establish the emotional bond now. A strong attachment is the best insurance that the baby will thrive with another caretaker after the mother returns to work.

Siblings

The birth of a new baby and the consequent "dethroning" of the prior child are major adjustments that siblings experience in a variety of ways, depending on age and individual temperament. According to several studies, the key factor in helping an older child adjust to the birth of a new baby is getting the older child involved in infant care. This can take the form of helping parents get diapers out of the diaper box and bottles from the refrigerator, discovering ways to entertain the infant, and perhaps learning to help feed the baby. While the primary focus of the mother inevitably will be on the newborn, taking the time every day to be with the sibling, preferably alone, is extremely important and reassuring. Parents are faced with a real challenge in trying to devote enough time and attention to both children, however. Many mothers find feedings an ideal time to invite the older child to sit beside them and read a story. It is also important to try to get visitors to pay attention to the sibling (some parents keep a supply of small gifts on hand for the sibling to receive when the baby is showered with presents), to prevent feelings of being left out.

Nonetheless, ambivalence and mood fluctuations in the relationship between the siblings are quite typical and likely to continue throughout their lives. For this reason, an infant should never be left alone with another young child, even a very secure one, because the older child could inadvertently (or deliberately) injure the infant. Hostility on the part of the older sibling is so common as to be normal; even if the toddler seems to want to kill the baby, this should not come as a surprise.

At first the older child may show signs of "regression" by wanting to return to diapers, to use a bottle, to crawl, or to breastfeed. Parents should not show alarm at these acts, which will quickly pass. Calling attention to some of the things that the older child does—such as being able to eat ice cream or build block towers—will reinforce the child's pride of age and accomplishment. Rather than condemning or punishing the older child for showing anger, parents can help defuse it by helping him or her verbalize feelings—saying, for example, "Sometimes that baby cries too much, doesn't she?" or, "It's hard when you want Mommy to play with you and she's so busy with the baby, isn't it?"

Pets

Despite some parents' romantic notions about children and pets "growing up together" and baby animals making cute playthings, it is not a good idea to introduce a new pet into the household with a new baby. Not only will it mean additional demands on the parents' time to care for, train, and discipline the pet, but there is a danger that either the pet or the baby will inadvertently or deliberately hurt the other. The addition of a pet, especially a young one, is best left until the child reaches age three or four.

On the other hand, many babies are born into households where pets already reside. Although nervous, untrained, or aggressive animals can be dangerous, and choices will have to be made, there is no reason to get rid of a good-tempered animal because a baby has arrived. There are, however, safety precautions that parents can take to protect both the newborn and the pet, and they should start before the baby arrives. They can, for example, teach a dog to follow them whenever they leave a room. Once the baby arrives, the dog will stay with the parent and not linger unattended in the baby's room—or any room where the baby may be sleeping. This may be a better practice than banishing the dog from the baby's room and setting up a situation where the dog feels its territory has been challenged.

Pet owners can also establish a place for the dog or cat to eat undisturbed by a toddler. Encroachments on a pet's food or feeding place are likely to provoke confrontations.

Like an older brother or sister, a dog or cat will be very curious about the new arrival and, if pushed aside or banished from the baby's presence, can show overt signs of jealousy. This is especially true of a pet who has been, in a sense, an "only child." Pet owners would do well to recognize this and treat the animal as one would treat an older sibling. One way to reduce potential conflict is to allow time for a thorough introduction. The cat or dog should be allowed to sniff the baby without being restrained. The parent can hold the baby or even better, if he or she feels comfortable doing it, kneel on the floor, place the baby on a blanket alongside, and allow the pet to approach freely.

Cats do not, old wives' tales aside, jump into cribs to smother babies. They do so out of curiosity and because they like to curl up next to something warm. Placing netting over the crib will eliminate this, if parents find it a concern.

As a general rule, children should not be left alone with pets, especially dogs, until they reach school age. Even a gentle pet with whom the baby has established a good relationship can snap if startled out of a sound sleep or playfully mauled by a child.

One final note of caution: Flea collars contain a toxin and should not be used on dogs or cats if there is a child in the house.

Safety

The entire house should be "baby-proofed" before the baby arrives and periodically thereafter as each stage of development brings new dangers into reach. (For more specific information, see chapter 14, Ensuring Your Child's Safety.) The most immediate safety concerns and practices include:

Car Seats. A young child should never ride in a car—not even on the way home from the hospital—without a safe car seat. Seatbelts are not safe at this age and car beds are not conveyances for an infant riding in an automobile. There are newborn car seats as well as convertible types that can be used later on for toddlers; newborns ride facing backward, and their heads may be supported with special liners or a rolled-up blanket wrapped around them. (See chapter 1, Before the Baby Is Born.)

Falls. Although not yet self-propelled, the baby is surprisingly mobile when placed on a high surface. For this reason, parents need to guard against falls. An infant should never be left alone on a bed or changing table. And an infant seat should not be placed near the edge of a table or a countertop: Flailing or kicking babies can propel themselves onto the floor.

Scalds and Burns. The thermostat on the hot water heater should be set no higher than 130 degrees F., and preferably at 120–125 degrees F. A parent should always test the water temperature before bathing the baby, and the baby should never be held directly under the tap in case the temperature changes. It is foolhardy to drink a hot beverage while holding a squirming baby—a spill could severely burn tender skin. The crib should not be placed against a radiator. If a baby is fed from a bottle, the bottle should never be warmed in a microwave oven, which may create hot spots that can cause severe burns.

Smothering. Pillows (no matter how small) can cause smothering and should never be placed in an infant's crib. Likewise, plastic bags (such as trash bags and dry cleaning bags) should not be left near the baby.

DAILY LIFE

AT FIRST THE MOST ordinary demands of infant care, such as bathing and diapering, can loom as impossible tasks, causing parents who previously considered themselves competent and successful in life to wonder whether they are not in fact quite the opposite. In time, however, these tasks become not only less daunting, but they also provide many opportunities to enjoy touching and interacting with the baby.

Breastfeeding

Whether or not a mother plans to breastfeed in the long term, nursing as soon as possible after delivery is the best thing for both mother and baby. The early nursing provides the baby with colostrum, which is rich in protective antibodies. The hormones released by the breastfeeding process help the mother's uterus shrink to its nonpregnant size. For mothers who do intend to breastfeed, frequent early nursings help bring in the milk.

Breastfed babies eat more often and have more bowel movements than bottle-fed babies, so much so in fact that feeding and stooling may seem to be continuous at first. On the bright side, they are much less likely to get diaper rash, and their stool has a far more pleasant odor than that of formula-fed infants. At two to three weeks the baby may seem to be incredibly hungry—this is often a growth spurt. In order to keep up her milk supply and her energy, the mother should drink more liquids and get more rest as the baby feeds more. It is best to breastfeed exclusively for the first three to four weeks. This ensures a good supply of milk and prevents the problem of nipple confusion, which may occur in some babies. (See chapter 4, Nutrition in the First Year.)

Breastmilk Substitutes

A mother who does not wish to breastfeed should ask the pediatrician which formula is appropriate for her baby. Cow's milk should be avoided for at least the first six to eight months, to prevent allergy problems.

Although some pediatricians believe there is no need to sterilize feeding equipment, most parents feel more comfortable boiling the bottles and nipples for the first six months. Many parents find it convenient to wash nipples, rings, and bottles in the dishwasher although this probably weakens the nipples, making them soft and likely to stick closed, preventing the flow of milk. In any case, it is extremely important to be sure that all milk is thoroughly cleaned out of the feeding equipment to prevent illness. Infants can also be fed with a cup and spoon, which eliminates the bother of bottles as well as the tendency of the baby to become emotionally attached to a latex nipple. At five to six months they can begin to drink from a cup.

Babies who are formula-fed have the same needs for warmth and closeness as their nursing counterparts. For this reason, it is essential that they be held close during a feeding, rather than left to suck from a propped bottle.

Burping

After feeding, a baby should always be burped in order to expel any excess air that may have been ingested along with the breastmilk or formula. Otherwise the air can cause discomfort and regurgitation. To expel the air, the baby can be held upright against the mother's or father's chest, looking over the shoulder and patted or rubbed gently on the back. Some babies respond better to being held in a sitting position on a lap, while their backs are gently rubbed. In either case, there is no need to thump the baby on the back; rubbing or patting will suffice. Because the baby is very likely to spit up a little milk along with the air, it is wise to drape a cloth diaper or towel over the shoulder or lap. Babies who spit up a lot may be carried for 15 to 20 minutes after the feeding. Soft baby carriers ("Snugli's") are particularly useful for these babies.

Thrush

The baby frequently gets a white coating on the tongue and the sides of the mouth, commonly assumed to be thrush. However, if the coating can be scraped off, it isn't thrush and is not a cause for concern. True thrush is caused by a common household fungus called candida or monilia, which frequently overgrows in the mouth. While thrush may cause some mild discomfort, it is not serious and can be treated with an antifungal medication.

Bowel Movements

The first bowel movement, called meconium and usually a dark greenish-black in color, should be passed within 36 hours of birth. Breastfed babies average three to six stools a day, although there is a great deal of variation from one child to another. Their stools are usually yellowish in color, loose, and have a sweet-sour odor. The stools of formula-fed babies tend to be firmer and darker in color, with a stronger odor. They usually are less frequent (from one to four a day, or even every other day), as the protein in formula takes longer to digest and clear the stomach. As parents change their baby's diapers, they become familiar with the pattern and will be able to detect any sudden variations in color or consistency, which are signals to call the doctor.

Babies strain and turn red when passing larger or firmer stools. This is normal; however, if blood is seen in the stool, the practitioner should be called.

Diapering

Whether to use cloth or disposable diapers is a personal choice. There is no evidence for doctors to advocate the use of either cloth or disposable diapers; the choice of diapers should therefore be based strictly on convenience, cost, and preference. Most parents find disposable diapers far more convenient than the cloth type, although they are more expensive.

Some babies need to be diapered more frequently than others; a few pass such loose stools that mothers change them right in the middle of a feeding. Prompt changing of wet and soiled diapers is the most effective way of preventing diaper rash.

To change the diaper, lay the baby down on the back and carefully clean the buttocks and anal area with a diaper wipe or a soft paper towel soaked in water (a squeeze bottle at the changing table is convenient). Place the clean diaper under the baby and fasten the tapes or pins, taking care not to make them too tight (you should be able to slip two fingers in easily). It is best to avoid powders, which may be inhaled by the baby; however, if desired, ordinary cornstarch is both safe and inexpensive.

Regardless of which diaper is used, many babies develop a diaper rash during the first months of life, especially a formula-fed baby or one that has frequent diarrhea. It is no longer believed that diaper rashes are due to ammonia. Urine and stool irritate the skin and pave the way for a skin infection with candida, a yeast found in the gut.

A baby who develops a mild case of diaper rash should be changed often and kept as dry as possible. Air exposure is helpful in preventing and treating diaper rash. Letting the baby go without a diaper, or fastening the diaper loosely and putting the baby in a playpen or on any washable surface often improves the condition. Before the baby goes to sleep, the parent may also try applying one of the over-the-counter ointments containing petroleum jelly, vitamin A, or zinc oxide. Plastering the baby's buttocks with creams and lotions should be avoided, however, as these are likely to block the skin's exposure to air.

If despite these measures, the rash gets worse, it is advisable to call the doctor, who will prescribe a cream for this yeast. The doctor should also be informed if another type of diaper rash with blisters develops, as it is due to a bacterial infection that must be treated medically.

Rubber pants worn over cloth diapers may also prevent air circulation and should be avoided if the baby has diaper rash. If leaky diapers are a problem, using two cloth diapers at a time may help. Some parents of little boys find that disposable diapers absorb more if used "backward" (with the tabs fastened from front to back).

Babies should never be left alone on a changing table even for a second—they are surprisingly skillful at flinging themselves off.

Carrying the Baby

Recent research suggests that babies who are carried in a soft baby carrier (such as a "Snugli") show greater security and are able to develop stronger attachments later in life. Soft carriers hold the baby snugly against the mother's or father's chest, leaving both hands free, and make traveling and even routine errands much less of a bother. Many parents find that the baby fusses less and falls asleep more easily in a carrier than in a carriage or stroller, which may be used later when the baby is too heavy to carry comfortably. Some parents even use the carrier in the house to quiet a fussing baby or simply to keep the baby close at all times.

A minor disadvantage of carrying babies this way is that the extra body heat can make it uncomfortable for the parent and baby in warm weather. An alternative, for young babies, is a sling (such as a "Pleat Seat") that is worn over one shoulder and rests the baby on the opposite hip, requiring one hand for support.

As babies grow heavier, it becomes difficult to carry them on the chest. Older babies like being carried on the back, for which a soft carrier or aluminum-frame backpack can be used.

The Umbilical Stump

The newborn will come home with the umbilical stump painted with a dye. The stump will dry out and fall off within one to two weeks. In order to keep the stump dry, the diapers should be fastened below the stump and the base of the stump cleaned two or three times a day with an alcohol pad. When the cord falls off it is common to see slight bleeding from the base of the umbilicus. This is of no concern and should cease in two to three days. Another common problem seen after the stump falls off is a small fleshy growth called a granuloma, which frequently needs to be cauterized by the physician with a silver nitrate stick. Any foul smell or reddening in the area around the umbilical stump should be reported to the doctor, as should bleeding that continues beyond three days.

Bathing

Babies should be kept clean at all times, not only for cosmetic reasons, but to prevent infections and decrease the likelihood of rashes. The timing of the bath can vary according to household needs and the baby's response to being bathed. Although most babies enjoy baths and find them relaxing, some infants do not. These infants may also find it difficult to adjust to other new experiences.

If the baby protests the bath, keep in mind that infants like to be handled firmly. They are usually not fond of being naked, and prefer to be dressed and wrapped. It is not advisable to bathe a baby who has just been fed—not because of the traditional fear of stomach upset—but because doing so increases the chances that the baby will stool in the bathwater.

Tub baths should be delayed until the stump of the umbilical cord has fallen off. The newborn can be sponge-bathed or washed with the hands. Special care should be taken in washing and drying the face, neck, behind the ears, buttocks and genitals, and especially the folds of the skin. The skin should be washed with mild soap or baby shampoo and patted dry with a soft towel, and the hair brushed to prevent "cradle cap" (patches of scaly, greasy-looking crust on the scalp). If the eyes are swollen or appear infected, they can be wiped gently with a clean, damp cotton ball, which then should be discarded. Clean the outside of baby's ears but never put anything (such as a cotton swab) inside them.

Once the baby is ready for tub baths, use a plastic dishpan, infant tub, or oversize sponge seat made especially for babies to avoid the back strain of having to bend over the bathtub. Have all the necessities on hand—soap, towel, clothes—so that there is no need to leave the baby alone in the water even for a second. Remember: Infants can drown in less than an inch of water.

The newborn's skin tends to peel for three to four weeks, starting on the trunk and ending on the arms and legs. This peeling does not necessarily indicate dry skin. Most babies have cradle cap, a scaly rash on the scalp, during the first two or three months of life. Daily shampooing is recommended. In general, oil or lotions on the baby's skin are not recommended because they usually clog the pores and make the skin break out more. This is particularly true on the face and scalp, which are prone to rashes in the first two months of life.

To clean a baby girl's genitals, use a soft cloth and lukewarm water. No special care is needed to clean a boy with an intact penis; do not attempt to retract the foreskin to clean underneath. To clean a circumcised boy, protect the healing area with a piece of sterile gauze coated with petroleum jelly or an antibacterial ointment; call the doctor immediately if there are signs of redness, swelling, bleeding, or pus.

There is no need for a full bath every day, although parents and baby may enjoy the skin-to-skin contact and both may find the routine convenient and reassuring. Washing the hair, face, and buttocks ("topping and tailing") can be substituted for a full bath on busy days.

Nail Care

The baby's nails, which are brittle and thin, should be kept trimmed, as babies tend to scratch their faces easily. The nails should be cut every fourth day or as needed, with nail clippers or blunt-nosed scissors, whichever is more comfortable for the parent. Many parents find it easier to trim the nails while the baby is asleep and the hands are relaxed and open. Mothers of very active babies sometimes bite off their babies' nails—a safe, if unesthetic, practice.

Noise

Parents who tiptoe around while the newborn is napping, take the phone off the hook, and post signs asking visitors not to ring the doorbell usually live to regret it. Keeping the home quiet is a very effective method of teaching the infant to require quiet, which is bound to become a nuisance. Babies are perfectly capable of sleeping in the midst of all kinds of noise; when they're tired, they will fall asleep. If the baby has siblings, there is no reason to hush them up during the baby's nap—in fact, such a policy is bound to exacerbate hostility between them. Awake, the baby will be happiest in the midst of family activities.

Swaddling

Newborns, fresh from the confinement of the womb, seem to feel secure when they are snugly wrapped. To swaddle a baby, lay a square receiving blanket on the bed so the corners correspond to 3, 6, 9, and 12 on the clock. Fold the top point (12 o'clock) down toward the center about six inches. Place the baby on the blanket so the head is above the top fold. Fold one corner across the baby and then fold the bottom up. Pull the remaining corner snugly and smoothly across the front, ending just behind the opposite shoulder.

For the first three or four weeks, babies should be swaddled each time they are placed in the crib or bassinet.

Dressing the Baby

Babies should be dressed with the same amount of clothing as parents would dress themselves—not more, not less. They can control temperature from birth and suffer heat and cold as adults do. Their hands and feet normally tend to feel cool; this does not indicate that they are cold, as long as the rest of the body is warm. If anything, babies have a higher metabolic rate than adults, a fact suspected 50 years ago by Dr. Rusty McIntosh, a pediatrics professor at Babies Hospital of The Columbia-Presbyterian Medical Center, who was often criticized for his habit of taking his own minimally clothed babies out in New York's Central Park in cool weather.

To make sure that the baby is not overdressed, check the head. When babies are hot, their heads sweat even though their hands and feet may be cool. Babies are very sensitive to heat, and overdressing can cause a heat rash called prickly heat. In this condition little red pimples appear mostly in the neck and upper trunk. Oiling of the skin will make prickly heat worse. The baby should be bathed often and kept cool.

Premature babies do have trouble regulating their body temperature, but full-term newborns can do it well. One exception: When the temperature outdoors is less than 70 degrees F., a baby should probably wear a hat, as 40 percent of body heat is lost through the head and babies don't have much hair to keep them warm.

Laundry

New baby clothes should be washed before they are worn in order to rinse out excess dyes that might irritate the baby's skin. It is also important to rinse clothes thoroughly (perhaps using the washing machine's rinse cycle twice) to remove any residual detergent. To preserve flame retardancy in infant sleepwear, use only detergent, not soap (such as Ivory Snow), and be sure the detergent is thoroughly removed.

Crying

Although at first a baby's crying is baffling and far too frequent for most parents' comfort, in time they come to distinguish between the various cries and to understand what each one means. A short cry, for example, may mean the baby is passing gas, or is about to urinate or have a bowel movement. Babies also cry out of hunger, wetness, boredom, tiredness, or the need to be held close. For the technology-minded who wish to calm a crying baby, there are recordings of sounds heard in the womb, as well as battery-powered toys that reproduce the mother's heartbeat. If an infant is soothed by the sound of the hair dryer or vacuum cleaner, parents can make recordings of these sounds. But in most cases, the best approach is just to hold the baby close. The baby is often soothed by being held close to the parent's chest, carried in a soft carrier, or swaddled in a blanket (see sections above on Carrying the Baby and on Swaddling). A warm bath may also help.

Some babies love being placed on their stomachs across the parent's lap for a massage. Others do best with motion—a cradle, rocking chair, wind-up swing, carriage, or stroller (inside the house or out), or a ride in the car. Even a baby who is not hungry has a strong need for nonnutritive sucking, which can sometimes be satisfied with a pacifier. And although babies do love touch, some extremely sensitive infants may respond negatively to too much handling and stimulation; it is important to learn when to let the baby rest.

Sometimes the problem is gas buildup, which can be alleviated by burping or carrying in the baby carrier after feeding. If the mother is nursing, she may wish to try eliminating dairy products for two weeks to see if the baby has an allergy to them that is causing the gas. Generally, a nursing baby can tolerate the same foods the mother can tolerate. Spicy foods, for example, should not be a problem for the baby if they cause the mother no distress. But a specific allergy can create problems and the mother may have to experiment with eliminating and then adding back certain foods. Similar problems in formula-fed babies may indicate an allergy to milk and the parent should discuss with the pediatrician the use of soy- or other non-milk-based formula.

If the baby's crying persists, check with the doctor. Illness, such as an ear infection, may be the underlying problem.

QUESTIONS NEW PARENTS OFTEN ASK

Should I worry about the baby's spitting up? New parents are often unprepared for how messy babies are—at both ends! All babies spit up, but they vary in terms of how much food they ingest, how much air they take in during a feeding, and how much comes back up afterward. The baby may appear to be spitting up more milk than he or she really is, because it is mixed with saliva and gastric juices. If the baby seems to be spitting up large amounts of milk or if vomiting is forceful or projectile, call the pediatrician.

In most babies, the valve at the entrance to the stomach is not very well developed, and in some infants it is very poorly developed, so that there is a tendency for food to come back up. Holding the baby upright and over the shoulder, or in a front carrier, for 10 to 20 minutes after a feeding will keep the baby leaning slightly forward, making it easier for the gas to be expelled; the "bubble" will be uppermost, causing less fluid to come up. In addition, a baby in this position will feel comforted and relaxed, which contributes to a reduction in spitting up.

Breastfed babies tend to spit up less because no air is mixed with the milk, as it may be in bottle feeding, and because they only take in as much milk as they need; the commonest reason for vomiting in the newborn is overfeeding.

Why does the baby get hiccups? As new mothers may remember from pregnancy, babies often hiccup. This happens most often after a feeding, when they tend to take in air, and is not a cause for alarm. Parents can try burping the baby or continuing feeding for a few more minutes.

What can I do to soothe a colicky baby? Child development experts are still mystified about the causes of colic, or the inexplicable and seemingly endless crying of some babies every evening (not to be confused with the crankiness most infants and children tend to exhibit around dinnertime). There is some evidence that it is related to stress in the family environment. Although some nursing mothers tend to blame themselves for the colic, it is actually less common in breastfed babies, and continuing to nurse is likely to be the best strategy.

Maintaining a peaceful environment at feeding times and in general—no mean feat with a colicky baby in the house—will probably help minimize it. A colicky baby needs even more caring and support than the average baby. Although there may be a link between the mother's use of mind-altering drugs during pregnancy and an irritable personality in the infant, babies are born with personalities, and some are probably born irritable and colicky. Ultimately, there is little a parent can do to eliminate colic, but carrying the baby in a soft carrier seems to help and should be done as often as possible. Some babies respond to being carried over your arm, stomach down, with the head in the crook of your elbow. (For other suggestions, see section on crying.)

Why does my baby have a stuffy nose? In the wintertime, most artificial heating systems cause dryness, and any environment below 30 percent humidity is stressful to the human respiratory tract. The thermostat should not be set above 68–70 degrees F., and the relative humidity should be 30 or even 40 percent. A humidifier can be very beneficial, but it must be kept clean. Houseplants, if they are watered regularly and especially if they are placed on a tray filled with pebbles and water, are another way of getting humidity into the air. Pans of water on the radiators can also help.

Babies can suffer the same allergies as adults, whether or not there is a family tendency. Consequently, with the arrival of a newborn it is more important than ever to try to maintain a clean environment in the home, eliminating as much as possible sources of dust and places where dust and dander can gather. (See chapter 31, Allergies).

Exposure to cigarette smoke is also harmful to infants and children. No one should smoke in the presence of a newborn. Secondhand smoke can expose children and adults to carbon monoxide levels that are more than twice as high as the maximum set by the government for industry exposure, also driving up the heart rate and blood pressure. The effects are more concentrated in the tiny lungs and smaller bloodstreams of babies and young children. There is evidence that hospitalization and respiratory problems in general are markedly higher among children whose parents smoke.

What can I do to prevent sudden infant death syndrome (SIDS)? Despite widespread media coverage, SIDS (also known as "crib death") is actually a rare event, and no clear cause has been established for it. Parents can rest assured that researchers draw a clear distinction between SIDS and smothering, and there is no need to fear sleeping with the baby or putting the baby to sleep on his or her stomach.

Should I give my baby a pacifier? Babies' sucking needs vary enormously. Some babies want to breastfeed for several years, others voluntarily give it up after eight or nine months. Likewise, some babies and not others seem to take to pacifiers. Babies whose oral needs are fully satisfied during the first few months of life seem to have a decrease in oral needs later on. If a baby needs to suck, parents should support that need and not worry about it. Thumb-sucking and pacifiers are virtually unknown in cultures where infants are breastfed on a very frequent schedule and children are usually breastfed through toddlerhood. Because extended nursing is impractical for most American mothers, they may find that the baby continues to have unsatisfied oral needs which can be met by a pacifier. In this case, an orthodontic-type pacifier is perfectly fine. Thumb-sucking during the first year is probably not harmful to the teeth. If it continues for a few years it may cause changes in the dental arch, but these are usually reversible once the child stops sucking. In any case, there is not much that can be done about it at this age, nor should there be, since most children will grow out of it.

What is a healthy pattern of weight gain? Newborns tend to lose weight in the hospital, sometimes as much as 10 percent of their birthweight. After that, they tend to gain six or eight ounces a week during the first three months, but small babies gain more while large ones usually gain less. Despite the popular image of the "bouncing baby" as healthy, it is important that infants not be overfed, as some research suggests that this may lead to a lifelong tendency toward obesity. Breastfed babies rarely gain too much weight because they take in just as much as they need. Formula-fed babies, however, may tend to be overweight; in such cases, the pediatrician will usually suggest a change in the amount or strength of formula. When comparing the baby's weight gain to that on the growth charts in books or at the pediatrician's office, keep in mind that the charts are based on typical gains of formula-fed babies. Nursing babies may gain more slowly, and mothers should not interpret this as a sign that they are failing to provide enough milk.

When will the baby sleep through the night?

Babies who sleep through the night the day they come home from the hospital are something parents brag about; the usual pattern, however, is that infants wake up as often as every one to three hours. Even after three months many babies do not sleep all the way through (sleeping through the night is generally defined by parents of infants as midnight to 5 A.M.). Breastfeedings are likely to take place quite frequently during the first weeks—as often as every hour or hour and a half. But maximum breast-feeding during the early weeks usually will pay off in a secure baby who will settle into a much better sleep pattern within the first two or three months—able to go for three or four hours or more between feedings. (However, there are exceptions: babies who are successfully breastfed yet continue to want night feedings until four or five months.) Meanwhile, it is important for parents to take the opportunity to sleep during baby's naps. Fortunately, infants average 18 to 20 hours of sleep a day, though some sleep as little as 10 hours and others up to 23 hours.

During these early weeks, it is most convenient for the parents and most comforting for the baby for all three to sleep in the same bed or at least for the bassinet to stay beside the parents' bed. If the baby sleeps beside the mother (as is the norm throughout most of the world), nighttime nursing can be accomplished with a minimum of fuss. There is no need to worry about rolling over on top of the baby. Many mothers find it comfortable to lie on the back or side with the baby resting in the crook of one arm.

For some parents, however, the irregular breathing of a newborn proves to be a major interrupter of their own sleep. In such cases, it is probably advisable to move the baby into a separate room.

In order to help the baby develop a dark-light cycle, try keeping the room bright during the day and wake up the baby every two or three hours during the day for feedings. Giving a bath in the evening may stimulate the baby to stay awake longer and then sleep better during the night.

UNSOLICITED ADVICE, OLD WIVES' TALES, AND FADS

NEW PARENTS ARE SUBJECT to unsolicited advice from grandparents, neighbors, friends, and even strangers. Sometimes the advice is common sense, but often it is outdated, a matter of personal preference, or just plain wrong. Among the most common warnings are:

- "Babies should be fed only every four hours or they'll become spoiled." Mothers who are nursing on demand are often admonished by their mothers and mothers-in-law that this accustoms the baby to frequent "dining." The concept of feeding every four hours came in with bottle-feeding, because cow's milk and cow's-milk formulas are nutritionally constituted to satisfy the baby for four hours between feedings. Mother's milk is not. The norm for breastfeeding during the first weeks of life is every hour or two. In fact, by feeding frequently, breastfed newborns are helping their mothers build up an adequate milk supply. Their own tiny stomachs are unable to hold large stores of milk that would keep them going for hours—mainly because mother's milk is easily digested and thus does not remain in the stomach for long.

- "Unless you want a spoiled brat, you've got to learn to let the baby cry." Studies show that babies who are picked up when they cry tend to cry less as time goes by, unlike those who are left to scream for hours on end.

  Picking up a baby immediately when crying starts does not encourage crying, although waiting until the crying continues to the point where you can no longer tolerate it does. Picking up the baby immediately is responding to the reason for the crying, which is perfectly appropriate. After all, crying is the only way babies have of expressing hunger, pain, tiredness, or the need to be cuddled. In time they will learn to communicate in other ways. But if they are picked up only after they've cried for a good while, they learn that only by crying can they get the attention they need.

- "Bringing the baby to bed with you sets a bad precedent." In most parts of the world, it is unheard of for an infant to sleep apart from the mother. There is a natural progression: the baby goes from being within the mother's womb to being on the parents' bodies. A baby who feels secure will be ready to separate when the time comes. One that feels lonely and rejected is far more likely to be clingy later on. In the long run, "contingent responsiveness"—not letting a baby cry, feeding often, allowing the baby in bed with you—more than pays off by producing a secure, happy child who is able to separate and able to relate to other adults.

  In terms of convenience, many parents find that having the baby in bed is the simplest way to handle the newborn's frequent night feedings. When the baby has settled into a pattern of sleeping for three to five hours between feedings (usually at three to six months), he or she can be moved to a crib.

- "In order to raise an intelligent baby, you need to provide a wide variety of stimuli, from educational programs to toys that teach." Achievement-oriented parents often worry that their child will fall behind unless they embark on a rigorous program of training and stimulation when the baby has scarcely seen the light of day. But during infancy, the most important stimuli are the parents' touch, smiles, and voices, which all help to produce a baby who is responsive to —and positive about—the surrounding world. Parents should talk or sing to the baby while going about daily tasks such as feeding, changing, and bathing. Touching the baby's body gently will help the baby become oriented to the world and to understand his or her own body, which is the first important step in cognitive development.

It is not just the mother who provides stimulation, of course; it is the family environment as a whole. The best learning experience of all for the baby is to be part of the family. This is facilitated when the baby is carried around the house or placed in an infant seat in the center of family interaction. Common household objects provide stimulation for the senses. Objects of interest should be held 10 to 12 inches from the baby's eyes. The baby should be offered the chance to experience the smell of things in the house—the various ingredients that go into dinner, for instance.

When the baby gets tired of this stimulation, sleep usually will come naturally, but parents should watch for signs of stress, such as an averted gaze, pursing of the lips, tightened fists, curling toes. Babies have a need for rest as well as for stimulation.

Toys such as crib mobiles can be fun for the baby and provide practice in visual "tracking," but there is no need to invest in a set of Beethoven flashcards at this tender age. Ideally, parents learn from their babies and encourage them to develop naturally, rather than pushing them. Even during these early weeks, when the baby is only beginning to raise the head, it is important to keep this approach in mind; otherwise, as time goes by, there is an unfortunate tendency (usually inspired by what we hear from neighbors and friends, or what we read in books) to decide just when the baby ought to sit up, ought to crawl, or ought to walk, and then to try to push the baby toward an artificial norm.

First babies are especially at risk for being taught, whereas later children have a better chance to learn at their own pace.

3 The Role of the Father

Kenneth Katz, M.D.

INTRODUCTION

FEW EXPECTANT FATHERS can fully anticipate their new role before the first baby arrives. But then, the same can be said of their wives. Paternal ignorance about gestation and its implications is not unusual even today, a time when many men are attending childbirth preparation classes.

At first the husband may be preoccupied with the emotional excitement of "my wife's going to have a baby." And this is not inappropriate, because pregnancy is an experience that both wife and husband should enjoy. More and more, husbands are not only enjoying their wife's pregnancy, they are participating in it.

As the pregnancy progresses, becoming obvious to the world, and the father first feels the baby move, the realization of his new dual roles of husband and father may come to the fore.

The birth of every child in a family has its own meaning and importance, but the arrival of the first is very special. For the father, there may never be another experience in life that compares with that moment when he first holds his baby in his arms. For fathers who are present in the delivery room, it is truly a magical experience to participate in the birth and hold the baby almost immediately after it is born.

A generation ago, fathers were viewed as "needless spectators" and barred from even attending, no less participating in, the delivery of their children. In the last 15 years or so, hospitals have changed and are urging fathers to participate in the birth process. Most large hospitals now offer childbirth classes and urge fathers to attend. Some are even offering postpartum classes for fathers, and in many communities support groups just for fathers are being formed, to help them adapt to their new role.

The first few hours of fatherhood naturally are filled with concern for the welfare of the mother and the new arrival. But it is also a time when the father feels tremendous pride in the realization that his procreative role has finally resulted in the birth of a baby.

The initial flush of fatherhood comes immediately after the baby is born. But the full impact may not become obvious until after family and friends have been called, the mother and baby are home, the support of the maternity nurses is no longer available at the push of a button, and the father is on his own.

For most fathers, in spite of all the planning, the first few days may seem like a constant dash between the supermarket, the pharmacy, the mother's side, and the baby's crib. With all the excitement and confusion that accompanies the baby's arrival home there is little time or energy to contemplate the consequences of parenthood. The hectic pace settles down gradually, but during that time the father has a specific role to play: providing both moral support and practical help.

THE CHANGING ROLE OF THE FATHER

THE ROLE OF THE FATHER has changed considerably in the past decade, in both the amount of time he spends and the kind of involvement he has in child rearing. The change often has been attributed to the women's movement, which raised questions about the legitimacy of fixed roles, but men, too, have questioned their traditional role. Economic demands and changing family patterns, particularly the demise of the nuclear family, have exerted influence on the transition. Even popular culture, reflected in the 1979 film *Kramer vs. Kramer*, is thought by some to have had a hand in the change. In that movie, the hero's forced conversion from workaholic to primary parent made strong involvement in parenting acceptable to many men.

Perhaps the best illustration of the changing role of the father is seen in its portrayal by child-care expert Dr. Benjamin Spock. In the 1968 edition of his classic book, *Baby and Child Care*, Dr. Spock characterized the father's role by saying: "A man can be a warm father and a real man at the same time . . . Of course I don't mean that the father has to give just as many bottles or change just as many diapers as the mother. But it's fine for him to do these things occasionally. He might make the formula on Sunday."

Just eight years later, in the 1976 edition of the book, Dr. Spock says: "I think that a father with a full-time job—even where a mother is staying home—will do best by his children, his wife and himself if he takes on half or more of the management of the children (and also participates in the housework) when he gets home from work and on weekends."

Bringing the baby home does not make a father out of a husband. Fatherhood is a challenging role and one that requires patience and planning (see box), but the key to enjoying fatherhood is an understanding of the concept of parenthood. Fathers do not exist in isolation—they are one half of a set of parents.

Many first-time fathers believe that the roles of the two parents are mutually exclusive or that fatherhood is distinct from motherhood. But social scientists, and many fathers, no longer feel that this

---

PLANNING FOR FATHERHOOD

There are no universal guidelines for preparing for parenthood or fatherhood today because each couple enjoys a unique relationship. But the following suggestions may help the expectant father during pregnancy:

- Learn about pregnancy and infancy through books, by talking to other parents, and by spending time around infants and toddlers.
- Identify household chores and divide the responsibilities.
- Know how to, and expect to, change diapers, bathe, and feed the baby.
- Start the search for potential babysitters. If the mother is only planning a brief maternity leave, the choice of child care is a major decision. (For more information, see chapter 16, Child Care.) Even if she is not, it is wise for both parents to plan to spend some time apart from the newborn, even an hour or two, in the first several weeks.
- Begin controlling the amount of time spent on work-related activities; and if possible, limit overtime work. Setting aside "baby-time" even before the baby arrives will help in managing time after the arrival.
- Get names of local pediatricians from the gynecologist, family doctor, and other parents.
- Arrange business schedules to make time for the doctor's visits during pregnancy. This will set the stage for making pediatrician visits after the baby is born.

In short, the father should get involved in every aspect of the pregnancy. This will not only enable him to better help his wife during pregnancy and labor, but it will also help overcome any natural feelings of being left out.

---

is true. Other than the mother's biological capacity for gestation and breastfeeding, there are no significant differences between the two parents.

Some experts challenge the value of interchangeable roles for the mother and the father. Their concern is that a baby, brought up in a family where the roles of the two parents are not distinct, may end up with two mothers or two fathers. But in a society that is headed toward a nonsexist norm and struggling with rising divorce rates, a more salient factor may be the effects of a single-parent versus a two-parent household, rather than a concern about two mothers or two fathers.

Couples, however, do not (or should not) bring

children into their lives to make a social statement. But parents do pass on their beliefs and values to their children, and in that process both parents make choices, not always consciously, that influence their child's future.

BECOMING A FATHER

EVEN THOUGH FATHERHOOD is not materially different from motherhood, there are a variety of emotions that are peculiar to fatherhood. The way in which new fathers cope with their feelings affects both the baby and the mother.

Many fathers seem to be as involved in the pregnancy as their wives and cannot wait for the baby to arrive. Others seem to neglect the pregnancy or to be indifferent to it. At another extreme are those who seem to be totally overwhelmed by the idea of parenthood and who may feel threatened by the unborn child. In fact, most fathers feel all of these emotions at one time or another. Every pregnancy and birth brings with it a variety of emotional surprises, for both the wife and the husband. Even the most committed fathers will confess to certain fears about pregnancy and childbirth, but these are normal.

To help overcome his fears, a new father should ask himself three questions:

- Does he understand the mother's physical and emotional condition once she and the baby are home?
- Does he understand the baby's needs?
- Does he feel capable of feeding and caring for the baby by himself?

It would take a "super father" to answer yes to all three questions; what is important is finding the answers.

THE MOTHER'S NEEDS

TYPICALLY, THE NEW MOTHER experiences a sense of relief that the pregnancy is over and, along with the joy of motherhood, some doubt and anxiety about her ability to care for the baby. A father who understands what the mother is going through, both physically and emotionally, can be a great source of help and support.

Physical Changes

The effects of pregnancy on a woman's body do not end with the birth of the child. The return to normal often takes more than a month, even when the pregnancy and delivery have been without complications. Postpartum discharge of a bloody substance called *lochia*, the residual blood from the site of the placenta, usually lasts four to five weeks, but may continue for up to eight weeks. The bleeding may be followed by a sticky white discharge that gradually disappears.

Oxytocin, a hormone that controls the flow of milk for breastfeeding, also produces postpartum uterine contractions that help the uterus shrink back to its normal size. The contractions may cause cramping for the first three to five days after delivery.

Other hormonal changes may produce hair loss and hot flashes, accompanied by profuse sweating. The sweating, along with what may seem an unusual frequency of urination, helps the body lose excess fluid.

If the mother has had an episiotomy, it will take several weeks before the incision is completely healed and the tissue strong again.

A cesarean delivery is the equivalent of major abdominal surgery and the recovery process usually lasts four to six weeks, while the mother regains her strength, the incision heals, and muscle tone returns (with the help of exercise).

Breastfeeding can also be a cause for discomfort. Until the milk supply is fully in and the baby is nursing regularly, there may be some soreness and swelling. Sucking comes naturally to the baby, but breastfeeding—although partially instinctive—is learned and can sometimes be clumsy and frustrating for the mother at first. Some mothers become discouraged; encouragement from fathers may help them relax and succeed at breastfeeding.

Fatigue

Fatigue is a natural part of the recovery process after labor and delivery. Add to that the demands of caring for the infant on a 24-hour basis and it is no wonder that this is the number-one physical complaint of new mothers. Lack of sleep can exacerbate the stress the mother may be feeling in her new role, as well as delay the shrinking of the uterus to its normal size. Nightly interruptions can mean that she is missing rapid-eye-movement (REM) sleep, the time when the emotional problems of the day are often worked out through dreams.

Emotional Aspects of Recovery

Some degree of postpartum depression (the "baby blues") is a normal and almost universal aspect of childbirth. Most women experience a feeling of anticlimax three to five days after the euphoria of the birth. It appears to be primarily a function of hormonal changes, combined with fatigue and the stress of new responsibilities. Typically a woman feels that she can no longer cope and that she just wants to cry and sleep. Even if she thinks she is coping she may be subject to sudden emotional surges when tears seem to well up at the slightest provocation—or for no reason at all. She may feel that she has made a mistake and that she was not meant to be a mother; she may resent the baby and then feel guilty for doing so. Her resentment may stem from the enormous amount of care the baby requires or (perhaps unconsciously) from the fact that the attention she received from her husband and family during pregnancy has now shifted to the baby. Some mothers are trapped by their own self-imposed need to watch constantly over the baby.

This period is particularly hard on a woman who is used to being in control of her life, doing things according to a schedule, and accomplishing each day what she sets out to do. Now she may find, especially if she is breastfeeding, that the baby wants to be fed every two hours or, perhaps worse, erratically, and that between feeding, changing, bathing, and laundry the days fly by without any intellectual satisfaction. If she is accustomed to being surrounded by colleagues, she may also feel isolation from adult company.

The majority of women are able to cope with postpartum depression and find that it lasts but a few days to a few weeks. However, about 7 percent of new mothers suffer a more debilitating depression in which they are unable to handle their responsibilities toward the baby, or for that matter, toward themselves and their partners. About 1 in 500 suffers the most extreme form of baby blues, puerperal psychosis, which requires professional help and sometimes hospitalization. No case of depression should be allowed to continue more than a few weeks without intervention—counseling and, if prescribed, medication.

For most women, however, the only intervention necessary is understanding and support from husband and family, adequate rest, and regular respite. Besides providing moral support and sharing chores, the father may have to intervene with visitors who overstay or well-meaning parents and in-laws who offer unwanted advice or attempt to take charge of the household.

Even an hour or two to nap or read, take a walk, or phone an old friend, or soak leisurely in the tub without worrying about the baby's cry—can be a great restorative for a new mother. The father can provide this respite by taking the baby for a walk or taking charge of the baby's bath while the mother relaxes. This also gives him valued time alone with the baby.

THE BABY'S NEEDS

THE NEWBORN PERIOD is one of the most profoundly helpless states of human life. Ironically, infants have a strong survival instinct and do not know that they are helpless. Babies' needs are simple and are sometimes summarized as the Four C's: calories, cuddling, clothing, and cleanliness. Their responses at this point are primarily negative reactions to discomfort: of hunger, of being wet or cold, of intestinal gas; and a positive reaction to comfort—of being held reassuringly by a parent.

The more complex concepts of love and trust are alien to a newborn or even a month-old baby. But a hungry infant, held close by the father or the mother during feeding, can experience satisfaction. The infant also can associate the feeling of satisfaction with the visual closeness of the parent's face. Fathers who provide attention to the infant's needs help the baby develop a sense of reliance on both parents. Ultimately they enjoy the rewards of the infant's reactions.

A new father who is not entirely comfortable with the idea of caring for the baby may find it easier if he realizes that a baby's "needs" are rather limited and that the baby's "wants" are practically nonexistent.

Fathers who have participated in the baby care classes offered by some hospitals, or discussed the newborn's daily schedule and needs with a pediatric nurse, will be better able to participate in caring for the baby and to exert a calming influence in what may be an emotionally confused state of affairs. But whether they have attended class or not, there is no substitute for experience. Many fathers, even enlightened ones, believe the myth that mothers instinctively know how to care for infants and fathers lack this instinct. They would do well to observe other fathers and to put more trust in themselves.

Another common problem is the "delicate baby syndrome." Fathers, more so than mothers, are apt to believe that babies are easily hurt, and so are afraid to care for them. Actually babies are quite resilient, even at an early age. They have to be handled gently, but they should be handled with confidence. Perhaps the best way for a father to overcome the "delicate baby" syndrome is simply to hold the baby and take care of it under the watchful eyes of a maternity nurse or an experienced mother or father.

Carrying the baby in a soft baby carrier around the home or on walks is an activity the father can share in right away.

THE FATHER'S NEEDS

FATHERS WHO UNDERSTAND the mother's and the baby's needs, and who feel capable of caring for the baby, will soon realize that fatherhood can be a rewarding experience. But, like the mother, the father can experience doubts about himself and his new role. For most fathers the negative feelings about fatherhood are only temporary.

The father may feel as if he is choreographing a three-dimensional tightrope act: allowing the mother to gain confidence in caring for the baby, developing his own confidence, and preserving enough energy for both parents to resume their adult relationships in the context of a family. When the balance is allowed to swing heavily in favor of any one of the three dimensions it is almost inevitably at the expense of the other two.

A father who constantly watches over the mother's actions may deprive her of a reassuring vote of confidence and leave her wondering if the baby has taken her place as the main focus of her husband's affection. On the other hand, if a father delegates the entire responsibility to the mother, he risks making an already difficult task completely overwhelming for her—and misses out on the emotional satisfaction of caring for his child.

Just as the mother may feel as if all the attention is focused on the baby, the father may feel left out when the mother's day is devoted almost exclusively to caring for the infant. This is particularly so when the mother is breastfeeding, but it need not be. The father can help by fetching the baby from the crib, burping, changing, and holding him or her afterward, and returning the baby to the crib. Once breastfeeding is well established (after six to eight weeks), he can also give the baby relief bottles, day or night, either with formula or breastmilk expressed earlier in the day and refrigerated for later use. If the mother is planning to return to work within two to three months after the birth, it is a good idea to accustom the baby to drinking from the bottle as well as the breast. This also allows the parents to begin to enjoy occasional evenings out.

There are moments when the father may even experience a twinge of resentment toward a newborn, and more so if the mother is having difficulty or complications during the postpartum recovery period at home. The tendency is to blame the infant for the mother's problems. When the father realizes that he is no longer the sole focus of his wife's love and attention, he may find himself competing with the baby. Reminding himself that he is first a parent with inherent obligations and responsibilities and second a father with emotional ties is the best way for him to overcome feelings of resentment.

Whether they are feeling insecure, jealous, or ambivalent, fathers should be candid about their feelings. Most of these feelings disappear over time and are replaced by a special relationship that develops between the father and the baby called bonding. The degree of influence that any adult has on a child depends on the attachment that the child forms with the adult and the frequency and duration of time they spend together. Generally, the younger and therefore more dependent the child, the greater the influence the adult has.

By the end of the first two weeks, most fathers will have resolved their emotional conflicts and have begun to develop positive attitudes about child rearing, child care, and managing new responsibilities around the house.

The first well-baby visit to the pediatrician should be scheduled for two weeks after mother and baby come home from the hospital but may be later, after three or four weeks. If at all possible, the father should accompany them to the pediatrician's. When both parents participate in caring for the child, they are more likely to ask more and better questions about the infant's development and well-being. The father can take responsibility for developing the list of questions to be asked of the pediatric nurse and doctor.

BECOMING A COUPLE AGAIN

FOR A TIME, so much of their day revolves around fulfilling the needs of a helpless little being that couples often forget they have a relationship unto themselves that needs nurturing. Some new parents believe that once they become a "family" they will never be a couple again. This is not so. As difficult as it may be emotionally, new parents need to spend time alone together away from the baby. Short respites are important both physically and psychologically for both parents, but especially for the mother. Even to take a leisurely walk through the neighborhood provides a refreshing break.

Separation will ultimately be easier on both parents and child if the habit is established by the third or fourth month. The separations need not be long—two or three hours may be sufficient. If the mother is breastfeeding, she may begin to get uncomfortable as the next feeding time approaches. She might express milk before leaving, for use by the babysitter as a relief bottle.

In the first several weeks, the mother may show little interest in resuming sexual relations. Fatigue, the emotional weight of her new responsibilities, and the recovery process may prevent her from even thinking about it.

Vaginal intercourse should not be resumed until the cervix is closed and normal mucus secretion has returned. Otherwise there is a danger of infection. In the majority of women, this takes about four weeks, but it can only be confirmed by a physical examination. For this reason, gynecologists recommend waiting until after the first postpartum checkup (usually scheduled for four weeks after delivery) to resume intercourse. By this time, the tissue underlying the episiotomy, if there was one, will have regained its strength as well. Nevertheless, libido may lag behind physical recuperation, and many women prefer to wait a few weeks longer. (Women who deliver by cesarean section usually resume intercourse within the same amount of time whether or not they experience any of these problems.)

Initially the vagina, which understandably has been stretched by the birth process, may be rather tight. Fear of injury may cause the woman to tighten it even more. When intercourse is resumed, it should be slow and gentle for the first few times. Extra lubrication with a product such as K-Y jelly may be necessary. If pain or burning persists, the mother should see her doctor, as this may be an indication that the episiotomy has not healed or that vaginitis unrelated to the pregnancy is present.

MANAGING HOUSEHOLD RESPONSIBILITIES

IF NEW PARENTS feel they can afford help with household chores, now is the time to invest. Even if they cannot afford to have someone clean on a regular basis, they might consider hiring a teenager to take care of shopping and other errands. Or a relative may be willing to come help with the household for the first week or two (baby care is best left to the parents).

For those parents who do not have these options, there are two others: to decide that the house can go without cleaning until things settle down or to divide up the cooking, cleaning, laundry, shopping, and bill-paying chores, if they do not already do that. Taking care of an infant is an around-the-clock job, leaving the primary caregiver with little energy for anything else. The father should be willing to pitch in, making simple meals (or bringing them home), doing the laundry and the grocery shopping, and at least keeping the bathroom and kitchen clean. It is not unreasonable to expect that this should continue even after he returns to work.

RETURNING TO WORK

PATERNITY LEAVE that lasts for more than a week or two is unusual in this country. Fathers generally return to work long before the mother does, leaving the responsibility of caring for the baby to the wife for 10 hours or so each day.

For his own peace of mind, the father can do the following to be sure that both mother and baby are safe:

• Prepare a list of all essential telephone numbers, such as the pediatrician, the gynecologist, a neighbor or a friend who lives close by, and the local emergency number. (The mother should have a similar list, as well as the numbers of the father's business associates.)

• Remember to call home each day, but not too often.

• Make sure that the home is safe and secure.

• Prepare a new schedule for taking care of the baby.

The father now has 10 hours of baby-free "adult time," while the mother becomes the sole caretaker of the infant for those hours. He should plan his evenings and weekends so that he can spend time alone with the baby, giving the mother some adult time, too.

Providing for the family is an appropriate function for the father (as it is for the mother, if she chooses), but this has to be balanced with the new demands being placed on the father's time and emotional energies. The mother, after taking care of the baby and the household all day, may not be particularly interested in goings-on in the workplace. The father, on the other hand, should be aware that both mother and the baby need attention in the evenings.

Fathers who work long hours for professional and financial advancement and to provide the best of everything for the family may eventually realize that they have done so at the expense of the family. They may regret sacrificing time that can never be regained. Those who only begin to pay attention to their offspring in mid-childhood, when they are "interesting" and "companionable," usually find it is too late to have a real influence on the child's development and to understand the person inside the child.

Infants grow rather rapidly, and for the child to have a meaningful memory of growing up with both parents it is important for the father to include the child in the daily "to do" list. There is a cliché among working parents: the quality of time spent with a child is always more rewarding than quantity. It is a way by which working parents rationalize being away from their children for eight or ten hours a day, but it has some validity. The quality of time *is* at least as important as the quantity, if not more so. A schedule serves as a guide in managing time for work, play, and family fun, with the ultimate objectives of strengthening the bond between the father and child.

THE GROWING BABY

DURING THE FIRST SIX MONTHS the baby's physical and emotional needs change rather rapidly, and the parents' role changes accordingly. A schedule devel-oped to take care of the baby six weeks after birth is no longer relevant. Feeding and caring for the baby has now become a routine task both for the father and the mother, and that should provide more time to play with the baby and enjoy the baby's reactions to playful behavior. Because the baby now needs food less frequently, it is possible for parents to assign feeding responsibilities by blocks of time, such as mornings, afternoons, evenings, and, if need be, nights. It is not necessary to assign feeding and changing responsibilities on the basis of "equal time." Both the father and the mother can now be flexible.

Together, fathers and mothers can derive a tremendous amount of joy and pleasure in watching the baby grow. By six months, the baby's routines are more or less established, and the parents now have an opportunity to fully resume their adult relationship, with and without the baby's presence. A six-month-old is obviously not as overwhelming as an infant, and at this time both parents can easily return to individual interests, such as hobbies or sports. A quiet evening, after the baby has gone to sleep for the night, is a more frequent occurrence. It also becomes a reward and a time for the parents to catch up with their lives.

4 Nutrition in the First Year

Allan S. Cunningham, M.D.

INTRODUCTION

ONE WOULD THINK that new mothers should almost instinctively know what and how to feed their babies, but there is probably no other aspect of caring for a newborn that worries parents more or about which they ask as many questions. And the worries do not necessarily disappear as the child grows older. Should I breastfeed or use a formula? Is my baby getting enough? Too much? Should the baby have vitamin and mineral supplements? If so, what kind and how much? When should solid food be started? What should it be? These are but a few of the more obvious questions that every new parent asks.

For the large majority of babies, the answers are straightforward and simple: Breastfeed exclusively for the first six months. When the baby is six months old, gradually begin adding solid foods and some water to go with them, while continuing to breastfeed until the baby is nine months old. Avoid formula or cow's milk until the baby is no longer breastfeeding.

Admittedly this is the ideal, and many mothers can follow this routine with ease and pleasure. But there are many exceptions and some controversies. If there were not, this chapter could end here. No two babies are exactly alike. Mothers have their own needs that must be considered. So do fathers. An almost infinite number of variables and circumstances can affect the baby's feeding process. There is only one cardinal rule: The parents are in charge. Doctors, nurses, neighbors, grandparents, sandbox mothers, and others are full of advice. So are manufacturers of infant formulas. The advice may be well meant and even sound, but parents should not lose sight of the fact that it's *your* baby. Don't assume that someone else knows what is best for you and the baby. Learn as much as you can, listen to the advice, and then decide what course is best in your own particular situation.

Above all, remember that this should be a joyful process for parents and infant alike. It is only natural that all new parents feel a bit nervous and uncertain. Getting a new baby off to the best possible start is undoubtedly one of life's most important undertakings. Still, we should take care not to make the process deadly serious; feeding a baby is fascinating and fun. As confidence builds, a sense of adventure takes over. Granted, the adventure may wear a bit thin when you are wakened by a hungry wail at 3 A.M., but no one ever said parenthood is all roses (and every rose has its thorns).

This chapter is intended to provide the basics of

sound early childhood nutrition. No single guideline will work for every baby and situation, but with the right information parents can make the best choices for them and their baby.

NUTRITION BEFORE BIRTH

SOUND INFANT NUTRITION begins even before conception; the nutritional status of the mother determines in large measure the health and nutritional needs of the baby after birth. In the best of circumstances, the mother should enter pregnancy near her ideal weight and in good health. She should not be anemic or have other nutritional deficiencies; if she does, these should be diagnosed and treated before attempting pregnancy. She also should have completed her own growth; a growing adolescent must make a special effort to provide adequate nutrition for both herself and her baby.

Of course, we do not live in an ideal world; not every pregnancy is carefully planned, and large numbers of women embark on motherhood with less than optimal nutritional status. In the United States, tens of thousands of teenagers become mothers every year, making this one of our most common sources of problem pregnancies. *Still, most of the babies born under these circumstances are normal and healthy.* The fetus is often described as a voracious parasite who will take what it needs from the mother's body. To a degree, this is true. But numerous studies have documented the fact that adolescent or poorly nourished mothers have a much higher than normal incidence of frail, low-birthweight babies. For example, babies born during famine conditions tend to be much smaller than those born when food is plentiful. Anemic mothers will have babies who are also anemic or have very low iron stores. On the other hand, excessive protein also produces small babies.

A number of pregnancy complications also are related to nutritional status. Preeclampsia, or toxemia of pregnancy, is more common among women who are markedly overweight or underweight. In addition to low-birthweight babies, adolescent mothers have a higher than average incidence of toxemia, prematurity, prolonged labor, and infant mortality. Factors other than nutrition play their part here—for example, smoking, drugs, stress, and so forth, but any mother who wants to ensure the best chances of having a healthy baby will pay attention to her nutrition, beginning from the time she starts planning her pregnancy until she stops breastfeeding. (Of course, although pregnancy and breastfeeding are a woman's most nutritionally demanding times, good nutrition should be a life-long endeavor, and not confined to particular life stages or circumstances.)

A woman's needs for nutrients increases during pregnancy and breastfeeding (see table 4.1), but the increase may not be as great as once believed. British research recently suggested that a mother needs 300 extra calories daily only during the last month. The average need through pregnancy is 70 extra calories per day. She should eat a variety of foods from all four food groups (see table 4.2, next page). Almost all pregnant women worry about gaining too much weight. At one time, women were cautioned to hold their weight gain to 10 or 15 pounds in the belief that this would minimize the risk of toxemia and other complications. We now know that, for most women, a 20–30 pound weight gain is consistent with normal pregnancy and a healthy baby. Also, it is not the total weight gain as much as an abrupt gain in the third trimester, as well as overall poor nutrition, that increases the risk of toxemia.

Under very close medical supervision, a markedly overweight woman may be able to get away

Table 4.1 **RDA'S DURING PREGNANCY AND BREASTFEEDING†**

(The following is adapted from the National Academy of Science 1980 Recommended Dietary Allowances, and are for a woman 5'4" tall who weighs 121 pounds.)

Nutrient	Nonpregnant	Pregnant	Nursing
Calories	2,100	2,400	2,600
Protein (gm)	44	74	64
Vitamin A (RE)	800	1,000	1,200
Vitamin D (mcg)	7.5	12.5	12.5
Vitamin E (mg)	10	12	13
Vitamin C (mg)	60	80	100
Folic acid (mg)	0.4	0.8	0.5
Niacin (mg)	14	16	19
Riboflavin (mg)	1.3	1.6	1.8
Thiamin (mg)	1.1	1.5	1.6
Vitamin B6 (mg)	2.0	2.6	2.5
Vitamin B12 (mcg)	3.0	4.0	4.0
Calcium (mg)	800*	1,200	1,200
Phosphorus (mg)	800	1,200	1,200
Iodine (mcg)	150	175	200
Iron (mg)	18	Supp**	18
Magnesium (mg)	300	450	450
Zinc (mg)	15	20	25

* Most experts now recommend that this be increased to 1,000–1,500 mg per day.
** Increased requirement cannot be met by ordinary diets, therefore supplementation is recommended.
† See text.

with a more modest weight gain than one whose weight is normal. But pregnancy is no time to skimp on calories and nutrients, or to try to lose weight. In a nutshell, the average woman should aim to satisfy her hunger and thirst with a variety of wholesome food and beverages. (More specifics of nutrition during pregnancy are discussed in the *Columbia University College of Physicians and Surgeons Complete Guide to Pregnancy*.)

Table 4.2 **DAILY FOOD GUIDE DURING PREGNANCY AND BREASTFEEDING**

	Servings per Day		
Food Group	**Usual Diet**	**During Pregnancy**	**During Nursing**
Protein	2	3	3
Dairy Foods	2 cups or equivalent	4	4
Starches Cereals/ Pasta/Breads	4	4	4
Fruits/ Vegetables	4 or more	4 or more	4 or more
Fats/Oils	1 to 2 tablespoons	2 tablespoons	2 tablespoons
Total calories	1,700–1,900	2,000–2,100	2,200–2,400

Adapted from *Nutrition During Lactation* by Frances Stout, M.S., RD, presented at conference on "Strategies for Successful Breastfeeding," held at Beth Israel Medical Center, New York City, April 24, 1985.

THE FIRST SIX MONTHS

Breastfeeding

There is universal agreement that breastmilk is by far the best food for normal full-term babies during their first six to nine months of life. In recent years, a growing number of mothers have responded to this fact and are electing to nurse their babies. In the early 1970s, for example, about 95 percent of American women bottle-fed their babies; today, half or more of mothers breastfeed. In our enthusiastic support for breastfeeding, however, we should not imply that mothers who must bottle-feed cannot do so with relative safety. Also, there are times when breastmilk must be supplemented. Premature babies, for example, have special nutritional needs. Although they do best when given their own mothers' milk, this may not be sufficient. Many will require special formulas or nutrient supplements to make up for the in utero growth and development they missed by being born too early.

Nutritional Quality. First and foremost, breastmilk is what nature intended for newborn human babies and no commercial formula has been able to equal, much less improve on it. Breastmilk provides virtually every nutrient, in the proper balance, that a baby needs for the first few months of life. Although advances have been made in attempting to come up with formulas that duplicate breastmilk, differences remain. There also is much that we still do not know about infant nutrition which makes it difficult, if not impossible, to come up with formulas that are exact substitutes for breastmilk.

As breastfeeding continues, the milk's composition changes somewhat. For the first few days, it is mostly colostrum, which is higher in protein and lower in sugar and fat than later breastmilk. Colostrum has a laxative effect and is thought to stimulate the newborn's bowels to begin functioning. It is also high in antibodies, which are important in giving the baby immunity against infections. After the first week or so, the volume of colostrum decreases, and by the tenth day the mother will be producing complete breastmilk. As time goes on, the milk will contain less protein and more carbohydrate and fat. The quantity also increases to meet the increasing needs of the rapidly growing baby.

The composition of breastmilk also changes during the course of the day and even during each session of nursing. Breastmilk produced early in the day tends to have more fat than that later on. When the baby first starts feeding, the breastmilk is bluish, watery, and high in protein and carbohydrate. As the breast begins to empty, the milk is higher in fat, which quickly satisfies the appetite and seems to signal the baby that it is about time to stop nursing. This change in the breastmilk's composition is thought to be nature's way of controlling appetite and regulating weight gain.

Protective Effects. Before birth, babies live in a protective, sterile world, but then they are suddenly thrust into an environment where they are exposed to a variety of microorganisms and other potentially harmful substances. Fortunately, the body has a complex, marvelously efficient immune system designed to protect it from outside invaders. In babies, however, this immune system is not fully developed, and the newborn must still depend upon its mothers' protective mechanisms. Colostrum is rich in immunoglobulin A, a type of antibody that helps protect against invading germs. Mother's milk has a number of other substances that protect a baby against disease. Although the mechanisms of protection are not completely known, the results cannot be overemphasized. For example, recent studies have found that most bacterial meningitis in young infants could be prevented by breastfeeding. This adds to what we already know about the protection breastfeeding provides against gastrointestinal and respiratory disease in infants.

The protective effects appear to extend far beyond infancy and childhood. A number of chronic disorders, including diabetes, celiac disease, lymphatic cancers, inflammatory bowel disease, asthma, and allergies, are less common among older children or adults who were breastfed as babies. Researchers are finding a lowered incidence of a certain kind of liver disease, chronic lung disorders, heart disease, and obesity among people who were breastfed. Breastfeeding may be especially important for babies who have a family history of diabetes, heart disease, and other serious, chronic conditions.

Almost every baby can tolerate breastmilk. In contrast, cow's milk allergy is one of the most common allergies seen in babies, but sensitivity to breastmilk is exceedingly rare, if not nonexistent.

Babies are not the only ones who seem to derive long-term health benefits from nursing. Breastfeeding in the early postpartum period helps promote uterine contractions, which helps prevent hemorrhaging. This is one reason nursing mothers find they regain their figures quicker. Breastfeeding also helps a woman lose the extra weight she gained during pregnancy. The risk of osteoporosis is lower in women who have nursed a baby and breastfeeding also reduces the risk of breast cancer in premenopausal women.

Mother-Baby Bonding. Women who breastfeed describe a unique feeling of closeness to their babies. Of course, women who bottle-feed also can derive the bonding and pleasure that comes from holding and cuddling their babies. Still, there is something very special about feeling a baby at the breast and knowing that you alone are sustaining that wonderful new little person.

Convenience and Economy. Breastfeeding does not require any measuring or mixing of formula, sterilizing bottles, heating, or other preparation. Breastmilk is always available, sterile, and the right temperature. It is also more economical than formula—an important consideration for anyone on a tight budget. It is indeed unfortunate that so many women in Third World countries have succumbed to the promotional efforts of Western formula manufacturers and are electing to bottle-feed instead of

following their traditional practice of nursing. The women mistakenly think that formula-fed babies will grow up to be like their counterparts in the United States. In practice, however, this has led to a marked increase in malnutrition and infant mortality. Often, underdeveloped countries lack a sanitary water supply and babies are exposed to a much higher risk of infections. Also, many of the women cannot afford adequate formula, so they end up overdiluting it to make it go further, which results in undernourishing the baby.

Getting Started

Although breastfeeding is the most natural and convenient means of feeding a baby, many women are unsure as to how to go about it and uncertain that they are doing all the right things. Ideally, preparation for nursing begins before birth. Obviously, the mother should consume an adequate diet that provides the nutrients needed for her growing baby.

For most women, the breasts themselves do not need any special preparation. Those with inverted nipples may need to "pull them out" or wear special shields to help them protrude. Women with thin, fair skin—the kind that sunburns easily—seem to have increased problems with sore, cracked nipples. This often can be prevented by "toughening" them before beginning to nurse. (See figure 4.1.) During pregnancy, a woman can rub the nipples with a terry towel. She can also tug and roll each nipple between the thumb and her fingers. Unless a woman has very dry skin, there usually is no need to rub the breasts with cocoa butter or other ointments, as is sometimes recommended. The breasts' Montgomery

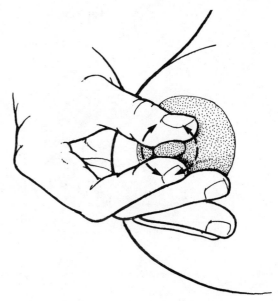

Figure 4.1. **Conditioning the Nipples for Breastfeeding.**

glands—the little yellowish bumps that are located over the areola—provide adequate lubrication. Some women also rub creams or ointments into their breasts in the mistaken notion that this will prevent stretch marks. The creams may soften the skin, but they will not prevent stretch marks. These usually fade with time after the baby is born, although they do not disappear entirely. The stretch marks also occur in mothers who never breast feed.

The breast is a glandular organ marvelously engineered specifically to produce milk. (See figure 4.2.) Each breast contains about 20 lobes arranged in spokelike fashion around the nipple. The lobes branch into clusters of lobules, which look something like tiny bunches of grapes. The grapelike structures are called *acini*, and these are the milk-producing glands. A network of ducts carry the milk from the lobes to the nipple. The pigmented area surrounding the nipple, the areola, house the Montgomery glands. The nipples contain erectile tissue,

which makes them stand out when stimulated or exposed to the cold.

Very early in pregnancy—at about the time of the first missed period—a woman's breasts become enlarged and somewhat tender. Many women can tell that they are pregnant simply by observing these early signs, which are due to the hormonal changes. As the pregnancy progresses, the breasts become more swollen but the early tenderness disappears. The areola enlarges and darkens. During the last trimester, there is often increased nipple discharge, generally a clear or milky fluid that is sometimes tinged with a drop or two of blood. This indicates increased glandular activity as the breasts are readied for milk production.

As term approaches, the breasts become more engorged and the nipples may begin to secrete colostrum—the forerunner to breastmilk. The actual manufacture and release of breastmilk is controlled by an efficient hormonal system. As soon as possible after the baby is born, he or she should be placed at the breasts and allowed to suckle. This suckling signals the pituitary gland to release oxytocin hormone. This is the same hormone that causes the uterus to contract during labor. It also prompts the muscles in the milk ducts to contract and let down or release milk to the nipple. The breasts are very sensitive to even a small increase in oxytocin. Many mothers find that hearing a hungry baby's cry, or sometimes simply thinking about the baby, will stimulate the release of a few drops of milk. Another important pituitary hormone, prolactin, is needed to actually produce the milk. It is the high levels of prolactin during breastfeeding that keep the ovaries from resuming their function, a sort of natural (albeit unpredictable and therefore unreliable) birth control to enable the mother to concentrate her full resources on her baby.

Before the baby is born, it is a good idea for the mother to learn about the techniques of breastfeeding. Unfortunately, many health professionals neglect this important aspect of prenatal education, so the woman herself may need to bring up the subject. Most prenatal or labor-preparation classes include instruction on breastfeeding. Many hospitals also have a nurse who is experienced in helping new mothers get off to a good start in breastfeeding. All pregnant women, even those who think they may not want to nurse, should at least avail themselves of these resources. Some mothers decide to breastfeed after the baby is born.

Most experts agree that the sooner the newborn baby is allowed to nurse the better. Most hospitals now ensure that nursing begins within the first hours after birth. If there are no problems, the newborn can be put to the breast immediately after de-

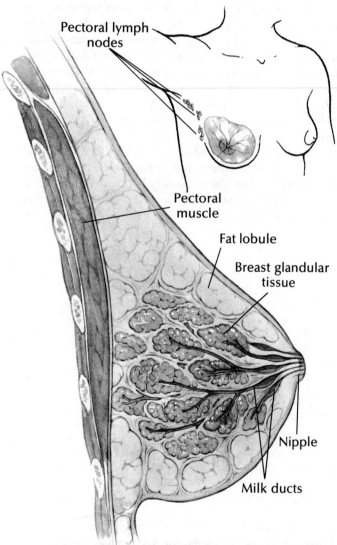

Figure 4.2. **Anatomy of a Normal Breast.**

Pectoral lymph nodes

Pectoral muscle

Fat lobule

Breast glandular tissue

Nipple

Milk ducts

livery. These early efforts are very important to both the mother and baby. Studies have found that the baby's sucking reflex may be strongest shortly after birth. Someone should be on hand to show the new mother how best to position herself comfortably and to make sure the baby can grasp the nipple properly. The baby should have the entire nipple and much of the surrounding areola in the mouth, which will enable the infant to suck properly and also prevent milk from leaking out. If the breasts are large and heavy, the mother may need to position her fingers near the baby's mouth to keep the baby's nostrils clear and to allow proper breathing while nursing.

In the first nursing session, the baby should be switched to the other breast after three or four minutes. This is done by gently removing the nipple from the baby's mouth and repositioning the baby on the other side. A nurse should be on hand to help the mother do this the first few times, and to check that the baby is sucking well. Most babies are alert and hungry almost immediately after birth, but some are tired and need a bit of prodding to suckle. In unusual circumstances, such as babies born with a cleft palate or other congenital defect, breastfeeding may be impossible. In these situations, a mother can still provide the breastmilk for her baby, but it will need to be expressed and fed via a special bottle.

During the first 24 hours, the baby should be kept at the mother's side and allowed to nurse as often as he or she wants, preferably every two or three hours. This stimulates the breasts to produce more milk. The baby should nurse on both sides to help ensure good milk production and also to help prevent nipples from becoming overly sore or cracked. If the breasts are engorged or sore, warm or cool compresses may help. In between nursing sessions, the breasts should be kept dry. Exposing them to the air or positioning a lamp a few inches away so that it provides dry warmth also help. Some women find that they are more comfortable wearing a bra that provides adequate support, even while in bed. The bra should not have a plastic nipple lining, which prevents the escape of moisture and can actually worsen the soreness. The bra also should not be too tight as "binding" prevents adequate breast stimulation and turns off milk production. In fact, firm binding of the breasts was once used to halt milk production.

Proper positioning of the baby also helps prevent nipple soreness. Each woman should find a position that is comfortable for her and that provides the baby good access to the breast. Some women prefer to nurse lying down; others are more comfortable sitting up with the baby cradled in the arms. A roomy rocking chair is ideal, and many maternity hospitals now have them in their rooms.

Although breastfed babies do not swallow as much air as bottle-fed infants, they still should be "burped" after each feeding to minimize discomfort from gas and also to discourage spitting up.

Almost always, breastfeeding is well established within ten days to two weeks. Some mothers leave the hospitals nursing like a pro, but many need more time and encouragement. Many communities have volunteer organizations, such as chapters of the La Leche League, that can provide help to women who are having problems. Local chapters can be located through a doctor, hospital, telephone book or by writing: La Leche League International, 9616 Minneapolis Avenue, Franklin Park, IL 60131, phone (312) 455-7730. In addition, mothers can now seek consultation with members of the International Lactation Consultant Association (ILCA). Ask your doctor for a name of one of these consultants, or write: ILCA, P.O. Box 4031, University of Virginia Station, Charlottesville, VA 22903.

Common Concerns

Many nursing mothers worry that their babies are not getting enough to eat or that their milk is not providing proper nutrition. These worries are usually without foundation. If the baby nurses regularly (normally, six to twelve times daily), which may be anywhere from every two to four or five hours, is growing at a normal rate, and has at least six wet diapers a day, chances are he or she is getting enough to eat. The presence of regular stools is also reassuring during the early weeks. Babies nurse at different rates—some babies are full after eight or ten minutes, while others may want to linger for a half hour or longer.

A mother's milk supply is determined in part by how much her baby consumes. Mothers of twins find they have no trouble nursing two babies, and there are some women who have successfully nursed triplets—a full-time job that is admittedly beyond the call of duty! "Good" babies who sleep most of the time, nurse only three or four times a day, and are growing slowly, if at all, are not eating enough. These babies are lazy or very sleepy and may need to be wakened and stimulated to nurse more often. On average, new babies are nursed eight times during a 24-hour period. In general, breastfed babies eat more often than those who are bottle-fed.

As the baby grows and requires more food, the mother's milk supply increases. On the average, babies double their birthweight in the first four or five months of life, and by their first birthday will weigh three times what they did at birth. A baby tends to grow in spurts rather than at a steady pace of so many ounces every week. During a growth spurt, a baby will nurse longer and more vigorously, emptying out the breasts' reserve supplies, which signals the body to increase total milk production. Many new mothers are alarmed when their babies go through their first growth spurt, and suddenly start wanting to nurse more often and longer. They misinterpret this hunger as a sign that the baby is not getting enough to eat, and many start giving supplementary bottles at this time. These extra bottles are not necessary; in fact, they should be avoided. The extra nursing stimulates the breasts to increase milk production to fulfill the baby's extra demands.

In general, a baby requires 45 to 50 calories per pound per day. As stressed at the beginning of this chapter, for the first four to six months of life, babies get virtually all the nutrients they need from breastmilk or from reserves built up before they were born. Fluoride, a mineral that helps prevent tooth decay, is not passed in breastmilk, and many pediatricians recommend supplements beginning sometime during the first six months. Some pediatricians also recommend vitamin D supplements, especially if the baby is not exposed to sunlight. In the past, iron supplements were often recommended, but this is no longer considered necessary for the majority of babies. Full-term babies are usually born with enough iron reserves to last until they are six months old, at which time they can get extra iron from fortified cereals and other foods. Although these supplements may be recommended as a sort of insurance, the average healthy baby who is breastfed can do very well without them. If a mother questions whether her baby needs supplements, she can ask her pediatrician if they are being recommended for a specific reason peculiar to her baby, or simply as a matter of course.

Formula Feeding

Although the vast majority of mothers can breastfeed exclusively for three to six months, there is a small number—estimated at 1 to 5 percent—who are, for a variety of reasons, unable to nurse their babies. In addition, there are a few women who simply do not make enough milk for their babies and need to supplement with formula feeding, including some who have had breast surgery that has removed some of the glandular tissue. It should be noted, however, that the large majority of women have no difficulty producing adequate milk, and, contrary to popular belief, breast size has no relationship to the quantity of milk produced. Small-breasted women can make just as much milk as those who are large-breasted.

Of course, there still are a large number of women who would prefer not to breastfeed and some who must work outside the home. Many working mothers are able to nurse when they are home, but this requires commitment, organization, and help. Then, too, women who are determined to provide milk for their babies even though they are working can do so by expressing milk from their breasts every four hours or so. The milk can be frozen and used to feed the baby in the mother's absence. The regular expression of milk provides the stimulation needed to maintain milk production. A woman should talk to her employer or supervisor, explaining that she is still providing milk for her baby, and that she needs a few minutes of privacy two or three times during the day and a place where she can keep the milk cool until she goes home. Most employers are understanding and will make the needed time and place available. The milk can be expressed either by hand or with a breast pump.

Most infant formulas are based on cow's milk, which has been modified to make it easier for a baby to digest. Typically, formula is made from reconstituted skim milk or a mixture of skim milk and electrolyte-depleted whey protein. Lactose, or milk sugar, is added; the fat is made up of a mixture of vegetable oils, usually soy, coconut, corn, oleo, and safflower oils, which are easier to digest than the butterfat in cow's milk. Babies who are sensitive to cow's milk or who cannot tolerate lactose may be given a formula based on soy protein. There is no clear agreement as to what formula is best for babies. Generations of babies have been fed homemade formulas based on whole or evaporated milk without major problems. For the first four months or so, commercial formula is preferred. In general, infants should not be given skim milk because it does not provide adequate fat and calories for proper growth and brain development.

Regardless of what formula is used, it should be prepared according to instructions. Commercial formulas come in three forms: ready-to-use bottles or cans, which should not be diluted; concentrated, which should be diluted according to instructions (usually one part formula to one part sterile water); and powdered, which should be mixed with sterile water, according to instructions.

Common Questions and Problem Areas

How often should a baby be fed?   In general, newborn babies should be fed a minimum of six to eight times a day, and some hungry breastfed babies will want to eat more often. At one time, there was considerable debate as to whether a baby should be put on a strict feeding schedule early on, or be fed on demand. Today, pediatricians agree that for the first four or five months, babies should be fed when they are hungry, or on demand. This does not mean that every time a baby cries he or she is demanding to be fed. Babies cry for many reasons other than hunger: to be changed, to get attention, for exercise, or simply because they want to. Parents quickly learn to distinguish a hungry cry and to act accordingly.

As a baby grows older, he or she can go longer between feedings. Mothers should avoid the urge to quiet a fussy baby by feeding; food should not be used as a pacifier or a substitute for attention and cuddling. By the same token, some babies do not cry very much, even when they are hungry. A mother should be concerned about a young baby who wants to eat only four or five times a day and is not gaining adequate weight. These babies may not be getting enough to eat, even though they do not seem to be hungry and seldom cry. Some should be wakened every three or four hours and fed.

How often should a baby have a bowel movement?

This varies greatly from baby to baby. On the average, a breastfed newborn may have several bowel movements a day, which can range from soft to watery. They are generally odorless or slightly sour and the color ranges from pale yellow to dark green. Formula-fed babies have smellier stools and are more apt to become constipated. Many mothers, especially those who are breastfeeding, become alarmed when their babies do not have a daily stool. It is not uncommon after a few weeks for breastfed babies to go several days, or even a week or more, without having a bowel movement. If the stools are soft and passed without undue straining, the frequency is not important.

As a baby grows older, bowel habits are likely to change. The newborn who had six or eight stools a day may suddenly go two or three days without any. Stools that were watery may become firmer or vice-versa. Often, these changes are misinterpreted as diarrhea or constipation, and the baby's diet is manipulated accordingly. Real diarrhea is characterized by watery (not just loose), frequent stools. Streaking with blood or mucus may occur, and these are warning signs that should be reported to a doctor. Even if a baby has diarrhea, feeding should continue. It is important that a baby with diarrhea receive adequate fluids to prevent dehydration. In general, breastfed babies should continue to nurse. For some babies, regardless of feeding method, professional advice may be necessary to specify feedings or decide if medical treatment is necessary.

Chronic diarrhea is less serious than the acute type. Often there is no specific cause for the frequent, loose stools, in which case the condition is referred to as "nonspecific diarrhea." Onset of the diarrhea often coincides with a change in diet or in the diet of the breast-feeding mother. The diarrhea could be a sign of an allergic sensitivity to the food, or the child's gastrointestinal tract may be unable to properly absorb the food. (See chapter 23, Gastrointestinal Disorders, for a more detailed discussion.) Nonspecific diarrhea is seldom life-threatening; typically the child continues to grow and is otherwise healthy. The diarrhea may come and go. Although there is some debate about this, teething may be accompanied by loose stools.

What if the mother gets sick?

Breastfeeding usually can continue through a minor infection, such as a cold or flu. Mothers often worry that they will pass the germs on to the baby in the breastmilk, but this is not how these microorganisms are transmitted. The baby will be exposed to the virus simply by being in contact with the mother, and breastfed babies are protected, although this is not absolute or foolproof. Mothers must still wash their hands, avoid sneezing on the baby, and take other common-sense precautions. More serious infections, such as tuberculosis, may require that breastfeeding be stopped. Similarly, the use of some drugs is contraindicated during breastfeeding. (See tables 4.3 and 4.4 on drugs to avoid while breastfeeding.)

If the mother is hospitalized or too ill to breast-

Table 4.3 **DRUGS THAT SHOULD NOT BE TAKEN WHILE BREAST-FEEDING***

Drug	Effects on Baby
Amethopterin	Possible suppression of immune system.
Bromocriptine	Suppresses milk production.
Cimetidine	May suppress gastric acids in baby; inhibits drug metabolism and stimulates central nervous system.
Clemastine	Drowsiness, irritability, refusal to feed, high-pitched cry, neck stiffness.
Cyclophosphamide	Possible suppression of immune system.
Ergotamine	Vomiting, diarrhea, convulsions.
Gold salts	Rash, inflammation of kidney and liver.
Methimazole	May interfere with thyroid function.
Phenindamine	Hemorrhage.
Thiouracil	Decreased thyroid function.

(Note: Some pediatricians add other drugs to this list. In general, not enough enter the breast milk to cause harm to the baby, but there may be special circumstances that contraindicate their use. Hence, ask your doctor's opinion if in doubt about any medication or substance.)
* Recommendations of the Committee on Drugs of the American Academy of Pediatrics, 1983.

Table 4.4 **DRUGS THAT REQUIRE TEMPORARY CESSATION OF BREASTFEEDING***

Drug	Recommended Alteration in Nursing
Metronidazole	Discontinue breastfeeding 12–24 hours to allow excretion of drug.
Radioactive dyes	Radioactivity present in milk; prior to studies, mother should express and freeze milk for baby, and continue expressing milk even when not nursing to ensure continued production, even though this milk should be discarded. Consult specialist in nuclear medicine to determine when milk can be used.
Gallium-69	Radioactivity in milk present for 2 weeks.
Iodine-125	Risk of thyroid cancer; radioactivity present for 12 days.
Iodine-131	Radioactivity present for 2–14 days depending on study.
Radioactive sodium	Radioactivity present for 96 hours.
Technetium-99m, 99m TC macroaggregates, 99m TC O₄	Radioactivity in milk for 15 hours to 3 days.

* Recommendations of the Committee on Drugs of the American Academy of Pediatrics, 1983.

feed, at least temporarily, she should discuss her options with her doctor. If it is likely that the illness will be short-lived and the mother wants to continue breastfeeding, she can request that her breasts be pumped periodically so that she continues making milk and will be able to resume nursing after she recovers. If there are no contravening circumstances, such as the presence of potentially harmful drugs, the expressed breastmilk can be given to the baby.

What about jealous siblings? Many mothers give up breastfeeding because it is upsetting to an older brother or sister. They may be overly concerned about sibling rivalry and resentment to begin with, and putting up with an obviously jealous toddler who picks the baby's feeding time as an opportune moment to demand attention proves too much and they resort to bottle-feeding. There is no one solution that works in every instance. The approach often depends upon the child's age. For example, explanations and reasoning usually do not faze a young toddler but may work with an older child. Understandably, a sibling will feel that the new baby is an unwelcome intruder and will fear that his or her place will be usurped by the newcomer. Finding special times when the mother can be alone with the older child is important and reassuring. Involving the sibling in the baby's care also may help. This is also an area in which the father can take the lead by spending more time with the older child.

Are there other roles for the father? Very often, fathers of breastfed babies feel left out and even somewhat resentful. In this era of enlightened fatherhood, in which men are expected to assume a more nurturing role than in the past, many new fathers are ready and willing to do their share in caring for the new baby. Psychologically they are not prepared to stand by while their wives spend several hours a day breastfeeding. Of course, there also are the more deep-seated sexual connotations; subconsciously a man also may resent the fact that the baby is taking his wife's breast—and the sexual pleasure it embodies—from him. Both of these feelings are natural and should be recognized. Women may derive a certain amount of sexual pleasure from breastfeeding, but this does not imply that they have lost interest in their husbands. Of course, feeding is not the only aspect of caring for a newborn. Fathers may participate in many ways. Some couples find that having the father help with the late night feedings—perhaps getting up, changing the baby, and bringing him or her to the mother to feed in bed—allows both to participate. Some mothers express a bottle of milk during the day that the father can give during the night, allowing the woman to get some much needed sleep and giving the father a turn at feeding.

When will the baby start sleeping through the night? Again, this varies greatly from baby to baby. Some can go through the night when they are one or two months old, others will still want a night feeding when they are nine or ten months or even older. In the latter instance, waking up during the night is more of a habit than a need for food. Professionals and laymen both have advice, but it is usually not scientific. As hard as it may be for the parents, simply letting the child cry may be the only way to get out of the night-feeding pattern. Obviously the baby should be checked to see if he or she needs changing or if there is some other problem. If all is okay, the baby will eventually stop crying and everyone will be able to get some sleep.

Parents are often horrified at this suggestion, thinking that it is cruel to ignore a baby's cries. But eventually the child must learn how to conform to the family's schedule, which does not include getting up in the middle of the night for a meal or simply a play session. Some mothers persuasively argue that they cannot bear to hear the child cry and will continue to get up. There is no proven harm in either approach. Practical compromise and patience is the prudent policy.

Do breastfed babies have less colic than those who are bottle-fed? Old wives think so, but this has not been demonstrated scientifically. A certain number of babies develop colic, no matter how they are fed. If there is an association to diet, it may well be linked to a sensitivity to the protein in formula or cow's milk. A nursing mother with a colicky baby may try eliminating cow's milk and milk products from her diet. This is sometimes quite helpful.

When can mother expect some "time off"? Caring for a new baby is a full-time job, and one that most mothers find rewarding and full of pleasure. Even the mother who works or has full-time help at home invariably finds excuses to "do for her baby." But no matter how determined a woman is to do it all, there will be times when she wants a break. Even a woman who is breastfeeding every few hours can arrange for an occasional break or evening out. Some breastfed babies do not take kindly to a supplemental bottle, even if it contains mother's milk, unless they have become accustomed to a rubber nipple in the first couple of months of life. After breastfeeding is well-established, a mother can express milk to fill a bottle and use this for a feeding. The baby may protest the nipple at first, but if he or she is hungry, it will not take long to figure out that food comes in more than one container.

Are pacifiers acceptable? Pacifiers have been given a "bum rap," but for no good reason. In fact, there are instances in which pacifiers are beneficial. Some babies want to suck all the time, and if they are allowed to feed to their hearts' content, they end up overeating. Giving these babies a pacifier will satisfy their desire to suckle and keep them from becoming obese. Contrary to popular belief, allowing a baby to suck a pacifier or thumb will not destroy the mouth or cause an overbite. Mothers usually understand the value of a pacifier; the main objections come from grandparents, aunts, and nosy neighbors, none of whom have any real responsibility in determining what is best for a baby. Obviously a hungry baby should not be given a pacifier in place of food, but there is nothing wrong in letting a sated baby suck a pacifier or a thumb. In many ways a thumb is better than a pacifier—it is always available, does not get lost, and a baby cannot choke on it. Well-meaning grandmothers often scold a child for sucking his or her thumb; in such instances, the mother should intervene on behalf of the child and the thumb.

Is it necessary to heat a bottle? Conventional wisdom seems to hold that babies like warm bottles, but there is no sound evidence to support this, or to document that warm milk is any more digestible than formula or milk that is room temperature or even right out of the refrigerator. In fact, many babies seem to prefer cool milk to that which is warmed. A word of caution: If the bottle is heated, it always should be tested to make sure that the contents are not too hot. Also, avoid warming bottles in a microwave. This may be convenient and fast, but microwaves can heat the contents to the boiling point even though the container may feel cool to the touch. There also have been reports of babies being burned by exploding plastic liners that are used in some types of bottles.

Is it necessary to sterilize bottles and formula? Most of the formula sold in the United States has been heat treated and is safe, so long as it is refrigerated and used in a reasonable amount of time. Most water supplies also are safe; exceptions are surface water or water from some wells. If there is any doubt at all, this water should be boiled. As for bottles, nipples, caps, and other such equipment, many experts advise that they be sterilized for the first three months, although it must be admitted that the advice is arbitrary and may be unnecessary. Some dishwashers have a heat cycle that will sterilize bottles and other items. Or they can be sterilized by boiling. All bottles and other equipment used in preparing the formula or feeding the baby should be washed in hot, soapy water and thoroughly rinsed after each use. Before using again, the bottles, nipples, caps, and nipple collars should be placed in a pot of water and boiled for five minutes. After the water has cooled, they should be removed with tongs (be careful not to touch the nipples in particular). A day's supply of bottles can be done at one time, then be filled and stored in the refrigerator. Care should be taken to wash the tops of canned formula before opening.

These are but a few of the common questions that arise in the first few weeks or months of feeding a baby. New parents should not hesitate to seek guidance from their pediatricians or family physicians. These physicians expect parents to have many questions, and answering questions and reassuring parents are among the more important aspects of these medical specialties.

Introducing Solid Foods

Questions about when and how to introduce solid foods into a baby's diet are second only to questions about breast- or bottle-feeding. Again, this is an area in which there is considerable conflicting advice and controversy. Twenty years ago many pediatricians advised starting some solid foods at four to six weeks of age, or as soon as a baby was well established on a feeding schedule. Then there was a shift away from early solid foods, on the theory that the extra food increased the risk of later obesity. Today many experts still advise waiting until the baby is four to six months old, especially if the mother is breastfeeding.

Actually, the question of when to start solid foods depends a good deal upon the baby. Some babies are ready for solid foods at a month to six weeks of age. It is the rare bottle-fed baby who gets no solids before two months. This is more likely to be true of formula-fed infants than those who are breastfed, and there are advantages to variety to compensate for nutritional shortcomings of the formula. Breastfed babies usually can wait longer, and since they get all the nutrients they need for the first few months of life from breastmilk, there is no need to rush.

In any event, even babies who are exclusively breastfed should begin getting some solid foods by the time they are six months old, and earlier if they seem to be very hungry. If circumstances permit, continued breastfeeding as solids are added, at least until the baby is nine months old, is ideal. By this age, a baby is developed enough to sit at the table and have three meals of solid foods a day with the rest of the family—which is the ultimate goal. The baby can then be weaned from breastmilk and switched to regular cow's milk. Naturally, babies and mothers can do nicely if nursing continues after nine months.

It is important to note that some babies who require more calories will need solid food by the time they are three months old, or even earlier in some instances. Despite fears of overfeeding, most babies know how much to eat—when they have had enough, they will simply stop, and when they are hungry, they will cry until fed. Some babies are naturally on the chubby side and others are naturally thin; parents should not become preoccupied with trying to alter a baby's natural build. So long as the weight is within the normal range for the baby's height and age, parents should not worry about the child being over- or underweight.

In introducing solid foods, start with one at a time and let the baby become accustomed to each before introducing the next. There are no iron-clad rules as to the order that should be followed. Many pediatricians recommend starting with rice cereal, and after the baby is eating cereal, strained fruits and vegetables can be added. Babies naturally prefer sweet foods; mashed bananas, apple sauce, or pears are common "starters." Carrots, squash, peas, and beans are favored first vegetables. By six or seven months of age, the typical baby will be eating a total of two or three tablespoons of cereal (rice and oatmeal are the best), fruits, and vegetables four or five times a day. Water, fruit juices, and whole cow's milk may also be given, especially if the baby is weaned from the breast. Formula-fed babies usually start drinking other fluids even earlier.

Strained meats are among the last of the strained foods to be added. Many pediatricians recommend waiting until the baby is nine months old before introducing eggs. As the baby's chewing reflexes develop and hand-mouth coordination improves, bread sticks, crackers, O-shaped dry cereals, and other finger foods may be added. This is an important prelude to learning how to self-feed, and babies should be encouraged to try finger foods. Obviously, a baby should not be given objects he or she can choke on, but even without teeth, most babies can "chew" a variety of finger foods.

Although commercial baby foods are convenient and popular, by the time babies are six or seven months old, most can eat mashed or pureed table food. Babies tend to prefer bland foods, so it is a good idea to go easy on spices. There are, however, many exceptions, including cultural differences. Some babies almost seem to inherit their parents' love of extra-hot Indian or Chinese cuisine, while others will spit out anything that tastes of onion, garlic, pepper, and other herbs or spices. It is not necessary to add salt to a baby's food.

Adverse Food Reactions

Food allergies and intolerances are fairly common in babies and young children. If a food produces any untoward symptoms—a rash, wheezing, coughing, diarrhea, or other gastrointestinal upsets—it should be stopped immediately. Foods that most commonly produce allergic reactions include cow's milk, eggs, corn, citrus fruit, wheat, barley or rye gluten, nuts, chocolate, and seafood. Sometimes a food can be reintroduced at a later date; if it again produces symptoms, do not offer it for several more months. Nuts, whole or in pieces, and popcorn should not be given until at least the age of three. Not only do nuts have a high allergic potential, but they also can cause choking.

Food intolerances should not be confused with allergies, although some of the symptoms may be similar. An allergic reaction involves the immune system, whereas an intolerance entails inability to digest or absorb a food. For example, some babies are unable to tolerate lactose; others cannot digest breads or cereals (a characteristic of celiac disease); and still others lack the enzymes needed to break down fats. Often children with malabsorption disorders fail to grow properly, even though they may consume large quantities of food. Any suspected food intolerance should be evaluated promptly by a doctor who is experienced in this area.

THE NURSING MOTHER'S DIET

MYTHS ABOUND AS TO WHAT a mother should or should not eat while breastfeeding. In general, a nursing mother's diet is quite similar to what she consumed while pregnant. The vitamin content of a mother's milk reflects her dietary intake and will be adequate with a varied diet and normal amounts of food. Vitamin supplements are usually not necessary for the nursing mother (or her baby), although the vitamin K given to babies in most hospital nurseries is a sensible precaution against bleeding in the newborn. Rickets can result from a deficiency of vitamin D, but this is now rare in the United States. Vitamin D is produced by mothers and babies themselves when exposed to sunlight. There may be a problem if a baby is exclusively breastfed for longer than six months and gets little exposure to sunlight. (This is more likely to occur in black babies whose skin does not absorb as much sunlight.) In such instances, vitamin D supplements may be needed.

A nursing mother may need more calories than normal, but this is open to debate. Much has been written about the need for extra food during pregnancy and lactation—the standard recommendation advises an extra 300 to 500 calories a day. Is this really necessary? Probably not. As noted earlier, British scientists have found that pregnant women normally consume an average of 70 extra calories a day—the equivalent of an extra slice of bread or scant glass of skim milk. Their pregnancies are normal; they have generous fat storage for later breastfeeding, and their babies are of normal birthweight. As a matter of fact, both British and American researchers have found that excessive protein and calorie consumption may be harmful to the baby and lower birthweight.

If this seems confusing or contradictory, it may help to understand three facts that are not widely known: First, many standard dietary recommendations are based on purely theoretical considerations and have not been tested in a truly scientific manner in normal circumstances. Second, the organizations that publish recommended dietary allowances actually increase the recommendations above their average calculations to accommodate the needs of people whose requirements may be above average. The result is that the standard RDAs are actually excessive for many people. Finally, this practice has been based on the general assumption that too much is better than too little. We are now learning that this assumption may be incorrect.

In this context, a few words are needed regarding calcium and osteoporosis. Common sense—and some theorizing—suggests that mothers need extra calcium during pregnancy and lactation to protect their own bone structure while providing for their babies' growth. But some more of those "contradictory facts" have recently come to light. Older women with osteoporosis are actually less likely to have borne children and nursed their babies than women without the disease. Moreover, experimental animals who receive large amounts of calcium when they are young lose excessive amounts from their bones in old age. These observations cannot be ignored, particularly since some of the foods recommended for their calcium content are unpleasant—or even harmful—for some mothers and their babies. For example, many mothers are nauseated by milk and other dairy products, particularly during pregnancy. Furthermore, even when mothers eat milk products without discomfort, they may cause constipation, anemia, and leg cramps. Sometimes infants are born with an allergy to cow's milk and other milk products because their mothers consume excessive quantities during pregnancy.

Variety and moderation are the key elements in formulating a diet for a nursing mother. She should consume a variety of wholesome foods from the four basic food groups and beverages to satisfy hunger and thirst. In many respects, the diet for breastfeeding should be a continuation or, in some instances, an expansion of what the healthy woman ate during her third trimester of pregnancy.

Substances to Avoid

In addition to concerns over providing adequate nutrients for a breastfed baby and her own needs, a nursing woman also should be aware that a number of potentially harmful substances can pass through her body to the baby. Breastfeeding mothers should avoid large amounts of alcohol and caffeine, both of which pass into breastmilk. An occasional alcoholic drink or cup of coffee or other caffeine-containing beverage probably will not harm the baby, but it's probably not a good idea to drink it just before breastfeeding. Nicotine also passes into breastmilk, as does the most active ingredient in marijuana—neither should be used while breastfeeding. There is also evidence that babies who inhale secondhand tobacco smoke have more respiratory problems and other illnesses than babies who are not exposed to smoke.

Medications also may pass into breastmilk and some may be harmful to babies whose liver and kidneys are still immature and not readily able to break them down. Tables 4.3 and 4.4 list those that should be avoided while breastfeeding. If in doubt, a mother should consult her pediatrician about specific medications.

A number of environmental toxins, such as DDT and polychlorinated biphenyls (PCBs) appear in breastmilk and may be harmful to the baby. Women exposed to such chemicals in the environment or workplace may want to have their breastmilk analyzed. If in doubt, check with your local or state health department or regional Environmental Protection Agency.

Intestinal Gas

It is popularly believed that eating onions, cabbage, beans, or other foods that produce intestinal gas will have a similar effect on the baby. There is no good evidence to support this, but if a baby invariably seems uncomfortable and fussy after a nursing mother has consumed a particular food, it may be a good idea to eliminate it from her diet.

Food Allergies

Some pediatricians and allergists caution mothers to avoid foods that are highly allergenic during the last trimester of pregnancy and while breastfeeding, especially if there is a strong family history of allergies, asthma, and other allergic disorders. Included on the list are peanuts, egg whites, and possibly shellfish and cow's milk.

SUMMING UP

GETTING A BABY OFF to a good nutritional start is one of the most important aspects of parenthood. Ideally the mother should plan for her baby's nutritional status even before getting pregnant, and continue by eating a balanced, healthful diet throughout pregnancy and breastfeeding. Common sense, moderation, variety, balance—all are key elements in ensuring a good diet for both mother and baby. This chapter has provided the basics for good nutrition in the first year; in the next chapter, nutritional guidelines for the toddler through preschool years will be discussed.

5 Nutrition for Toddlers and Preschoolers

Allan S. Cunningham, M.D.

INTRODUCTION

ALTHOUGH MOST PARENTS begin to feel more secure about feeding a baby as the child graduates to solid food and self-feeding, remember that good nutrition throughout the early years is important to proper growth and development. And during these vital early years, the child forms important lifelong eating habits. Toddlers quickly develop very definite food preferences and also learn that what they will or will not eat can gain a parent's undivided attention. They also observe the way other family members eat and are just as quick to emulate bad habits as good ones. In this chapter we will review the nutritional needs of the growing child and also outline a practical, common-sense approach to fostering sound eating patterns.

CHANGING NUTRITIONAL NEEDS

DURING THE FIRST YEAR of life, the typical infant triples his or her birthweight. After the first birthday,

the growth rate slows considerably, and it will take the next four to five years for weight to double. On the average, toddlers gain five to ten pounds annually during their second and third years, and preschoolers gain even less rapidly, at an average rate of three to five pounds a year. As during the first year, growth comes in spurts—the child will suddenly add a couple of inches in height, and then have a period of very little skeletal growth. During this "resting period," the youngster will gradually put on weight to catch up with the previous spurt in height. This pattern will be repeated throughout the early growing years.

A child needs some 50 essential nutrients to ensure proper growth and development as well as body repair and maintenance. These nutrients are the same ones required by adults, but the amounts vary (see table 5.1). Since no one food provides all the needed nutrients, it is important that a child's diet provide a variety of foods from all four food groups (see table 5.2).

Vitamin/Mineral Supplements

The routine use of vitamin and mineral supplements is not recommended, despite the fact that they are

Table 5.1 RECOMMENDED DIETARY ALLOWANCES FOR BOYS AND GIRLS AGES 1 TO 6

	Age and Size	
Nutrient	1–3 years 29 lbs., 35 ins.	4–6 years 44 lbs., 44 ins.
Calories	1,300	1,700
Protein (g)	23	30
Vitamin A activity (R.E.)	400	500
Vitamin D (mcg)	10	10
Vitamin E activity (mg alpha T.E.)	5	6
Vitamin C (mg)	45	45
Thiamin (mg)	0.7	0.9
Riboflavin (mg)	0.8	1.0
Niacin (mg NE)	9	11
Vitamin B6 (mg)	0.9	1.3
Folacin (mcg)	100	200
Vitamin B12 (mcg)	2.0	2.5
Calcium (mg)	800	800
Phosphorus (mg)	800	800
Magnesium (mg)	150	200
Iron (mg)	15	10
Zinc (mg)	10	10
Iodine (mcg)	70	90

	Provisional Recommendation	
Nutrient	Age 1–3	Age 4–6
Vitamin D (mcg)	15–30	20–40
Biotin (mcg)	65	85
Pantothenic acid (mg)	3	3–4
Copper (mg)	1.0–1.5	1.5–2.0
Manganese (mg)	1.0–1.5	1.0–2.5
Chromium (mg)	0.02–0.08	0.03–0.12
Selenium (mg)	0.02–0.08	0.03–0.12
Molybdenum (mg)	0.05–0.1	0.06–0.15
Sodium (mg)	325–975	450–1,350
Potassium (mg)	550–1,650	775–2,325
Chloride (mg)	500–1,500	700–2,100

Prepared by Food and Nutrition Board, National Academy of Sciences—National Research Council, Washington, D.C., 1980.

Table 5.2 HOW TO USE BASIC FOOD GROUPS

Foods Included in This Group Are:		Serving Sizes			Daily Servings	Nutrients Supplied
		1 Year	2–3 Years	4–5 Years		
Milk and Dairy Products	4 servings daily in the amounts recommended from a variety of foods listed in this group					
	Milk, yogurt, and milk-based soups; cottage cheese	¼–½ c.	½–¾ c.	¾ c.		
	Custard, milk pudding, and ice cream (served only after a meal)	2–4 T.	4–6 T.	6 T.	4	Calcium Riboflavin Protein
	Cheese (1 oz. = 1 slice or a 1-in. cube)	⅓–⅔ oz.	⅔–1 oz.	1 oz.		

Table 5.2 **HOW TO USE BASIC FOOD GROUPS** (continued)

Foods Included in This Group Are:		Serving Sizes			Daily Servings	Nutrients Supplied
		1 Year	2–3 Years	4–5 Years		
Meat and Meat Alternatives	4 servings daily in the amounts recommended from a variety of foods listed in this group					
	Beef, pork, lamb, fish, and poultry; liver (every two weeks)	1 oz.	1½ oz.	4 T. or 2 oz.	2	
	Eggs	½	¾	1		Niacin
	Peanut butter	2 T.	3 T.	3 T.		Iron
	Cooked legumes, dried beans, or peas	¼ c.	⅜ c.	½ c.	2*	Thiamin
	Nuts	no servings	¾–1 oz.	1–1½ oz.		
	* use additional servings of red meat, fish, or poultry if 2 servings of peanut butter, nuts, or legumes are not eaten daily					
Fruits and Vegetables	4 servings daily in the amounts recommended from a variety of foods listed in this group					
	Vitamin C Source Fruits, Vegetables, and Juices Citrus fruits, berries, melons, tomatoes, peppers, cabbage, cauliflower, broccoli, and potatoes	¼ c.	¼ c.	¼ c.	1	Vitamin C
	Vitamin A Source Fruits and Vegetables (deep green and yellow) Melons, peaches, apricots, carrots, spinach, broccoli, squash, pumpkin, sweet potatoes, peas, beans (green, yellow, and lima), and Brussels sprouts	1–2 T.	3–4 T.	4–5 T.	1	Vitamin A
	Fruits	⅛ c.	¼ c.	½ c.		
	Vegetables	1–2 T.	3–4 T.	4–5 T.	2	
Breads and Cereals	4 servings daily in the amounts recommended from a variety of foods listed in this group					
	Whole grain, enriched, or restored breads	½ slice	¾ slice	¾–1 slice		
	Cooked cereals, rice, and pasta;	¼ c.	⅓ c.	½ c.	4	Thiamin Iron Niacin
	Whole-grain or fortified ready-to-eat cereals	½ oz.	¾ oz.	1 oz.		
Fats/Oils	Butter, margarine, oils, mayonnaise, and salad dressings	1 tsp.	1 tsp.	1 tsp.	3	This group is a significant source of fats, for which there is no U.S. RDA
	(1 tablespoon = 100 calories)					
Other Foods	Jams, jellies, soft drinks, candy, sweet desserts, salty snacks, gravies, olives, pickles, and ketchup	USE IN MODERATION			NO AMOUNT RECOMMENDED	This group is a significant source of fats, for which there is no U.S. RDA

This chart has been adapted from: Endres, F., and Rockwell, R., *Food Nutrition and the Young Child*, St. Louis, 1980, C. V. Mosley Co.

widely promoted and many parents look upon a daily vitamin pill as insurance against possible dietary shortcomings. Some vitamins, especially thiamine and B_{12}, are promoted as appetite and growth stimulants—both claims that have no basis in fact. Many parents also have the mistaken notion that megadoses of certain nutrients—particularly vitamin C—can help prevent colds and other ailments. Again, there is no scientific evidence to support these claims and, indeed, megadoses of any nutrient, including vitamin C, can be harmful. When taken in amounts greater than the body needs for normal functioning, vitamins or minerals take on the property of drugs with the same potential for adverse side effects as any medication. Most parents would not give a child powerful drugs without a physician's guidance; unfortunately, the same cannot be said for vitamins and minerals. There is probably no other area in which people indulge in more self-treatment, very often without need or proper understanding.

Not uncommonly, grandparents are the primary promoters of unneeded supplements. In the past some important nutrients were lacking in many youngsters' diets, but this is no longer true. For example, iron deficiency once was relatively common among babies and young children, but today's widespread fortification of cereals, bread, and other foods have made additional supplements unnecessary. In recent decades, national nutritional surveys have not found any major vitamin or mineral deficiencies among the general population; where problems exist it is among the economically disadvantaged or in isolated instances of neglect or abuse. In these instances, the problem is more likely to be an insufficiency of food, rather than a lack of specific vitamins or minerals. A varied diet that includes adequate amounts from all four food groups will provide all of the vitamins and minerals needed for growth and development. A possible exception is fluoride in areas in which this mineral is not added to drinking water.

In unusual circumstances, a child may have a metabolic disorder, numerous food allergies, or other diseases that require a restricted diet. These youngsters may require vitamin or mineral supplements to make up for what is lacking in their diets, but these are exceptions and not the rule. (See chapters on specific disorders later in this book.)

Over- and Underfeeding

With the marked slowdown in growth, a young child's appetite naturally diminishes to prevent overeating. Also, after the first birthday, the baby's stomach and digestive system are developed enough so that very frequent feedings are no longer necessary. Most toddlers do nicely on three meals and perhaps a couple of snacks a day. Unfortunately, many parents (and grandparents) misinterpret these natural changes in growth rate, appetite, and reduced food requirements as hallmarks of "a poor eater." They worry that the child is not eating enough or becoming finicky, and will try to urge the youngster to eat more than is needed. Very often sweets are used as a bribe: "Eat all of your vegetables and you can have a cookie" or, "Three more bites and you can have dessert."

Conversely, we have a growing number of young parents who are overly preoccupied with slimness and the possible links between diet and heart disease or other serious health problems. Since the parents are constantly warned to cut down on fats and cholesterol and to count calories, they mistakenly think these dietary principles should be extended to their young children. For example, we see parents who limit a young child's consumption of eggs or switch to skim or low-fat milk, thinking that this will help ward off later heart disease. There is no evidence that such dietary restrictions at such an early age help, except in very unusual circumstances. But curtailing important nutrients, including fats, at an early age can interfere with proper growth and result in serious nutritional imbalances.

As a general rule, if a child is growing within the normal ranges on standard height and weight tables and is otherwise active and healthy, he or she is getting enough to eat. If the day's meals include a variety of foods in the portions suggested in table 5.1, it's a good bet that the child is also consuming a nutritionally balanced diet. Of course, such assurances will not completely allay an anxious parent's worries about what a young child is or is not eating. Sadly, the stereotype of the anxious mother imploring a balky toddler to "please eat" is all too real. We know that nutrition is important and it is only natural to be concerned that a growing child is well nourished. Still, it is also important to find a middle ground that is comfortable for both parent and child, and not to let mealtime become a test of wills —a battle that an obstinate toddler or preschooler invariably wins!

LEARNING TO EAT

DURING THE FIRST YEAR, the typical baby's diet consists primarily of milk, either from the breast or from a bottle, along with pureed or chopped foods added in increasing variety and amounts after the first few months. Well before the first birthday, the baby will begin to show interest in a greater variety of food and in learning to self-feed instead of simply being fed. Babies naturally put almost anything they can grasp into their mouths and will try to chew it. Finger foods—crackers, O-shaped and other dried cereals, pieces of fruit, cooked noodles or macaroni, or any other item that can be grasped and does not pose a danger of choking—are important for several reasons. A baby needs to learn to chew at an appropriate age, and this varies from child to child. Some babies will begin "gumming" food in an adult chewing pattern when they are only seven or eight months old, while others may not be ready for this until they are a year or more. Begin offering finger foods as soon as a child can cope with chewing and swallowing small pieces of semisoft foods. This provides an opportunity to experience more texture than pureed or chopped baby foods, and encourages chewing, even without an appreciable number of teeth.

Self-feeding is almost as important a milestone toward independence as the first step. At this point, don't worry about table manners. By definition, learning to eat is a messy process. It takes time and patience to master using a spoon; even the toddler who can manage to get food onto a spoon and the spoon to the mouth is likely to give up after a few tries and revert to using fist or fingers instead. It's the trying and feelings of accomplishment—and not the mashed potatoes or cereal in the hair or on the floor—that are important.

Frequently a baby's desire to self-feed may exceed his or her coordination. A toddler may decline to be spoonfed, but will also become very frustrated by not being able to adequately grasp and pick up food from a dish or highchair tray. Typically a baby develops a palmar grasp before being able to use his or her fingers. The palm or even entire fist will be dipped in the food and the baby will then suck or lick it off. Before long, however, the fingers will become coordinated enough to allow a pincer grasp, and the youngster will begin picking up bits of food and experimenting with a fork or spoon.

Playing with food is very common during this stage of learning to eat, and although it can be messy and drive parents to distraction, it should not be overly discouraged. Toddlers need to explore and experiment—playing patty cake with applesauce or squeezing mashed potatoes through the fingers are learning experiences that should not be denied. If a youngster is allowed to explore food in many ways, he or she is more likely to accept—and enjoy—it. Wait to teach proper table manners until after a child has mastered a pincer grasp and can ade-

quately handle a spoon. Even then, don't expect that spills and accidents or toying with food will abruptly end. Instead of getting upset over messes and the poor manners, try to focus on the more positive aspects of learning and growth. The expression of sheer exhilaration on a young child's face when he or she manages to get food from a plate to mouth unaided is a joy in itself. Rest assured that neatness and decorum will come in their own good time, especially if the youngster has good models to follow. In the meantime, distress over spills can be minimized by placing a plastic sheet under the highchair or placing the chair in an area where the floor is easy to clean.

Of course, providing easy-to-use utensils and manageable foods can make self-feeding easier for parents and child alike. A child may not be able to manage a knife until age three or four, but will still want to try. Don't discourage the trying, but you can also avoid needless hassle by cutting foods into bite-size pieces. Spoons and forks should be smaller than adult-size, with handles that are easy to grasp and wide bowls to facilitate scooping up food. Start with plastic or nonbreakable cups and dishes, and even then, don't be upset if most of the food ends up on the highchair tray. Even if a child can chew, tough or fibrous foods like steak or similar meats can be overly challenging. Pieces of chicken, fish, meatloaf, or hamburger are more manageable and better choices for a young child.

Catering to What Kids Like

Even at a very early age, children have very definite food preferences and strong ideas about what is and is not acceptable. As stressed earlier, food should not become an object of bribery, nor should mealtime become a test of wills. Still, every mother knows that feeding a stubborn toddler can be trying. At times it seems that *yuckie* is the most used word in a young child's vocabulary, and many parents make the mistake of presenting a youngster with too many alternatives. Parents need to find the middle ground between being dogmatic about what a youngster eats and caving in to every whim. Patience, imagination, and loving firmness can go a long way in fostering good eating habits without placing too much emphasis on a particular like or dislike. Sometimes a food that is rejected as "yuckie" can be transformed into a "yummie" by suggestion or presentation. A bowl of oatmeal with a smiling face made from raisins or bits of fruit may be much more acceptable than the same cereal served in a more ordinary fashion. There also are a number of physical characteristics that make foods more acceptable. These include:

Temperature. As a general rule, young children prefer food that is at room temperature, rather than hot or cold. Often a toddler will poke and stir ice cream or other cold food until it turns into a soupy mess or blow on a cup of hot chocolate or soup until it is lukewarm. Fixing a child's plate and pouring milk a few minutes before mealtime will give the foods a chance to reach the acceptable temperature before the meal begins and will head off an excuse for rejection.

Texture. Children tend to prefer foods that are soft and moist to those that are dry or fibrous. For example, a soft bread or mashed potatoes are often preferred over a coarse (albeit more flavorful) bread or a baked or boiled potato. This may be because moist, soft foods are easier to chew and swallow. In addition, a young child does not produce as much saliva as an adult, and this may be another reason why soft foods are preferred.

Quantity. Small portions served on a child-sized plate are not as daunting as larger ones. It is best to start with a small serving of even a favorite food; seconds can be offered if the first portion is finished, but avoid urging a youngster to eat more than he or she really wants.

Color. A plate that has one or two bright colors—orange carrots, a few green peas, a bit of red apple—is more appealing to the eye and appetite than one that is a study in white or beige. But don't go overboard—inedible garnishes or foods in odd shapes or colors are just as apt to be rejected as ones that are too pale.

Flavor. Bland foods are more likely to be accepted than those that are spicy or have strong natural flavors. Children tend to be particularly sensitive to flavors, and can tell immediately if the milk is beginning to turn sour or if the potatoes were scorched a bit. Onions, cabbage, and other strong-flavored foods may be more acceptable if cooked in such a way as to make them more bland. For example, vegetables that are boiled or cooked in a soup may be preferred to those that are lightly steamed, even though the latter may retain more nutrients. When introducing strong-flavored foods to a youngster, it may be better to start with the less-flavorful boiled version; after the child is used to the mild version, you can try other preparation methods.

Familiarity. When it comes to food, most toddlers and preschoolers are creatures of habit, and they prefer the tried and true to foods that are novel or new. Since variety is crucial in structuring a nutritious diet, it is important not to let a youngster get "hooked" on a limited number of favorite foods.

Involving a child in food shopping or preparation often makes trying a new dish more appealing. When introducing a new food, offer a small portion and avoid making a production if it's rejected. Above all, don't try to bribe or force a child to eat a new food. This places undue importance on the food, and may well lead to a permanent aversion to Brussels sprouts, broccoli, or whatever is being introduced. Saying something like: "Maybe you'll try a little next time" is more apt to bring eventual acceptance than comments like, "You don't know what's good for you" or, "You can't have any dessert unless you eat your broccoli first."

Sugar and Sweets. Babies are born with a strong preference for sweet-tasting foods, and there is no evidence that the "sweet tooth" diminishes with age. Still, catering to this natural preference can lead to tooth decay and the rejection of foods that are not sweet. Despite Mary Poppins's advice that "a spoonful of sugar makes the medicine go down," sweets should never be used as a reward for good behavior or a bribe to eat less appealing foods. At one time or another, all of us have been tempted to "give in" and use food as a reward. Buying a candy bar or cookies to halt a tantrum in the supermarket may save Mother the embarrassment of wheeling an unruly toddler around, but it also sends the child an unfortunate message that he or she not only can get away with bad behavior but will be rewarded for it as well. In such a situation, a firm no gets your message across, and while it's no fun to have a child misbehave in public, he or she will quickly learn that such tactics don't work and aren't really worth the upset.

Including a sweet—a piece of fruit, pudding, a cookie, or other such dessert—as part of the meal minimizes the harmful effects of sugar on the teeth and also is an appropriate way of satisfying a natural food preference. Some pediatric nutritionists suggest putting the dessert on the plate with the rest of the food, rather than saving it for the end of the meal. If dessert is the "best" part of the meal, a child may be tempted to save room for it by skimping on the main courses, and then asking for extra dessert because he or she is still hungry. Alternatively, using dessert as a reward for eating everything on the plate encourages overeating. Candy, cookies, and other such sweets should not be used as snacks, since they increase the exposure of the teeth to cavity-causing sugar and also substitute low-nutrition, high-calorie foods for more nutritious items such as cheese, vegetable sticks, or fresh fruit.

Salt. Many foods, including milk and many vegetables, contain small amounts of natural sodium, and most commercial foods contain varying amounts of added salt. Thus, it is not necessary to add any salt to the diet. Since salt is an acquired, rather than inborn, taste, a child who has not been exposed to salty food will not miss it. At one time salt was added to many commercial baby foods, not because the infant needed it, but because mothers who were accustomed to the taste of salted foods found them more pleasing to their palates and assumed the same was true for their offspring. Baby-food manufacturers have since discontinued adding salt to their products after widespread adverse publicity linking early sodium intake to an increased risk of later high blood pressure. Although the link between sodium and high blood pressure has not been proved except for people with an inherited tendency to develop it, experts still recommend that salty foods be avoided in early childhood. A young child who becomes accustomed to liberally salted foods may find it very hard to break the salt-shaker habit later in life.

Snacks. Many of us look upon snacks as "junk food time," with little importance in overall nutrition. Actually, snacks can be as important as regular meals in establishing good eating habits and obtaining needed nutrients. Timing is important—a snack should be offered in midmorning, midafternoon, and perhaps before bed. A snack should be timed to ease hunger without killing appetite for the next meal. Getting too hungry and then gobbling up everything in sight fosters poor eating habits and, all too often, a lifelong weight problem. Many adults fall into the habit of skipping breakfast, having very little lunch, and then gorging themselves in the late afternoon and evening. They may think they eat very little because most of the day is spent hungry; in reality, many will consume more calories in the latter part of the day than in three regular meals and a couple of well-timed snacks.

Enough time should lapse between the snack and the previous meal that a child will not be tempted to skip the main course at lunch, for example, because he or she knows that a more favored food will be forthcoming soon at snack time. Similarly, a snack should not be served so close to the next meal that the child will not feel hungry. The timing of the next meal also dictates how much food should be offered. If dinner is going to be late, then a larger-than-usual snack may be appropriate. Similarly, if the youngster is late coming in from an afternoon at the playground, and dinner is going to be served in an hour or so, a lighter snack will ease the immediate hunger pangs yet not kill the appetite for the main meal.

Snacks are an added opportunity to provide foods with nutritious value. (See table 5.3 for suggestions.) Parents also can use snacks to introduce new foods—an assortment of fresh vegetables and a cheese dip are both nutritious and fun to eat, and provide an opportunity to offer something new.

Table 5.3 **HEALTHY SNACKS FOR YOUNGSTERS**

Following are suggested snacks that can be offered to toddlers and preschoolers as part of their overall diet:
- Bread or crackers (graham, soda, or other low-fat varieties)
- Corn or bran muffin
- Cheese or bits of meat
- Fresh or canned fruits
- Dried banana chips, apples, raisins, and other fruits
- Yogurt (with fresh fruit)
- Raw vegetables (plain or with cottage cheese or yogurt dip)
- Milk, custard, ice cream, or pudding
- Dry cereal (as finger food)
- Unsweetened fruit juices
- Animal crackers, ginger snaps; other low-fat, low-sugar cookies

SOLVING COMMON PROBLEMS

MANY SO-CALLED FEEDING PROBLEMS really are not problems at all, but instead are natural stages of development or normal "testing" of parental authority. A common-sense approach can solve most of these so-called problems before they become real difficulties. Following are some common examples:

Food Jags. All toddlers and preschoolers go through stages in which certain food preferences or eating rituals seem to take on a life of their own. They may arrange foods in a certain manner on their plates or eat them only in a specific order. A peanut butter sandwich may be the only acceptable food for lunch or cereal must be served in a specific bowl if it is to be eaten. These are natural phases, and so long as they don't get out of hand, they usually are harmless and will pass with time. If a food jag is interfering with good nutrition by severely limiting the amount or variety of food consumed, avoid catering to the whim without making it seem you are concerned. This may be easier said than done, but a firm, matter-of-fact approach usually can prevail. For example, many problems can be avoided simply by not letting a youngster dictate his or her menu for regular family meals, but allowing choices, within reason, for snacks. Instead of asking: "What would you like for lunch," simply decide what you consider an appropriate menu and serve it. Thus, if little Johnny comes to the table and takes one look at what is on his plate and demands a peanut butter sandwich instead, say: "This is what we are having for lunch today—I'll fix a peanut butter sandwich for your snack after your nap." You will not be giving in to his demand for a different lunch, but you also are not denying his preference for a favorite food.

Dependence on the Bottle.

Some babies are ready to give up a bottle (or breast) as soon as they can drink from a cup; others may want to have a bottle, especially at certain times of the day, until they are two or three years old. A good deal depends upon the individual child and how the bottle is being used. For example, if the toddler is skimping on meals and still relying on a bottle for most of his or her nutrition, it is time to give it up. On the other hand, if a toddler wants a bottle at snack time or the comfort of having a bottle at nap time or just before going to bed, there probably is no harm being done unless, of course, he or she is allowed to sleep and continue sucking the bottle. This causes a pooling of milk in the mouth, and constant contact of milk sugar with the teeth, resulting in a particular pattern of tooth decay. Remember, juice also is high in natural sugar and can have the same results. If a baby or toddler cannot fall asleep without sucking something, a pacifier, bottle of water, or thumb are acceptable alternatives to a bottle of milk or juice.

Difficulty in Chewing.

Occasionally we see children two or three years old who balk at eating any food that requires chewing. They will gag on even lumpy applesauce or will eat only milk or pureed foods. In rare instances, the child may have a developmental problem that interferes with proper chewing and swallowing patterns. More often, however, the problem can be traced to delaying introducing lumpy-textured foods during the first year. If not encouraged to learn how to chew and swallow at the proper time, the youngster can become overly dependent on milk and pureed foods. As time goes by, the toddler may become increasingly resistant to new foods. In such instances, parents must be firm in gradually substituting regular food for the pureed baby foods. This is one reason why many experts encourage mothers to mash up regular table food for babies instead of relying on the convenience of commercial pureed baby food.

Countering the TV Commercials.

Each year, several billion dollars are spent on television food advertising, and the bulk of these messages are directed to children. Anyone who has watched after-school or Saturday morning cartoons knows that almost as much time is devoted to selling sugar-coated cereals, soft drinks, and fast foods or snacks of dubious nutritional value as to the exploits of cartoon heroes. One seldom sees commercials for milk, fruit juice, vegetables, and other foods that are mainstays of a nutritious diet. The effects of all this child-directed advertising quickly become apparent simply by visiting a supermarket and observing parents with young children in tow. Invariably the child will plead for a certain cereal, soft drink, or snack food because of appealing TV commercials or offers. One rarely witnesses the same sort of pressure to buy vegetables, fruits, unsweetened cereals, and other more wholesome foods.

One of the most effective ways of countering child-oriented food commercials is to watch television with the children and point out the ways in which food manufacturers are trying to manipulate them. Even very young children do not like to think others are trying to "make them do something," and helping a child see through the hype can foster healthy skepticism. Parents also can use shopping trips as mini-nutrition courses of their own: "Here's the fruit juice—it has more vitamins and minerals than soda, so we'll buy that instead" and so forth.

Refusal to Eat.

Even very young babies quickly sense that they can get a parent's undivided attention to eating or not eating, as the case may be. Toddlers can be very adept at manipulating parental concerns about what they eat. "I'll eat all my dinner if I can stay up to watch TV," or, "Tommy's Mommy doesn't make him eat broccoli" are common refrains. Very few young children will actually go hungry, although they may spend hours sitting over a cold bowl of oatmeal or a soft-boiled egg in a test of wills. Ignoring inappropriate eating behavior and steadfastly refusing to let the consumption of a certain food become an issue usually will forestall such eating problems. A firm, reasonable response is all that is needed: "Eating dinner has nothing to do with staying up late to watch TV, but we can tape the program so you can watch it tomorrow," or, "I'm not Tommy's Mommy and broccoli is the vegetable we are having at this house tonight" should be enough to end such discussions. At any rate, don't be drawn into lengthy arguments; if a certain food is not eaten after a period of time, remove it from the table without further comment.

Before concluding that a youngster is not eating, parents should make sure that they are not in some way sabotaging mealtime. Is the atmosphere really conducive to eating? Is the atmosphere warm and friendly? Or are you saving up the day's grievances to air when everyone is seated around the table? Do you pay attention to each other, or silently gulp down food so each person can move on to other activities? It is important for parents to realize that their attitudes and food habits have a tremendous influence on their children's eating behavior. If mealtime seems to be turning into wartime between parents and children, it may be well to look closely at adult eating habits to see if they are the source of the problem.

NUTRITION AND SPECIFIC DISEASES

Overweight

Despite the fitness boom and our preoccupation with slimness, our children are fatter than ever. In fact, obesity is by far the most common nutritional disorder in the United States. Although we tend to think of it as an adult disease, 10 to 30 percent of American children are obese. A recent Department of Health and Human Services study found that American children of the 1980s are significantly heavier than youngsters in the 1960s. They also are in poorer physical condition than past generations —a study of 18,000 American children by the Amateur Athletic Union found that almost two-thirds of the children surveyed could not pass a basic physical fitness test.

There is no one definition of what constitutes obesity (see table 5.4). Generally a weight that is 20 percent or more above what is considered ideal for age, sex, and height is classified as obese, but experts disagree as to what should be the ideal weight for a child. From a practical standpoint, a youngster who looks too fat can be assumed to be overweight, bearing in mind, of course, that not all babies have the

same build and some are normally stocky while others are lean.

Obesity has an impact on both physical and psychological health. It is linked to an increased risk of several serious adult diseases, including high blood pressure, heart disease, adult diabetes, and some forms of cancer. To a child, the psychological burden of being fat can be particularly devastating, especially when growing up in this society that prizes slimness. Fat children often have poor self-images; they also are subject to teasing and ridicule by their peers, and frequently find themselves sitting on the sidelines instead of joining in active games. Of course, inactivity adds to the weight problem; in fact, studies by Dr. Jean Mayer, nutritionist and researcher, found that overweight children often do not eat as much as their slender counterparts, but that they were far more sedentary.

Obesity is a complex disease whose cause is not fully understood. It appears that both genetic and environmental factors may be involved. Overweight parents are likely to have children who are also overweight—perhaps due to an inherited tendency to metabolize food more efficiently. These children require fewer calories and do not need to eat as much as normal-weight individuals to produce the same amounts of energy. Thus, people with a genetic tendency to gain weight have to be particularly careful about overeating. But the family diet cannot be overlooked because, in the final analysis, weight gain is a direct result of eating more food than the body needs for its day-to-day activities, no matter what the underlying cause. (See table 5.5.)

It is well known that lifelong weight problems very often start in childhood—an overweight child is likely to grow into an obese adult, and he or she

Table 5.4 **MEAN WEIGHTS AND HEIGHTS OF BOYS AND GIRLS FROM AGES 1 TO 5**

Age	Girls		Boys	
	Weight (lbs.)	Height (ins.)	Weight (lbs.)	Height (ins.)
1 year	21.5	29.2	22.2	29.5
2 years	26	34.2	27.2	34.2
3 years	31.0	37.0	32.2	37.2
4 years	35.2	40.0	36.8	40.5
5 years	39	42.7	41.2	43.2

Source: National Center for Health Statistics, Department of Health, Education and Welfare.

Table 5.5 **HOW MUCH IS ENOUGH?**

Children's caloric needs vary greatly due to changes in appetite, activity, growth, and weight gain. When estimating calorie needs, a good rule of thumb is to begin with a base of 1,000 calories and add 100 calories for each year of age.

Age	Daily Calorie Requirement
1 year	1,100 calories
2 years	1,200 calories
3 years	1,300 calories
4 years	1,400 calories
5 years	1,500 calories
6 years	1,600 calories

This system for determining can only be used for children ages 1 to 6. Also, remember, these are only averages. Caloric requirements will vary with each child.

will also have difficulty maintaining weight loss. Two things happen when youngsters gain excessive weight—they develop many more fat cells (adipocytes) than those whose weights are normal, and these cells grow bigger as extra fat is stored. The fat cells may shrink in size if weight is lost, but they never disappear. (Adults who gain weight also appear to add extra fat cells, but not as many as during childhood; for them, weight gain is reflected mostly in increased size of the individual cells.)

Parents of an overweight child should seek the help of a doctor or qualified nutritionist before putting the youngster on a weight reduction diet. Care must be taken not to restrict calories too much, which can interfere with normal growth and development. Except in very unusual circumstances, the goal is to cut food intake only enough to slow down the rate of gain, rather than actually losing weight. Eventually the stored fat will be used for growth. Increasing physical activity also is vital since this will help control appetite, burn up extra fat, improve muscle tone and fitness, and promote a more positive self-image.

Helping an overweight child requires special sensitivity on the part of parents, grandparents, and other family members. An overweight child needs to be assured that he or she is loved as a person, and that size has no bearing on that love. Parents need to take care not to add to a child's negative self-image by registering disapproval of size or eating habits. Nor should parents make the situation worse by encouraging an overweight child to eat or by having fattening food on hand.

Overcoming a child's weight problem should involve the entire family. Above all, don't expect the child to diet alone—watching other family members indulge in ice cream, candy, potato chips, and other high-calorie (low-nutrition) foods while munching on a carrot stick is too much to ask of even the most motivated person. Earlier cautions about using food as a reward or an incentive are particularly important when it comes to helping an overweight child. Many parents and grandparents also tend to confuse food with love and nurturing. Many unwittingly add to the child's problem by tempting him or her with favorite foods, encouraging a second or third helping, going out for a high-calorie treat. Such actions may be motivated by love, but the end result is detrimental. Food should be thought of as fuel—something that the body needs to run properly—and not as a token of affection, reward, or security blanket.

This also may be a good time to take a hard look at the entire family's eating habits. Are the parents and siblings also overweight? If so, this is a good time to gradually overhaul the family diet, substituting high-nutrition low-calorie foods for more fattening items. Avoid crash diets or fad weight-loss schemes. Following such a regimen may get rid of unwanted pounds, but it also can lead to serious nutritional imbalances and growth problems for children. And "going on a diet" implies that eventually you can go off it and revert to your former (fattening) way of eating. It's far better to put the entire family on a sound eating program that will last for life, rather than a few weeks or until short-term weight-loss goals are achieved.

An observant parent can spot a child's most vulnerable times for overeating and help by providing satisfying low-calorie foods at those times. For example, if a preschooler spends hours watching TV and munching on whatever is handy, you can help in two ways: first, find a more active pastime than watching TV, and second, discourage eating while viewing or provide low-calorie snacks, such as vegetable sticks. Serve small portions at mealtimes and don't urge seconds (if a child asks for a second helping, make sure that it is small or suggest that he finish his entire meal and see if he is still hungry).

A family exercise program will also benefit all participants, but especially the overweight child. Try to find enjoyable family activities that are not focused on a meal. Going on a hike or bicycle outing, visiting a museum, or playing a game are possible alternatives to a restaurant outing. Remember, too, that children and adults alike may turn to food to ease boredom, overcome feelings of insecurity, or overcome frustration. Determining why a child is overeating and taking corrective measures can forestall poor eating patterns.

Food Allergies

True food allergies in which there is an immune system response to a specific substance or antigen in a food probably are not as common as people think. Also, contrary to popular belief, there is considerable doubt among experts that hyperactivity, tantrums, and behavioral problems are caused by allergic reactions to additives or specific foods.

Still, we know that allergic reactions can cause a variety of symptoms, including wheezing, asthmatic attacks, sneezing, running nose, and other respiratory reactions; diarrhea, vomiting, stomach cramps, and other gastrointestinal symptoms; hives, itching, rashes, mouth sores, and other skin reactions; headache, dizziness, and in severe cases, an anaphylactic collapse. Food allergies occur most often during infancy, and are most likely among children whose parents have allergic disorders.

Diagnosing a food allergy can be difficult because of the wide variety of symptoms, and also the fact that they may not occur immediately after eating. Sometimes a reaction can be delayed for hours, or even days. Frequently, a child will outgrow the allergy, and foods that once produced symptoms can later be tolerated without problems. A variety of tests are used to diagnose food hypersensitivity, but the most effective is an elimination diet. (See chapter 31, Allergies.)

Any food can cause an allergic response; the most common offenders are listed in table 5.6. Sometimes the response may be altered or eliminated by the manner in which food is processed. For example, a child allergic to cow's milk may be able to tolerate evaporated milk, which has been altered somewhat in the canning process. And sometimes the response is not to the food itself, but to contaminants, additives, and other hidden ingredients.

Table 5.6 **COMMON FOOD ALLERGENS**

Most Common	Common
Cow's milk	Chocolate
Egg whites	Oranges
Wheat	Strawberries
Fish	Tomatoes
Seafood	Corn
Nuts	

The best approach to treating a food allergy is to eliminate the offending substance from the diet. This can be difficult if the allergy is to corn, wheat, milk, or other items that are frequently "hidden" in a number of unlikely processed foods. Before severely limiting a child's diet, parents should make sure that the youngster is, indeed, allergic to the food. Not uncommonly, a child is put on a very restricted diet without adequate testing and proper diagnosis, only to later learn that he or she is not allergic to the suspected food. Remember, too, that many children spontaneously outgrow allergies, and foods that once provoked a response often can be reintroduced without problems at a later age. Also, allergies may be dose-dependent. For example, a child who is allergic to chocolate may be able to tolerate a small, infrequent helping, such as a piece of cake at a party. But having an entire chocolate bar or chocolate every day or two may provoke a response. Obviously, extra care must be taken if the child has a serious allergic-related disease, such as asthma. (For a more complete discussion, see chapter 31, Allergies.)

Iron Deficiency Anemia

As noted earlier, nutritional deficiency diseases are relatively uncommon in this country. But among very young children, iron deficiency anemia is the one seen most often in this country. Most affected are children between the ages of six months and three years, although it increases again during adolescence (especially among girls who have heavy menstrual periods).

Anemia is characterized by a low level of hemoglobin, the pigment-containing portion of the red blood cell that transports oxygen. The most common type of anemia is caused by iron deficiency; other causes include blood abnormalities such as thalassemia, infection, chronic diseases, or deficiencies of folic acid, vitamin B_{12}, and certain other nutrients.

Under normal circumstances, a full-term baby is born with enough iron to last through the first four to six months of life. Breast milk and cow's milk are low in iron, so the baby calls upon its iron reserves for the first few months of life. As formula or iron-fortified cereals and other solid foods are introduced to the diet, the baby is able to replenish iron stores. But there are exceptions. An infant fed fresh cow's milk may have hidden gastrointestinal bleeding, which increases loss of iron and can lead to anemia. An iron-deficient diet or other circumstances (i.e., hookworm infestation, gastrointestinal disease, etc.) also can result in anemia. In most instances, diagnosis and treatment with diet and iron supplements will reverse the anemia. (See chapter 24, Childhood Blood Disorders, for a more complete discussion.)

Other Miscellaneous Diseases

There are a number of disorders that are either caused by nutritional factors or have an effect on diet and metabolism. These include diabetes, cystic fibrosis, inflammatory bowel disease, various malabsorption syndromes, chronic diarrhea, and infection, among others. These are discussed in chapter sections dealing with the specific diseases.

DIET IN THE PREVENTION OF DISEASE

INCREASINGLY, DIET IS BEING LINKED to some of our most serious diseases, including heart attacks, cancer, high blood pressure, strokes, and adult diabetes. Many medical researchers are convinced that these are progressive diseases that may start during childhood. Thus, the big question is: Can disease be prevented by diet? In some instances, the answer appears to be "maybe," but there are still many unknowns. Most pediatric nutritionists caution against widespread and drastic changes in the way we feed our children in the hope of preventing adult diseases. On the other hand, there are researchers who feel this is overly conservative, and that some changes are warranted. We prefer to take a middle ground, urging that moderation, variety, and common sense prevail.

Heart Disease

Heart attacks remain the leading cause of death in the United States, claiming more than 600,000 lives a year. Most heart attacks are caused by atherosclerosis, the buildup of fatty deposits in the coronary and other arteries. The large majority of heart attack deaths occur in later life, but atherosclerosis is a progressive process that begins in the early years. Autopsies done on young men killed in both the Korean and Vietnam wars have found that a large number already had significant fatty deposits in their coronary arteries. Fatty streaks, a forerunner of the atherosclerosis, have been found in blood vessels of very young accident victims.

No one knows what actually causes atherosclerosis, but high blood cholesterol is a major factor. Americans of all ages tend to have blood cholesterol levels that are higher than those found in nonindustrialized countries with a correspondingly low incidence of heart attacks. Many factors contribute to high blood cholesterol, including a genetic predisposition. But diet, especially one high in saturated fats, excess calories, and high-cholesterol foods like egg yolks, whole milk, and other animal products, is probably the major cause of high blood cholesterol.

At what age should people start to pay attention to diet and cholesterol? The National Cholesterol Education Program, a government-coordinated effort to increase diagnosis and treatment of high cholesterol, has issued recommendations for adults (anyone whose blood cholesterol is over 200 mg/dl should follow a cholesterol-lowering diet with more extensive treatments if this is insufficient), but its recommendations for children have not yet been announced. The American Heart Association recommends that all people over the age of two consume no more than 30 percent of daily calories from fats, and that no more than 10 percent of calories should come from saturated fats. The American Academy of Pediatrics and a number of pediatric nutritionists take issue with these recommendations, arguing that 40 percent of calories from fats is a more realistic and healthful recommendation for young children.

At this time, there is no convincing evidence that severe restriction of fat in a child's diet will prevent atherosclerosis, except in unusual circumstances. Some children are born with a disease called familial hyperlipidemia; their livers manufacture an abnormal amount of cholesterol and other blood fats. These children have very high cholesterol levels, and unless treated at an early age, many have heart attacks in their teens or even earlier. Obviously for these children a strict cholesterol-lowering diet is important. Such a diet also may be important for children with a strong family history of early heart attacks, and who already have borderline high cholesterol. But for the majority of children, a moderate diet that is low in saturated fat, but with enough other fats to ensure proper growth and development, is a prudent course.

Unfortunately many parents today think that advice intended for them should be applied to their young children. Even babies are being fed skim milk and overly restricted low-fat diets. Growing babies and young children need the concentrated calories in fat for growth; eggs, meat, cheese, and other foods that perhaps should be limited in an adult diet also are needed by young growing bodies. Common sense should prevail—obviously a diet made up of fatty hotdogs, luncheon meats, ice cream, and other foods high in saturated fats is not in a child's best interest. But neither is one that is inappropriately restricted in the hopes that it may prevent a later heart attack.

High Blood Pressure

Another controversial area involves the question of salt and high blood pressure. Over the years, our high-salt diet has been linked with an increased risk of developing high blood pressure, or hypertension —the leading cause of strokes and also an important risk factor in heart attacks. One out of five adult Americans has high blood pressure, and children whose parents have the disease are likely to develop it themselves.

As noted earlier, salt is an acquired taste, but once acquired, it is hard to break. By giving babies and young children salty foods, they are likely to develop a taste for it and reject unsalted foods. Since we get more than enough salt in a normal diet, many experts feel there is no need to introduce it in a young child's diet. Still, it has not been proved that a high-salt diet actually causes high blood pressure or that withholding salt from a child's diet will prevent later hypertension. Again, moderation appears to be the best advice. Cutting down on salt certainly will do no harm, but it is not necessary to be obsessive about ferreting out every source of hidden salt in a youngster's diet.

Cancer

Numerous population studies have identified diet as a possible link to some cancers, but again, we lack absolute proof that a specific food can actually cause a certain cancer. There are more than 100 different kinds of cancer, and we know very little about what causes any of them. It is clear that smoking or chewing tobacco increases the risk of a number of cancers. Alcohol also increases the risk of some cancers. Animal studies have found that pesticides, saccharin, and certain other contaminants or additives increase the incidence of cancer, but it has not been proved that this applies to human beings.

Population studies have attributed a protective effect to certain foods or nutrients, including dietary fiber, selenium (a trace mineral abundant in our food supply), beta carotene (a precursor of vitamin A), and cruciferous vegetables such as cabbage or broccoli. Similarly, foods that are smoked, charred over a high heat, or preserved by salt pickling or with nitrites are linked to an increased risk of cancer. A high-fat diet also appears to increase the risk of cancer.

Although firm evidence is lacking that diet can either cause or prevent cancer, a prudent course would be to minimize those foods or additives that are linked with an increased risk and to provide moderate amounts of those considered protective. The American Cancer Society suggests a varied, prudent diet very similar to that recommended by the American Heart Association: high in complex carbohydrates, with low to moderate amounts of protein, fat, salt, and sugar. Limit consumption of cured, smoked, or charred foods, but include citrus fruits, dark green or yellow vegetables, and frequent servings of cruciferous vegetables in the diet. As for artificial sweeteners, dyes, and other additives that are not really needed, many nutritionists advise that you either avoid or limit them, especially in a child's diet. They have not been proved harmful, but they also do not serve any real purpose, so why take even a minimal risk if there is no benefit?

VEGETARIANISM AND OTHER ALTERNATIVE DIETS

IN THIS CHAPTER, we have concentrated mostly on what is considered "the typical American diet." But what is typical varies greatly according to region of the country, cultural background, social and economic status, and parental preferences. Some alternative diets are well-balanced and will provide more than adequate nutrition for a growing child. Others can be dangerous and result in serious health problems or even death. In adapting any alternative diet for young children, it is important to remember that their needs are different from those of adults if they are to experience normal growth and development.

Vegetarian Diets

With careful planning, a vegetarian diet can provide all of the essential nutrients needed for growth and development. At one time, a vegetarian was looked upon as being a bit odd; today, we recognize that a vegetarian diet can be more healthful than the steak, French fries, and apple pie fare touted as the "all-American diet."

There are a number of variations of vegetarian diets, and some, particularly the partial, lacto-ovo, or lactovegetarian, are more appropriate for children than the stricter, more limited vegan regimens. But with proper guidance, even a strict vegan diet can be tailored to meet the needs of a growing child. For example, a soybean milk fortified with vitamin B_{12} (which is found only in animal products) is an easy alternative to cow's milk. Calcium and iron can be obtained from a variety of plant sources.

To provide adequate protein for growth, a vegetarian diet must be carefully balanced with specific combinations of vegetable proteins. Tables 5.7 and 5.8, on the next page, list combinations that form complete proteins and practical examples.

Fad Diets

Every few months it seems, we encounter yet another "revolutionary new diet" that claims to improve athletic prowess, magically melt away unwanted pounds, prevent heart attacks, cure cancer, improve intelligence, add years to one's life—to name but a few of the promised "miracles." After a few weeks or even months on the best-seller list, most of these fad diets disappear, only to be replaced by yet another fad. As a general rule, any diet that makes a sweeping promise—easy weight loss, cure for hyperactivity or chronic disease—should be suspect. Exceptions are special prescription diets, such as those that have been developed for diabetes or high cholesterol, and these should not be confused with unproved fad diets. Some of the more popular fad diets of recent years follow.

Natural or Organic. A number of popular nutrition writers such as the late Adelle Davis popularized the notion that "natural" or "organic" foods are

Table 5.7 **HOW TO MATCH VEGETABLE PROTEINS**

Food Group	Some High-Quality Combinations
All Grains and	Milk and dairy products Eggs
Rice and	Legumes Soybeans and wheat Sesame seeds Peanuts and soybeans and wheat Spinach and cauliflower
Wheat and	Legumes Soybeans and rice Soybeans and sesame seeds Soybeans and peanuts Spinach and broccoli
Corn and	Legumes Cauliflower and potatoes Soybeans and sesame seeds
Legumes and	Milk and dairy products Eggs Rice Barley Oats Millet
Beans and	Wheat Corn
Soybeans and	Rice and wheat Wheat and sesame seeds Peanuts and sesame seeds
Peas and	Sesame seeds and brazil nuts
Seeds and nuts and	Milk and dairy products Eggs

Table 5.8 **SAMPLE VEGETARIAN DISHES**

Vegetarian chili with rice
Pea soup with corn bread
Black-eyed peas and rice
Broccoli-noodle casserole
Vegetable lasagna
Omelet with vegetables
French toast
Pizza
Lentil pot pie
Vegetable stroganoff
Bean tostadas
Baked zucchini, tomato, and rice casserole
Broccoli-cheese baked potato
Macaroni and cheese
Hummus (chickpea and sesame paste) and pita bread
Egg foo yung
Green peppers stuffed with rice and tomato

more healthful than those grown with artificial fertilizers or processed with preservatives or other additives. They are often marketed as "health foods," with the implication that other foods are not healthful. These "health foods" are sold in special shops or supermarket sections, usually at prices considerably higher than their regular counterparts. Not uncommonly, a family will pay extra money for these foods without realizing they are not getting fair value. This is especially unfortunate if the family has a limited food budget.

Although it is desirable to eliminate pesticides and other potentially harmful substances from the food supply, so-called "health foods" generally are not any more nutritious than items stocked in ordinary supermarkets or food shops. In fact, some "health foods" are not as healthy as regular items: notable examples are unpasteurized milk and cheeses, which can harbor dangerous bacteria. Very often, a careful check of the labels will reveal that high-priced items in health-food stores are exactly the same as much lower-priced regular foods.

Many health-food proprietors double as "nutrition counselors," advising parents on what they should feed their families. Some of the advice may be quite harmless, but all too often these usually unqualified counselors promote things like megadose vitamins and mineral supplements and diets that are inappropriate for growing children. As a rule, it is far better to follow the nutrition advice of your pediatrician or qualified dietitian or nutrition counselor, and to steer clear of "Health-food" promoters.

Feingold Diet. This controversial diet claims that "hyperactivity" is caused by certain food additives, especially dyes, flavorings, salicylates, and preservatives. A number of regular foods, such as apples, tomatoes, oranges, and grapes, also are eliminated from the diet. Dr. Benjamin Feingold and his followers have reported considerable success in treating hyperactive children with this diet, but a number of controlled scientific studies have failed to duplicate their achievements. Still, a National Institutes of Health consensus conference noted that the Feingold diet provides adequate nutrition and, after careful evaluation by a physician, a trial of one or two months on the diet was reasonable. The major problem with this is a tendency to begin eliminating other foods from the diet if the expected results are not achieved on the Feingold regimen. If parents are determined to try the Feingold diet, they should not try additional modifications without consulting their pediatrician or qualified nutritionist.

Zen Macrobiotic and Other Cult Diets. The Zen Macrobiotic diet is a strict eating system that is supposed to help its practitioners achieve heightened spirituality. The diet goes through 10 progressive stages in which an increasing number of foods are eliminated. For example, babies usually are fed a mixture of sesame seeds, brown rice, beans, and grains—a regimen deficient in calcium, vitamin B_{12}, iron, calories, and other important nutrients. Following an extreme macrobiotic diet can lead to serious nutritional deficiencies and even death, and it certainly should not be considered for young children.

Fad Formulas.   From time to time, fad formulas are developed and promoted as being "more like mother's milk" than regular commercial ones. A recent example was the barley water formula, made from barley water, corn syrup or honey, and whole milk. The formula was promoted by a religious group and fed to some babies, mostly in California. After a number of these babies developed serious growth problems, nutritional analysis found the formula seriously deficient in iron and vitamins A and C. Similarly, formulas have been made from nondairy creamers, resulting in serious protein deficiency in babies fed them.

FORMING GOOD LIFELONG HABITS

As STRESSED THROUGHOUT this chapter, there is no rigid diet that should be consumed by all children.

A varied diet drawn from all four basic food groups should provide all of the nutrition needed for growth and development. Although many parents think that a child should eat differently from the rest of the family, in reality what is good for the youngster is likely to be just as appropriate for adults. It certainly is not necessary to plan two different menus.

Unfortunately many adults have developed poor food habits—they prefer a diet made up mostly of meat, fast foods, white bread, coldcuts, and sweets, with very few vegetables, starches, or fresh fruits. Understandably a person who is accustomed to this kind of diet may not find it easy to switch to what is more appropriate for a child. Still, since children tend to want to eat what they see on their parents' plates, now may be a good time to make a concerted effort to modify the adult diet to one that is more healthful for both them and their offspring.

A child who learns to enjoy a wide variety of foods and how to cut down on fats has a better chance of escaping the more common adult nutrition-related problems. Even a very young child can be taught to trim the skin from chicken and fat from meat and to enjoy vegetables without globs of butter or rich cream sauces. Good nutrition is not complicated, and it should not be equated with dullness or deprivation. Learning to savor the natural flavor of many foods at an early age will give a youngster a headstart on forming good eating habits that will last for life.

6 If Things Go Wrong

Stanley James, M.D., and
John M. Driscoll, Jr., M.D.

INTRODUCTION

AT BIRTH INFANTS are thrust from a warm, protected home into a bright and cool, air-filled environment in which they must immediately fend for themselves. Every year, millions of babies make this dramatic transition without incident. Even after a pregnancy labeled "high risk," the odds are good that a baby will make a rapid and normal adjustment in the delivery room. When things go wrong, it is often because phases of this biological transition are delayed or require outside assistance.

Forces pushing on the infant's chest during delivery help clear the fluid-filled lungs. *Surfactant*, a natural detergent produced during the last trimester of pregnancy, is then activated and it coats the lung's tiny air sacs. The stress of labor leaves the newborn slightly *hypoxic*, or oxygen-deprived, providing an added stimulus to the respiratory centers in the brain to continue the breathing movements begun in utero. After the first deep breaths inflate the lungs, the surfactant keeps the air sacs from collapsing between subsequent breaths.

Before birth, the placenta fills the blood with oxygen and the fetal heart circulates it through the rest of the body, largely bypassing the immature fetal lungs. Once the umbilical cord is cut, the newborn must circulate the blood through the lungs to pick up oxygen. Blood vessels in the lungs expand when the first breath is taken. At the same time, in the uterus, the temporary blood vessel that was used for bypass of the lungs, called the ductus arteriosus, begins to close.

To measure how well the baby is making these transitions in the first crucial minutes after birth, doctors perform an Apgar evaluation, named after its developer, Virginia Apgar, the noted Columbia Presbyterian Medical Center anesthesiologist. At one and five minutes after birth the baby is rated on five signs that indicate whether sufficient oxygen is reaching the brain and other tissues. Each sign is scored 0, 1, or 2, and the ratings are added to determine the baby's Apgar score (see table 2.1). The Apgar score is not a measure of intelligence—a normal score of 6 or 7 at one minute and 9 or 10 at five minutes simply indicates that the baby is normally handling the transition between womb and outside world. A score below 6 indicates moderate to severe distress, alerting the delivery team that the baby may need help in getting air into the lungs.

As soon as a baby is born, the nose and mouth are gently suctioned to remove any fluids blocking the airway. The umbilical cord is clamped and cut. A baby that has trouble taking initial breaths is put on a warming table and quickly dried with warm towels, a procedure that may stimulate breathing. If the newborn continues to have trouble, a health professional will intervene, delivering air to the lungs at a slightly increased pressure. Air from a squeezable bag will be gently forced in and out of the baby's lungs through a mask placed over the nose and mouth. If this does not stimulate the newborn's own breathing motions, a small, flexible tube is inserted through the mouth into the trachea (the windpipe leading to the lungs). The bag is pumped by hand until breathing begins or it is determined that the infant requires a respirator to supplement or completely take over breathing. If needed, the respirator is then attached to the endotracheal tube already in place.

While in the delivery room, the baby is briefly examined for visible birth defects, abdominal masses, or apparent blocks in the digestive tract, as well as heart and lung problems.

THE TRANSITIONAL CARE NURSERY

IN LARGE HOSPITALS, infants who are in difficulty from the moment of birth or those who have no obvious problems but who may be at risk for complications are admitted to the transitional care nursery. In this setting there are sufficient numbers of nurses and physicians to facilitate close monitoring and to handle emergency procedures should they become necessary. In smaller hospitals, there may not be a separate nursery, but the baby will be closely watched and evaluated for possible transfer to a better equipped facility.

Equipment in the transitional nursery includes isolettes, respirators, monitoring devices, and transport modules that can provide oxygen and maintain the infant's temperature during the initial care and subsequent transfer to an intensive care unit.

The mother's medical history often determines whether an infant will go first to a transitional care nursery. No matter how healthy they seem at birth, infants usually are sent for a period of close monitoring if their mothers are under age 15 or over age 40 or have a history of:

- Toxemia, preeclampsia, or eclampsia
- Diabetes
- Cardiac or pulmonary disease
- Hypertension in pregnancy
- Drug addiction
- Fever or evidence of infection
- Rh negative blood type with history of previous sensitization
- Many previous births
- Any major medical or surgical complications

The transitional care nursery is also the first stop for infants who:

- Have meconium (intestinal material) present in the airway at delivery
- Are born by cesarean section
- Weigh less than 2,250 grams (5 pounds)
- Weigh nine pounds or more
- Are large or small for their gestational age
- Have one or more unusual physical features that might suggest underlying medical problems

Usually a newborn will only stay in the transitional nursery for four to eight hours' observation before being transferred to the regular newborn nursery or to an intensive care setting. Some hospitals use the transitional nursery as a longer-term home for premature infants who need special monitoring but who do not have respiratory problems requiring a respirator.

THE NEONATAL INTENSIVE CARE UNIT

A NEONATAL INTENSIVE CARE UNIT (NICU) provides sophisticated equipment and staff with special training to sustain life and closely monitor the medical condition of sick or high-risk newborns. Not all babies admitted to a neonatal intensive care unit are seriously ill—many just require a short period of careful observation until doctors are convinced that all their vital systems are functioning properly. Other infants are completely dependent on respirators and other life-sustaining equipment.

About 12 in every 100 newborns are sent to a special neonatal unit. Health professionals should inform parents at the time of admission why their newborn is being placed in the unit. (Table 6.1 lists the most frequent reasons.)

Table 6.1 REASONS FOR ADMISSION TO A NEONATAL INTENSIVE CARE UNIT

- Weight of less than 1,500 grams (about 3 pounds, 5 ounces).
- Require breathing assistance.
- Inhaled amniotic fluid containing meconium (a material present in the fetal intestinal tract).
- Are in distress, as indicated by a low Apgar score (less than 4 at 1 minute or 7 at 5 minutes).
- Were asphyxiated (deprived of oxygen) during birth.
- Show signs of infection.
- Were injured during birth.
- Have an abnormally fast heartbeat.
- Have a serious birth defect.
- Have experienced seizures in the newborn period.
- Have recurrent or persistent low blood sugar.
- Will require much surgery (other than circumcision) in the first month of life.
- Were exposed to cocaine, heroin, methadone, significant quantities of alcohol, or other addictive drugs before birth.
- Have congenital heart disease.

At first sight, a neonatal intensive care unit can be frightening, especially to parents already anxious about the medical condition of their baby. Many of the babies in neonatal intensive care are born prematurely, some weighing less than two pounds and looking very fragile indeed. Add to this a forest of wire and tubes and the beeps and bells of monitors and respirators, and it is no wonder that parents are daunted. But most soon learn that these units are not run by technology but by a caring staff who create a warm, comforting, and humane atmosphere in which babies receive medical care that is remarkable in its ability to support even the tiniest and sickest of infants. In most hospitals, parents are encouraged to participate in this care as much as possible, with staff suggesting ways in which they can nurture their infants even through the maze of technology. (See box, Myths and Fears About the Neonatal Intensive Care Unit, later in chapter.)

The Neonatal Health Care Team

Part of the intensity of a neonatal unit is in the sheer number of staff involved with each infant. For every one to four infants, there is a nurse around the clock with special training in newborn care. In addition to standard nursing procedures, these nurse-specialists are trained and experienced in resuscitation, starting IVs, readying an infant for transport, understanding laboratory and monitor readings, and placing a breathing tube in a baby's windpipe. Practical nurses and nurses' aides with special infant training perform routine aspects of care.

Although the private pediatrician the parents have selected may stay actively involved, the physician in charge of neonatal intensive care is a *neo-natologist*, a pediatrician who has completed advanced training and received certification in neonatology by a professional board. Working under the neonatologist will be *fellows*, licensed pediatricians gaining experience toward their neonatology certification, as well as medical residents, who have completed medical school and are now receiving an additional three years of training in pediatrics.

A host of specialists routinely see children in the neonatal intensive unit. They include:

- *Respiratory therapists* are specialists in handling respiratory equipment and assisting infants with breathing difficulties.
- *Lab technicians* and *X-ray technicians* perform specific tests, although the physician will interpret the results.
- *Physical therapists* evaluate infants' behavior and development and design stimulation and activities for infants who will have a long stay in the unit.
- *Pediatric consultants* may be called to help diagnose and treat problems within their medical specialty. These include pediatric cardiologists, surgeons, radiologists, geneticists, neurologists, anesthesiologists, nephrologists, and ophthalmologists. (See chapter 19, How to Find a Specialist.)
- *Neonatal social workers* assist families coping with the fears and new experiences that are part of having an infant in the intensive neonatal unit. They are also available for counseling about financial and family problems and to help families gain access to community resources.

Special Equipment and Procedures

All the daunting, high-technology equipment of the neonatal intensive care unit serves three simple purposes—round-the-clock monitoring of an infant's condition, assisting breathing and other body functions that aren't yet working properly, and promptly diagnosing and treating any illnesses and medical complications.

Monitoring the Infant's Condition

Temperature. Newborns, especially when small and sick, need an environment of constant warmth and moisture to help maintain a normal body temperature of 98.6 degrees Fahrenheit (or 37 degrees Celsius). Infants are kept either in an open container heated by radiant lamps or in an enclosed incubator (isolette). The incubator is a warm Plexiglas unit that protects the baby from drafts and temperature changes. Completely opening an incubator can chill a very vulnerable newborn, so nurses and parents usually reach in through small portholes to touch the infant.

A thin probe (wire) is taped to the baby's abdomen. This hooks to an electric thermometer in the isolette that, like a very delicate thermostat, provides adjustment of the environment to the baby's changing temperature needs.

Blood Tests. Blood must have enough oxygen to keep the baby's tissues alive and functioning, but an overabundance may be harmful. Carbon dioxide must also be present in the right balance to keep the baby's blood from becoming too acidic. Several times a day—or several times an hour in a very sick newborn—a sample of blood is drawn to test for the level of these blood gases. This sample must be taken from an artery, the oxygen-rich blood on its way out from the heart to the rest of the body. Doctors may draw the sample from small arteries in the infant's wrist, foot, or scalp.

Sometimes a small catheter (tube) is inserted into the aorta through an artery in the umbilicus (belly button), where there are no nerve endings. This *umbilical artery catheter* can be left in place to draw blood samples, to record blood pressure continuously, and to administer fluids. The umbilical artery catheter will be withdrawn as soon as possible because of the risk of introducing an infection or seriously disturbing blood flow, resulting in blood clots in the legs, kidneys, or intestines. Some centers prefer to use catheters in small peripheral arteries for monitoring.

Frequently tests are performed on a blood sample collected after a heelstick. The baby's heel is warmed so the tiny capillaries dilate and more blood flows to the area. After cleansing, a tiny prick will be made and the blood collected in slender capillary tubes. Because heelstick blood samples can sometimes provide misleading information on blood gases, this technique is not relied on when very precise measures are essential, as they are during the baby's first day and if supplemental oxygen is being given.

An important new technique, *transcutaneous monitoring*, measures blood gases through the skin, but under some circumstances these readings may not always be as accurate as direct tests, so blood drawing is still needed occasionally. To protect delicate skin and to maintain accuracy of measurements, these monitors are repositioned frequently.

New "micro-methods" of blood testing are crucial in the NICU. These allow accurate blood testing with a sample only 1/10 to 1/50 the volume usually taken in adults.

Heart and Breathing Rates. Electrodes, usually taped on the chest, are connected by thin wires to a TV-style monitor that displays the baby's heart and breathing rates. An alarm sounds if breathing stops (apnea) or heart rate slows down (bradycardia), changes that require immediate medical attention. The alarm can be frightening but it will sound in time to prevent harm to the baby and it does not necessarily mean there is a serious problem.

Blood Pressure. Also displayed on a monitor is the infant's blood pressure. If there is a catheter in place in the umbilicus or other artery, an attachment can take direct pressure readings. A baby in the neonatal intensive care unit without a monitor may wear a small plastic blood pressure cuff around the thigh or upper arm to obtain these readings.

Weight. Babies in neonatal intensive care units are generally weighed once a day. Weight is usually recorded in grams (1 pound equals 454 grams) and is plotted on a growth curve that gives the normal standards for a given length of gestation. It is normal for the baby to lose 10 to 15 percent of birthweight during the first few days of life, and there are always going to be temporary weight fluctuations. A general growing trend is the most important sign.

Each infant's formula intake is recorded in milliliters (30 milliliters equal 1 ounce) and urine output is measured or estimated by comparing the wet and dry weights of the baby's diapers.

Medical Support Systems

Respiratory Assistance. Much of the equipment in the unit is for providing oxygen and breathing assistance to sick newborns. Inside the isolette is a moist, oxygenated atmosphere, but the oxygen can

FEARS AND MYTHS ABOUT THE NEONATAL INTENSIVE CARE UNIT

- **Myth:** Most babies in the neonatal intensive care unit don't live.

    Facts: In the past, a baby born weighing three pounds was simply not expected to live. Today, more than 90 percent of infants born weighing between two and three pounds survive. Of those weighing only one to two pounds at birth, 50 to 70 percent may survive. All of these infants require intensive care, and their first several weeks of life are often filled with medical problems. However, with good obstetrical management, delivery at a tertiary hospital, and the immediate availability of required newborn care, there is a high probability of survival with a reasonable prospect for normal development.

- **Myth:** In the neonatal intensive care unit, babies are saved who have permanent brain damage and would be better off dead.

    Facts: More than two decades ago, half of the infants born weighing less than three pounds had either neurologic or intellectual impairment. With improvements in care, the probability of neurologic or intellectual impairment has declined to the point where only about 15 percent of infants born prematurely have subsequent handicaps. Even though they may have specific motor handicaps, frequently cerebral palsy, many of these infants will function normally within society.

    It is rare for a premature infant to have an intellectual deficit without an accompanying motor deficit. When significant mental retardation is a premature infant's major problem, it can usually be attributed to congenital or adverse events very early in fetal development—not to the premature birth.

- **Myth:** Babies can become blind or deaf in the neonatal intensive care unit.

    Facts: Most low-birthweight infants who survive have normal sight and hearing. Very premature infants *are* at risk for blindness from a disease called retinopathy of prematurity (ROP). For years, oxygen given in the nursery was believed to be the basic cause of this blindness, but it is now known that the disease is primarily related to the immaturity of the retina at birth. With the increasing number of low-birthweight infants who survive, there are more children with minor signs of retinopathy of prematurity. However, the number of children who develop blindness from ROP remains low.

    Deafness is infrequent in premature infants, and it is usually unrelated to medical problems that occur in the nursery. It is more likely today, however, that an infant's deafness will be diagnosed while the baby is still in the neonatal intensive care unit. An increasing number of states require auditory screening, either prior to discharge from the unit or early in life, as part of the organized follow-up program for the low-birthweight infant. With early diagnosis and referral to appropriate agencies, hearing-impaired infants can be helped to develop normally.

- **Myth:** Medical staff in the neonatal intensive care unit don't like having parents around.

    Facts: In the modern neonatal intensive care unit, participation of parents is not only welcome—

be better regulated and supplied in higher concentration when given in a clear plastic hood that fits around the baby's head. Inside the *oxygen hood*, an analyzer indicates just how much oxygen the baby is receiving.

Babies whose tiny lung sacs tend to collapse (see Respiratory Distress Syndrome, later in this chapter) are given a steady flow of pressurized air to keep the lungs slightly inflated all the time. Called *continuous positive airway pressure* (CPAP, pronounced see-pap), this technique is capable of delivering air containing from 21 to 100 percent oxygen. Several methods of delivery are effective, including prongs or tubes into the nostrils, or a mask over the nose and mouth. The advantage of CPAP is that the baby can make his or her own normal breathing motions and an endotracheal tube may be avoided.

Sometimes a machine must temporarily take over breathing completely, usually for an infant who is extremely weak or whose brain does not send regular signals to breathe. A tube is inserted down the windpipe and a respirator takes over breathing. As with CPAP, a measured amount of warmed, moistened, oxygen-rich air is given under enough pressure to keep the lungs partially open at all times. The pressure is varied rhythmically to simulate inhalation and exhalation.

An infant with an endotracheal tube will not make sounds when crying, because the tube is inserted between the vocal cords. In some units, the baby may be initially given drugs that paralyze the breathing muscles temporarily so the infant doesn't fight the respirator-induced breathing pattern. The medications, curare or pancuronium (Pavulon), render a baby unable to move but still able to hear and feel. As an infant is weaned from the respirator, the it is expected. In the past, parents were not allowed into the unit because of concern about infections. Now, parents are involved in the care of their infants from the moment of birth until the day of discharge. Wearing clean gowns over street clothes and rigorous attention to hand washing minimizes the risk of infection. Most units have 24-hour-a-day visitation for parents and grandparents as well as arrangements for sibling visits.

● **Myth:** If a baby needs the neonatal intensive care unit, it usually means the mother did something wrong during pregnancy.

Facts: Apart from complications arising from drug addiction, if an infant is born with an unanticipated problem, whether it is prematurity or a medical or surgical problem in a full-term infant, the parents may be overcome by feelings of guilt, anger, rejection, and hopelessness. All of these feelings are normal and must be dealt with by both the mother and father with the assistance of medical staff.

It is rare that an infant's problem bears any relationship to something that the mother did during her pregnancy. We still know little about the specific events that trigger the onset of premature labor. Most congenital anomalies stem from unexplained problems in the fetus's organ development very early in the pregnancy.

● **Myth:** The noisy environment of the neonatal intensive care unit is harmful.

Facts: The neonatal intensive care unit is definitely abuzz with noise and activity during the day.

Studies of sound levels in newborn intensive care units reveal noise levels that are well within the safe range. In fact, the common presumption that the uterus is a quiet place is not true; the average number of decibels that a fetus is exposed to in utero is approximately 70, which is the same background sound level in today's neonatal intensive care unit.

Researchers continue to examine the long-term impact of light, sound, and sensory bombardment. Ultimately, these studies may result in changes in the physical design of the units.

● **Myth:** Babies are experimented on in the neonatal intensive care unit.

Facts: Much of the progress in survival and well-being of low-birthweight infants has been the result of research that originated in laboratories and then proceeded to research projects in university neonatal intensive care units. The highest standards of neonatal clinical care must include simultaneous research—without it, progress would cease. However, research does *not* mean experimentation. Most clinical research involves asking constructive, critical, and practical questions about the day-to-day care of infants.

Today, all clinical research projects are approved initially by divisional and departmental committees and subsequently at the university level, where consumers participate in the approval process. No infant can be entered into a clinical research project without prior signed approval of the parents.

machine is set for fewer and fewer breaths per minute, and in between these respirator breaths the baby's natural breathing can take over.

Nutrition. A premature or sick newborn is often unable to safely nurse or receive feedings by mouth. When the newborn is struggling to breathe or just to stay alive, circulation is diverted away from the digestive system to other vital organs. If nourishment is introduced into the digestive tract too early it will not be digested and a serious injury could occur, with subsequent infection.

Intravenous feedings, through a tube or needle inserted into an artery or vein, deliver fluids, sugar (glucose or dextrose), and protein during the first few days of life. The umbilical catheter (see above, under Blood Tests) is often chosen to deliver nourishment and medication. Sometimes an IV is in-

serted into a vein just under the skin, using small plastic catheters. To hold the IV safely in an arm or leg, the limb is held immobile with a padded splint. Often, to allow free movement of arms and legs, the IV is inserted in a scalp vein. While these *superficial IVs* are good for giving simple fluids, the delicacy of these veins prevents them from being used to draw blood for testing, or to deliver more concentrated medications and nutrients. When a superficial IV is in use, nurses watch carefully for swelling that might indicate that the needle has shifted slightly and fluids are leaking into surrounding tissues instead of entering the vein. When this infiltration occurs, the IV is quickly removed and the fluid is allowed to absorb into the tissues.

For intravenous feeding, a larger vein lying deeper beneath the skin is used. Thin tubing, called a *central line,* is inserted into the vein using a percutaneous needle. Less often, an incision, called a *cut-down*, is needed to place an IV in a deep vein. This is done under local anesthetic. A central line is less likely to shift or to disrupt circulation than other types of IVs, but close monitoring for signs of infection is necessary.

Gavage feeding is giving formula directly into the stomach through a tube. A more complete formula of protein (already broken down into simple amino acids for easy digestion), fats, vitamins, and minerals, and sugar water can be given for prolonged periods, providing nutrition complete enough to keep an infant growing.

The gavage tube is inserted through the nose and threaded down into the stomach. If vomiting is a problem, the tube may be passed beyond the stomach with the tip ending in the upper intestine.

Gavage feeding starts with very small quantities of plain sugar water, usually less than a teaspoon at a time. If the infant tolerates the feedings, larger amounts of breastmilk or a more complex formula are gradually added until the infant is taking more than an ounce of formula every two to three hours. Infants can make sucking motions with the nasogastric tube in place and, as practice for nursing, they may be encouraged to suck on a pacifier while a feeding is being given. For the smallest infants, formula is given continuously in smaller amounts, using a pump.

Infants may demonstrate their readiness to suck by attempting to suck on the tube. When the baby is allowed to nurse, the small amounts given are usually supplemented by tube feeding for many days. Feeding by suckling requires coordination of swallowing and breathing. Parents may be able to give the baby a first bottle, but doctors may want to monitor the infant's breathing and heart rate closely during suckling.

Bloating of the abdomen and failure to move undigested food past the stomach are common difficulties following the first gavage feedings. The stomach contents may occasionally need to be emptied through the feeding tube.

The diagnosis and treatment of specific illness and complications will be discussed later in this chapter.

Regionalization and Transfer

In the 1970s, as part of an effort to prevent infant deaths and improve the medical care of very sick newborns, a system called *regionalized neonatal care* was developed. Under this system, certain hospitals, designated Level III or tertiary care centers, were outfitted with the most sophisticated equipment and highly trained personnel. High-risk mothers and newborns from a defined geographic area are accepted for treatment, even if the delivery is elsewhere or the primary physician is not part of their staff. Level III care is usually found at major medical centers or hospitals where more than 3,000 babies are delivered each year. Smaller community hospitals (designated Level I) offer regular newborn care, while larger community hospitals (Level II) provide specialized transitional care for relatively healthy premature babies and infants needing a temporary close watch. Innovations in neonatal care, and the regionalization system, are credited with a 40 percent drop in infant mortality in the United States over the last decade.

Women who are at high risk to deliver a baby needing intensive care are encouraged to deliver at a hospital with Level III facilities. Yet, even with greater awareness of risk factors, it is estimated that 40 percent of cases needing the neonatal intensive care units can't be predicted. Women who have chosen a small community hospital or delivery at a non-hospital site may suddenly find their baby must be transported to a hospital with a more sophisticated Level III nursery.

When a newborn must be transferred, a doctor-and-nurse pair will often serve as the transport team, stabilizing the baby before transfer and accompanying the child on the trip. Paramedics with newborn training assist in the actual transport, which may take place in a fully equipped ambulance, van, helicopter, or airplane. Parents should be provided clear, written information on the neonatal unit where their baby will be admitted. Physicians, nurses, and the parents will all participate in deciding whether transfer is the best choice for a baby, as all must consent before transfer takes place. Whenever possible, parents are encouraged to see and hold their infant before transfer, especially if the Level III hospital is far away.

Many hospitals encourage the father to follow the transport team to the new hospital and spend a few hours getting acquainted. The staff will explain the baby's condition and treatment plans. Often, they will provide a photograph of the baby in the new surroundings for the father to take back to reassure the baby's mother.

Several medical procedures may be required to ensure a safe transfer. These include:

- Blood tests for oxygen and glucose levels.
- Chest X ray.
- A tube placed into the infant's stomach.
- A tube placed in the baby's windpipe and assisted breathing.

- Prongs placed in the infant's nose and respiratory assistance, i.e., CPAP.
- An intravenous line and, in the sickest infant, an arterial line.

COMMON REASONS FOR A SHORT STAY IN A NEONATAL UNIT

Asphyxia

Asphyxia occurs when there is too little oxygen and too much carbon dioxide in an infant's blood at delivery. A severe disturbance in oxygen/carbon-dioxide balance inhibits the function of the brain and other organs and is one of the reasons a baby fails to breathe spontaneously at birth.

Asphyxia may be caused by a variety of factors operating before and after delivery. Before birth, maternal or fetal factors such as maternal hypotension or a blocked umbilical cord, may inhibit the flow of blood to and from the placenta. After birth, asphyxia may be caused by lung immaturity, airway obstruction, and various birth defects that prevent lung expansion. In some cases, painkilling drugs given to the mother during labor and delivery may reduce a baby's ability to breathe independently, increasing the risk of asphyxia.

Infants with significant asphyxia often have abnormal breathing patterns, loss of muscle tone, poor sucking and feeding, and sometimes seizures. Long-term concerns are that an infant may have sustained permanent brain damage from lack of oxygen, resulting in cerebral palsy or hearing loss.

Asphyxiated infants are treated with prompt resuscitation and oxygen support. The oxygen/carbon-dioxide levels in the blood are closely monitored while the medical staff remains alert for the onset of related medical problems. If the period of asphyxia was brief and muscle tone returned to normal in a few minutes, there is a very good prognosis.

Meconium Aspiration

At birth the intestines contain *meconium*, a greenish-black material that will be passed in the first few days. In about 10 percent of deliveries, meconium passes into the amniotic fluid before birth. Its presence in the fluid, called meconium staining, is more likely when there is fetal distress, or if infants are delivered significantly past the due date or are undersize for their weeks in the womb. It is rare in premature infants.

Meconium in the amniotic fluid can be aspirated by the infant during labor and delivery, resulting in breathing difficulties and pneumonia. When meconium staining is present, the delivery team will suction the newborn's mouth and nose. If meconium is thick and present in a large amount, it will be suctioned from the windpipe before the infant is resuscitated. In general, these efforts should take no longer than one to two minutes, but is the most severe cases, it may take longer. After resuscitation, the stomach contents will also be suctioned to reduce the risk of later aspiration.

In most infants with meconium staining, only a tinge of the substance is found in the fluid and none found in the airways. Their breathing will be normal and the health team will have little special concern. When there is significant meconium staining, particularly if the Apgar score reveals evidence of a difficult transition, the infant's vital functions will be monitored carefully in the transitional nursery and, in extreme cases, in the neonatal intensive care unit, with special attention to any signs of developing pneumonia or other infection.

Transient Tachypnea

Tachypnea is an increased breathing rate, defined as more than 60 breaths per minute in a newborn (the normal newborn breathing rate is about 40 breaths per minute). Transient tachypnea is a temporary breathing problem, sometimes called respiratory distress syndrome Type II or wet lung syndrome. It occurs most often in infants born by cesarean section and full-term infants who may have slight distress at birth but who are easily resuscitated. The infant might arrive in the nursery in good condition and able to breathe well while stimulated. A few hours later, however, the infant might strain with each breath, have trouble clearing fluid from the lungs, and have poor cough, gag, and swallow reflexes.

Infants with transient tachypnea require supplementary oxygen and may need oxygen delivered under pressure (CPAP) or a respirator. As the name implies, transient tachypnea is only temporary (lasting several hours to three days) and the outlook for the baby is very positive.

Maternal Diabetes

One in every hundred babies is born to a mother with preexisting or gestational diabetes. With proper care of the mother and fetus during pregnancy, almost all babies born to diabetic women will be normal and healthy. Because the newborns are at special risk for some complications, women are usually advised to deliver in a hospital where the newborn can be specially observed in a transitional care nursery or spend a day or two in the neonatal intensive care unit.

Infants of diabetic mothers who are not managed well during pregnancy are often larger than expected for their gestational age, and may be obese. They are at risk for several complications, including respiratory distress, jaundice, a low level of sugar or calcium in the blood, congestive heart failure, prematurity, blood vessel clots, and sepsis (blood infection). However, even with perfect management, the incidence of certain birth defects (such as heart and skeletal malformations) has not changed. Parents should know within a few hours if any of these complications has emerged and what special medical care their infant will require.

Birth Injuries

Although improved obstetric techniques have decreased the problem, some infants will sustain some sort of injury during delivery. Most are mild and heal without any special intervention, and temporary observation in a special nursery setting is the only treatment needed.

Bruising or abrasions over the presenting part of the baby are relatively common, especially if the infant was large for the size of the pelvis or if forceps were used. Traumatic deliveries, involving sudden changes in pressure on the infant's body, may result in temporary red spots.

Swelling or blood accumulation over the presenting part of the infant's skull are not infrequent, but rarely require any treatment except a careful watch for infection or jaundice during the five to ten days before swelling disappears. When there is unusual swelling, the medical team may recommend an X ray to rule out a skull fracture. This is a rare occurrence, as the infant's skull is pliable because the bones of the skull have not yet joined. Simple skull fractures require no special treatment.

Nerves are sometimes compressed or traumatized during delivery, resulting in temporary paralysis that mimics some birth defects. Treatment is generally to protect the body part from injury, provide physical therapy to preserve the movement of joints and muscles, and to rule out permanent damage or any other underlying causes of nerve damage. The most common nerve injuries are to the facial nerves, the brachial nerves of the arm and, rarely, the phrenic nerve (which controls diaphragm movement).

The bone most likely to be fractured during labor and delivery is the clavicle (collarbone). The fracture is rarely complete and may not be noticed until several days following birth. Generally no treatment is required. Fractures occasionally are sustained to the humerus (long bone of the upper arm), nose, jaw, and femur (thigh bone). Fractures in newborns generally heal rapidly and without complications.

Injuries to external organs—eyes, ears, and genitalia—during difficult deliveries are usually mild and heal without specific treatment. When internal organs are injured, which happens very rarely, early detection of a problem is crucial. Infants who show signs of shock, anemia, irritability, or abdominal distension after a difficult delivery and without an obvious cause, will be examined carefully for damage to the liver, spleen, and adrenal glands.

NEONATAL PROBLEMS REQUIRING LONGER-TERM CARE

Prematurity and Intrauterine Growth Retardation

Infants with low birthweight may have been born too soon, born too small, or both. Infants delivered before 37 weeks of gestation are called preterm, or premature. Birthweight will depend on the number of weeks in the womb—about 1,200 grams after 29 weeks and 2,000 grams after 34 weeks.

Infants who are small for the number of weeks spent in the womb are said to have *intrauterine growth retardation* (IUGR). Using standard growth curves for length and weight, a pediatrician will designate an infant as small for gestational age (SGA) if weight falls below that of 90 percent of all infants at that age. With the use of sonographic information, retarded growth is often diagnosed before birth.

The infant's proportions help physicians determine when and why growth was slowed during pregnancy. If the infant's body is in proportion but uniformly tiny, it is likely that growth retardation started early in pregnancy. The reason may be as innocuous as an ethnic or familial predisposition to smallness (the mother's birthweight and adult size are good indicators). Growth retardation starting early in pregnancy can also result from maternal smoking, chronic maternal hypertension, inadequate food intake, prenatal infection (see TORCH infections), chromosomal disorders (such as Trisomy 13 and Turner's syndrome), or maternal drug addiction.

When growth is impaired late in the third trimester of pregnancy, weight is affected more than length or head circumference—hence a full-term infant may appear long and skinny. Sometimes called prenatal malnourishment, failure to gain weight in later pregnancy may be caused by any condition that restricted blood or oxygen flow to the fetus:

- Placental problems
- Maternal high blood pressure
- Multiple births
- Poor nutrition
- Drug, alcohol, and tobacco use
- Toxemia

Undersize infants may have some of the problems associated with prematurity and are particularly prone to asphyxia, low blood sugar, high hematocrits (excessive numbers of red blood cells), and difficulties regulating body temperature. Small-for-age infants are also known for being fussy and reacting differently to parental attempts to feed and comfort them. Before the baby is discharged, parents may find it helpful if a professional demonstrates soothing techniques and special methods of interacting with the infant.

Respiratory Distress Syndrome

Formerly called *hyaline membrane disease*, respiratory distress syndrome (RDS) is the most life-threatening aspect of prematurity. It occasionally affects full-term infants and about 35 percent of premature infants, including nearly all infants weighing less than 1,000 grams.

The lungs of many premature infants are immature and lack the natural, detergentlike lubricant called surfactant. Surfactant keeps the lung's tiny air sacs (alveoli) from collapsing and sticking together on exhalation. Lacking surfactant, the newborn must reinflate collapsed lungs with each breath. Rapid or difficult breathing with a heaving chest, flaring nostrils, and grunting noises are signs of extraordinary breathing efforts that may be evident during the first few hours after birth.

Although the infant uses a tremendous amount of energy attempting to breathe, too little oxygen enters the bloodstream. Treatment for respiratory distress involves breathing support and ensuring appropriate amounts of oxygen in the blood until the newborn is able to produce enough surfactant and to breathe regularly without assistance. More than 85 percent of infants survive respiratory distress syndrome.

RDS and its treatment may result in complications, including pneumothorax, bronchopulmonary dysplasia, and subglottis stenosis.

Bronchopulmonary dysplasia (BPD) is chronic lung damage and scarring following treatment for respiratory distress syndrome and other respiratory disorders, particularly with ventilation under high pressure. When lung damage occurs, dependence on the respirator or supplementary oxygen can last for several weeks or months, until enough healthy lung tissue develops. Asthma medication, such as theophylline, may be given to open up the airway. Diuretics such as Lasix may be needed to counter fluid buildup in the lungs. If fluids must be restricted, physicians will want to ensure that all fluids taken by the infant are rich in nutrients, and supplements may be added to breastmilk and formula.

Some infants with bronchopulmonary dysplasia are discharged from the hospital while still receiving oxygen and may require respiration care at home. Throughout infancy, this condition may result in an increased chance of pneumonia and bronchitis, wheezing and labored breathing, difficulties feeding and gaining weight, irritability, and an enlarged chest.

Fortunately, a considerable amount of lung tissue is formed after birth. Although treatment of bronchopulmonary dysplasia can be difficult and discouraging, lasting for many months, the ultimate outlook for normal breathing and activity is good for many of these infants.

Treatments for respiratory distress are continually being refined to reduce the complications of bronchopulmonary dysplasia. According to a recent study, dysplasia is less common where support for breathing difficulties (by means of a mild airway pressure together with supplementary oxygen) is started soon after birth, where use of muscle relaxants is avoided, and where those in charge of respiratory support for the unit have expert experience.

Subglottis stenosis is a scarring and narrowing of the windpipe from prolonged use of an endotracheal tube. The infant may breathe noisily or with difficulty. A *tracheostomy*—an opening in the neck surgically created to insert an artificial breathing tube lower in the windpipe (past the vocal cords)—can be used to treat or prevent subglottis stenosis when mechanical ventilation is required for prolonged periods. The tracheostomy is surgically closed when no longer needed, in the most severe cases after more than three years.

Pneumothorax, or collapsed lung, occasionally occurs when air is given under pressure and leaks through the delicate lung tissues into the chest cavity. This medical emergency is treated by inserting a tiny tube between the ribs to draw out the air between the lungs and chest wall, thus allowing the lungs to reexpand and the air leak to close.

Intraventricular Hemorrhage (IVH)

Bleeding into the ventricles, the fluid-filled cavities in the center of the brain, affects nearly half of infants born before 34 weeks of gestation. Numerous blood vessels are present in this rapidly developing area of the brain, and the premature infant's vessels are fragile and liable to bleed.

Bleeding into the ventricles ranges from mild to severe. With the extent of the bleeding visualized using ultrasound, it is graded I to IV:

- Grade I   Bleeding is in a small area confined to the vessel-rich area of the central brain called the germinal matrix. This is also called a *subependymal hemorrhage* because it does not break through the ependymal membrane that lines the ventricles.
- Grade II   The ependymal membrane ruptures and bleeding extends into the ventricles.
- Grade III   The ventricles are filled with blood and expanded, pushing on surrounding brain tissue.
- Grade IV   Blood in the dilated ventricles ruptures into the surrounding brain tissue or bleeding occurs directly into the brain without involving the ventricles.

Occasionally, bleeding is so rapid and extensive that the infant goes into shock, coma, and death.

Intraventricular hemorrhage may be diagnosed using ultrasound imaging or CT scan. Resorption of blood after the bleeding takes about two to three weeks with severe hemorrhage (grade III and IV). Treatment during this time is aimed at preventing hydrocephalus, the most common complication of IVH. Most infants with grade I and II hemorrhage have no complications.

Hydrocephalus (Acquired)

A buildup of fluid in the ventricles, hydrocephalus can occur if the lining of the brain becomes inflamed or irritated from the presence of blood, if clots of blood obstruct the normal flow of the cerebrospinal fluid, or following meningitis. It also occurs in relation to congenital anomalies. Preventive measures may include spinal taps to remove fluid and to relieve the pressure, or medications that may temporarily reduce the amount of fluid produced. (See section in chapter 28 on hydrocephalus.)

Blood can also irritate the brain tissue, causing *seizures*, which are disturbances in the electrical discharges in the brain. In a newborn, symptoms of seizures are twitching, jerking movements, apnea, abnormal eye movements, and rapid changes in skin coloration. Other causes of newborn seizures are asphyxia, trauma, low blood sugar, infection, drugs, or other metabolic disturbances. Anticonvulsants (usually phenobarbital) are used to control seizures while the underlying condition resolves or is treated.

With routine ultrasound testing on all infants with birthweights below 1,500 grams, it has become evident that intraventricular hemorrhage is relatively common. Mortality and complications from brain bleeds were previously thought to be quite high. It is now known, however, that the outlook for an infant with a Grade I or II bleed is comparable to infants without this complication. The likelihood of complication for Grade III is approximately 40 percent—some require treatment for hydrocephalus. With a Grade IV bleed, the chance of death or residual brain damage is significantly higher than in other newborns of the same weight, with at least 75 percent of the infants who survive having some complication.

Patent Ductus Arteriosus (PDA)

While the baby is in the womb, all the oxygen in the blood is supplied by the mother. In fetal life, blood bypasses the lungs through a temporary blood vessel called the *ductus arteriosus*. This vessel connects the aorta and the pulmonary artery, the two main vessels that leave the heart, allowing a large amount of circulating blood to return to the placenta for oxygenation. Within the first day or so after birth, this vessel closes off. In many preterm and some full-term infants, the ductus remains open (or patent) for much longer, allowing some blood to continue to bypass the lungs or to flow back into the lungs. This eventually puts serious stress on the heart and lungs. A patent ductus is the most frequent cardiac problem in premature infants, occurring in about half of those with a birthweight below 1,500 grams.

Infants with a patent ductus have a characteristic heart murmur and may develop excess fluid in the lungs, difficulty breathing, and heart failure. The ductus often closes spontaneously; sometimes fluids are restricted to relieve stress on the system until this happens. Indomethacin, a nonsteroidal antiinflammatory medication commonly used for arthritis, is given to some infants to help the ductus to close. Approved for this use since 1984, indomethacin has saved thousands of infants from early surgery. If it doesn't work, or if jaundice, bleeding, or kidney problems contraindicate its use, surgery may be needed.

Surgery to correct the patent ductus does not involve the heart itself, just suturing and cutting off the useless vessel. No residual heart problems are expected in infants born with patent ductus arteriosus. (For more information, see chapter 21, Childhood Cardiovascular Disease.)

Infection

Either before or after birth, newborns normally may be exposed to bacteria and viruses that may cause infection. Undiagnosed maternal infection is increasingly suspected as an important cause of premature labor. Intrauterine infection is suspected whenever a mother is running a fever at the time of delivery, there is a prolonged or difficult labor, or the protective membranes surrounding the fetus have ruptured more than 24 hours prior to delivery. The most common signs of infection immediately after birth include breathing difficulties, rapid heart rate, or poor muscle tone.

A newborn, particularly a premature infant in the neonatal intensive care unit, is at a disadvantage in fighting infection. Disease-fighting antibodies, normally passed from mother to child in the last weeks of pregnancy and through breastfeeding, may be missing. A fragile newborn's skin is also less protective. Once in the nursery, an infant may become more vulnerable to infection as a result of treatment methods and procedures required by their illness. Careful medical nursing care minimizes these risks. An estimated one out of fifteen premature infants develop an infection while in the neonatal intensive care unit.

In the nursery, infection must be suspected whenever an infant is not doing well. Nonspecific symptoms, such as a change in feeding habits, abdominal distention, vomiting, irritability, excess sleepiness, low or high temperature, diarrhea, and changes in breathing and heart rate, will trigger medical tests for infection, called a sepsis workup. Usually the tests' results will be negative. (See table 6.2.)

When an infant is born with signs of intrauterine infection (growth retardation, small head size, enlarged liver or spleen), a TORCH test may be ordered. TORCH is an acronym for the chronic intrauterine infections that can harm the fetus.

- *T*oxoplasmosis is a parasite found in undercooked meat and in cat feces. Most people are exposed to toxoplasmosis during childhood, causing either no symptoms or a flulike illness. The danger comes if a woman has her first exposure to toxoplasmosis during pregnancy, when it can cause severe brain and eye damage in the fetus. Early diagnosis and treatment of an infected newborn can prevent the damage from increasing.

- *R*ubella, preventable by immunization, is a mild childhood illness that can be devastating to the fetus if the mother contracts it during pregnancy. Affected infants may have congenital rubella syndrome, which can include mental retardation, deafness, blindness, and congenital heart defects.

- *C*ytomegalovirus is very common and most people are exposed before adulthood. If a pregnant woman contracts it, her baby may have multiple birth defects and mental retardation.

- *H*erpes infection can infect a child before labor or during delivery if genital sores are present. It can be disabling and life-threatening to the newborn.

Infections in the newborn can be very serious, necessitating a prolonged stay in the neonatal intensive care unit while antibiotics are administered and supportive care given to prevent dehydration and to sustain cardiorespiratory function. Antibiotics must be administered through an IV tube when infants are very sick or small or have poor circulation, or if the infection is in the brain and spinal column.

Pneumonia is a common newborn infection that can masquerade as respiratory distress syndrome. An X ray or cultures of a sample of fluid from the lungs may be needed to make the diagnosis. Although antibiotics can only help if a bacteria is causing the infection, they are usually started right away, before the results of culture tests are available. Breathing may be supported until the infection clears.

Infection in the blood, called sepsis, is treated by antibiotics and, in some of the sickest infants, with exchange transfusions. All body systems, including temperature regulation, breathing, and circulation, may require support while the baby recovers.

Table 6.2 A TYPICAL NURSERY WORKUP FOR INFECTION

Following are some of the more common procedures:

- Looking at specially treated blood or urine under a microscope to detect the presence of bacteria (blood or urine smear or Gram stain).
- Growing cultures of blood or urine in the laboratory for several days to identify bacteria and to test which antibiotic is most likely to kill it (culture and sensitivity).
- Analysis of numbers and types of blood cells, which may indicate that the infant is fighting an infection (complete blood count).
- Analysis of a urine sample obtained by inserting a needle directly into the bladder (suprapubic tap), made necessary because a clean-catch sample is impossible in an infant and analysis of urine from a catheter can be misleading because of germs on the tube itself.
- Analysis of spinal fluid obtained by inserting a needle between two of the lower vertebrae (spinal tap) while the infant is held in a curled position. The fluid is examined for protein, sugar, blood cells, and bacteria which may indicate meningitis, an infection of the brain and spinal column.

Seizures or a tense fontanel, the soft spot between the skull bones, will lead doctors to suspect meningitis, an infection of the brain and spinal column that can be caused by bacteria or viruses. It is the most serious infant infection, carrying a risk of death or permanent brain damage. Several weeks of intensive care and antibiotics may be needed.

Necrotizing Enterocolitis (NEC)

Necrotizing enterocolitis is a severe inflammation of the intestines that occasionally occurs when feedings are started in an infant who has been seriously ill. During the premature infant's struggle to stay alive, the blood is shifted toward the brain and other vital organs and away from the digestive tract. Use of an umbilical catheter, while necessary, also means less blood flows to the intestines to nourish the tissue there, and this tissue may simply be unable to function when feedings are begun.

If undigested milk remains in the intestine after an early feeding, inflammation and infection can occur. Symptoms of NEC are abdominal distention, vomiting that may contain bile, bloody stools, an increase in milk remaining in the stomach, and an overall worsening of the infant's condition. Diagnosis is confirmed by X ray.

When necrotizing enterocolitis occurs, treatment is aimed at preserving the intestinal tissue and may include deflating the intestines (using suction applied to a nasogastric tube) and administering antibiotics. A close watch is kept for air in the lining of the gut or a perforation of the intestine that can be life-threatening. If perforation occurs or seems likely, surgery may be performed to relieve pressure and to remove any dead areas of intestine. An ileostomy or colostomy may be performed, in extreme cases, so the digestive tract can empty temporarily into a bag outside the body. A few months later, the healthy ends of the digestive tract can be surgically rejoined.

Recuperation, even without surgery, usually means an additional two weeks of IV nutrition, followed by small, dilute feeding trials with a nearly digested formula. If the enterocolitis has been severe, special formula may be necessary for several months. Some infants with the most severe form of the disease, in whom a large segment of the intestine has been removed, form a group with a "shortgut" syndrome. At present it is not known how long they will require special feeding.

Jaundice

Until an infant's liver begins to work properly, bilirubin (a normal breakdown product of red blood cells) can build up in the body, causing the yellowish tinge referred to as jaundice. Because high bilirubin levels are toxic to brain tissue, an infant with this condition will be placed naked under fluorescent lights. The ultraviolet radiation converts the bilirubin into a form that is nontoxic and more easily eliminated from the body. During phototherapy, the infant's eyes will be covered to prevent damage. Most infants with jaundice are cared for in the regular nursery and are moved to the intensive care unit on rare occasions.

If phototherapy is not sufficient to reduce the bilirubin concentration to a safe level, an exchange transfusion may be given. (See section later in this chapter, When an Infant Needs a Transfusion.)

Addiction to Drugs

Almost all drugs readily cross the placenta, exposing the fetus to two types of potential damage. Developing organs may be permanently damaged by the drugs (such as occurred with Thalidomide) or the newborn may suffer life-threatening withdrawal symptoms following fetal exposure to addictive substances.

Infants born to heroin-addicted women are likely to have had their growth stunted in utero, and consequently to be low-birthweight and small for gestational age, with proportionately small heads. The chance of stillbirth is increased. More than half the infants born to heroin-addicted mothers are themselves addicted, and they begin to show withdrawal symptoms within the first few days of life. Withdrawal symptoms can include irritability, jitteriness, tremors, a high-pitched cry, sneezing, yawning, vomiting and diarrhea, sweating, muscle spasms, and sometimes seizures. Addicted newborns are treated with sedation and fluids to prevent dehydration. Symptoms of withdrawal may last four to six weeks. Following withdrawal, infants may continue to show abnormal behavior patterns and learning problems, and frequently they will have trouble fighting infections during the first year of life. Infants born to IV-drug-abusing mothers are also at high risk for AIDS (see next page).

Methadone, a synthetic morphinelike substance that is used in heroin treatment programs, also causes withdrawal symptoms in 70 to 90 percent of newborns exposed in utero. Unlike those exposed to heroin in utero, these infants are usually born larger but are more likely to suffer neonatal seizures. Infants withdrawing from fetal methadone exposure may require up to four months of sedation.

Cocaine is associated with an increase in miscarriages, stillbirths, fetal strokes, premature labor, and premature separation of the placenta (abruptio placenta, a medical emergency for both mother and fetus). Although large studies are not yet available, physicians know that cocaine-exposed newborns are small for their gestational age. Cocaine also may be associated with malformations, including a serious defect in development of the abdominal wall. Withdrawal symptoms after cocaine exposure include seizures, irritability, and jitteriness. Infants who survive the neonatal period may be at increased risk for sudden infant death syndrome, and they appear to have residual behavioral and learning problems.

Chronic alcohol exposure during pregnancy may result in a variety of symptoms that have been labeled fetal alcohol syndrome. Growth is stunted before and after birth, and the baby's head is disproportionately small. Characteristic facial features include small eyes, a thin upper lip, and receding chin. Mental retardation and heart and joint defects may be present. Withdrawal symptoms in an alcohol-exposed newborn may include irritability and tremors, gaps in breathing (apnea), and seizures. Treatment for withdrawal includes sedation and treatment of seizures.

Infants showing signs of possible withdrawal are immediately given a urine test to screen for the presence of several commonly abused drugs.

AIDS

AIDS (acquired immune deficiency syndrome) is a progressive, and ultimately fatal weakening of the immune system caused by the human immunodeficiency virus (HIV). Infants born to HIV-infected women may be exposed to the virus in the womb or at delivery. Infants infected with the AIDS virus usually appear to be normal at birth but may be sickly and, after a few months, will show failure to thrive and gain weight, diarrhea, swollen lymph and salivary glands, and frequent infections. Many HIV-infected children are developmentally delayed.

The possibility of HIV infection is considered in infants born to mothers who are known to be infected or who are members of a high-risk group—IV drug abusers, prostitutes, and sexual partners of IV drug abusers, bisexual men, or men with hemophilia who may have received contaminated blood products before the blood screening test became available in 1985. Because of the wide range in health status among those infected with HIV, a mother can appear to be healthy, but can bear an infant who will subsequently develop AIDS.

There is currently no definitive test for HIV infection in the newborn. If the mother's blood has antibodies indicating prior exposure to the virus, these will be present in the baby's blood for several months, whether or not the infant is infected. Infants who seem to be infection-prone should be promptly treated and tested for other causes of immune deficiency. HIV-infected children require aggressive treatment for the most common infections. If HIV infection is suspected, live virus vaccines (such as mumps, measles, and polio) will not be given.

Congenital Malformations

About 2 percent of infants are born with some type of malformation, an abnormality in the body's structure that has medical or cosmetic significance for the newborn. A body part may be duplicated, such as extra fingers or toes; missing, such as a shortened arm or cleft lip or palate; or improperly formed, such as a clubfoot, a heart defect, or open spine (spina bifida).

Physicians also make note of minor malformations in newborns—insignificant physical traits that are only remarkable because they are found in less than 4 percent of infants. The presence of three or more minor malformations, which may be of no medical consequence themselves, indicates that there may be an underlying medical problem or that a specific diagnosis should be considered. For example, most people have two deep creases running horizontally across their palms, neither crease going all the way across. A single deep crease extending entirely across the palm is labeled a simian crease. It is found in about 3 percent of all newborns but in about half of children with Down's syndrome. Other minor malformations noted at birth are umbilical hernia, birthmarks, and unusual ear shapes or hair patterns.

Malformations in a newborn can occur for a variety of reasons, such as infection during pregnancy, a chromosomal defect (missing or extra material in the genetic blueprint), or a combination of environmental and hereditary factors. A genetics consultation is usually arranged to aid in diagnosis, counseling, and treatment planning for a malformation. (See chapter 3 in *The Columbia University College of Physicians and Surgeons Complete Guide to Pregnancy* for a description of a genetics consultation.)

Retinopathy of Prematurity (ROP)

In premature infants, the capillaries and cells of the retina (the portion of the eye that receives visual images) are still growing and have not yet reached its edges. In very tiny and sick infants who require high concentrations of oxygen for survival and prevention of brain damage, these tiny blood vessels constrict and stop growing. After oxygen levels return to normal, they begin to grow again—but often in an abnormal pattern. These vessels are fragile and vulnerable to bleeding and formation of scar tissue in the eye. Scientists once believed that this constriction was caused by the presence of oxygen alone, but they now consider the cause primarily to be related to extreme prematurity.

Residual eye damage from retinopathy of prematurity can include nearsightedness, partial loss of vision, or complete detachment of the retina and resulting blindness. Retinopathy occurs, to some extent, in about 35 percent of infants weighing less than 1,500 grams. Although more than 75 percent of premature infants have no evidence of retinopathy, those who have received oxygen therapy are routinely tested by an ophthalmologist to detect retinal damage.

The smallest infants are the most vulnerable to retinopathy. Some have retinal damage without having received oxygen therapy.

WHEN AN INFANT NEEDS A TRANSFUSION

AN INFANT HAS ABOUT 1½ ounces of blood for each pound of body weight. Loss of blood can send the infant into shock, with low blood pressure and rapid pulse and breathing. This can happen at birth if there is damage to the placenta or the umbilical cord, or if there has been exchange of blood between twins or between mother and infant prior to delivery. When there is a medical emergency from low blood volume, a transfusion should be given, ideally within 15 minutes. Blood is usually administered through the vein in the umbilicus; a pump may be used to hasten the blood's delivery.

In emergencies, blood for transfusion may be taken from a donor with O negative (a universally compatible blood type) or sometimes from the mother or the placenta. In nonemergency situations, instead of whole blood, red blood cells or platelets may be administered separately to counteract anemia or clotting problems. Premature infants are likely to receive several simple transfusions of red blood cells during their hospitalization.

Exchange Transfusions

Sometimes an infant who is severely anemic or who has a dangerously high bilirubin level (from serious Rh or ABO blood group incompatibility) that does not respond to phototherapy (see under Jaundice, earlier in this chapter) requires blood to be exchanged for healthy blood from a donor. Less commonly, exchange transfusions are suggested to remove drugs or other toxins from the blood or to help fight an overwhelming infection.

In an exchange transfusion, care is taken to keep the baby's total volume of blood constant throughout the procedure. In very sick infants, for example, about 5 cc (or 100 drops) of the baby's blood will be removed and 5 cc of donor blood given through a tube placed in the vein of the umbilical cord. Over and over again, for about an hour, these tiny quantities will be exchanged and will remove in whole or in part the damaging antibodies and bilirubin. Naturally, as the exchange transfusion proceeds, part of the blood that is drawn out will be donor blood. To ensure that enough fresh blood stays in the infant, the total volume exchanged will be twice the total blood volume. Some infants will require more than one exchange transfusion.

During the exchange transfusion, the baby will be monitored very closely to check blood chemistries and to make certain that the minute fluctuations in blood volume are not overtaxing the heart. Possible complications include shock, heart rhythm abnormalities, blood chemistry alterations, infection, or the introduction of air or blood clots into the blood vessel.

A *partial exchange transfusion* can be used to adjust the concentration of red blood cells in the infant's blood. If red blood cells are too concentrated (polycythemia), portions of the infant's blood can be exchanged for donor plasma. If severe anemia is present, portions of blood can be exchanged for concentrated packed red cells.

When an infant needs a blood transfusion of any type, parents are concerned about safety and cost. There is a very small risk of contracting hepatitis, cytomegalovirus, or the AIDS virus from a transfusion, but advanced and stringent screening procedures for donors and blood have reduced the risk substantially. The availability of blood products depends on donations. If someone in the family has donated blood, a credit to receive blood may already be present. If an infant requires many transfusions, the family may be asked to find donors in the infant's behalf.

WHEN AN INFANT REQUIRES SURGERY

LIFE-THREATENING MALFORMATIONS may necessitate emergency surgery in the newborn. Blockages in the gastrointestinal tract, congenital heart defects, a hole in the diaphragm, or defects in which portions of an infant's nervous system or internal organs are exposed to the air are problems that may need surgical intervention. With skilled pediatric surgery and anesthesia, the newborn infant can undergo surgery with no greater risk than an older child. For some procedures, such as a hernia operation or even an operation involving opening the abdomen or chest, the infant may be perfectly comfortable and free from pain with sedation plus local anesthesia.

WHEN AN INFANT DIES

WHEN AN INFANT DIES, it is a tragedy experienced and mourned as deeply as the death of an adult. Unfortunately, society often fails to recognize the extent of parents' attachment when there is a miscarriage, stillbirth, or infant death. The grief can be especially difficult because parents lack a lifetime of consoling memories of their child.

Decisions made at the time of an infant's death can haunt parents for years. Often what seems like the sensible and least painful decision at the time may turn out to prolong uncertainty and grief. Parents and physicians who have been through the experience offer these suggestions and options for other parents:

If possible, be with a dying baby. Usually, health professionals know ahead of time when medical intervention has nothing left to offer. Many nurseries offer a special, private room where parents can cradle and be with their dying infant. Holding the baby, with tubes removed and away from the glare of the neonatal intensive care unit, may provide the sweetest memories and expressions of the parent/child connection in the infant's brief life. Medical personnel stay close by to offer any needed assistance. Baptism and visits from loved ones may be arranged.

Name the baby. A name confirms forever the baby's reality and many parents find it easier to talk about a baby later using the name. If a name was selected during the pregnancy, parents may wish to use it or to choose a separate name.

See the baby after death. Time alone to say goodbye, perhaps to dress the baby in special clothing or have friends or clergy visit, can be very meaningful. Although it is extremely painful, many parents feel it is nevertheless an important first step in accepting the reality of the infant's loss. If a baby dies after transport to another hospital, the staff can arrange for the mother to view the body and hold the baby if she wishes. Hospital staff should respect parents' wishes, whether it is to spend just a few minutes or several hours with the body. Even after the body is taken to the morgue, it is not too late to request time with the baby.

Save mementoes of the baby's life. Many remembrances are available at parents' request, including photographs, ID bracelets, printouts from monitors in the neonatal unit, clothes, footprints, sonogram pictures, or a lock of hair. Many hospitals keep several items with a baby's permanent medical record that can be given to parents later. At many hospitals, photographs are routinely taken of infants who die because many parents later request the pictures.

Avoid tranquilizers if possible. Instead of a restful calm, many parents find that tranquilizers merely make them feel dopey and confused, blunting their ability to cry and express their anguish. Sometimes a sedative is needed at bedtime.

Plan a ceremony to mark the baby's death. A simple ceremony, whether a memorial gathering of involved staff and close family in the hospital or a full religious funeral, is meaningful to many parents. Hospitals and many funeral homes offer options for an infant memorial that are far less expensive than an adult burial and that allow greater participation by the parents.

Request an autopsy. Often the autopsy report is the only source to answer parents' lingering questions about the exact cause of an infant's death. It can also provide information that is reassuring and helpful in planning any future pregnancies. Except under circumstances when an autopsy is required by law, the decision is the parents'. Parents should discuss fully with health professionals what the autopsy will entail and specify any limitations or religious considerations before they sign an autopsy permit.

Discuss the death with other children in the family. Parents are unable to hide their grief, and they may find that they react in an atypical way to their other children for many weeks. Explaining the sadness, and giving children the chance to express their feelings and fears, is less upsetting to children than not discussing the loss.

Announce the birth and death. Some parents choose to inform nonintimate friends and acquaintances in a combined birth and death announcement.

Take advantage of professional help. The natural grief process after the death of an infant is a physical, emotional, and marital strain. Counselors are available in many areas, as are support groups of other bereaved parents. Some hospitals have a counselor who specializes in perinatal bereavement, while others can make referrals to local groups and professionals.

When an infant is stillborn or dies in the neonatal unit, the doctor remains available to the parents for many months. Thoughts, questions, and problems in coping with the tragedy can be discussed openly. Results of the autopsy and other tests can be reviewed and parents can participate in the medical team's review of their baby's case. Health professionals realize that shock and grief hampers people's ability to comprehend and remember information. They anticipate that parents may need to ask the same questions many times.

WITHHOLDING TREATMENT FROM A SERIOUSLY ILL NEWBORN

THE MEDICAL TEAM and parents sometimes come to the painful realization that additional medical treatment for a seriously ill newborn is no longer beneficial or even kind. Sometimes death is inevitable and further intervention may cause unnecessary pain or prevent the parents from holding their child and privately sharing final hours. In other cases, the prognosis for an infant's future is grim—most commonly when injury, malformation, or extensive bleeding has severely damaged the brain.

Making the decision to withhold treatment from an infant is agonizing. While the medical staff may have studied the outcome of many other infants with similar medical problems, it is often impossible to be certain about the prognosis for an individual baby.

Parents are recognized as the persons best able to represent the infant and family needs in decision making. Procedures are usually available to sustain an infant's life so that decisions need not be made hastily. Parents should be offered information on the full range of treatment options and possible outcomes. They may wish to have the opportunity to discuss fully the situation with medical personnel, outside consultants, counselors, other parents who have faced a similar decision, and religious advisers.

When life support or heroic therapy is discontinued, palliative therapy to relieve suffering—including feeding, medication for pain, and sedation if needed—can continue.

Parents may disagree with medical personnel and with each other about the best treatment for their infant. If parents do not wish to withdraw life supports or if they are unable to participate in decisions about a proposed surgery or other medical intervention, physicians will feel obligated to continue life supports and pursue every reasonable treat-

ment. If parents do not wish to continue a therapy that the medical team feels is beneficial, a third party may be asked to enter the discussions as an advocate for the infant.

There has been much publicity about "Baby Doe" cases, in which the government has tried to influence medical decision making after parents and physicians decide to forgo treatment for a handicapped infant. "Baby Doe" cases usually involve situations in which the prognosis is highly variable and unpredictable (such as infants with open spina bifida) and situations in which surgery would clearly be lifesaving but would not alter the child's underlying handicap (such as Down's syndrome).

As the law currently stands, parents and physicians have unquestioned authority to forgo treatment if it is of uncertain value or if it is clearly futile. When the treatment is of clear benefit (such as surgery to remove an intestinal obstruction), the law requires that an infant's underlying handicap—unless it is a fatal condition—not be considered in the decision. Life-and-death decisions are made every day in intensive care units and attempts to second-guess the parents and medical team have been few and largely unsuccessful. Attorneys and sometimes ethicists are available to counsel health professionals and parents making decisions regarding seriously ill newborns.

PARENTING IN THE NEONATAL UNIT

BEFORE THE WIDESPREAD use of antibiotics, parents remained outside the nursery at most U.S. hospitals and viewed their sick or premature infants through a glass barrier. As recently as 1970, only one-third of premature nurseries allowed parent visitation. With better understanding and treatment for infections, and growing respect for the primary role of the parents in a baby's ultimate health and development, most nurseries are now open to parents 24 hours a day.

Preventing Infection. Though no longer a barrier to visitation under most circumstances, infection remains a legitimate concern of caretakers of sick and premature infants. Before touching the baby, parents are asked to scrub—washing hands and arms and scrubbing under the fingernails with an antibacterial soap. A sterilized gown, tied in the back, should cover street clothes during visits. Sometimes a mask will be suggested.

Parents should not enter the nursery if they are

feeling ill or show any signs of an infectious disease, including diarrhea, sore throat, cough, fever, nasal congestion, or open sores. If in doubt about whether a visit is safe, they should ask a physician or nurse. Toys and clothing brought to children must be absolutely clean and easily washable.

Visitation rules concerning siblings differ from hospital to hospital, but children should not visit if recently vaccinated, exposed to a contagious disease, or showing any signs of infection.

Missing Early Bonding. During pregnancy, mothers usually anticipate a very special moment of greeting and bonding with the new infant shortly after birth. Not infrequently, this early interaction is impossible because of the medical condition of infant or mother, leading to concern that a critical phase in the relationship may have been missed. Fortunately, no single encounter is paramount in a complex human relationship—and there is no evidence that absence of this early bonding causes any problems. After all, before that moment labeled "bonding," the mother has already nourished and held the infant close inside her for many months. And there were no devastating ill effects on children born during the decades when mothers were routinely anesthetized during delivery and infants were whisked off to the nursery before their mothers awoke.

Stimulation. A rich sensory environment beginning early in life has been documented as beneficial to infant growth and development. Premature or sick infants are no exception—they have fewer lapses in breathing and steady weight gain when they are talked to, touched, rocked, and cuddled. Although the following suggestions have not been proven conclusively, many health professionals find that they can be effective.

The sense of touch is the most mature at birth and is often the easiest means to comfort and show love to a sick or premature baby. Gentle touching, stroking, and massaging can be very soothing to the baby. From prenatal life, the infant is accustomed to the firm support of the uterine muscles. Thus, being cradled between adult hands may be more comforting to the infant than lighter touches on the arms or legs. It is possible to hold and even rock an infant who is in an incubator. Some nurseries place infants on a water bed or use a rocking device within the incubator to provide constant touch.

While in the womb, the infant becomes accustomed to hearing the mother's voice. Talking to the baby during a visit may provide a soothing, human sound to counteract the noise of nursery machines. Health professionals understand the value of gentle talking or singing and encourage parents to communicate with their infants in this way, although at first it may seem awkward or embarrassing to converse with a nonresponsive baby. Sometimes a tape recording of a mother's voice or sounds simulating those in the womb may be used between visits.

Touching and talking to an infant at the same time may help the developing nervous system to integrate these two types of sensory input. At first, however, an infant may only be ready for one type of sensation at a time—touching or talking or seeing, but not all three at once. Each baby has a unique way of responding to overstimulation and letting caretakers know when their best efforts are a little too much. Where a full-term, healthy infant may begin to cry, a less mature infant may show overload by turning pale, suddenly changing heart or breathing rhythm, starting or going limp, looking exhausted or distressed, or simply turning away.

When an infant becomes distressed, attempts at comforting by jostling or talking can be futile. It does not mean the parent has made a mistake in interacting with the baby—simply that the infant needs a rest and will respond better later.

An infant's special skills and responses to interaction are often assessed using the Brazelton Neonatal Behavioral Assessment Scale. Parents can benefit greatly by watching as a specially trained health professional administers the scale and explains his or her actions and the baby's response. This helps parents appreciate the baby's repertoire of behaviors, understand the subtle ways the baby is trying to communicate, and learn which types of socializing or consolation may be most suited to their baby's individual needs.

Visual responses are often the last ones to develop in a premature baby, particularly when the infant's eyes are kept covered for many hours as phototherapy is given (see under Jaundice, above). Face-to-face contact with the baby during visits is an important start of visual communication. A newborn finds the human face more appealing to look at than any inanimate object.

Breastfeeding. The benefits of breastfeeding, especially in helping the baby develop immunity to infection, are increasingly appreciated in neonatal units. Expressing milk and bringing it to the nursery is a positive and unique contribution a mother can make to her infant's well-being at a time when she may feel that the nursing staff have taken over her baby's care. Many neonatal unit babies are eventually able to breastfeed.

If she wishes to breastfeed, a woman should discuss it as soon as possible with the neonatologist, who will review her medications and give instructions for collecting and transporting breastmilk under the most sterile conditions possible. In some hospitals, women with a premature or seriously ill infant are routinely given drugs to dry up their milk, with the idea that engorged breasts will merely serve as a painful reminder of the child's condition. Regardless of hospital practice, a woman who strongly desires to breastfeed should insist that she be helped to do so even if the infant's condition requires a delayed start.

Caring for Parents. When things go wrong in the birth of a child, parents must cope with a bewildering bombardment of information, choices, and fears. During this difficult period, parents need support and counsel to deal with their own disappointment and complex emotions. It is expected that parents will wonder how they can love and nurture a baby that is so different from what they expected. Conflicts and stresses within the family, the marriage, and the workplace should not be set aside and ignored, but parents should seek help in dealing with them.

While an infant is receiving round-the-clock care in the neonatal unit, it is a good time for parents to explore their feelings, talk to other parents, receive financial advice, and take part in activities that will heal and support them for the challenges ahead.

DISCHARGE FROM THE NEONATAL UNIT

EVERY DAY IN the unit is geared toward the baby's eventual discharge. As the infant is weaned from various pieces of equipment and parents can play a greater role in caretaking, the health team is thinking ahead toward discharge.

The next stop before an infant comes home may be the semi-intensive or intermediate nursery, a less intense environment where growing preemies and other neonatal-unit graduates can spend more time with their parents. It may be frightening at first to see the baby away from the staff and the monitors that parents have come to rely on to ensure the baby's well-being. It is an especially difficult transition when the shift in nurseries means moving back to a local community hospital and away from staff members parents have grown to trust.

Prior to discharge, parents will take increasing responsibility for caring for the baby, with staff nearby to help while they build skills and confidence. Some hospitals offer a "nesting" program in which the mother can stay in the hospital and be the child's primary caretaker for a few days prior to discharge.

Medical preparation for discharge includes completion of neonatal screening tests, tests of hearing and vision and, on rare occasions, a 24-hour recording of heart rate and breathing to anticipate any problems with apnea. A formal discharge conference may be held so the neonatologist can review the baby's progress and any special care needs. At this point, parents should be informed about problems that require continuing concern and observation.

Even experienced parents need special preparation to take home an intensive care graduate. Parents should be comfortable with their child's reactions and special needs during bathing, feeding, and diapering. The nursing staff should help parents observe and become familiar with their infant's breathing pattern, medication schedule, and use of any special equipment. Often, a health professional will visit the home to observe and assist with care of a tracheostomy, colostomy, or respirator. Some hospitals, believing that all people should know CPR, routinely train parents in infant CPR before discharge.

Parents may also want a few days to rest and take care of themselves before the responsibility of home care. This is a time when speaking with the neonatal unit social worker or other parents can be very reassuring.

HOME CARE AFTER THE NEONATAL UNIT

A PREMATURE INFANT, or other neonatal-unit graduate, may need weeks or months of special care after discharge. Some frequent concerns or problems are:

Temperature. Without the insulation provided by a layer of fat in term infants, as well as a poorer ability to adjust body temperature, an infant weighing less than eight pounds needs an environment that is comfortably warm (at least 70 degrees and without drafts). Arms and legs should be covered unless it is very warm.

In very hot weather, the baby can be helped to keep body temperature normal by dressing lightly (diaper and T-shirt).

Anemia. A drop in the number of red cells occurs in all infants during the weeks after birth, in premature infants at about 8–12 weeks. If the baby received a transfusion in the hospital, or lost blood because of hemorrhage or frequent blood sampling, anemia is likely. During this period of rapid formation of new red blood cells, it is important that the infant has an adequate supply of iron. Premature infants will require iron supplementation for the first year.

Anemia may underlie symptoms of pallor, listlessness, rapid heart rate, and irritability.

Respiratory Problems. All infants get colds—premature infants and those with previous respiratory problems are even more susceptible. Preventive measures include:

- Not permitting many different people to handle the baby
- Not allowing visitors with colds or coughs
- Not smoking

Treatment of the infant with an upper respiratory infection centers around easing breathing so the baby can feed and sleep as normally as possible. Use of a vaporizer, positioning the infant with head slightly up so that secretions can drain, and unclogging the nostrils with a special syringe are often very helpful. Antibiotics and analgesics are usually not necessary.

Parents should contact the pediatrician if the infant's temperature rises above 100 degrees or if they are concerned.

Infections of the middle ear (otitis media) are common in children. They are likely to occur when the eustachian tubes become clogged with mucus or milk during a cold, and bacteria accumulate. An infant should be seen by the pediatrician if any of these signs of ear infection occur while the baby has a cold—fever, irritability, rubbing at the ear, and refusal to feed.

With a lower respiratory infection, an infant may have recurrence of breathing problems from neonatal care days. If wheezing, heaving chest, rapid breathing, and a bluish tint to the skin are evident, parents should call the pediatrician immediately.

Apnea. The overwhelming fear of many parents is that their infant will stop breathing. It is common and harmless for infants to briefly stop breathing for 5 to 10 seconds. If a lapse in breathing lasts more than 15 seconds, or is accompanied by a dusky skin coloration (bluish tint around eyes and mouth), the baby may need some stimulation to start breathing again. Calling the child's name and gently jostling is usually sufficient stimulus to the respiratory centers to initiate breathing again.

If even vigorous stimulation does not work, help should be summoned immediately while CPR is administered to the infant. The pediatrician will make note of the pattern of apnea spells (mostly during sleep? while eating?) and help decide whether an apnea monitor will make life at home safer and less frightening.

An apnea monitor usually sounds an alarm when breathing movements cease for more than 20 seconds. It is frightening and confining for parents to remain alert for the sound of the monitor and to know that a CPR-trained adult must be within earshot of the infant at all times. A recent controlled trial of apnea monitors showed that they did not reduce the incidence of sudden infant death syndrome (SIDS).

Irritability. Following discharge from the neonatal unit, it may take several weeks for the infant to adjust to home life. After a world of noise and lights, the baby may seek quiet or may not be able to tolerate an unstimulating environment. An eating-and-sleeping pattern takes time to develop. Understandably, parents may have trouble interpreting the infant's needs, because the infant does not give clear signals. Rarely, an infant may cry up to six hours a day.

Although crying demands attention, sometimes sick infants become irritated by overstimulation. Instead of rocking or talking to the irritable baby, removing some stimulation (light, motion, or noise) may have a calming effect. On the other hand, the baby who begins to cry "for no reason" may be showing boredom or a readiness to play.

Growth and Development. Even when the baby's age is calculated from the due date (instead of the actual birthdate), a premature infant is likely to be smaller and less developed than other newborns when discharged from the hospital. Some babies have a rapid period of catch-up growth; a few remain small throughout childhood.

In development, infants cannot be pushed to catch up. Offering companionship and comfort will allow the baby to develop at his or her own pace. The pediatrician or developmental specialist can often show parents ways to play with their baby that encourage social, language, and motor development.

OUTLOOK FOR THE FUTURE

RECENT INNOVATIONS in the neonatal intensive care nursery have improved survival and lowered complication rates and at the same time have allowed a more natural interaction between infant and parents. In one experimental system, monitoring sensors are placed in a belt worn around the baby's chest. Rather than being transmitted to a monitor screen by wires, the temperature, heart, and breathing rates are transmitted via radio signal. Parents can rock and carry the infant around the nursery without concern about wires and without sacrificing second-by-second monitoring of the baby's vital signs.

For respiratory distress syndrome, much research has focused on surfactant, the lungs' natural lubricant that keeps the tiny air sacs (alveoli) from collapsing between breaths. Some scientists have extracted the natural surfactant from calves' lungs while others have attempted to manufacture a substitute surfactant mixture of proteins and fats. Some research has focused on understanding what triggers the production of surfactant during pregnancy, so that the signal could be given earlier when a preterm birth is anticipated. Although the technique is still investigative, high-risk infants given surfactant appear to show better survival rates and require lower levels of supplemental oxygen.

New experimental machinery called extracorporeal membrane oxygenation (ECMO) is used in extreme life-and-death situations when an infant suffers heart or lung failure. In this system, originally designed for use in adult open heart surgery, the blood is circulated into the oxygenation device rather than through the lungs, and there it picks up oxygen before being sent to the rest of the body. The therapy raises the survival rates for certain lung disorders to about 80 percent. It is usually needed for about three to six days. So far, this type of oxygenation therapy seems to have the most value in treating infants with persistent fetal circulation (in which the blood doesn't flow to the lungs), diaphragmatic hernia (in which pieces of the intestines are in the chest cavity so the lungs have no room to expand or develop), and severe meconium aspiration (in which the lungs are contaminated before birth).

7 When a Child Goes to the Hospital

Penelope Buschman, R.N., M.S.

INTRODUCTION

HOSPITALIZATION IS A significant event in the life of a young child. Whether it is for emergency care, elective surgery, or planned medical evaluation and treatment, the experience cannot help but have an impact on the impressionable child and on the concerned parent.

For the young child, the hospital is a strange and stressful environment where strangers poke and prod, performing procedures that are often painful, where there is an unusual focus on body parts and functions, where adults speak in terms difficult if not impossible to understand, and where the child's normal routine is abandoned.

Not surprisingly, children often experience marked behavior changes during and after a hospital stay, changes that range from withdrawal to aggression to a heightened fear of death or mutilation.

Parents can do a lot to lessen the trauma of hospitalization for a young child. Much depends on their recognizing and successfully coming to grips with their own fears so that their energies can be devoted to preparing the child to go to the hospital,
supporting the child emotionally during the stay, and participating in the child's care and recovery.

If the parents understand hospitalization from a young child's perspective, they can prevent or at least mitigate some of the negative effects.

THE YOUNG CHILD'S EXPERIENCE OF HOSPITALIZATION

Emotional Issues

Although most parents are understandably anxious about hospitalizing their child, it is important that they recognize that a certain amount of anxiety is contagious. Children are acutely sensitive to the moods of their parents. If the parent conveys extreme anxiety, the child will sense it and become more fearful. Naturally parents cannot be expected to hide behind cheerful masks. On the contrary, it would be confusing for the sick child to see a euphoric parent. While it is not harmful for the child to know that a parent is upset and to see tears, for the sake of the child the parent should try to remain as confident and as reassuring as possible.

The young child is totally dependent upon the parents; many have never been separated for a single night. When hospitalized, the child is suddenly thrust into a confusing place where strangers hover about, where the senses are bombarded by blaring intercoms and strange smells, and where the only thing predictable is the unpredictable. The parents represent a life raft in this stormy sea of confusion.

Separation Anxiety. This is commonly felt by the young child during hospitalization. If the parent leaves the room for even a moment, the child may cry and cling desperately upon the parent's return. The full-time presence of a parent or at least a trusted friend or family member can go a long way toward quelling this fear.

Fear of Mutilation. The fear that something bad might happen to their bodies is often experienced by young children during the hospitalization. Even something as seemingly inconsequential as a finger prick may represent to the child a mutilation of the body. The child knows there is now a hole in his or her body and wonders what will prevent the blood from seeping through. The parent, in this case, can comfort the frightened child by recalling a time when the child's finger was pricked at the pediatrician's office and how a bandage was used to cover the tiny hole. The parent should emphasize that the procedure is quick and in a short time the finger will be all better.

Even though parents can prepare a child for certain events in the hospital, there is not much they can do to shield the child from fantasies, which during this stressful time can be quite vivid. It is, however, important to recognize that actual fears and fantasy are intertwined. Above all, any fears should not be dismissed as trivial.

Fear of Death. Children, especially those over age three who may have experienced and been affected by the death of a family member or pet, are subject to this fear. It can be manifested in various ways: Some children may verbalize their fear, while others may, for example, refuse to sleep because they are afraid they will not wake up.

Again, the parent should try to reassure the child. One way for the parent to do this is to talk about all the things the parent and child will do together when the child returns home. If the child wishes to talk about death, the parent can listen carefully, even though it may be difficult. The child may ask if he or she will die because grandfather

died when he went to the hospital. In this case, the parent should explain that grandfather was very old and sick but that the child is young and the doctors are going to fix the hurt so that the child can go home soon.

In the case of a terminally or critically ill child, the subject of death comes up often. Again, there are no hard and fast rules. Some children may discuss death in the abstract, while others ask point blank whether they are dying. Others express their fears through play or artwork. The most important thing the parent can do is to be sensitive to what the child is saying and to provide opportunities for the child to talk about fears.

Cognitive Issues

Ages Two to Four Years. The preschool child, even a very intelligent and verbal one, has a limited capacity to understand what is happening in the hospital.

It is difficult for the very young child to understand any but the simplest and most concrete explanations. Simple drawings of body parts to be fixed may be helpful, however.

Children in this age group have a limited ability to understand the concept of time. Therefore, it is better not to talk about the length of the hospital stay, but rather to stress that mother or father will be there with the child.

Nor should a parent go into much detail about a surgical procedure. A young child will have no idea of what an appendectomy is, but will understand the notion of having something fixed. If, for example, the child is to undergo an evaluation, talking about going to the hospital for some tests is meaningless. Tests are not part of a preschooler's experience. Rather, a parent might explain that the doctors in the hospital are going to check the child's body all over to find out why his or her tummy hurts. A special toy, a stuffed animal or doll, might be used to illustrate the parts of the body to be studied or repaired.

Ages Four, Five, and Six Years. The child in this age group can understand more than his younger counterpart, which opens the way for a somewhat more detailed explanation. Books (recommended at the end of this chapter) are often helpful in preparing the child for hospitalization. Moreover, children this age usually are familiar with the names of body parts as well as simple medical tools that might be used in the hospital. Their concept of time also is better developed.

These children have a global concern about

their bodies and are particularly fearful of damage to their genitals. They also have a newly developing conscience and a sense that nothing happens by chance. Hence, they may believe that the hospitalization is the result of something they have done wrong. This is enhanced if the hospitalization is the result of an illness or injury incurred while disobeying the parent, as in the case of a child who has been warned about climbing trees, does so anyway, and breaks a leg.

Parents should try to be sensitive to these feelings, providing realistic information and abundant reassurance.

Telling a child to "be good and you'll get better," is well meaning but not very helpful. Children this age feel responsible enough for their condition without tying recovery to behavior.

Intertwining of Emotional and Cognitive Issues

The child's perception of the hospitalization is as important as the experience itself. For example, parents may be astonished at how easily their child has undergone abdominal surgery. Then they see the child become upset when blood is drawn. How, they wonder, can someone who has endured major surgery without a tear fall apart at the prospect of a prick on the finger? Children sometimes focus all their anxiety on one particular thing, however innocuous it may seem to an adult. A blood test or the insertion of a rectal thermometer may be seen as an invasion of the body and a true threat.

Sometimes even after returning home the child focuses on that unpleasant and seemingly minor part of the hospital stay. The repeated blood test may be far more important than any other part of the experience.

Common Coping Behaviors. *Regression* is common in the hospitalized young child. Children may lose a newly acquired skill, such as when a recently toilet-trained child reverts to bed-wetting during a hospitalization. Parents should accept regressive behavior as a normal and temporary reaction to hospitalization and should not lecture or shame the child.

Withdrawal is sometimes seen when a very sick child is too weak or frightened to interact.

Aggression may be directed against the hospital staff or even the parents, especially if the child is fearful and feels overwhelmed or abandoned.

Being "too good" is manifested in the form of total compliance. Children who obey unconditionally generally do so out of a fear that something worse will happen to them if they do not do as they are told.

It should be stressed that these are commonly seen and transient behaviors and are no cause for alarm. (For information on the effects of chronic illness on development, see box, Effects of Chronic Illness on Development.)

PREPARATION FOR HOSPITALIZATION

Planned Hospitalization

Parents often ask how to prepare their child to be hospitalized. Usually it is advisable to begin gradually, first by talking to the child about the impending hospitalization. Books are an important tool in this preparation. A couple of weeks before the admission the parent may want to read to the child a book such as *Curious George Goes to the Hospital*, which introduces preschoolers to the concept of hospitalization. (This may be an especially good choice for children who are already familiar with the Curious George character.) Prior to admission the parent can introduce more specific books and discuss their contents simply with the child. (See the list at the end of the chapter.) When choosing a book, however, the parent should make sure it is appropriate for the child's age and not so graphic as to frighten the youngster.

Sometimes showing the older preschooler a simple drawing of the body part to be fixed may help. A parent is the best judge of what will benefit the child. Some children are fascinated by a description of how things work in the body; others may be frightened.

Most children's hospitals encourage families to visit prior to the actual hospitalization. A facility's failure to do so may be an indication that it is not geared toward the needs of the child, and parents should question whether their child might be better served elsewhere.

For most children a tour of the unit where they will be staying is helpful because it makes the hospital seem more familiar. On such a tour a child may be shown a room similar to the one where he or she will be staying. The child may be allowed to examine simple hospital equipment, and there may be an opportunity to meet a nurse who will be involved in the child's care.

Reactions vary following a visit. Some children are talkative and excited, others do not want to talk about the hospital immediately but may ask questions or make comments about it during the days following the tour. Some children cry and need extra comforting. But for the most part, the experience is beneficial and painless, provided the parent accompanies the child and the introduction is geared to the child's age.

A day or two before admission to the hospital the parent and child can begin packing. Now is not the time for new pajamas or toys. Older, more familiar belongings provide comfort. Items should be limited to toothbrush and toothpaste, pajamas and slippers, a familiar blanket or pillow or both, and a few favorite toys, books, and games. The parent can always bring additional books, toys, or clothing later.

Unplanned, Emergency Hospitalization

Most important for the young child when the hospitalization is unplanned is the continued presence of the parent. This is a particularly difficult time because the child is ill or injured and the parents are upset.

Moreover, in an emergency, discussion of the child's condition and treatment usually takes place in the child's presence, making it imperative that the parent translate that information into language the frightened child can understand. The parent should provide simple, reassuring, and honest explanations such as, "Yes, the blood test will hurt, but only for a short time, and I will be with you."

If the child asks a question the parent cannot answer, the parent should not be afraid to ask the staff to help.

WHAT TO EXPECT DURING HOSPITALIZATION

ALTHOUGH HOSPITAL routine and rules vary, most follow these general procedures:

Admissions. The pediatrician or specialist is responsible for scheduling the hospital admission. It is advisable, however, for the parent to call the admissions office on the day of scheduled admission to be sure that a bed is available. In general, admission will be mid- to late afternoon on the day before a surgical procedure is scheduled, or earlier if tests are to be performed first. If the test or procedures require special dietary routines, this may affect admission time.

Diet. A pediatric nurse will usually meet with the parent during the admission to ask about food preferences, eating rituals, and method of eating (finger food or spoon). Many hospitals provide menus from which the parent can choose the child's meals. If the child is not being fed intravenously or a special diet (such as liquid or bland) and the parent wants to bring food treats for the child, this should be discussed with the nurse first. Often hospitalized children will have a poor appetite, even for their favorite foods.

Roommates. Unless the child has a contagious disease or is particularly susceptible to infection, he or she most likely will have one or more roommates. Most hospitals try to group children by age, but this is not always possible. For the most part, children enjoy the presence of another child.

Sleeping Arrangements for Parents. Some hospitals provide a cot in the child's room, while others have reclining chairs. A parent should seriously question the wisdom of using a hospital that provides neither, as it implies a lack of commitment to parental presence.

Activities. Many hospitals have playrooms; some offer school instruction for children whose stay will be extensive. Television sets are readily available, and some hospitals offer special children's programs on closed circuit or videotape players in a playroom setting. Sometimes parties are scheduled for children hospitalized during birthdays or holidays. Parents can inquire at the nurse's station about a hospital's activities.

Family Visits. Visiting hours vary from hospital to hospital, and from service to service within the hospital. Generally parents are welcome at any hour, but visits are more limited for other family members. Young siblings may require special permission to visit. A parent can discuss the possibility of a sibling visit with the nurse in charge of the floor or with the pediatrician. The benefit of the visit to the patient should be weighed against any potential adverse affects to the sibling: the possibility of exposure to infection or increased anxiety if the child is too young to understand the hospital environment or what is happening to the patient.

Staff. The doctor responsible for the child's admission will direct the child's care. This is usually the child's pediatrician, but may be, for example, a pediatric surgeon. If another physician is in charge, the pediatrician generally will still be involved, and often is the best person to provide information to the family.

Day-to-day care will be provided by experienced pediatric nurses. Not only are they familiar with diseases and disorders that commonly afflict children, but they are experienced in caring for young patients and in dealing with the concerns of parents. Parents may feel more comfortable asking questions of the nurses and should not hesitate to do so.

Children hospitalized in a teaching facility will be seen by residents—physicians training to be pediatricians or pediatric specialists. These physicians will provide much of the child's medical care, carrying out orders from the admitting physician under the supervision of a medical school faculty member. A parent whose child is in a teaching hospital should not be surprised to find several faculty members, residents, and perhaps social workers, physical therapists, and other hospital staff members gathered in the child's room discussing their child. Called "rounds," this procedure is simply a way of acquainting the resident staff with the child's care.

PARENTAL PRESENCE DURING HOSPITALIZATION

ONLY WITHIN THE past 15 years have most pediatric hospitals allowed parents to stay with their children throughout the hospitalization. In fact, most encourage it. An increasing number of even the most critically ill children in intensive care units are today getting the benefit of continuous parental support and comfort.

Those parents who have the luxury of a planned admission for their child should question their physician and the hospital's admitting staff about the rooming-in policy for parents, the availability of cots, bathrooms, showers, and parent resources such as support groups and social services.

Parents should not be timid about asking questions that pertain to their child's care. Moreover, they should be reasonable, but assertive, about their desire to stay with their child whenever possible. Obviously a parent will not be allowed to witness the child's surgery. However, if the parent feels confident in his or her ability to hold up during a test or other nonsurgical procedure, the parent should request to stay with the child.

Parents should continue to parent throughout the hospital stay. This means participating in the child's care as much as possible, whether it be bathing, diapering, playing, or taking a temperature. Children simply feel more comfortable when their needs are met by parents rather than strangers. When the care must be administered by a nurse, the parent can still maintain an active role by simply holding the child's hand, stroking his or her forehead, and being otherwise reassuring.

Sometimes it isn't possible for a parent to remain with the child. In this case the child should be told that the parent has to leave but will return.

The child's nurse should be apprised of anything that will influence care, such as food or medication allergies, food preferences, names for body parts and functions, developmental milestones, and favorite toys and activities.

Finally, it is important that the child be allowed to express openly his or her feelings without fear of being shamed (the older preschooler is acutely sensitive to shame). The child may select a favorite nurse, a child-life specialist (see below), or a parent as a confidant. It is not necessary, admirable, or healthy for a young child to be brave. That is the parents' task.

Sometimes a parent will say to a child who cries upon seeing the nurse, "Don't cry. I won't let her touch you." This puts the nurse in a difficult position. Parents should avoid setting up an adversarial relationship between the child and hospital staff. Instead, the staff should be presented as caring, knowledgeable, and trustworthy "helpers."

Most pediatric hospitals offer "child life" programs designed to help children deal with fears and experiences during hospitalization. Child-life specialists who have completed an undergraduate degree program and intensive training in the therapeutic use of play, provide safe, familiar, and comfortable play areas for pediatric patients. They also teach and encourage positive ways of dealing with the stresses of hospitalization and help children verbalize their concerns through supervised play and art projects. These specialists are a helpful resource for the parents as well.

RETURNING HOME FROM THE HOSPITAL

PARENTS CAN EXPECT one or more of the following to occur in the days or weeks following hospitalization:

Sleep Disturbances. The child may be restless, may awaken frequently during the night, and may have night terrors. These are different from nightmares (which are frightening "bad dreams"). Night terrors are sudden attacks of panic that interrupt sleep, causing the child to remain afraid and confused for many minutes without awakening fully. Parental reassurance is important.

Regression. A gentle coaxing back to the way things were prior to hospitalization often is successful. Sometimes parents may ignore behavior such as baby talk, and sometimes additional attention is necessary for a while.

Appetite Changes. These may take the form of a change in food preferences, diminished appetite, or

THE EFFECTS OF CHRONIC ILLNESS ON DEVELOPMENT
Candace Erickson, M.D.

Chronic illness can have far-ranging effects on both the family and the child. It affects the child in different ways at different stages of development. Children with chronic illnesses often require additional parental awareness and support to master the challenges of each stage. What follows is an explanation of how a chronic illness can interfere with normal development and how the parent can intervene to encourage the appropriate mastery at each stage. (For a short summary of normal development, see chapter 12, Emotional and Intellectual Development.)

Effects on Infants and Very Young Children

At this age, chronic illness interrupts the child's sense of the predictability of the environment and his or her internal sensations and responses to the environment. It also disrupts the parents' ability to bond in several ways. Parents grieve the lost "healthy" child and, because the chronically ill child does not give the parents normal reinforcement, they find it more difficult to develop confidence in their ability to nurture.

Illness can lead to hospitalization, which can mean separation from nurturers. It can restrict physical movement that is essential to the child's development. The illness itself can limit the child's movement either by enforced immobility due to braces, casts, armboards, confinement to bed, or fatigue. It can also restrict the child's physical movement indirectly, through the parents' overprotectiveness.

It is difficult for a constantly ill child to understand that things are under control. Parents, made uneasy by the child's illness, have trouble communicating a feeling of predictability to their child. Instead, they communicate their own insecurity.

Parental Intervention. With a chronically ill infant, the parent can add stability by developing regular routines. Patterns—where waking, feeding, bathing, dressing, playtimes, naptimes, and bedtimes happen as much as possible in the same order and at the same time from day to day—increase predictability by establishing a rhythm of daily life. Small rituals such as rocking or singing lullabies before bed also help the child learn to anticipate what is coming next.

Parents should work with the medical staff to ensure consistency when medical procedures are being done. For example, if a specific treatment always takes place in a certain room or the child is always placed on a special pad or the health care professional or parent always wears a certain apron, the child learns that the procedures only occur when these special things are present and he or she needn't fear that every approach by an adult will result in pain. This helps confine anxiety to specific situations and associations, so that the child does not live in constant fear of another "attack."

Anxiety also can be reduced if pain and other symptoms are treated as adequately as possible. The parent should not assume that because the child does not verbalize pain it is not being experienced.

Parents need to anticipate the child's negative reactions to the illness, such as irritability or difficulty in eating. At these times, they should try to understand that the child is not manipulating or rejecting them. They should make a special effort to appreciate the child's positive attributes.

Parents must recognize that, despite the child's need for professional care, doctors and nurses are not substitutes for parents and cannot provide parental love. A parent's loving presence is a child's most important coping mechanism. Attention to the child's medical needs is also a way in which parents care for their child and assure healthy development. When the care is successful, so are the parents.

Parental support is especially important when the child is hospitalized. To lessen separation and the disruption of predictability, parents should, if at all possible, stay in the room with a young child who must be hospitalized. If the hospital makes no provisions for rooming-in, parents should consider another hospital.

Parents also need to develop a realistic understanding of the child's limitations and then encourage the child to fully explore the world within these limits. While encouraging the child, they must be realistic about their expectations and learn to accept their sadness that limitations may be required. Parents need a forum to express this sadness, whether it be with the child's pediatrician, a counselor, or friends and family.

Effects on Toddlers

For the toddler, pain, immobility, hospitalization, medication, dietary restrictions, and other limitations prohibit the mastery over his or her body that normally would be appropriate at this age. Ill children often must go back to being fed or wearing diapers, which thwarts their developing feelings of mastery.

Parents of an ill child may be reluctant to set appropriate limits. They may be both overly protective and permissive. This deprives the child of the consistent parental guidance that helps him or her incorporate limits and establish self-control. Parents may also have difficulty establishing realistic expectations of the child because of the illness: They may expect more than the child realistically is able to do. This repeated inability to accomplish goals damages the child's self-esteem.

Chronically ill children at this egocentric stage are likely to believe that they cause their own illness and the bad things that happen as a consequence of it.

Parental Intervention. Parents should allow—indeed, encourage—the child to master as much as possible by him- or herself. They should establish guidelines with the pediatrician about appropriate behavioral limit-setting. They should not hesitate to seek the doctor's support as they work through difficult situations, such as when a child refuses to take necessary medicines or learns to use a physical symptom to avoid limit-setting or gain attention. They should also seek their pediatrician's advice about realistic expectations for the child's development and mastery, based on age and specific illness. This will prepare them to help the child succeed without being overly demanding. With the doctor, they can determine areas in which the child can succeed, and then they can reward that success with excitement, warm gestures, and praise.

The child needs to be continually confronted about the imagined view that he or she is the cause of the illness and reassured that this is not true. Parents should take care to avoid such statements as "You are going to make yourself sick" and "It is your own fault."

Effects on Preschoolers

Just as limitations caused by illness inhibit a younger child's mastery over the body, they now may prohibit mastery of the environment. The child may be infantilized and overprotected in social situations, which limits his or her ability to develop social mastery with adults. The child gets many negative cues that relate to the illness and not just to social boundaries. This "bad" illness becomes inherently a part of the child over which he or she feels little control.

Heightened body awareness and concern for body integrity at this stage may make some diagnostic and treatment procedures very threatening.

Preschoolers still see themselves as the cause of events relating to the illness, commonly stated in terms such as "If you go out without a coat, you will get sick." They may develop belief rituals, inventing

explanations for things that happen. Then, when things don't work as they imagined, their sense of structure is abolished. They may also have a limited view of the illness, identifying it as only one symptom. If that symptom disappears or is brought under control, they do not understand why restrictions and medications are continued.

Parental Intervention. Parents should encourage mastery in every area possible. Socially, they should arrange for interactions with supportive adults and peers. They must be sure, however, that other adults recognize the child's abilities and limitations so that they neither overprotect nor expect too much of the child.

Care must be taken not to label the illness as bad. Parents might acknowledge that it hurts, is uncomfortable, difficult, and so forth, but not that it is bad. They should help the child to understand both the cause and effect as well as the symptoms of the illness. They must never label the child as bad because of the illness and they should watch for any indication that the child is thinking this. If he is, they must help him understand that he is not bad and has in no way caused his own illness.

In consultation with the child's pediatrician and other physicians involved with the case, parents should see that invasive procedures are limited as much as possible without jeopardizing diagnosis or treatment. When such procedures are necessary, the parent should be sure that the child gets a careful age-appropriate explanation of what will happen and should elicit feedback from the child. Play is a very useful mechanism for exploring and working through problems.

Chronic illness in childhood interacts with the developmental demands placed on children and parents in a variety of ways. With young children in particular, the parents provide the child's major coping resource. It is therefore important that the parents recognize and work through their own reactions to their child's illness, so that they can be emotionally available to help the child deal with his or her reactions. Parents need to be aware of the potential emotional as well as physical consequences of an illness, and work with the child's health care providers to minimize the negative impact of the illness and use it instead as an opportunity for growth. They must not forget that the child's illness can affect the whole family, including siblings, and they must weigh all of these factors in working with the doctors to develop the most appropriate treatment program for their child.

SUGGESTED READINGS

A Doctor's Tools, Kenny DeSantis, 1985, nonfiction. (Ages 2 to 6)

This is a photograph picture book of common tools used in the doctor's office, including a stethoscope, blood pressure cuff, thermometer, and blood lancet. It describes how the tools are used and what they feel like. While the book does not describe hospitalization, children will come in contact with these tools while hospitalized.

Curious George Goes to the Hospital, Margaret and H. A. Rey, fiction. (Ages 2 to 6)

This is a good introduction to some of the routines and procedures a child *may* encounter during hospitalization. Since many young children are familiar with the Curious George series, they are immediately interested.

The Little Engine That Could, Watty Piper, fiction. (Ages 2 to 6)

This is not a book about hospitals, but Piper's little engine that says, "I think I can, I think I can . . ." can give a sense of control to a child and provide incentive to try.

I Have Feelings, Terry Berger, 1971, nonfiction. (Ages 2 to 12)

This is a photograph picture book of children experiencing common feelings such as shame, anger, pride, loneliness, or shyness. While this book is not about hospitals, it does give names to these feelings children may have during hospitalization.

A Visit to the Sesame Street Hospital, Deborah Hautiz, 1985, fiction. (Ages 2 to 8)

Grover has been having sore throats lately and needs to have his tonsils out. On the advice of his doctor, Grover, his mother, Ernie, and Bert visit the hospital to find out what to expect. The tour includes a pediatric hospital room, playroom, X-ray room, and operating room. The book does *not* include information about what will happen to Grover or about his feelings.

Emergency Room—An ABC Tour, Julie Steedman, 1974, nonfiction. (Ages 2 to 10)

Using the alphabet, different hospital emergency-room equipment is shown in black-and-white photographs.

A Hospital Story, Sara Bonnett Stein, 1974, nonfiction. (Ages 3 to 10)

Jill needs to have her tonsils out. Black-and-white photographs show Jill being admitted, going to surgery, and returning home. Developed in cooperation with the Center for Preventive Psychiatry in White Plains, New York. This book is an excellent resource for handling questions and discussions.

(Compiled by Barbara Joslyn, R.N., and Carmel Mahan, Child Life Manager, Babies Hospital, Columbia Presbyterian Medical Center.)

---

even outright refusal to eat, especially if the child is upset or angry. This usually is temporary and it is best if the parent refrains from putting too much emphasis on eating.

Heightened Sense of Body Vulnerability. This is understandable, considering what the child has been through. A scraped knee, once virtually ignored, suddenly is cause for alarm. The child becomes acutely aware of the most minute cut or bruise. The parent need only stock up on bandages and offer comfort.

Play. The fears and experiences associated with the child's hospitalization may be reflected in play. The child may become more aggressive, acting out the hospital experience. It is up to the parent to encourage this play, helping the child channel the aggression in a way that is not harmful to others.

Parents should take heart that the above behavioral changes usually are temporary and subside within a week or two. In the meantime, the best course is to offer reassurance and to allow the child the opportunity to talk about his feelings. The child's nursery school or daycare center should be informed about the hospitalization so that the teacher can be alerted to the possibility of aggressiveness or other changes in behavior. If after two weeks the child is still having problems, a visit to the pediatrician may be helpful.

SUMMING UP

HOSPITALIZATION LEAVES its imprint on the young child. It may mean that the next visit to the pediatrician is marred by a tantrum. Or it may simply make the child feel proud and important. Whether the positive or negative, a hospital stay is never a neutral experience; its influence is felt. Though potentially traumatic, hospitalization can be weathered if the child is not overwhelmed by anxiety. The experience, in fact, can be one of growth for both parent and child.

8

The First Year

Matilde Irigoyen, M.D.

INTRODUCTION

THE BABY's first year sets the stage for a childhood of steady growth and development. Each event that occurs during this time—the baby's first smile, the first time the baby sits up or pulls to stand, the first word—represents an intricate set of accomplishments. Parents can view these "firsts" as a series of one-time special events offered to them in advance of the first birthday. The child will continue to grow and develop, but never as much or as rapidly as in the first year, the most extraordinary year in the human life after birth.

The baby's physical growth during the first year after birth follows a remarkable pattern. (See figures 8.1–8.4, next page.) From an average birthweight of 7½ pounds the baby triples in weight by the first birthday, to 22 pounds. From an average height at birth of 20 inches, the infant grows to more than 29 inches at 12 months. The circumference of the head increases from 14 inches to 17½ inches, and the size of the brain from about one-fourth that of an adult to three-fourths its adult size.

Development, which is programmed into the infant's nervous system, is a continuous life process from conception to maturity. The sequence in which all children develop is the same and follows a head-to-feet direction. Infants first control the head by achieving control of the neck muscles. Control of the spinal muscles follows, and the baby is then able to roll over, then sit, then creep or crawl, and finally walk. The baby achieves good control of the hands before being able to control the feet, and is able to play with toys before being able to walk.

The sequence of these developmental milestones is well defined. (See figures 8.7 and 8.8 later in the chapter.) Before the baby reaches a particular milestone, the previous landmark is fully mastered. This implies not just doing it, but doing it well. For example, most babies can be propped into a sitting position by five months of age, but it is only by eight months that most infants will have achieved excel-

BOYS: BIRTH TO 36 MONTHS
PHYSICAL GROWTH
NCHS PERCENTILES[a]

[a]Adapted from: Hamill PVV, Drizd TA, Johnson CL, Reed RB, Roche AF, Moore WM: Physical growth: National Center for Health Statistics percentiles. AM J CLIN NUTR 32:607-629, 1979. Data from the Fels Research Institute, Wright State University School of Medicine, Yellow Springs, Ohio. © 1982 ROSS LABORATORIES

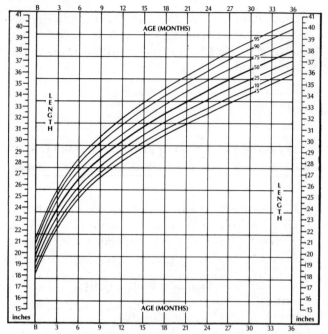

Figure 8.1. **Growth in Length of Boys.**

Figure 8.2. **Growth in Weight of Boys.**

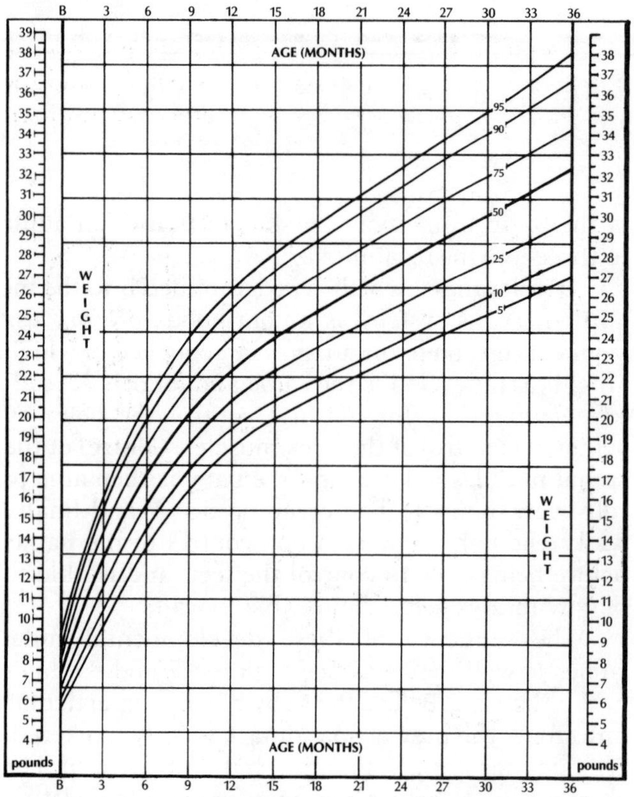

BOYS: BIRTH TO 36 MONTHS
PHYSICAL GROWTH
NCHS PERCENTILES[a]

[a]Adapted from: Hamill PVV, Drizd TA, Johnson CL, Reed RB, Roche AF, Moore WM: Physical growth: National Center for Health Statistics percentiles. AM J CLIN NUTR 32:607-629, 1979. Data from the Fels Research Institute, Wright State University School of Medicine, Yellow Springs, Ohio. © 1982 ROSS LABORATORIES

GIRLS: BIRTH TO 36 MONTHS
PHYSICAL GROWTH
NCHS PERCENTILES[a]

[a]Adapted from: Hamill PVV, Drizd TA, Johnson CL, Reed RB, Roche AF, Moore WM: Physical growth: National Center for Health Statistics percentiles. AM J CLIN NUTR 32:607-629, 1979. Data from the Fels Research Institute, Wright State University School of Medicine, Yellow Springs, Ohio. © 1982 ROSS LABORATORIES

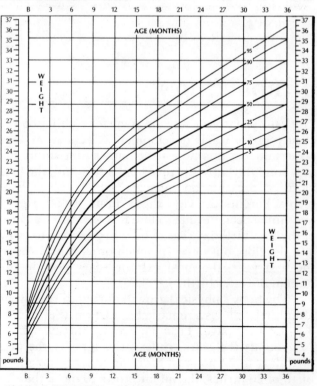

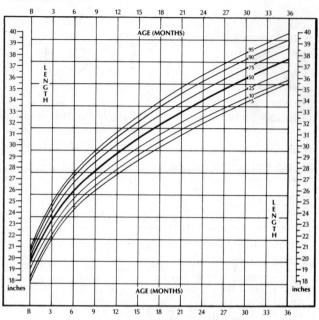

Figure 8.3. **Growth in Length of Girls.**

Figure 8.4. **Growth in Weight of Girls.**

GIRLS: BIRTH TO 36 MONTHS
PHYSICAL GROWTH
NCHS PERCENTILES[a]

[a]Adapted from: Hamill PVV, Drizd TA, Johnson CL, Reed RB, Roche AF, Moore WM: Physical growth: National Center for Health Statistics percentiles. AM J CLIN NUTR 32:607-629, 1979. Data from the Fels Research Institute, Wright State University School of Medicine, Yellow Springs, Ohio. © 1982 ROSS LABORATORIES

lent sitting balance. Only after this has happened will the infant be ready to achieve the next milestone: standing.

Although the sequence of development is programmed, the rate at which development occurs varies from infant to infant. Every baby must sit before walking, but the age at which babies learn to sit and walk varies considerably. The rate of development depends on the maturation of the nervous system and cannot be advanced by training. If a baby is not ready to walk, training will not make him or her walk earlier. This holds true for milestones throughout life, such as talking, reading, and riding a bicycle. This readiness cannot be determined simply by age. Each child develops and learns at an individual pace.

The rate of development is often uneven; the baby may be actively learning a skill in one area and there might be a slowdown in the progress in another area. "Areas" refer to the different aspects of development, such as language, social interaction, and motor skills. A baby at one year of age may be so busy learning to talk that walking might be deferred. Likewise, babies who are very active and are walking by nine months may be too busy exploring the world to concentrate on the acquisition of verbal skills.

Although training will not help achieve milestones before the baby is ready for them, practice will improve performance of the skill acquired. Love, stimulation, and encouragement by the parents are crucial to the baby's development. Babies without nurturing wither and become uninterested in their environment. Babies who are loved and encouraged in their performance will progress to their full potential.

GROWTH AND DEVELOPMENT

Reflexes

Babies at birth are universally endowed with a variety of "primitive" reflexes, which they slowly outgrow by the third month of life. For example, when stroked at one side of the mouth, a baby will root, or turn the head in that direction with open mouth. (See figure 8.5.) This reflex enables the newborn to find the nipple and feed. Likewise, when the lips are touched the baby sucks. When a finger (or nipple) touches the roof of the baby's mouth, the sucking reflex intensifies. The gag reflex helps protect against choking.

A newborn will grasp a finger that touches the palm of the hand, and will hold on with surprising strength while being pulled into a sitting position. (See figure 8.6.) This grasp reflex also applies to the feet: the toes turn down to grasp the finger that touches them.

An infant who is "startled" will throw arms and legs open, stretch out the neck, cry briefly, and then quickly bring arms and legs together as in an em-

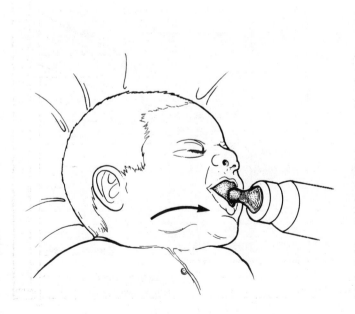

Figure 8.5. **Rooting Reflex.**

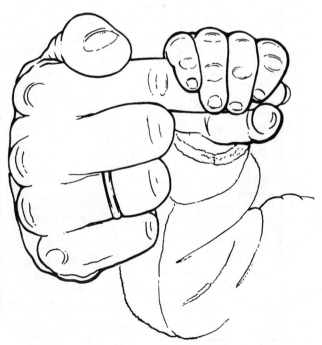

Figure 8.6. **Grasp Reflex.**

Figure 8.7. **Developmental Milestones—Boys.**

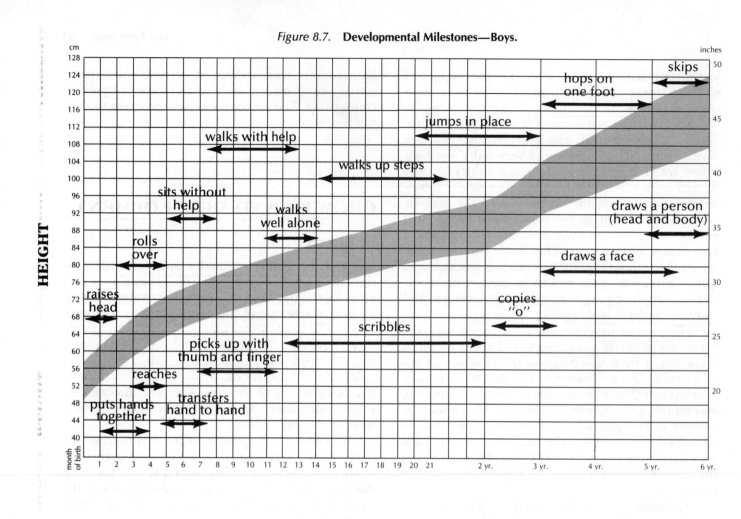

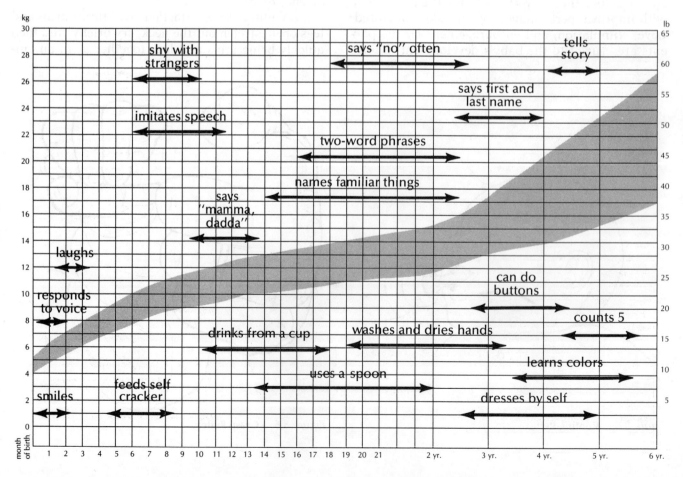

Figure 8.8. **Developmental Milestones—Girls.**

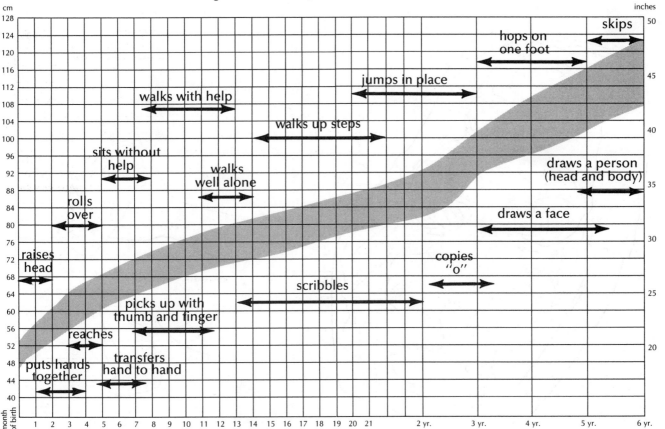

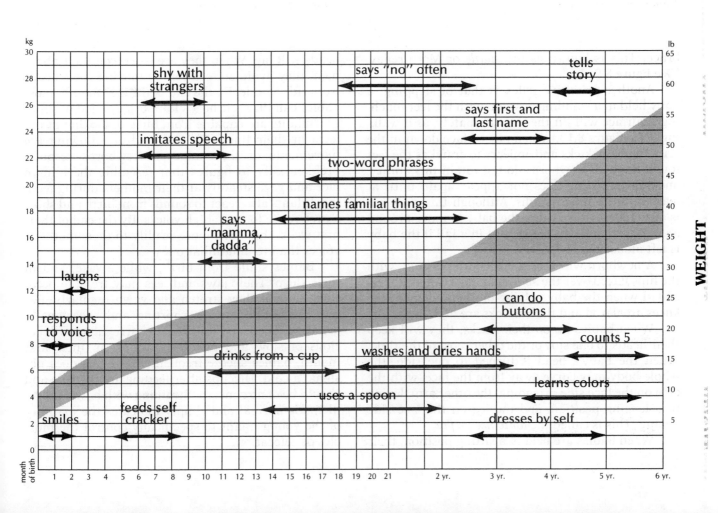

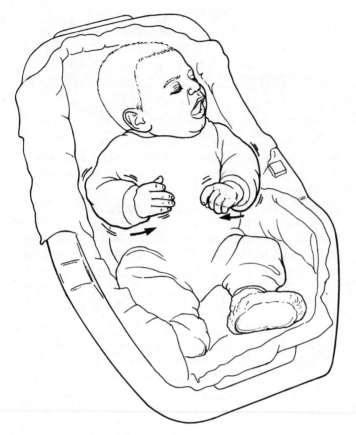

Figure 8.9. **Moro Reflex.**

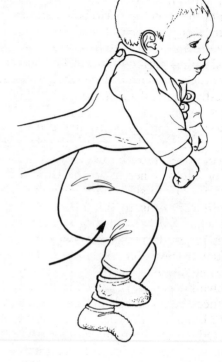

Figure 8.10. **Stepping Reflex.**

brace. This is known as the *startle* or Moro reflex. (See figure 8.9.)

Another primitive reflex is that of stepping: a baby held in a standing position with the feet touching a surface will lift the feet alternately, as if walking. (See figure 8.10.) When placed face down in the crib, the baby kicks and appears to crawl as the feet touch the bed. Newborns do not retain this ability, and real crawling does not appear again until at least seven to nine months. Although this crawling is only reflex, it can cause the baby to move around a great deal and can even result in a fall if the baby is left alone on a bed.

A newborn will keep a curled-up position, with the hips flexed over the abdomen. This can be appreciated when the baby is lying on the abdomen: the knees are flexed and the buttocks are high in the air.

When babies lie on their backs, they will keep their heads to one side or the other most of the time. When the baby's head is turned to one side, the whole body may curve away from the face, with the arm on the face side extending, the other arm flexing in a fencing position, and the leg on the face side flexing. This is called the *tonic neck reflex*.

When babies are held in a sitting position, their heads will lag. When they are placed on their abdomen, they avoid suffocation by moving their heads from side to side. By the end of the first month, most babies can lift their heads for a brief period of time.

Infants are capable from birth of looking at objects in their lines of vision and of following the movements of these objects. Newborns respond preferentially to figures that resemble the human face and gaze steadily at their mothers during feeding. Infants also react to sounds from birth and show a preference for soft, high voices. By the end of their first week, they turn more readily to their mothers' voices than to unfamiliar ones.

Babies smile from birth, while awake, and in their sleep. Their jaws and legs may tremble occasionally, and they stretch and yawn regularly. Babies are usually noisy, snorting and occasionally grunting. Their breathing is often irregular, with periods of slow and fast respirations. In their first month, babies sneeze frequently, but this does not signal a cold. Hiccups after feeding are the rule and should be of no concern. Straining with bowel movements is normal and simply indicates the inability of the young infant to specifically control the muscles of defecation.

Sleep

Although newborns appear to sleep some 14 to 18 hours a day, many times they lie with their eyes closed without sleeping, in a drowsy state. The duration of the sleeping periods is variable, depending primarily on the type of feeding. Breastfed infants feed more frequently than bottle-fed infants; thus their sleeping periods tend to be shorter and more frequent. One-month-old infants will have a "long" four-to-five-hour sleep period each day, not necessarily at night.

How the baby is positioned during sleep is primarily determined by cultural patterns. In European countries, most babies are put to sleep on their sides or backs, whereas in the United States, most babies are put to sleep on their abdomens. There is no right or wrong to this choice. Startling is less likely when the baby sleeps on the abdomen. Spitting-up is also decreased in most babies by the prone (face-down) position. Although some parents are concerned about a baby spitting up and then choking during sleep, this is extremely unlikely, as the tonic neck reflex keeps the baby sleeping with the face to one side, whether lying on the abdomen or back. Other health considerations may affect the decision on a baby's sleeping position. If the baby's feet show any indication of pigeon toeing (the doctor can check for this), it is better to have the baby sleep on the side. Sleeping face-down might reinforce the foot deformity by keeping it in the wrong position for 12 to 18 hours a day.

The Second Month*

The second-month baby already has a more rounded appearance. The average weight is 10½ pounds and the average length is 22 inches. At this age, the baby should have a checkup and receive the first set of immunizations. (See section on immunizations, later in this chapter.)

During the second month an acnelike rash, whiteheads, and red pimples may develop on the baby's cheeks. This rash comes and goes spontaneously, gets worse with crying and oiling of the skin, and resolves without treatment.

In some babies, a fullness is noted in the belly button, particularly with crying and straining. This fullness is due to an umbilical hernia, a condition in which the abdominal muscles are not yet lined up in the middle. Umbilical hernias rarely cause any problem and are outgrown by the majority of children by the time they reach school age. Bandages

---

* For a description of the first month, see chapter 2, Caring for the Newborn.

are of no help and might irritate the skin.

If the baby has wry neck, a condition that makes the head tilt to one side, then the doctor will not only recommend exercises, but might advise having the baby sleep on one side or the other to prevent the head from becoming misshapen.

The baby in the second month focuses the eyes distinctly and is able to follow objects and faces, probably as far away as eight feet. Infants at this age love mobiles and are fascinated by bright colors. They turn to voices and are able to distinguish the mother's voice in a noisy room.

Babies usually cry more in this month than in the first month, and most of the fussy crying takes place in the evening (see Crying and Colic, under the section Common Health and Medical Concerns in the First Year). They can usually stay awake longer after feeding, and they begin to learn ways to quiet or soothe themselves. They will discover their hands and frequently find pleasure in sucking their fingers.

The baby's increasing social awareness is evident. At around six weeks of age most infants reach a major milestone: the social smile. Parents and siblings compete to see who can make the baby smile faster. To everybody's delight, the baby now makes cooing and vowel sounds.

By the second month the family begins to adjust to the new baby. Infants at this age are more regular on their feeding schedules. Sleeping after the evening feeding usually stretches, at times to seven to eight hours a night.

The baby's position is not so curled up, and already some straightening of the legs is evident. When placed on the abdomen, the baby is able to lift the head to get the chin up. This may be done repeatedly, but the head can't be kept up long. In a sitting position the head lag is less. The "primitive" reflexes are still present, but slowly begin to fade. The baby startles less; "walking" is not so easily elicited. The "grasp" reflex persists until the age of about eight weeks and is slowly replaced by an active grasp.

The Third Month

In the third month, the baby becomes the joy of the house—smiling, gurgling, and cooing at everybody, and loving to be talked to endlessly. For many parents, the baby suddenly becomes a little person, one that they can talk to and play with. The baby has now developed the ability to interact with the world and is very responsive. As soon as the parent comes over to the baby to say hello, the baby will focus on the eyes, smile immediately, stretch the arms, and wiggle the entire body excitedly. When talked to, the baby will coo and squeal with pleasure. And when picked up and played with, the baby laughs and wants more of it.

Babies in their third month begin to show an understanding of the environment. Until then, they express all their needs by crying and expect instant satisfaction. For example, if hungry, they cry until the nipple or bottle is placed in the mouth. By the third month, a hungry baby may start out by complaining, and only begin to cry after a while. Then, when the mother arrives, the crying stops and the baby waits patiently for the mother to get ready for the feeding. This new ability to postpone gratification represents a level of comprehension and trust that a younger infant does not show. Parental consistency and nurturing help in the development of this behavioral achievement.

The baby's development in the motor area shows that he or she has lost most of the primitive reflexes. The head muscles are stronger and the head lags less when the baby is propped. In a sitting position the baby shows a curved back and the head bobs intermittently.

Another area of advancement is that of eye-hand coordination. Babies discover their hands in the second month, but it is in the third month that they become fascinated with them. They can now bring both hands together. When offered a toy, the baby will reach but frequently miss. When an object is placed in the hand, the baby will hold it and take it to the mouth. Mouthing becomes a joyful experience, one that must be viewed as an exploratory activity and should not be confused with teething.

Most babies sleep through the night by this age, awakening occasionally for a feeding. In the daytime, two or three naps are common.

The Fourth Month

By the end of the fourth month of life an average baby will weigh 13 to 14 pounds and measure 24½ inches. The baby's appearance will be more rounded, with plump cheeks and dimples on the knees and the elbows. The head is usually rounded and the scalp may have less hair than at birth because many babies shed it during the first few months of life. The baby's skin is now smoother and the rashes that kept appearing on the baby's scalp and face during the first three months are gone. At this age the baby should get a checkup and receive the second set of immunizations.

During the fourth month of life the infant continues to show increased awareness of the social environment. At this age preferences may be already evident. The baby enjoys the constant company of the mother, but rejoices in the company of other children. Some mothers will even detect the baby's preference for one of the siblings: just the sight of this child will make the baby laugh and squeal with joy.

The baby has achieved at this age good control of the neck muscles. Now the baby enjoys sitting and will keep the head steady and turn to look in all directions. When babies are lying on the abdomen, they will lift the head and upper part of the chest by extending the upper arms. As they get tired of supporting the arms, they will make "swimming" movements with the arms and legs and rock themselves on the abdomen like a seesaw.

The fascination with the hands continues. By the end of the fourth month, the baby plays with the hands as if they were toys, grabbing objects with either hand, and then letting go of them as interest turns to another toy. The baby will continue to mouth all objects, and in doing so will drool. Sucking continues to be a very relaxing experience and the baby may often do it to fall asleep.

The Fifth Month

By this time the baby will not only readily recognize a familiar face but will stare at strangers with a puzzled look. This marks the beginning of what is usually called stranger awareness. Although all babies show it in varying degrees, from this month on into the toddler years, they will express it very differently: some will remain calm and serious and adjust to new faces or circumstances easily; others will panic and scream nonstop. If the infant should appear distressed by a new person or place, the parent should be comforting, staying close and allowing the baby time to get used to the new face or event. At their own speed, most babies will come to accept most people on their own terms.

During this month, babies will continue to experiment with sounds. Parents and siblings rejoice in these vocalizations and repeat them back to the baby. This is a rewarding response for the baby, who then continues to repeat the babbling with the new inflections. Babies also learn to reach out with their voices: when they want to be heard, they vocalize louder.

Babies in their fifth month are more agile physically. They will roll from the front to the back. They will raise the head and shoulders, arch the back and twist, give the body a kick or push with the legs, and roll over. They will also push with the legs, but are unable to get the abdomen off the floor yet.

The baby can now sit, playing, for a long time and will lean forward less and keep a straighter back when sitting. The infant seat is no longer safe because the baby keeps trying to sit up straight and may flip over. A baby held in a standing position will keep the legs rather stiff and may bounce up and down, lacking control. Although parents may be eager to put the baby in a walker, it is advisable to wait until the sitting balance is adequate, which usually happens by about nine months. Walkers do not speed walking, and they frequently cause accidents.

The five-month baby will grab anything within reach, examine it, and then take it to the mouth to complete the "exploration." Grasping is done with the full hand, as if the fingers were in a mitten. The baby now enjoys crumpling paper, making noise with a rattle, and holding the bottle during feedings. Babies in the fifth month will also start exploring themselves. They will take their feet to their mouths and poke at their faces.

Babies at this age continue to sleep through the night and frequently wake up early in the morning, full of energy and ready to play. Each night they go from light sleep to deep sleep several times. During these cycles, babies may make noises, toss, cry, or become semiawake. If parents rush to the baby during these periods of semiawakeness, they may set a pattern of night waking that is hard to reverse.

The Sixth Month

The average weight at the sixth month is 16 pounds and the average length is 26 inches. The baby's eye color is usually defined by this age. The soft spot near the top of the head is easily felt, and its size will decrease from now on. It is time again for a well-baby checkup and the third set of immunizations.

From this point on, babies show great individual variations in their development. More active, stronger babies will achieve the motor milestones earlier. Quieter, less active babies may concentrate on the development of fine motor and language skills.

Parents should not be concerned if what is described here for the average baby does not fit their baby, for each baby matures at his or her own pace and may show uneven progress. But if they feel that their baby is falling far out of line with the majority of babies the same age, they should talk to the physician, who will observe and examine the baby's reflexes and motions, and will order testing if appropriate. The diagnosis of developmental delay in an infant should be viewed with caution, because it is very hard at this young age to predict intelligence. It is only later in life, when speech is established, that more accurate evaluations can be done.

Infants at six months babble profusely, making vocal responses to their world. Although the babbling may include recognizable sounds such as "dada" and "mama," the baby has not yet given them meaning. The baby will react to a parent's tone of voice, being puzzled by an angry intonation, responding with obvious pleasure to a happy one.

By the sixth month most babies are able to sit briefly by leaning on their hands. On the floor or on the bed they are constantly active. Dressing them and changing their diapers can be a major chore because of the constant wiggling and rolling. Very active babies will begin to move forward and backward, pulling themselves along with their arms and hands while the stomach and legs drag on the floor. An active infant will also enjoy being held up under the arms and stepping from one foot to the other.

Fine-muscle development in the hands is demonstrated by the ability to pick things up and then drop them. This frequently becomes a game, one for which an older sibling may have more tolerance than a parent.

Nearly all babies are ready for solid foods at this age. (See chapter 4 on breastfeeding and early nutrition.) Not only can they hold the head steady and move it to all sides, but their tongue-thrust response is almost gone, which makes spoon-feeding easier. They are also very interested in food, and many times want to try what the parents or siblings are eating. They can also push the parent away when they do not want to eat anymore.

The Seventh Month

The baby can now sit with good balance without support. Many of the babies who were creeping earlier now begin to crawl on their hands and knees. Others scoot around on their buttocks. Some even begin to pull themselves up to a standing position, using furniture or the sides of the playpen for support. Standing may be frightening at first because they cannot reverse the process and sit down again.

The hands are now being used independently and without a clear preference for either one. Objects are transferred from hand to hand and toys are picked up with one hand instead of two. Banging toys together becomes a favorite game that reflects a new ability.

Joy in manual dexterity extends to feeding time. Babies at this age may prefer to feed themselves with their hands. Feeding time becomes playtime and babies enjoy handling and examining bits of food before eating them. Eating can become such a joyful experience that occasionally babies start rejecting the bottle. Parents should follow the baby's lead, and offer milk in a cup, or replace it with other milk products in the diet. This is a normal developmental stage and should not be confused with the baby suddenly not liking milk anymore: it simply means they like other food better.

Sometime between the seventh and the tenth month, babies start waking up and crying at night. The baby might settle easily into sleeping or might awaken briefly during a period of light sleep. If the parents readily respond to the first toss, the first cry, they will positively reward this behavior, and a pattern of nightly awakening may be established. It is best to let the baby go back to sleep without interfering, even if this means some crying. The company of a favorite toy or a pacifier may be helpful in soothing the baby, but parents should resist going back to the night bottle, for they will be paving the road for nursing-bottle decay (see section on teething later in this chapter). Learning to go back to sleep is part of growing up.

The Eighth Month

By now the vision is sharpening and works together with the hearing: the baby turns accurately in the direction of a sound or voice. Babbling consists of syllables like "ba," "ka," and "da," often in combination. The baby starts responding to his or her name.

Babies now enjoy interactive games such as peek-a-boo and love seeing their images in the mirror. A wide range of facial expressions, including frowns and grimaces, express the infant's emotions. Stranger awareness may be prominent and babies may become frightened and cry when confronted with an unfamiliar face. At this age, many babies adopt a favorite toy or blanket that must go with them everywhere. This is perfectly normal and a sign of growing emotional independence that parallels the increased physical ability.

The baby can now sit for long periods without support, and even those who have not yet learned to stand can bear their weight for a while when held upright. Most are very mobile by eight months and endlessly curious about the inside of cupboards and the "wrong" side of doors.

Many babies bring thumb and forefinger together in what is known as a pincer grasp. They will use this grasp to pick up a block, drop it intentionally, pick it up, and drop it again. With their sight and upgraded hand ability, they are able to pick up even minute things and put them into their mouths: it is important for parents to babyproof the house at this time if they have not yet done so.

The Ninth Month

An average baby this age weighs close to 20 pounds and measures 28 inches. The appearance of the nine-month-old is cherubic, for this is the chubbiest stage of normal weight in the entire human life. Mothers often cherish this appearance and wish their children would look like this forever, but from this moment on the growth rate decreases, and so does the appetite. This normal "fatness" evolves into the normal "slimness" of the young school-age child. At this time the baby should get another checkup.

Most babies at this age express anxiety when separated from their parents, and some of them become clingy and whiny when the mother leaves. Bedtime may also be an occasion for separation anxiety. Parents should not wait until the baby is exhausted to put him or her to bed: tired babies find it harder to unwind and fall asleep. It is better to establish a steady bedtime and sleeping routine and be firm about it. Babies will learn to fall asleep at bedtime just as they will master going back to sleep after awakening in the middle of the night.

Many infants can now get themselves from a lying to a sitting position and can also pull themselves to stand. The ninth-month baby has a perfect sitting balance and can now look at the abdomen and genitalia for the first time. Babies at this age love to poke at their belly buttons and genitalia. Exploration of their own bodies is normal behavior and should not be discouraged.

The Tenth Month

A ten-month-old baby will enjoy playing peek-a-boo and pat-a-cake, waving good-bye and imitating other gestures. The baby will be more cooperative for dressing and diaper changing, will respond to his or her name, and will understand no-no and bye-bye.

By this time, many babies are beginning to imitate sounds, which makes verbal communication and response more important than ever. Language may have two or four meaningful sounds.

A characteristic activity of this age is the development of rhythmic patterns such as crib rocking at bedtime. Thumbsucking, which the baby probably has been doing all along, is another example. These rhythmic body movements provide comfort and relaxation and the baby will resort to them to release tension when tired or sleepy. Sitting with a parent in a rocking chair for a while sometimes serves as a substitute.

Most ten-month-olds can pull themselves to stand and can bring themselves down again. At this age most babies can get themselves almost anywhere by their own brand of creeping, crawling, bear-walking, or sidewalking. Some already are climbing and can briefly stand on their own. A few start walking.

The baby's hands can now perform fine motor tasks. The index finger is used to poke and explore, the thumb and index finger to grasp and to pick up very small objects. While the baby will still test objects by bringing them to the mouth, this mode of learning decreases in favor of the use of hands and eyes.

The Eleventh Month

By 11 months, babies usually understand a number of words and can identify common objects that are named to them. Babbling continues, often at great speed and with varied inflection.

Babies at this age imitate behaviors. They will closely follow their mothers all day long and lay their hands on whatever she did: the TV controls, the broom, the magazine. They are loving, and they actively seek and show affection. They are now clearly aware that some behaviors bring parental approval and some do not. Babies should be praised and encouraged in their striving for autonomy and independence. Distraction is the best method for coping with unwanted behavior. Parents should try to be realistic and clear in limit setting, reserving "no-no" for behaviors that are potentially dangerous.

Most babies at this age are able to walk sideways while holding on to a support. Some babies will be walking and others will be briefly standing without help. With walking comes the need for shoes. Shoes for infants should be flexible, soft, and wide at the toebox, with a nonskid sole to decrease the likelihood of falls. Although ankle tops stay on longer, they prevent the foot from flexing, which is necessary to develop a good foot arch.

The Twelfth Month

The average 12-month-old girl will weigh 21 pounds and measure 29¼ inches; the average boy, 22½ pounds and 30 inches. Another checkup should be scheduled at this time.

The baby now loves to have an audience and will try to repeat behavior that has brought smiles and laughs from the family. He or she will meet the arriving parent with great joy: walking or crawling to the parent, arms stretched, face in a big smile, saying "mama" or "dada," to embrace and cling to the parent's legs. The baby will enjoy playing with a ball, looking at books with the parent, listening to music, and moving back and forth to a tune. For some, this time signals the beginning of the age of temper tantrums.

Language will consist primarily of gibberish and two or three words with meaning besides *mama*

and *dada*. Understanding has increased enormously and the baby recognizes many words by their sound. If the parent asks, "Where is the shoe?" the baby will start looking for it. One in four normal children will have no adult words (other than *mama* and *dada*) in their vocabulary until they are 16 or 17 months old. If, however, the child does not attempt to localize a voice, or fails to imitate sounds, there is cause for concern and the physician should be informed.

Approaching the first birthday, most children are taking at least a few independent steps, though when they want to get somewhere fast they drop into a crawl. The infant's steps will be unsteady and falls will be frequent, but the tears are usually of frustration and disappointment rather than pain; the infant will soon recover and start over.

MEDICAL CARE IN THE FIRST YEAR

Well-Baby Care

The first well-baby checkup should take place one to two weeks after birth. The schedule of visits from then on may vary from baby to baby, but in general they are every two months during the first six months of life and every three months during the latter part of the first year.

Regular well-baby visits give the doctor or nurse-practitioner an opportunity to check on the infant's growth and development, to do screening tests as needed, to identify possible problems, and to keep the vaccinations up to date. For parents, the visits provide the opportunity to ask questions and air their concerns.

One question parents frequently ask is whether their baby is growing normally. As long as the baby's growth follows a steady upward curve on the growth chart, the baby is growing properly, no matter what his or her size.

Growth charts are based on the patterns of growth of normal children, from birth to adolescence. They show the usual, and therefore the expected, gain in height and weight for boys and girls of average (50th percentile), smaller than average, and larger than average size. Usually a child will be at or near the same percentile for both height and weight.

The physician or nurse-practitioner measures the child's weight and height at each visit and records them on the growth chart. If, for example, a baby boy of 9 months weighs 17½ pounds, the doctor will locate 9 at the top of the boy's chart, circle the number, and follow the line down to the horizontal line at 17½. Another circle drawn where the two lines meet shows the baby's weight at the 25th percentile (somewhat below average). The doctor will then measure the baby's height: 27 inches. A line drawn downward from the 9 to the 27-inch marker shows that the baby's height, too, is at the 25th percentile. The baby's weight and height are thus within the normal range for his age. At 12 months, this baby, continuing at the 25th percentile, should weigh 19½ pounds and measure 28½ inches.

Head circumference is also checked at each regular visit. If the size of the head remains significantly small as growth proceeds, or if it increases rapidly in circumference, there is cause for concern.

Immunization

The goal of immunization is to protect the body from infectious diseases. Immunization may be active or passive. Active immunization or vaccination consists of the administration of a bacteria or virus that will stimulate the body's defenses against a specific disease, without causing any of the symptoms of the disease itself. To take the measles vaccine as an example: the vaccine—consisting of live treated virus that will not make the body ill—stimulates the production of antibodies against it. The antibodies react to the vaccine virus, inactivate it, and "remember" it. If in the future the measles virus itself invades the body, the antibodies will respond immediately, inactivate it, and expel it. The body has set up a specific defense against a specific contagious illness. The child is now immune to measles.

Some vaccines, such as measles and mumps, induce lifelong protection against disease. Others, such as diphtheria or pertussis, can only induce (or elicit) temporary protection, and repeat injections are needed to stimulate the antibody production to a protective level of immunity.

In contrast to vaccination, in which the body is stimulated to make its own antibodies, passive immunization refers to the direct transfer of preformed antibodies into the body. For example, infants are born with a supply of protective antibodies transmitted from the mother, so they have some level of protection against infections. These antibodies stay in the infant for only a few months, but by the time they disappear, the baby, appropriately vaccinated, has already produced a set of his or her own protective antibodies. Scheduling of vaccinations is determined in part by the presence of maternal antibodies in the newborn. For a vaccine to be effective, the level of maternal antibodies has to be low. If there are many antibodies against the organism in the vaccine, they will immediately neutralize the

organism, without giving it time to stimulate the immune system.

Another example of passive immunization is gamma globulin, or processed antibodies from the blood of immune donors, which is administered to the body following an exposure to certain contagious disease such as hepatitis.

Vaccinations in infancy and childhood follow established schedules. At two, four, and six months of age infants receive DPT (diphtheria, pertussis, tetanus) by injection in the thigh. Boosters (revaccinations) are given in the second year and before school entry. With the DPT vaccine some babies may have a slight fever and be irritable, usually within 24 hours. Acetaminophen at the recommended doses can be given every four hours. About half of babies develop some soreness and swelling where the shot was given. Sometimes a lump or "knot" may appear and remain a few months, but it eventually disappears; this should not be a cause for concern. Infrequently, more serious side effects, such as high temperatures, limpness, and seizures—usually febrile—may occur. These rare but frightening side effects are due to the pertussis (whooping cough) part of the DPT. For babies with a history of seizures, or for those suspected of having a problem of the central nervous system, the physicians may advise the DT vaccine (diphtheria and tetanus, no pertussis). Infants who suffered a severe reaction to the previous DPT vaccine should receive DT the next time. It should be kept in mind that pertussis is an illness that causes severe spells of coughing that interfere with feeding and breathing. Infants are more severely affected than older children and adults, and the disease may result in complications such as pneumonia and seizures or even death. Although the pertussis vaccine in rare cases may cause severe side effects, it prevents a significant number of deaths and brain damage among the babies who receive it.

The oral polio vaccine (OPV) is given with the DPT at two, four, six, and eighteen months. The oral polio vaccine is very effective and has virtually no side effects. It is given by mouth and, as some of the vaccine virus passes in the stool, it can spread from the vaccinated baby to those in close contact and might vaccinate them unknowingly. The oral vaccine very rarely (one in eight million cases) causes paralytic polio in the person who receives it or who gets it by close contact with recipients of vaccinations (one in five million). For this reason an infant known to have, or to live with someone who has, an immune deficiency condition, should receive inactivated polio vaccine (IPV), which is given by injection and requires booster shots. The inactivated vaccine may produce local pain and redness but no severe reactions.

Under special circumstances, additional vaccinations may be recommended for babies under one year of age. Infants born to mothers who carry the hepatitis B virus should receive the globulin and the vaccine at birth, and boosters of the vaccine at one and six months of age. Babies less than one who are exposed to measles should receive the globulin or the vaccine, depending on the age, with revaccination after 12 months. A flu (influenza) shot may be given to infants over six months old if they have a special health risk.

Premature infants follow the same vaccination schedules and no correction is made for prematurity. Vaccinations may be delayed in case the baby is ill with something more serious than a cold, or is taking a medication that may lower the body's resistance to infections. In case of delay in the immunization schedule, several vaccinations may be given at the same time.

COMMON HEALTH AND MEDICAL CONCERNS IN THE FIRST YEAR

Crying and Colic

An average baby cries for one to two hours a day at two weeks of age and more than two hours a day at six weeks. The amount of crying decreases from then on to about an hour a day by the tenth week. Crying patterns are greatly determined by the infant's temperament. At one extreme, the easygoing, quiet baby may hardly cry, whereas the difficult, demanding baby may cry and fuss many hours a day. It is also known that in societies where mothers carry their babies most of the time the babies cry little and colic is a rare event. Studies done in our society have confirmed this fact. When babies were carried in soft infant carriers for several hours a day, crying did not increase after the second week of life and colic was prevented.

Parents soon learn that their baby has different types of crying. There is crying that is due to hunger or discomfort, crying that indicates the need for attention and nurturing, and a fussy type of crying that has no obvious cause. Most of the fussy crying takes place during the evening and at night. In some babies, nothing that the parents do seems to relieve it and, as time goes by, it seems to happen every day and with greater intensity. This extreme fussy crying period, which usually occurs during the evening and is cyclic in nature, is referred to as colic. Babies with colic can cry nonstop for hours and seem to be in severe pain. Babies with colic grow at the normal rate and are in good health; most outgrow it by three months.

The cause for colic is not known. It can be seen in breastfed and formula-fed babies alike. Some doctors believe that if a formula-fed baby develops colic, it may indicate a milk allergy. Unfortunately, changing formulas rarely solves the colic. Carrying the baby during the colic and keeping him or her in motion seems to provide temporary relief. A recently marketed device, which simulates the motion of a car ride, can be attached to the baby's crib. Medications, particularly antispasmodics, have no role in colic and may cause severe side effects in infants. Home remedies, such as anise, fennel, or other herbal teas, have been associated with serious side effects and are not recommended.

Excessive crying and colic in an infant creates tension in the family, generates feelings of parental inadequacy, and makes parents constantly worry about their infant's health. Parents should take turns in caring for the infant, or find a good sitter so that they can take some time out. They should understand that they are not responsible for the condition and, although it may be wearing on their nerves, the baby is healthy and thriving.

If the tone or pattern of the crying changes, or if the baby has fever or looks ill, the physician should be consulted, for not all unexplained crying is colic.

Bowel Habits and Constipation

What is "normal" in bowel function varies from baby to baby. Most newborns move their bowels several times a day; for others, especially breastfed infants, missing one to five days may be part of the normal pattern. In older children, as many as three movements a day, and as few as one in three days, can both be considered "normal." It is also normal for a child who has a fever to have fewer movements than usual. Thus, deciding whether or not a child is constipated has less to do with stool frequency than with consistency or with a child's problem within his or her own pattern.

The consistency of the stools varies according to the diet the baby is fed. Most breastfed babies have loose, unformed, yellow to brownish-green stools, with pea-soup consistency, whereas formula-fed babies have yellow, firmer, and more formed bowel movements. A common myth is that iron-containing formulas cause constipation. In a controlled study, a group of infants was fed from birth formula containing iron while another group was fed the same formula without iron. The mothers, who were not told in advance whether the formula they fed their infants contained iron or not, reported no differences in bowel movements or type of gastrointestinal problems among their infants.

Another common myth is that straining in small infants is due to constipation. Newborns and very small infants often grunt and turn red in the face, and at times this accompanies bowel movements. This apparent straining is normal and should not be cause for concern.

A very young infant who passes hard stools may be given half an ounce of prune juice with half an ounce of water. If a young infant does not pass a stool for seven or more days, or if the stools alternate between hard and loose, the physician should be informed. The possible causes for the problem include a tight anal sphincter and aganglionic megacolon (Hirschprung's disease), a condition in which the rectum lacks adequate innervation and is not able to push the stools effectively. In order to rule out such conditions, the physician will examine the baby and occasionally will have to perform a rectal examination in addition to other tests.

Constipation in the older infant is characterized by passing hard and large stools, occasionally with blood. The blood in the stool comes from a tiny tear (fissure) in the anus, the result of passing a large hard stool that distends the rectum and anus excessively. Most cases of constipation can be handled by modifying the diet. The amount of fiber in the diet can be increased with cereals, vegetables, fruits, and stewed dried fruits. Limiting the amount of milk to a maximum of a quart a day will ensure a reasonable appetite for a more varied and balanced diet. Suppositories, enemas, and laxatives should only be used following a physician's advice.

Diarrhea

Frequent bowel movements are normal for many infants; some babies move their bowels after every feeding. Loose bowel movements may also be normal; breastfed infants tend to have looser stools than those of babies on formula. This normal looseness should be distinguished from diarrhea, in which the stools are very frequent and very watery, leaving a water ring on the diaper.

Like fever or vomiting, diarrhea is a symptom of an illness or disorder, not a disease in itself. The most common cause of diarrhea in infants in the United States is an infection of the gastrointestinal tract. Babies have fever and vomiting for one or two days, then develop frequent loose bowel movements. Most cases of diarrhea resolve on their own within five to ten days. In general, antibiotics and other "antidiarrheal" medications are not beneficial and are not recommended routinely.

The most common cause of gastroenteritis is a viral infection. Less frequently, diarrhea is caused by bacterial or parasitic infections. If the physician

suspects the presence of these infections—for example, if the bowel movements have blood or mucus in them—tests of the stools may be ordered.

The most common danger with diarrhea is dehydration, which is more likely to occur if fever and vomiting are present. Parents should be alert to signs of dehydration, such as decreased urination, dry mouth, lack of tears, and sunken eyes. Although most mild cases of diarrhea can be successfully treated by the parents at home, the physician should be called if the infant looks ill or dehydrated, or is less than three months of age.

Mild cases of diarrhea can be overcome with minor changes in the baby's diet. Breastfeeding should not be stopped, for it is usually well tolerated. Formula can be diluted with water to half strength for one or two days. This means adding a can of water to the ready-to-feed formula or three cans of water to the concentrated one.

If a baby develops a severe case of diarrhea or vomits frequently, it is advisable to stop all milk except breastmilk and to give an oral solution such as Lytren or Pedialyte, which come in ready-to-use bottles and can be purchased in drugstores. The oral solution can be given for up to 6 to 12 hours, when normal feeding should be gradually resumed.

Although acceptable for older children, juices are not recommended for infants with vomiting and diarrhea, for the high sugar content worsens the symptoms. The baby should be offered small but frequent amounts of the oral solution. If vomiting persists, using a spoon or a dropper, instead of a nipple, usually helps.

Feeding will increase the volume of stools, but withholding of milk and food deprives the baby of adequate nutrition. More emphasis should be placed on the overall well-being of the infant than on the stools themselves. Inadequate nutrition may lead to small, frequent, greenish, mucous "starvation stools" which resolve when the baby is put back on a regular diet.

Diarrhea that persists may be due to lactose intolerance, the temporary inability to digest the predominant sugar in the milk. When this is suspected, the physician may switch the baby to a soy-based or lactose-free formula. Other causes of persistent diarrhea include milk allergy and rare conditions that cause poor absorption of the nutrients in the gastrointestinal tract, among them cystic fibrosis, AIDS, and celiac disease (see chapter 23, Gastrointestinal Disorders).

Spitting-up and Vomiting

It is common for babies to spit up after feeding. Until about the sixth month of life, the entrance to the stomach is not tight enough to keep all the contents down, so some milk will head back up and spill out of the baby's mouth. This is called *gastroesophageal reflux* and is the most common cause of spitting up. If the baby grows normally despite frequent spitting up there probably is no cause for alarm.

Vomiting, on the other hand, is a symptom of many conditions, both trivial and severe. For example, two- or three-week-old babies who vomit forcefully and fail to put on weight should be brought to the attention of the physician, for they may have a pyloric stenosis. This condition involves a narrowing of the muscular valve at the stomach outlet and must be corrected surgically.

Sudden onset of vomiting may indicate gastroenteritis, an intestinal infection commonly caused by viruses. In this case, the vomiting is usually followed by diarrhea. The major risk of vomiting and diarrhea is dehydration due to loss of body fluids. (Dehydration is discussed under Diarrhea in this chapter.)

Less frequently, sudden onset of vomiting may be due to intussusception, a type of intestinal obstruction seen in babies. When there is obstruction, the vomit may look greenish and the abdomen may appear bloated and be painful when touched. These symptoms should be reported to the physician at once. Other causes of vomiting include food allergies, infections, chronic diseases of the liver and kidney, and some rare genetic conditions.

As a general rule, if the baby vomits and does not look right, the physician should be contacted.

Failure to Thrive

Failure to gain weight or height raises the question of whether the baby is "failing to thrive." Some infants, of course, are shorter and lighter than others of the same age, but if their growth is steady, there is generally no cause for concern. To determine whether a child is failing to thrive, it is necessary to review the measurements of height and weight over a period of weeks or months.

Failure to thrive during the first year of life is almost always related to inadequate nutrition. In affluent societies, this generally reflects a feeding problem of some kind, rather than actual scarcity. Occasionally errors are made in the preparation of the formula, such as diluting it too much. A baby who sleeps a lot and never cries might be fed less than needed because the parents are hesitant to awaken him or her. Other times parents who are overly concerned about obesity feed their babies less than needed to sustain growth.

An infant's emotional environment may also have a role in the lack of normal growth. If a mother is depressed, overwhelmed by work or personal problems, she may unknowingly neglect the baby emotionally and nutritionally. Sometimes there is a failure in communication: the baby is difficult and demanding and the parents cannot interpret the cues. Studies have shown that babies who receive little stimulation or nurturing become withdrawn and irritable and seem to lose interest in feeding.

Emotional deprivation leading to nutritional neglect accounts for about half the cases of failure to thrive in infancy. The diagnosis may be elusive, for most parents are usually not aware of the impact their own problems have on their young infants. On occasions, the diagnosis only becomes apparent after the infant is hospitalized and adequate growth is observed away from the home.

Less commonly, failure to thrive is associated with disease. Infants who have difficulty in sucking and are slow in their development might have disorders of the central nervous system. Babies who vomit a large amount after every feeding might have severe gastroesophageal reflux (see immediately preceding section on vomiting). Malabsorption problems, in which nutrients are not properly digested, are a further nutritional cause of failure to thrive. Chronic disorders of the heart, kidneys, lungs, and endocrine system may also be responsible for retarded growth.

Fever

The human body controls its temperature very carefully by means of an internal thermostat. Normal body temperature for children and adults ranges from 97 in the early morning to 100.4 degrees Fahrenheit in the evening. (See box, next page, on taking the baby's temperature.) Activity makes the temperature go up, and the body lowers it by sweating and making the skin turn warm in order to release heat by radiation. When exposed to a cold environment, the body keeps its internal temperature steady by cooling the skin and shivering, which makes the muscles generate heat. The presence of fever means that the body's thermostat has raised its temperature to a higher point than normal. Left alone, a fever will go as high as the thermostat meant it to go and not higher.

Heat stroke refers to a condition in which the body looses its tight control mechanisms and the temperature goes to 107 degrees F. or more. These extreme fevers may develop under special circumstances and are usually associated with dehydration. Heat stroke may be seen in a child whose brain does not regulate temperature or thirst well, or in a baby who is left in a closed car in the sun.

Fever is a symptom and can be seen in a large

TAKING THE BABY'S TEMPERATURE

The easiest way to take a baby's exact temperature is the axillary method (under the arm), using an oral or rectal thermometer. First the thermometer should be shaken down so that the mercury is well below the normal mark (by holding the thermometer at the high temperature end and snapping the wrist—best done over a soft surface such as a bed). The thermometer is then placed snugly in the baby's armpit for four minutes. Axillary temperature is usually one degree lower than rectal temperature. To measure the latter, dab the thermometer bulb with petroleum jelly and hold the baby face down across the lap with legs dangling. Insert the thermometer into the rectum about an inch, holding it between the fingers. Forcing the thermometer in may seriously injure the baby. Hold the thermometer in place for three minutes.

number of illnesses, such as infections caused by virus or bacteria, allergic reactions, or following vaccinations. There is no scientific proof that teething can cause fever. Often the fever is followed by a runny nose, cough, or diarrhea. When fever is the only symptom in a baby over three months who looks well, the parent may want to wait 24 hours before calling the physician, for the fever may just resolve itself. Even if it persists, the chances of making a diagnosis, for example an ear or throat infection, will be better after 24 hours. A physician should be called if the baby is less than three months of age, looks ill, or has any other disturbing symptoms, such as trouble breathing, a rash, or severe diarrhea.

Parents are always concerned about the risk of febrile seizures. Convulsions caused by fever are infrequent—only 4 out of 100 children will ever have one. Most of the time the seizure is the first indication that the baby has a fever. The height of the fever is not a crucial factor in the development of a convulsion, for it may occur when the fever is 102 degrees F. or less. Although they are frightening, in most cases febrile seizures are not known to cause brain damage. (For more information, see chapter 28, Neurological and Neuromuscular Disorders.)

In managing fever at home parents should follow the general principle of making the baby as comfortable as possible. Most babies seem to tolerate fever better than adults; in fact, fever in itself may be a healthy reaction of the body and helps fight infections. Medication usually is not necessary for a fever of less than 104 degrees F. unless the baby is uncomfortable or a physician advises it. If treatment is given, acetaminophen is preferable to aspirin, which has been linked to Reye's syndrome (see the section on Reye's syndrome, chapter 20). Although this disease is unlikely during the first year, it is prudent to avoid giving aspirin to young children.

If acetaminophen is given, it should bring the temperature down a degree an hour. A baby that seems cold should be wrapped and should not be given a cool bath at this point, for it will only cause discomfort and shivering. On the other hand, a baby who is hot, which indicates that the body is lowering the body temperature, should be undressed. Lukewarm baths at this point may be soothing. Bathing and sponging by themselves do not affect internal temperature very much. Sponging with alcohol may be dangerous, for it is absorbed through the skin and can poison the baby. Fluids should be offered frequently to prevent dehydration. Because the appetite might be decreased, the baby should not be forced to eat. With fever the bowel movements are less frequent, and this should not be confused with constipation.

Teeth and Teething

Although occasionally a baby is born with one tooth or more, the vast majority of infants cut their first tooth between the ages of five and nine months. The first teeth to appear are the lower central front teeth, followed in order by the upper central front teeth, the upper lateral and the lower lateral. By the time they reach their first birthday, most babies have six to eight teeth. In the second year, the first molars and the canines (pointed teeth) appear. The last four teeth, the second molars, usually come out by the first half of the third year. The permanent teeth begin appearing at six or seven years of age.

The age of teething is quite unpredictable. Teething early or late in life bears no correlation with growth or intelligence. Parents should not be concerned if their healthy infant has as few as two teeth at one year.

When the teeth cut the gum, occasional mild swelling and discomfort may result. Although crankiness and drooling might be evident, teething is a painless event in most babies. The belief that teething is the reason for most of the problems in babies has no scientific basis. Because six to eight baby teeth appear in the first year of life and close to twenty erupt by age two and a half, it is understandable that teething is blamed for almost anything that upsets the baby. The mouthing and drooling that starts at two months of age is normal and should not be attributed to teething, which rarely occurs at this age. Older infants may wake up and cry at night due to separation anxiety; teething should not be the scapegoat for this common problem. Likewise, fevers, colds, and diarrhea blamed on teething are caused by viruses and microbes.

In order to determine if teething is causing pain a parent can look at the baby's gum. If the color is pink and the ridge is sharp and does not hurt when touched, then teething is not the answer to any of the baby's problems. In contrast, if the gum appears swollen, bluish, or tender when touched with a finger, then teething is causing symptoms. Acetaminophen can be given to relieve the pain and the infant allowed to chew and suck. Frozen bagels or teether rings can also soothe temporarily. Teething medications containing local anesthetics are not recommended, for even in small amounts they can be toxic and cause seizures. Home remedies such as honey do not alleviate pain and may promote tooth decay. Honey should not be given to infants in any case, as there is a danger of botulism contamination in those under one year of age.

Once the teeth have erupted it is the responsibility of the parent to keep them healthy. At least once a day the teeth of a young infant should be cleaned with a washcloth. As soon as more teeth erupt, usually in the second year, a soft small toothbrush can be used. By establishing a daily routine, parents will be guiding the child toward a lifetime hygienic habit that will reduce plaque and tooth decay.

Also paramount to the prevention of tooth decay is fluoride. Studies have shown that fluoride given from early infancy helps make teeth (including the permanent teeth) stronger and less prone to decay. The easiest way to give babies fluoride is by giving them water if they live in communities where water has been fluoridated. Otherwise parents may want to check with their pediatrician about obtaining a prescription for fluoride drops.

Diet plays a major role in the health of the teeth. A particular problem of the young child is "nursing bottle caries." This particularly severe form of tooth decay affecting the upper front teeth is due to the practice of putting babies to sleep with a bottle of milk or juice. The sugar or starches in the bottle stimulate the bacteria that destroy the enamel of the teeth. The cavities are usually seen after the first year of age, but the process leading to teeth destruction starts in early infancy. Pacifiers dipped in honey or other sweets can also lead to the same problem.

Colds

Frequent colds are very common during the first year of life. They are usually mild and start with a low fever, followed by sneezing and a stuffy nose. There might be a cough, which sometimes is accompanied by wheezing, in which case it is called bronchiolitis. Colds can have complications such as pneumonia. If a baby with a cold looks ill, has a high fever (above 103 degrees F.), wheezing, a deep cough, trouble breathing, or an earache, the physician should be called.

A large number of viruses can cause colds. The body's response to any of them provides only a short-lived immunity, so a cold may be due to a new virus or to one that infected the system only months ago. The popular belief that chilling predisposes to colds has no scientific basis.

It is extremely hard to prevent exposure to cold viruses. The viruses causing colds are transmitted from person to person. The more people the baby is exposed to, the more likely it is for the baby to get a cold. This is why when children start daycare or nursery school they invariably start getting one cold after another.

Most colds are mild and can be easily handled at home. Stuffy noses are particularly bothersome to young babies because they have difficulty breathing through the mouth, and they get frantic when they have to nurse or suck. To relieve the bothersome stuffy nose, apply saline drops in the nose and then suck the mucus out with a nose bulb or syringe. A cold-water humidifier might help by keeping the air moist in the baby's environment. Most pediatricians do not recommend decongestants and nosedrops with medicine for babies under one year. Because colds are caused by viruses, not bacteria, antibiotics do not change the course of a common cold, although they are usually needed in the case of complications.

If there is fever and discomfort, acetaminophen can be given. Fluids should be offered frequently, and parents should try to make the baby as comfortable as possible. There is no benefit to overdressing or sweating. The infant should be bathed as usual, for baths can be soothing.

Ear Infections

Otitis media, or inflammation of the middle ear, is a very common illness among infants. Half of all children will suffer at least one ear infection before their first birthday. This high incidence is due to the fact that in children the eustachian tube, which connects the middle ear to the throat, is less rigid than in adults and therefore collapses frequently, preventing adequate ventilation and drainage of the middle ear. The middle ear, which lies behind the eardrum and contains three bones that transmit sound vibrations to the inner ear, becomes a closed chamber, trapping fluid that can easily become infected.

Otitis media usually follows a cold. An infant with otitis media may be feverish, crying, or just cranky. Sometimes the pressure in the middle ear breaks the eardrum and a yellowish discharge (pus) will be seen in the ear canal. The physician should be called when an ear infection is suspected. Using an otoscope, a thin tube with a magnifying lens and a light, the physician will see a red swollen eardrum. If there is a discharge, the eardrum will have a tear.

Ear infections are treated with antibiotics. In case of pain, acetaminophen may be given. If the condition fails to improve within 48 hours, the physician may recommend a change in antibiotic. Following an episode of otitis media, fluid in the middle ear may persist for several weeks, but it usually clears up by itself.

The major problem with ear infections, aside from the discomfort they cause, is that they may temporarily impair hearing. As soon as the fluid resolves, the hearing returns to normal. When fluid persists behind the eardrum for more than three months, it is advisable to check the hearing. If the hearing is decreased, the ear specialist might drain the fluid or insert little tubes in the eardrum to prevent the buildup of fluid. Babies who have recurrent otitis media may be given a low dose of antibiotics daily to try to prevent further infections. (For more information see chapter 26, Eyes, Ears, Nose, and Throat.)

Eye Problems

Many babies develop inflammation and discharge in the eyes during the first month of life, a condition called pink eye or conjunctivitis. In the very young infant, pink eye is frequently due to germs contracted in the birth canal. Pink eye in the older infant usually comes with a cold or an ear infection. All cases of conjunctivitis should be brought to the attention of the physician. Eyedrops may be all that is needed, but sometimes antibiotics will be prescribed.

Sometimes a baby seems to have a recurring case of pink eye. The eyes tear easily and the eyelids are stuck when the baby wakes up. This kind of lingering eye infection is due to obstruction of the tear ducts, tubes that drain the tears from the eyes into the nose. This condition is frequently outgrown. If it has not resolved by one year of age, the tear duct may have to be probed by an eye specialist in order to unplug it.

Strabismus, or crossed eyes, is another common concern of parents. It is normal for a baby's eyes to turn in or out temporarily in the early months of life. However, if the baby appears to have crossed eyes most of the time, or if the eyes are not steady by three months of age, the physician should be informed. Most cases of crossed eyes or wall-eyes are caused by imbalance in the eye muscles or by defective vision in one eye. If the baby gets accustomed to using only one eye, the brain can lose the ability to receive signals from the other eye. To force the baby to develop vision in the weak eye, a patch may be all that is necessary. Left untreated, the condition may require surgery or may be permanently disabling. (For more information, see chapter 26, Eyes, Ears, Nose, and Throat.)

Sudden Infant Death Syndrome (SIDS)

SIDS or "crib death" remains the leading cause of death for infants between one month and one year of age in the United States, accounting for one-third of all deaths in this age group. Nevertheless, although it is devastating to parents, SIDS is not as common as it would seem from the attention it has gotten.

SIDS usually affects babies between two and four months of age and rarely occurs after the age of six months. Typically a baby seems well, has no cold or other infection, is put to bed in the usual way, and the next time he or she is checked, is found dead.

The risk for SIDS is higher among certain groups, such as premature babies, infants with a low birthweight, and infants of adolescent mothers, among others. The risk is also increased among infants who suffer a severe life-threatening event: the baby may turn limp, dusky, stop breathing, or choke and require resuscitation.

The cause of this fatal disorder remains unknown and doctors are not even sure whether it is caused by one or many diseases. Home monitors to keep track of an infant's breathing are available, but their value is questionable at this time.

Parents are understandably distraught by a crib death. They may blame themselves, although no one can predict or prevent SIDS, and they may become overprotective of their other children. It is strongly recommended that parents who have lost a child to SIDS contact the National Foundation for Sudden Infant Death Syndrome, or one of its chapters, to get in touch with a parents' support group.

TRAVELING WITH THE BABY

TRAVELING WITH A BABY can be a pleasant experience for the family, as long as the baby is in good health and parents are adequately prepared for it. The first rule to follow is to get things organized beforehand. This applies to short outings to the doctor, for example, as well as to long trips. The following suggestions are meant to aid parents in organizing travel.

Health.   When parents plan an extended trip or a trip to a foreign country, it is advisable to check with the baby's physician first. A checkup and immunization update might help allay any anxiety. If the baby has any particular health problem, parents should ask the doctor to write a brief summary, which should be carried with them at all times. This will be of great help in the event the baby requires emergency medical care. In addition, the doctor may have advice regarding special immunizations or safety precautions needed for the travel destination. The local health department can be another useful source of information.

Clothing.   Parents should try to keep things simple from the start. Clothing should be easily washable and comfortable for the baby (such as stretch overalls, rather than clothes with elastic waistbands). Babies not only get annoyed at prolonged dressing sessions, but bulky or stiff clothes make them uncomfortable. Disposable diapers and wipes are convenient and should be packed along with plastic bags for the dirty diapers.

Feeding.   Breastfeeding is the safest and most convenient way to feed an infant during travel. If the infant is formula-fed, disposable bottles of ready-to-use formula are a safer and less messy choice than carrying home-prepared bottles for the trip. Warming the milk should not be a concern, for babies can be given room-temperature milk at all ages without ill effects. Bacteria can overgrow rapidly in milk or food, and as a general rule, whether traveling or at home, parents should refrain from prolonged feeding and should discard the milk or food an hour after the feeding starts. If the family is traveling to a foreign place where the safety of the water is questionable, it is advisable to refrain from using any water in the formula or the food for the baby, unless it is adequately sterilized. In such places, older infants should be given only commercial ready-to-feed baby food in addition to the formula, and spared from any table food.

Safety.   If traveling by car, the baby should ride in an infant car seat at all times. (On plane/car trips, car seats can be checked as baggage on the flight or rented with the car.) Most babies enjoy car rides and sleep comfortably. But parents should be realistic in their expectations. They may have to stop frequently and adjust the length of the trip to the baby's needs. If traveling on a warm day, parents should make sure to offer the baby plenty of fluids.

When planning an airplane trip with the baby, parents should try to get to the airport early. Parents with infants are generally allowed to board first. Most infants tolerate air travel well. Some doctors recommend withholding feeding or pacifiers on ascent because the air swallowed with the sucking will expand at higher altitude and might cause abdominal discomfort. Although it is a rare occurrence, if the baby has an ear infection, the eardrum may burst due to the increased pressure and a discharge will be seen in the ear canal. A plane flight may also set the stage for ear infections in babies who are prone to them. Nursing, bottle-feeding, or sucking a pacifier during the plane's descent appears to be beneficial in preventing ear pain.

9 The One-Year-Old

Harriet McGurk, M.D.

INTRODUCTION

THE SECOND YEAR is an exciting time for children and their parents. In a few short months, babies consolidate all they have learned in the preceding year, and then fling themselves into the toddler stage. Toddlers feel an urgent need to begin separating from their parents and asserting themselves as autonomous individuals. They push limits to define boundaries.

Thrilling advances in independence are interspersed with periods of anxiety and clinging, which can be puzzling for parents. Toddlers are growing up so fast that sometimes they seem to scare themselves.

The enthusiasm they bring to learning to walk is an example of the intensity of feeling that characterizes children at this age. The child's emotions are contagious and parents are caught up by their child's elation. When the child learns to walk, the parents' pride and pleasure makes up for the tinge of sadness they feel that they're no longer quite so needed in the physical sense. Later, when the 18-month-old worries about having gotten too far away and comes back to be held, only to squirm away when the parent tries to oblige, the parent may understandably feel confused, hurt, and angry. Antici-

pating these mood swings may help a parent keep his or her equilibrium, step back and decide when it is necessary to be rational, and remember the responsibility that comes with being the older and larger member of this dyad.

The job of parenting a one-year-old is different from and much more complex than the role parents worked so hard to master when they had an infant to care for. Before, they had to learn to anticipate, interpret, and respond to the primarily physical needs of a totally dependent little being. Now they are pushed into a greater awareness of who this little person *is*—not just a baby to hold and feed and play with, though this aspect remains important. Instead there is a real, increasingly separate person, determined to teach them more than they really wanted to know about basic human psychology, not just his own, but theirs as well.

The forces of nature driving the toddler's development sweep away many of the parents' ideas about propriety, privacy, and control. At times the child's struggle to mature becomes a struggle with parents, painful for both sides. Yet the rewards are great, for in the process of becoming themselves, children find and affirm their parents' selves.

In 12 months the child moves from a tottering, uncertain walk to a rather confident run; from a smattering of a few barely recognizable words and syllables to a vocabulary in the hundreds, often arranged into short telegraphic sentences; from self-centered, need-driven behavior to the beginnings of self-control; and from rudimentary thought processes to the start of true problem-solving and thinking. And while this year is an exciting one for parents, for children, intrepid explorers venturing boldly into the unknown, it is thrilling beyond compare.

PHYSICAL GROWTH AND DEVELOPMENT

PHYSICAL GROWTH between 12 and 24 months is much less dramatic than it was in the first year. The average child will grow about six inches and will only gain five or six pounds. Slower growth means fewer calories are needed, so appetite usually diminishes. In contrast, the child's increased mobility will mean a greater expenditure of calories for energy. The typical early toddler has a taller, slimmer, less babyish body and an indifference to food that results, not only from slower growth, but also from distraction by all the interesting things he or she would rather do. The head continues to be large in proportion to the body; by the end of the year, it will have reached almost 90 percent of its adult size.

Toddlers have a pronounced forward curvature in the spine (lordosis), creating a pot-bellied appearance that does not result from being fat. While any concerns about the child's spine should be brought to the attention of the pediatrician, forward curvature at this age is a normal part of the skeleton's growth.

Teething continues in the second year as 8 to 12 more teeth erupt, including the deciduous molars and the cuspids, bringing the total to between 16 and 20. There is no set order for the eruption of the teeth. While the molars are often last, in some children they may come before the cuspids. (See chapter 33, Childhood Dentistry.)

Motor Skills

The gross motor skills are those that involve the large muscles of the body, coordinating the arms and legs for such activities as crawling, creeping, walking, carrying, throwing, and kicking. Fine motor skills involve the use of the hands and fingers for the manipulation of small objects.

Gross motor development. During the first three or four months of the second year, most of the child's time will be spent practicing and mastering all the activities involved in moving around. Not only does the toddler exult in the pure joy of being able to move about, but these skills provide access to the strange and intriguing world that has so far been out of reach.

By the end of the first year, most children are adept at pulling themselves to a standing position and, holding onto successive pieces of furniture, have begun "cruising" the living room. Those who have not already progressed from there to the first tentative, unaided walking steps will generally do so now, by age 13 or 14 months. In the beginning, a child's walking form is unsteady, the legs far apart and the gait uneven. Mastery of walking depends not so much on practice but on how the neurological system matures. Early on, children find that carrying something helps them walk better by giving the arms something to do and helping to maintain balance. Later in the year, with an increasing confidence in walking, they will love pushing a cart or dragging a pull-toy behind them.

By their second birthday, toddlers will be walking with ease and will have progressed to exploring every known form of locomotion except skipping. They will run, trot, hop, jump, climb, and generally propel themselves forward, backward, up and down stairs and into every imaginable place. At first they will have little control running and some trouble stopping.

Play activities change as children's motor skills improve. At first they throw a ball with a simple underhand toss, soon progressing to overhand, using the whole arm. Eventually they are able to toss a ball into a basket on the floor with reasonable accuracy. At the first try at kicking a ball the child will often miss it or step on it and fall down. Later, he or she will be able to kick without falling and even have some control over direction.

Because all kinds of exploring become a passion during this year, safety precautions are crucial. Better-developed motor skills and increased problem-solving capacities allow the child to reach previously unreachable heights—kitchen counters, desktops, cabinets, and cupboards—and to explore the potentially dangerous contents of these places. As with most activities, the toddler's physical skill develops before judgment and attention to danger mature. Most accidents result not from lack of skill, but from poor planning, e.g., when toddlers use an object with wheels to climb on, or forget they are on the stairs when they decide to go to the next room. Parents who haven't already childproofed the house should do so now, and those who have should reassess their efforts in light of the child's new capabilities (see chapter 14, Ensuring Your Child's Safety).

Also, a child who can scale a sofa is likely to climb out of a crib, so it may be time to consider a junior bed with removable sides.

Stairs are a great attraction now and will take the better part of the year to conquer. After the first few exploratory encounters, the child will start practicing climbing up, one step at a time, and coming down on the buttocks. By 24 months or so, most children will be able to climb up and down unaided, but generally should not be trusted alone on the stairs until sometime in the third year. Until then, safety gates (not the accordion kind) should be placed at the top and bottom of stairs to prevent falls. The one at the bottom can be put a few steps up the stairs so that the child can enjoy some climbing without real danger.

Fine motor development.   With an improved ability to focus vision, the child will show increasing interest in smaller objects and details. One-year-olds explore everything within their reach, often needing to feel a thing with their mouths as well as their hands. By 14 months, most will have mastered a pincer grasp with the thumb and forefinger to pick up everything they find. As the year progresses, they will be able to hold and manipulate increasingly more intricate objects. They will enjoy practicing their new dexterity on objects that stack, fit together and snap apart, and fit inside one another.

Favorite activities include stacking cubes or graduated rings, putting things into containers then dumping them out again, and working the action of any hinged object—a book, a cupboard door, or a trash-can lid, for example. By the end of the year, a child will easily use crayons to scribble and may be able to mimic an adult's drawing of a straight line or perhaps even to draw a crude circle. At the same time, the right or the left hand will usually become dominant.

A great deal of fine motor play involves handling things to learn about the physical qualities of objects—their weight, size, feel, bounce, texture—and their relationship in space to each other and to the child's body.

INTELLECTUAL DEVELOPMENT

Curiosity and Exploration

When Shakespeare wrote "the world's mine oyster" he might have been picturing the 12-month-old. Poised to embark on a surprisingly systematic exploration of that oyster, the toddler's mood is con-sistently one of eagerness and optimism. Once walking has been mastered, the child moves on to running and climbing, and seems to be everywhere at once. Now a simple walk in the park means at least one game of "catch me," a teetering walk on a low wall (holding a parent's hand), a chase after a falling leaf or a pigeon, an attempt to scale the playground slide from the bottom, and a roundtrip at a run in the amount of time it takes the parent to walk once—all accompanied by squeals of delight. The toddler's exhaustion by bedtime pales in comparison to the parents'!

When toddlers aren't exploring with their feet, they do so with their eyes, hands, and mouth. Each new object they encounter will be scrutinized, then tested. Thorough testing determines each of the object's properties and functions (including some never considered by an adult). Thus, everything needs to be opened, closed, dropped, banged, poked, prodded, turned, twisted, knocked over, squeezed, rattled, and tasted, especially tasted. Because everything will be mouthed, if not chewed, parents should try to keep the child's hands and toys reasonably clean, and, as much as they can, suspend for a time their concern about germs and dirt. (The child may also mouth things to relieve the tenderness of teething, but that mouthing is not accompanied by the same delight as exploratory mouthing.)

Parents can facilitate this exploration by providing an environment that is safe—free of items that can hurt the child; childproof—free of items the child can hurt; and child-oriented—stocked with items of different shapes, colors, and textures that stimulate the senses and invite observation and testing.

Over the course of this year, the toddler will spend less and less time exploring and more and more time mastering whatever objects are encountered. For this reason it is important that parents continue to broaden the child's horizons—by trips to the grocery store, the park, the zoo, other people's homes—and, as fine motor skills develop, by giving the child new and more complex objects—especially things the parents themselves use—to explore and master. (For other suggestions, see the section on play below.)

Play as a Learning Experience

Although *play* is the word used to describe much of the activity of children, it has the wrong connotation. To an adult, "play" signifies that which is *not* work; to a one-year-old, however, play *is* work. Play is the practicing and perfecting of new skills and concepts. It is the child's version of thinking out loud. Much of a child's solitary play at this age involves experimenting with the laws of physics—practicing with objects, learning about his or her own body in space, or observing the results when objects are dropped, filled, or dumped.

Toddlers love to be busy, stirring and mixing, banging pots and pans, sweeping, hammering, giving bottles to dollies, pretending to talk on the telephone or drive the car. These activities are much more than simple fun and frolic for a child this age. Indeed, the child observed during play often appears very serious about what he or she is doing. This is how children learn about the world and their role in it.

Interactive playtime for a child is not limited to periods when parent and child sit and roll a ball back and forth, but happens all through the day. Cooking, shopping, and cleaning all provide opportunities for constructive play with a child, if the parent has the time and patience. Although toddlers can play alone for longer periods, they need interaction with an interested adult.

Often the most valuable play takes place in the kitchen. With the company of an adult doing household chores, most toddlers are delighted to tag along and make their own games. Given a few plastic containers of graduated sizes, wooden spoons, and a bowl, they are content to watch a parent cook and clean. They love to be in and out of the cupboards, to imitate the parents' activities, and, increasingly as the year goes on, they want to "help."

Imitation of parents extends to appearance, and toddlers enjoy dressing up like Mommy and Daddy. They can amuse themselves endlessly with a few old hats, shoes, aprons, neckties, scarves, and handbags, especially if they have an appreciative audience.

Toys. Many of the best toys are, like those items mentioned above, not really toys. Household and natural objects that can be used again and again in various play situations help stimulate creativity; toys with elaborate detail that can only be used in one way tend to be ignored. Children enjoy manufactured toys as well. The best ones are *simple* (a one-year-old doesn't care if the toy phone has a dial on it), *sturdy* (the child will be brutal), and *safe*.

Favorite toys for this age are toy telephones, a pretend car dashboard with steering wheel, balls of various sizes, straddle toys (wheeled vehicles or animals without pedals), blocks, push toys (shopping carts, lawn mowers, and baby carriages), pull toys (animals, wagons, wooden trains), dolls, and stuffed animals. Board books with their thick, stiff cardboard pages, are enjoyed by one-year-olds, who like to handle the books themselves and who should by this age have some quiet time looking at books with an adult. Toy banks (with coins too large to swallow)

and plastic containers that the child can stack or put things in are also popular.

At this age, children particularly enjoy lightweight toys that are overscale or large compared to themselves, but still easy to handle and carry. Examples are inflated plastic animals, big cardboard-brick blocks, and balloons. (Parents should be sure that when a balloon breaks, all the pieces are picked up and disposed of immediately, as they are a choking hazard.)

In the second half of the year, when mud pies hold universal fascination, their indoor equivalent—play dough—is a useful plaything that is relatively inexpensive to buy or easily made at home.

Complicated toys, with parts to piece together, or wind-ups such as jack-in-the-boxes, are generally beyond the scope of children this age. Most parents, eager for the child to enjoy what they consider a wonderful new toy, have experienced the disappointment of seeing the gift ignored while the child plays happily with the box and wrappings.

Toys to avoid include any with rough surfaces or sharp edges and toys that may expose such dangers once broken, as well as toys with parts that can be broken or bitten off. Since toys will invariably go in the mouth, any toy or toy part of less than 1½ inches in diameter poses a potential danger. Imported painted folk toys can be charming, but should be avoided until the child is not interested in chewing them, unless the parent can be sure that they have been painted with lead-free paint. (For more information, see chapter 14, Ensuring Your Child's Safety.)

Water and sand seem to hold universal attraction for children as early as 12 months. They will want to splash in any water they see—whether it's in a bathtub, toilet bowl, pool, puddle, or lake (which can pose safety problems and is yet another reason why children must be closely supervised at all times). Small plastic or rubber bathtub toys, especially ones that hold water, and the same set of graduated plastic containers they use in the kitchen will keep them happily occupied at bath time. In warmer months, water play can move outdoors with a sprinkler or small wading pool. A second wading pool makes an inexpensive sandbox (which should be covered when not in use to keep neighborhood cats from finding a use for it).

Books. One of the most pleasant things parents can do for their children, not only for their intellectual growth but for lifelong pleasure, is to introduce them early to books. As early as the first year, children profit enormously from hearing nursery rhymes and songs and being read to from simple books with big, clear pictures. By 12 months many will enjoy naming animals and other items in books and will soon develop favorites among their books that they want to read again and again.

Board books with simple pictures on thick pages are good beginning books for children. These books should not be costly, as one-year-olds can be quite destructive in their eagerness to explore. They will also enjoy tactile books such as *Pat the Bunny*, books with rhyming or repeating words such as *Goodnight, Moon*, and books with visual surprises like the fold-out pages of *Feed the Animals* or *Is Anybody Home?*

Parents should reserve some skepticism for the recent wave of didactic books for babies. These are obviously designed to teach a simple concept, one per book. The many good ones (e.g., the "Sesame Street" books) are simple and fun. The appeal of the characters and the sense of humor have their own value. Others, less skillfully done, are often boring or condescending.

The best books for children are still stories with layers of meaning that sustain them through many readings. Classics of children's literature have a connection to their culture and a sense of poetry. A good story develops a child's sense of anticipation and stimulates the imagination.

Thought

Developmental psychologists have proffered a number of theories to explain cognitive learning in children. Although they may not agree on how children acquire knowledge or intelligence, they agree that learning follows a specific pattern. Children may develop at different rates, but they pass through the same developmental stages in the same order, even across cultures.

Some of the most widely recognized theories of cognitive development are those of an early pioneer in the field, Swiss psychologist Jean Piaget. By closely observing his own three children as they grew up, he discovered much about how humans begin to think.

Piaget observed that if a toy is taken away from a child under eight months of age, who is then distracted for a few moments, he or she does not try to get it back. After observing a variety of experimental situations, he concluded that this happens because when the toy is out of sight, its existence is forgotten. But toward the end of the first year, the child develops the ability to hold an image or pattern in mind after the object (or person) disappears from view, a concept Piaget termed "object permanence."

As this concept is gradually refined during the second year, brief separations from the parent become easier to handle. Earlier, when the mother (or primary caretaker) left the room, the child had difficulty maintaining a clear image of her existing somewhere else. But as the child's ability to sustain a mental picture of her gradually matures, he will begin to feel more confident that when the mother goes away, she is somewhere else and will come back. For a toddler, this mental image is still quite fragile and cannot be sustained for more than a few hours under the best of circumstances. It is even less likely to allay separation anxiety during times of stress or illness. Playing peek-a-boo and going-away-and-returning games, and hiding things and finding them again, are part of this process, which will not be complete before the third birthday.

Piaget called the period from birth to 18 months the sensorimotor stage, when children's thoughts are not yet in words, but consist mainly of physical sensations, physical movement and observation of physical events and objects. These activities progress from primarily reflex actions of infants to trial-and-error to more systematic problem-solving.

During the second half of the year, one-year-olds are in transition between sensorimotor and symbolic thought. For example, a play block may represent a car. The most valuable symbols are the words toddlers use during this second year—mostly nouns, but enough verbs and adjectives to make meaningful, short sentences by the end of the year. Much of the talking toddlers do is really thinking out loud. Listening to them chatter to themselves, one can hear them develop reason. Symbols, especially words, give the toddler a powerful tool to expand the intellect. "Language" usually refers to what is said, but for the toddler, it is even more important as a tool for thinking.

Use of mental and verbal symbols begins to free the child from concrete objects and the present moment. This development allows the first stirrings of imagination, anticipation, and conversely, the ability to wait for short times. Children become more aware of cause and effect, and begin to solve problems by trying out solutions mentally rather than by acting them out physically. Now a child who wants to reach something on a high counter may well stop and consider more than one method of getting it down before selecting the one he or she hopes will work best. The problem is solved in the mind before the solution is acted out.

Language

The child's development of language is a remarkable and exciting process both to the child and the parents. For the child, it's part of the desire to join the world of his or her caregivers, to make sense of that world, and to voice feelings and wants. It is not merely an intellectual accomplishment, but a physical and a social and emotional one as well. Vocal exchange is an integral part of happy social and emotional interactions from the earliest months of life, leading naturally to the desire for language in order to imitate and communicate with others. In addition there is just the sheer need for self-expression—and a great joy in it—as any parent knows who has come upon a toddler happily babbling to himself.

In the first half of the second year, children become more attentive to language. They obey simple commands such as "Give me a kiss" and "Wave bye-bye." They will also be able to babble in sounds that are not yet words, but with intonations of a real conversation. They answer with baby talk when spoken to, and clearly grasp the idea of talking to communicate.

At about 18 months or so, the consuming passion of toddlers shifts from walking to talking. Their curiosity about language becomes focused; they will imitate words they are taught and repeat new words over and over. They will be fascinated by two people speaking, especially if the voices are animated.

The rate of language acquisition varies considerably among normal children and most dramatically so during the second year. While many children by two years of age speak in short sentences, some who are developing normally may have a more limited vocabulary. Inherent in the learning process is a child's ability to understand more than he or she can say. Children who babble for the pleasure of it, who vocalize when they mean to communicate, and who make sound effects are well on their way to speaking. A distinction should be made between language, the essential tool of the intellect, and clarity of speech, a more technical problem which calls for little or no attention during this year.

Parents who are attuned to their children communicate by gesture, expression, context, and so on. In a natural setting, such nonverbal communication may even be necessary for anyone to learn such a complex system as human language.

Children cannot be taught to speak, per se, but parents can create an atmosphere that encourages learning language. The best way to facilitate language development is by talking. For example, parents can simply name people and objects the child encounters in the course of the day, talk about what they and the child are doing, name body parts while they are dressing the child, point out sights on the way to playgroup, name items in the grocery cart, and so on. Most important, they can listen to the child and be responsive to the child's attempts to speak. This not only increases the child's opportunity to learn but creates an atmosphere in which language development is tied to social and emotional gratification.

It is a common misconception that a slow talker will catch up if he or she is among other children, and should be sent to nursery school. Actually, the opposite is probably true. Language is learned best from adults, not from other children, and can be expected to progress more rapidly in a setting where the child receives more exclusive attention from and has stronger emotional bonds with adults.

Toward the second birthday, a child's receptive vocabulary may include more than 300 words, and the speaking vocabulary may be well over 200. Nouns will make up the bulk of the vocabulary, but usually there will be enough verbs and adjectives to form sentences. Although most utterances will continue to be one-word summations (for example, "Bottle" means "Give me my bottle"), there is an ever-increasing use of the two-word sentence, in telegraphic form ("Want milk" or "Play ball") that will grow more elaborate through the end of the second year and into the third.

By the end of the second year, toddlers are ready to begin organizing a sense of time, to use words to remember and anticipate. Parents can help provide this structure verbally ("When we get to the park, we're going to see Patrick and Beatrix and their mother, Cynthia"). At bedtime, children love to help the parent recite a list of all the things they did that day, although they have little ability to remember which day was which. By no means should they be tested or pushed to produce an answer, or the fun and the benefit will be lost. In the same way children can understand a word before they can say it, they can follow an adult's thought before they can formulate it themselves, thus gradually learning to use language to help organize their perceptions and thoughts.

SOCIAL AND EMOTIONAL DEVELOPMENT

A MAJOR SOCIAL THEME during the second year is the start of a gradual evolution of the child's sense of himself as a person. This process depends a great deal upon the child's growing physical independence. Even more, it is intricately involved with the simultaneous process of beginning to separate emotionally from the mother, whom the child originally perceived as being a part of himself. The push and pull of the effort to begin separating will color the child's interactions with the parents throughout the year. The need to establish an individual identity and the fear of being held back or cut free too soon are expressed in the willfulness, negativism, clinging, and defiant independence that characterize the second half of the second year.

Play with Other Children

At this age, children still play with adults whenever possible, but are content to play by themselves for longer periods, as long as an adult is nearby. Even the most independent toddlers follow a pattern of exploring away from the parent, then returning periodically to check that he or she is still there, seemingly to confirm that his distance and independence have not endangered his security. If the adult shows interest or approval during these "refueling" visits by the toddler, the toddler is more likely to return to his play than if the adult is withdrawn or unavailable. In nursery school or playgroup situations, toddlers do feel a bond with the other children, and being among other children seems to expand their sense of who they are.

When two toddlers do play together, the play tends to be parallel. That is, they will both engage in the same or similar activity, and may sit near each other and be aware of each other's play, but they won't actually play together. Although there may be occasional interaction, it is not cooperation or collaboration.

Parents are often surprised at how aggressive children can be with their peers, hitting, pulling hair, grabbing toys away (regardless of who owns the toys). Although sharing can be enforced, the concept won't be internalized for at least another year. For this age child, duplicating toys or putting away the most popular ones will work better than trying to make them share.

Toddlers need adults nearby, at least intermittently involved, if they are to play safely with each other. It is probably a good idea to limit their play time with peers to an hour or two at a time unless it is their usual babysitting or daycare setting, where the familiar scene and routine make conflict less likely. If there is turmoil, an adult may enter the play and try to turn the game to a better course, or distract the combatants with other ideas or toys. Inevitably, however, no matter how hard one tries, there will be situations in which a cantankerous toddler will have to be physically removed.

Rapprochement

The joys of this age are many, but the important process of separation is never entirely smooth. The child makes forays into the world, then returns to the parent, only to leave again—in both the physical and emotional sense. The forays are fueled at first by the desire to practice locomotion, then by the opportunity for discovery. The child needs to share this excitement with the parents, and so the objects of discovery are brought back to them. The child takes pleasure in newfound freedom, but feels more anxious as he gains awareness of his mother as a person outside himself and of the reality of their separation. So periodically he returns to "refuel." The child may obtain this psychic nourishment by physically clinging to a parent until he or she feels ready to move on again or merely by making eye contact or hearing the parent's voice.

Psychoanalyst Margaret Mahler termed this ambivalent reapproach to the parent "rapprochement." Although it can be seen in varying degrees in a child aged anywhere from 15 to 24 months, it seems to reach a peak—called the "rapprochement crisis"—at about 18 months, when the conflicting demands for closeness and autonomy are most intense.

During this time, many of a child's favorite games consist of the compulsive repetition of certain simple acts. These cause such giddy laughter and are so insisted upon that it is obvious that they are serving some symbolic emotional function. For example, how many times past the fortieth or fiftieth in a day can the parent play "chase me, catch me, sweep me up, let me go" before realizing that child's excitement will never wane, and the need for this game must come from something more than a desire for attention or entertainment?

A classic example of the rapprochement crisis is the toddler who howls and wails if Mother leaves the room, then squirms out of the parent's arms when picked up. The child seems angry at the parent for being so needed. Some understanding of the process helps, but it is nevertheless an extremely trying period for parents, who are asked to help a clinging, whining child feel calm, confident, and beloved just when that child is the most unpleasant.

Separation anxiety may become particularly intense around 18 months. If the child is having difficulty at this stage, it is best to avoid leaving him if possible. It is common for parents returning from a day or more away to complain that after all that fuss, the child wasn't even glad to see them come home. This misunderstanding can be destructive. Actually, the toddler who turns his back and pretends not to notice when a parent returns is struggling with his anger and relief, and needs a little time to reorganize his feelings, which he has temporarily suppressed because they are too stormy for him to handle. Gradually the crisis subsides as the child matures and finds a comfortable distance from the parent, but the theme is repeated in different ways, for many years to come.

As the year progresses, certain objects associated with comfort may serve as symbolic substitutes for the mother. A security blanket or a favorite teddy bear may take on special importance. Pediatrician and psychoanalyst D. W. Winnicott describes this "transitional object" as an aid to the child in evoking the feeling of comfort and security that would in the past have required the mother's physical presence. The object serves not quite as a symbol, but as a magical talisman to protect the child in the transition from dependence to independence.

Negativism

As knowledge of the world grows, so do needs and desires. Physical mobility is the paradigm for independence, literally the ability to stand on one's own two feet. A sense of one's self as a separate person is the inevitable product of physical development. Any toddler who has mastered walking can figure out that it is possible to walk away. Scary as that is from the child's perspective, he or she can't resist trying it when someone calls. Exploring the limits and the bonds in relationships, trying to define one's self: this is the driving force of the period of negativism that is so prominent between 18 and 24 months.

When babies first begin walking, the happiness and excitement they feel at their liberation keep them delightfully cheerful. Their cheer is such a pleasure for the parents that they may fail to notice that the now constantly moving toddler is growing more oblivious to their wishes and increasingly intent upon his own investigations. Children at this age begin to lose tolerance for the constant interruptions and find that they must be quite firm with their parents if they are to stick to their agenda. They find it necessary to say *no* quite often, in some cases, almost constantly.

Whether the parents are strict or indulgent, the toddler will experience limits and frustrations. There are so many limits and so many daunting circumstances: small size, poor coordination, gravity, lack of language, the setting of the sun . . .

As the toddler's awareness of his or her small self in the world increases, relationships to other people develop in a similar way. Conflict is a kind of psychological exercise, defining who one is, what one can do, how effective are different strategies. It leads to a clearer sense of "you" and "I," which deepens the relationship with the parents.

At its peak, negativism is characterized by a child's across-the-board refusal to do just about anything the parents ask, especially if the child senses that they really want it done. In fact, the child often does just the opposite of what is asked. The refusal may be physical or verbal or both. At one-and-a-half, when toddlers are just finding that talking is the greatest thing since walking, their favorite word is "no." They will use it to answer every command, direction, or suggestion—even to refuse something they want to do.

Wise parents may find a way to acknowledge the "no" and then proceed without requiring a verbal agreement first. It is best to leave children room to give in without losing face. After all, they're just trying it out. They're not really dedicated to defeating parents personally. Especially to be avoided is a refusal to let toddlers change their minds ("I thought you didn't want to . . ."). In their sense of time, the "no" of five minutes ago is gone, and now is a new time. A child teased about changing his or her mind may be goaded into being more stubborn next time. This negative stage is trying for the child as well as the parent, and making decisions becomes hard for him. Even as he tries to push the parent away, he fears making them angry and losing their love.

Negativism becomes especially intense by the end of the year and may even lead to trying to hit a parent. The child should be prevented from doing so; otherwise his own anger seems too powerful and frightening. There should be a clear message that the parent can control him, and will help him control his destructive impulses when he is angry.

If a child plays happily with a babysitter or at nursery school and then has a tantrum soon after the parent gets home, it is not because the teacher or babysitter does a better job. It is more likely that the child, who had to be grown up and good all day, has been saving the explosion for the person he or she trusts most. With the parent, the child may relax, let go and act as babyish as he wanted to before, because he expects the parent to love him anyway and help him work things out.

Even the most patient parent will sometimes react with dismay, and often anger, at the provocative behavior of a toddler. Even if you could always keep your cool, never try to hurt the child back, and act as mature as you would like, it would be no help. Only with the full range of emotions can real intimacy develop. The toddler is a real person, who needs to feel parental anger and pain if the child is also to feel the pride and pleasure he or she gives the parents.

Discipline

Discipline is a crucial part of the socialization process and a major issue in parenting. Its purpose is to teach a child to have self-control in order to be able to follow the social and moral rules of our culture. It is also to help the child learn self-discipline, so he or she will be able to control the impulses that might interfere with becoming a successful, productive, attractive adult.

During the second year, when discipline begins to be an issue, parents find themselves examining their values and beliefs from an altered perspective and shifting to a more ambiguous, complex relationship with their child. The child is old enough to be willful, yet not old enough to be reasoned with. Because children can now walk and talk, parents sometimes forget that children are still very immature in their ability to truly understand and internalize the behavior and rules parents wish to teach. Parents should avoid reading too much into their child's motives for misbehaving. At this age, the ability to anticipate more than immediate superficial reactions is limited. Children still lack any real understanding of right and wrong.

Beyond a certain point, parents cannot accommodate their lives and household entirely to the child, but it takes maturity beyond the capacity of a toddler to anticipate that things may break or be spoiled by eager little hands. It may be possible for some families to have an area in which children are not allowed, but the living space shared with children should contain as little temptation for trouble as possible. Constantly scolding and threatening is frustrating and unpleasant for the parent. Children inevitably feel criticized on a personal and general level as they cannot distinguish between doing a bad thing and being bad children. Their self-confidence or sense of being admired by their parents is diminished by too much scolding; their happy mood and efforts to please may decline. Children who are constantly told *no* will either learn to ignore it, or may, in more extreme cases, suppress too many of the exploratory urges that keep getting them into trouble. (See box for alternatives.)

Inevitably there will be many occasions on which parents will need to say no, but they should choose a few that are most important. Although limits must be set, parents will need imagination to enforce them appropriately—neither always capitulating, nor insisting on winning every issue. A frustrated, angry adult may be tempted to try to establish absolute authority, to "show 'em who's boss." The outcome is a constant power struggle, and both sides lose.

Children at this age obey for two reasons: parents are bigger so they can enforce their authority and children want love and approval from people they love. Trying to control a one-year-old's behavior by punishment and force only promotes anger and guilt, which lead to more bad behavior. Constant scolding and criticism is a poor motivator for anyone, especially a small child who lacks perspective about himself. When criticized too much, a

---

PRACTICAL TACTICS FOR DISCIPLINING TODDLERS

Toddlers can't really be reasoned with, so parents of children this age often become quite adept at avoiding confrontations. The following are useful tactics:

1. Remove sources of temptation and danger from the child's environment. As much as possible, make your home "child proof" (see section on curiosity, exploration, and mastery, and chapter 14, Ensuring Your Child's Safety).
2. Use distraction. A one-year-old has a short attention span, so you may be able to engage his interest in something else, especially if he doesn't realize you are trying to distract him.
3. Offer alternatives. You will find that it is a lot easier to take the pearl necklace away from Sally if you first hand her wooden beads to play with.
4. Consider reverse psychology, which is logically well-suited to negativism. You may sometimes accomplish your goal by asking the child to do the opposite of what you want, or make a game of the yes-no reversal.
5. Avoid saying no. Try to phrase your admonitions in a positive way. A basic rule of behavior modification is "Say what you want, not what you don't want."
6. Remember that this little person who looms so large in your life is really immature and cannot yet be expected to internalize rules. Don't expect too much.
7. Try to step in as soon as you see trouble coming. British psychoanalyst John Bowlby sums up the ideal response as "friendly but firm intervention." He is referring to simple physical intervention before orders are given and defied.
8. Avoid asking if the child wants to do something that really is not negotiable. If, for example, you need to go to the grocery store, introduce the subject by mentioning something you want to buy. Don't say "Don't you want to go to the store?" if it isn't a real choice. A rebellious answer is guaranteed.
9. Compliment any shred of good behavior, even if you made it happen. Don't discuss a child's bad behavior very much with him or with anyone else when he is listening.

toddler feels unvalued and undeserving of love.

In disciplining, the parent ideally should strive for the most positive stance possible, giving the message that the child is a very good child who temporarily succumbed to temptation, but who tries to be good and who usually is good. The child's self-image is not very clear at this stage, and it is important to begin to teach the difference between who the child is and what the child does. Even the best children are naughty sometimes, and being naughty does not make them bad children. When parents show their children that they will still be loved, no matter how obnoxious their behavior, they are encouraging the child's confidence as a separate person, which lays the foundation for self-control.

When discipline is needed, it should be gentle but unambivalent, with sympathy for the child's point of view. Once a decision is made, parents should stick to it, making sure the child understands their resolve (children easily detect any sign of indecision). Yet, while consistency is important, rigidity is unnecessary—parents should feel free to change, bend, or stretch rules, if the situation calls for it. This age is not the time for a contest of wills. It's a good idea to back down sometimes and let the child win, especially if the issue is not that important. After all, the goal of effective discipline is not to make the child feel powerless. Indeed, what parents want to promote is the child's understanding of *responsibility*, which requires belief in power over one's own fate. Parents should be willing to reconsider an order that brings a heartfelt protest—on occasion the child may actually be right!

If parents are hurt by something the child has done, there is no reason for them to hide it. Children need to understand that disobeying their parents has consequences other than just being punished. They are beginning the long process of developing empathy for others and need to see a full array of the emotions they cause in others. In general, parents should try to be themselves, albeit their most gentle, generous, and patient selves.

There has long been controversy over whether parents should use spanking as a form of punishment. Some child development experts say it can, from time to time, be effective, but it must be administered with an open hand, not a belt or stick, and should never be used on the front of the body, especially the face. Most argue that it works no better than nonviolent punishment and that it may do harm by teaching violence.

A quick hand slap in response to finding the child in a dangerous situation may be appropriate, but even then, physical restraint and removal from the scene, accompanied by a firm *No!* imbued with all the emotion a parent will feel at such a time, is just as effective. Parents must be sure to reserve this tone of voice for only the most serious offenses, however. Children will pick up and respond to the emotional level of such prohibitions, but only if they haven't been dissipated by overuse.

Regardless of how they feel intellectually about corporal punishment, parents are not saints. There are very few who haven't on occasion lost their temper and swatted a bottom or smacked a wrist—and then felt guilty about it. They might be comforted to remember the views of George Bernard Shaw on the subject: "If you strike a child, take care that you strike it in anger . . . A blow in cold blood neither can nor should be forgiven."

Tantrums

Tantrums are outbreaks fueled by anger, frustration, indecision, and ambivalence. At this age, they are not motivated by a desire to manipulate the parent. They result in a child's total loss of control. The child weeps hysterically, throws things, throws himself to the floor, and may bang his head, hands, and feet.

These episodes are most frequent from about 18 to 30 months, occasionally recurring during periods of stress. They are usually impossible to interrupt, either by force or coaxing. If the tantrums occur at home, the best practice is to either leave the child where he is or carry him gently to his room and leave him alone to calm down.

If the child is really out of control, most parents are very upset by the child's real anguish. The best policy is to avoid getting drawn into the child's hysteria. Parents can express sympathy that the child feels upset but should try not to be impressed by the intensity of the tantrum. Sometimes parents are so disturbed by the child's overwhelming anxiety that they become angry and similarly upset and want to force the child to stop. This is a dangerous course. If they do find themselves getting drawn in they should make sure the child is not going to get hurt and then remove themselves from the scene, perhaps even take themselves out of earshot, until they feel calmer. If the parents can remain calm, it will help the child regain self-control.

Parents are usually most upset by tantrums that take place in public. These are harder to cope with because parents are so embarrassed that they cannot muster the aplomb with which they may manage the same situation at home. Swift removal from the scene may not always be feasible, but if it is possible to take the child outside for a few minutes to cool down, a change in location may help distract the child. It is also comforting to remember that most of the people staring at the scene are not feeling as critical as one might think—a lot of them are thanking their stars that it isn't them, and remembering a time when it was.

Physical restraint should be avoided, as it provokes more violence in the child, violence that then can threaten even the calmest parent's self-restraint. The one exception is where there is danger of injury. In this case, gentle restraint is necessary. (For more information, see chapter 10, The Two-Year-Old.)

COMMON CONCERNS OF PARENTS

Sibling Rivalry

Children in the second year of life are deeply engaged in their relationship with their parents. Their love is possessive and intense, their world view is egocentric and the loss of the baby's role if another baby is born during this year is intensely felt. In the long term, the advantages may make it all worth it, but at the time, parents should be prepared to give the toddler a great deal of support when a sibling is born.

The toddler does not need to be told too much about the baby's arrival before the last month or so of pregnancy. He or she should know there is a baby growing in Mommy's tummy and what arrangements are made for the time when Mommy goes to the hospital to have the baby, but the toddler can be spared the details. Some toddlers are proud and interested, but many will prefer to more or less ignore it. Parents should follow the child's lead. While the mother is in the hospital, the child should be taken care of by the father or other close family members and in the home if at all possible. If siblings visits are permitted, the toddler should be taken to see the mother and the new baby in the hospital.

Once the new baby comes home, parents and visitors should make every effort to give the child extra attention and not to fuss too much over the newborn in the older child's presence. Also, both parents should set aside some time each day to give undivided attention to the older child, including time out of the house. When gifts and special supplies for the baby are brought into the house, the parents should supply small gifts for the older child, too. As child psychologist M. Patricia Boyle explains, it is almost impossible for the child at this age to see that the love the parents feel for him is not diminished by being shared with a sibling. It will help if parents are very demonstrative of their affection with the older child, and they may even find a way to explain that the love parents feel is not a fixed amount, to be divided up among their children but that it grows with each child.

The most important part of a toddler's world is usually his relationship with his mother. That relationship is disturbed when the mother goes away to the hospital, and it is irrevocably changed when the baby comes home. Although most children manage well, some one-year-olds may be so hurt and angry at the mother that their behavior becomes even more provocative and negative than is expected at this age. Transient eating and sleeping disturbances are common. There may also be some regression: a child who has given up the bottle may now want it again, one who has achieved some manner of bowel or bladder control may lose it, and clear speech may slip back into baby talk. If the toddler regresses in an attempt to show that he or she is still a baby, too, and needs love, it is best to allow this for a while. The child can cuddle, imitate the baby, pretend to breastfeed, or drink from a bottle again without any lasting harm. At the same time, parents should show that they are proud of the child's "big boy" or "big girl" accomplishments, pointing out that the baby cannot yet do all these wonderful things.

Although most children manage to keep the worst of their jealous feelings submerged, it is not rare to encounter a toddler whose anguish at the change in roles in the family seems overwhelming. Realizing how betrayed the older child feels, the parents may have difficulty giving the baby as much affection and attention as the newborn deserves. They may find themselves cuddling the baby only in secret, when their firstborn cannot see and be wounded. Not only is this unfair to the baby and the parents, there is a menace in the idea that a parent can be unloving to a child, even a rival. Especially if the new baby was not planned, parents may feel so guilty toward the older child that they act as if the child has been wronged (as opposed to hurt), confirming the child's sense that the parents have done a bad thing and owe restitution. If the parents can put guilt behind them and decide that all the love they feel and their best effort really are enough, they may find that the toddler dwells less on misery and returns to his or her former pleasure with life.

Even the most well-adjusted child will feel some resentment, so there is always some potential for aggressive behavior toward the infant. The threat may be greatest from children who deny jealousy, but are excessively enthusiastic in their affection. The rules in this case must be clear and firm; hurting the baby simply cannot be tolerated. Any aggression toward the baby must be stopped swiftly and firmly and it is best not to tempt the toddler by leaving him or her alone with the baby.

A one-year-old who is the younger of two siblings separated by less than three years may become the aggressor, knowing that the older child usually gets blamed. Parents must be on the lookout for this ploy and be sure to give the older child some benefit of the doubt.

No matter what the ages and spacing of siblings, there is bound to be rivalry. Rivalry between children spaced less than three years apart can be a major source of stress in young families and should be taken into consideration by parents when planning a family. (For more information, see chapter 13, How Does Your Baby Fit In?)

Sleep

Difficulties with sleep are common during the second year. Going to bed seems to mean giving up all the fun and excitement of being alive. At this age children may fight to stay awake even when they are literally staggering with exhaustion. They also may object to being alone. Especially by the middle of the year, feelings of loneliness and the anxiety about separation can make trouble during the night as well as at bedtime.

For problems in going to bed, moving the nap to earlier in the day and increasing outdoor physical exercise may help. A bath before bed calms some children, although for others it may have the opposite effect. A treat for a bedtime snack may be used to ease the shift from playing to getting ready for bed. A routine of washing up, reading, cuddling, rocking, saying good-night to dollies and teddies, and tucking in may become a ritual the child depends upon to help him through the nightly separation ordeal. (For more information, see chapter 10, The Two-Year-Old.)

Even a child who seems to have settled down may call out after the parent leaves the room. It may be enough to answer without coming in. Usually the best way to deal with these tactics is more or less to ignore them. Using a fairly bright night light and leaving the door ajar help the child feel less afraid of being alone.

During normal sleep, children rouse periodically. They change positions, mumble or call out, and may awaken the parent without fully waking up themselves. Parents should wait a bit before responding, as answering or going in to the child's room may wake him completely. If the child really wakes up and calls persistently, they can try talking to him or her from the next room. Sometimes just hearing the parents' voices is reassuring enough to allow the child to go back to sleep.

A remedy many parents use is to let a persistent child "cry it out" for a few nights in a row, enforcing the idea that time in bed is nonnegotiable. If strictly applied, this eventually works for most children, although it may be as hard on the parent as on the child. It goes against the grain to refuse to respond to a crying child. If used this technique is best applied during the earlier part of the year, when the child feels relatively confident and free of anxiety. If the parents feel the child is really afraid or is overwhelmingly upset, it may be wiser to be patient for another few months. Although giving in does effectively end the use of that training technique for the time being, the parents must trust their own sense of whether their child is ready.

Under no circumstances will it be possible to completely avoid comforting the child during the night. Many pediatricians advise parents to return the child to the crib after comforting him or her, rather than taking the child into their own bed. While it is generally not a good idea to let the child sleep in the parents' bed, it won't hurt occasionally. If a child is used to starting and ending the night in his or her own bed, it will make it easier in the long run for the parents to get more sleep and more privacy.

Other experts feel there is no harm in letting the child come into bed with the parents, especially after five or six o'clock in the morning, an hour when many children are up for the day otherwise. Parents may enjoy the close, affectionate feelings of being in bed with their children; certainly the children will.

There is no easy answer for how to deal with a child's wish for company or comfort during the night. By the end of the year, many children begin having nightmares, which complicates the issue. In some cases, night waking is just a habit that can be successfully discouraged if the parent ignores it. In other cases, the child's anxiety is so strong that he or she will feel an overwhelming need for some kind of reassurance. After many trips to the child's room, an exhausted parent may give up and stay, or bring the child back to his bed. It is a trade-off: sleep now in exchange for more trouble getting the child to sleep alone later. It is not ideal, but it will not harm the child.

Fears

As irrational as a child's fears may seem to be, they actually follow a very rational progression that correlates with their stage of development. From 12 to 24 months, children tend to be quite fearless in physical ways, yet their greatest fear, separation from the parent, pervades most aspects of life.

Near the end of the year, children often develop fear of the toilet flushing and of the bathtub drain. Parents can deal with this by taking the child out of the room before flushing the toilet or removing the stopper from the bathtub drain. It is hard for an adult to realize that the child is afraid of being physically sucked down the drain. It may help to show the child the pipes and drains and to explain that he cannot fit through, but it will be months before he really understands that he is safe. When the child wants to, he should be allowed to drop paper in the toilet or to practice flushing it, and to use other kinds of water play to help master this fear.

All childhood fears have some basis. Children should not be teased, shamed, or forced to do what frightens them. On the other hand, it is impossible and undesirable for parents to avoid all potentially frightening situations or remove every possible scare from a child's environment. As child psychoanalyst Selma Fraiberg noted, even children raised on the "correct" fairy tales, with no bad monsters and dragons, dream of monsters under the bed and dragons in the closet. Dreams are a way for children (and adults) to relive the day and to deal with unresolved or frightening matters. (For more information, see chapter 10, The Two-Year-Old.)

Eating

During the second year, most children will complete the transition from the bottle to the cup. They will begin to handle a spoon and want to feed themselves. By the end of the year, they will be able to eat most of the foods their parents do. Parents can begin the transition by giving juices in a cup and using the bottle only for milk or water. The circumstances of bottle use can also be gradually restricted —for instance, no bottle in the park or in the stroller. If bedtime is not right after dinner, a bedtime snack may be substituted for the evening bottle. No bottles should be allowed in bed, as milk or juice pooling in the mouth during sleep can cause severe tooth decay.

As their fine motor skills improve and as they move toward independence, children will want to feed themselves. Toward the middle of the year, they may become more fussy about which foods they will eat, but these strong opinions are apt to change from week to week or even day to day. Extremely picky eating behavior (nothing but melon and cheese or peanut butter and crackers) does not usually appear before the second birthday.

The best course is to offer children a variety of foods and let them eat what they want. As long as they get something from each of the food groups— protein, fruits and vegetables, dairy, and grains and cereal—every few days, they will do fine nutritionally. What is important is autonomy.

Parental tastes shouldn't interfere with children's food choices. The child may like sweet potatoes even if the parents don't, or may enjoy dunking green beans in Jello—it doesn't matter. It is best to avoid salting a child's food to suit an adult's taste. Finger foods, such as cheese sticks, apple slices, string beans, and sandwiches cut in quarters, facilitate self-feeding.

Toddlers do not chew carefully, so their food should be cut in a way that avoids the possibility of choking. For example, grapes should be cut in half, and hot dogs should be cut lengthwise as well as across.

At this age, children love to handle their food, to feel it, smear it, and fling it around. Providing a variety of textures—creamy peanut butter, squishy applesauce, crunchy crackers, juicy peaches— makes the experience even more appealing.

If the parent serves a small amount at a time, it is easier for the child to handle, and a spill will not be a major disaster. While the child plays and feeds himself, the parent, using another spoon, will still do much of the feeding. If the adult can stand the mess and avoid rushing, the meal will be a success. Parents who try to prevent food play may find the child beginning to refuse food, even to the point of losing weight. Eating should be a casual, happy, social time. At this age, children think it is a great game to feed their parents, so both adult and child should wear clothes that are easy to wash. The child should eat in a place that is relatively easy to clean, with a cloth or some newspapers on the floor to catch the fallout.

Most parents of toddlers worry that their child is not eating enough. After the rapid growth of the first year, children normally do not need to eat as much because growth and weight gain are slower. Appetite may vary from week to week and from mood to mood, but the child will eat enough unless there is a great excess of anxiety or anger at meal time. As long as the pediatrician determines that the child is growing normally, then he or she is getting enough to eat. The most important rule for parents is to avoid showing that they care as much as they probably do about what or how much their children eat. Children should eat for themselves, because they are hungry, in order to grow, because food tastes good. It is a mistake to take a lot of trouble to prepare a special treat for a picky eater. At this age, that will be an invitation to refuse it. (For further discussion, see chapter 5.)

The small size and high activity levels of children this age make them naturally more suited to smaller, more frequent meals than adults. Meals at the table with other people are more often social occasions and should be supplemented by at least three snacks: midmorning, midafternoon, and before bed. Snacks may be adapted to wherever the child is playing—in the park, in the stroller, or on the kitchen floor.

At this age, children will imitate their parents in everything, including food tastes. If parents love junk food, they will have to reconsider their habits, save junk food for late-night snacks, or accept having their children eat it too.

Toilet Training

Before the advent of the diaper service and disposable diapers, parents had a greater incentive to free themselves of the diaper-washing routine as early as possible. In many families it is still considered a virtue to train a child early. This is unfortunate because not only is accelerated training more difficult for parents, but it can create problems for the child. Early training—before 18 months—has the potential to be upsetting and disruptive. Some toddlers, especially younger siblings, are so eager, they seem to train themselves. The general rule, however, is that the later one begins to toilet train a child, the more quickly and easily it will be accomplished. Children trained earlier tend to have more lapses of control during the following years than do children trained later.

Physically, the child generally gains some control of the sphincter muscle as early as 9 months and can cooperate voluntarily in training by 12 to 15 months. But most experts, particularly the pediatrician/writer T. Berry Brazelton, now believe that waiting until the child is at least 18 months, makes it a more positive experience. Generally, parents are advised to attempt daytime bowel control first, followed by bladder control and then finally nighttime control.

The child's readiness for training has a lot to do with psychological and social development. The stronger the child's sense of self, and the greater the craving for independence, the better prepared he or she is for toilet training. The potty can be introduced before 18 months, but the child may not show much enthusiasm before 24 months, or when the height of negativism is passing. Improved language skills at this stage make the child better able to understand the procedure, and improved motor skills give him or her greater autonomy in the process. Finally, the child by this age will have less ambivalence in his wish to please and imitate the parents.

Brazelton argues that the emphasis in toilet training should be on the child's accomplishment, not on the parents' victory. He calls his approach "child-oriented," leaving it to the child to signal when he or she is ready to start each successive stage of training. Children will indicate that they are

ready by showing awareness of their body's signals. They may gesture and squirm or grimace when they are aware of an impending bowel movement. Another sign of readiness is a surprising phase of fastidiousness: They want to be changed as soon as their diapers are wet or dirty, they may be distressed by dirty hands, and they start to show an interest in putting things in their proper places.

Before the child shows interest in being trained, parents can begin by placing a potty chair in the bathroom. They can teach the association with the toilet and explain that the chair is the child's own. When he or she begins to be interested, they can let the child sit on it (still clothed), play with the lid, and put objects into the bowl. At the same time, the child will probably be developing a keen interest in water play, which extends to playing in the toilet. While most of this should be redirected to other, more hygienic water play, the child can be allowed to toss bits of toilet paper and other harmless items into the toilet and to practice flushing.

Next, the child can be taken to sit on the potty, still fully clothed, at a routine time each day. The parent may be able to entice the child to stay by reading a story or offering a snack, but by no means should the child be forced to stay. If all goes well, the next step will be to have the child sit on the chair with diapers off. There should still be no attempt to time this to a bowel movement or urination; the idea is to just make the situation commonplace and routine.

Once the child is comfortable with this, he or she can be brought to the potty a second time each day. If this is done soon after a bowel movement, the child's diapers can be changed on the seat, with the contents of the diapers disposed of in the bowl. This is accompanied by an explanation of what the chair and toilet are for. Once this concept is understood and the signals of an approaching bowel movement learned, the child can be taken to the potty to "catch" it. It often happens that a child is frightened by some step in the procedure, usually by the parents' rush to catch the bowel movement. If this happens, it is best to temporarily stop training until the child is more relaxed.

In the next stage, diapers are removed for short periods of time and while the child is bare-bottomed, he is encouraged to play with and sit on the potty as he wishes. At this time, the potty chair can be put in the child's room or play area to make it easier. After the child begins to use the potty chair regularly, for both bowel and bladder functions, he or she can wear training pants for part of the day. This is a great reward, as they are much more comfortable than diapers. Achieving this—becoming more like an adult and receiving great praise from parents—can be very exciting for the child. Since the process can happen relatively quickly, it is worth waiting until the child is ready.

Staying dry during sleep requires a combination of physical maturity and subconscious motivation that are extremely variable in their development. Even without drinks at bedtime, some normal children may need a diaper at night as late as age four or five.

Throughout the process of toilet training, parents must recognize the child's accomplishment with appropriate praise and rewards. If the child becomes frightened or unduly anxious and destructive, training should be temporarily discontinued until the child is reassured. Especially with bladder control, lapses will be common. The child should be cleaned up without a fuss, and reassured that occasional accidents happen to everyone, and have no importance.

SUMMING UP

THE SECOND YEAR can be roughly divided into four quarters. In the first three months, learning to walk makes the toddler excited and cheerful as he explores his enlarging world with exuberance. The second quarter is a little quieter, as the youngster concentrates on refining these new motor skills. Around the eighteenth month, the child suddenly begins to wonder about being *too* independent. At this point, many children "reapproach" the mother, often becoming clingy and whiny. However, the need for independence and the pleasure of mastering new skills will continue to propel the child forward. Negativism, which is increasingly apparent throughout the last half of the year, is a way for the child to test limits and boundaries as he begins to develop a sense of himself as an individual.

10 The Two-Year-Old

Margaret Stillman, M.D.

INTRODUCTION

ALTHOUGH MOST CHILD-DEVELOPMENT EXPERTS consider that toddlerhood begins at 12 months, it is the two-year-old that epitomizes this active period. Two-year-olds are constantly on the go, using their increasing physical skills to explore and test their environment, and their burgeoning language skills to ask questions about it and then describe it, albeit in two-word sentences. If they seem to be always taking things apart, poking at them, dropping them, climbing on them, hiding inside them, it is not in an effort to exasperate their parents, but as a way of finding out how things are made, how they work, how they react to being prodded and poked, or how they look from the inside.

The major changes in this third year occur in the child's intellectual, social, and psychological growth. Growing verbal skills play a major role in his or her behavior and in relationships with others. There is a slow shift in focus from nonsocial activities (such as exploring and practicing motor skills) to social activities, including interaction and cooperation with peers.

Psychologically, the two-year-old begins to develop a greater sense of self, obvious in the increased use of possessives *my* and *mine*. The negativism of the previous year gradually disappears. The rapprochement crisis will also subside as the child comes to better terms with reality and feels more confident about increasing independence. Nevertheless, the struggle for self-control will continue. By the end of the year, the child will be able to take some measure of responsibility for his or her own behavior.

During this year, especially between two-and-a-half and three, children become better organized. They will be able to play by themselves from time to time and often they show the beginnings of judgment. Improved motor skills enable them to begin dressing themselves, although supervision is still needed. Their ability to manipulate objects improves, sometimes making it possible to put back together things that previously could only be taken apart.

Two-year-olds begin to lose interest in exploring the home, and instead will turn to the outside world, giving every new object and situation, once it has been found not to be threatening, a thorough going-over. They will be less concerned with observable characteristics of objects and more with what they are used for and how the pieces fit together, especially if they are objects used by the parents. Youngsters will now want to use them more and more as tools for other purposes. For example, a cup and spoon may be transformed into sandbox toys, and food may become an object of play as well as something to eat. This is the beginning of symbolic play, a milestone in the third year. Dolls and trucks will no longer just be carried around, hugged, or admired. Dolls will be scolded and fed bottles and trucks will be "driven," complete with sound effects.

The third year, while perhaps not as tumultuous as the previous one, nevertheless has its own share of excitement and challenge and, as the child's skills of reason and communication continue to improve, there is a growing sense of satisfaction and self-delight.

PHYSICAL GROWTH AND DEVELOPMENT

THE PHYSICAL GROWTH of two-year-olds progresses at a slightly slower pace than it did the previous year. Typically a child will add four to five pounds and grow three inches during this third year of life. The average two-year-old of either sex will be about 34 inches tall. For boys, the average weight is 28 pounds; for girls, 26 pounds. Both boys and girls will slim down slightly during the third year, but they will retain their protruding bellies until sometime the following year. Their facial features will be more mature, although their heads—nearly adult size—will continue to be large in comparison to their bodies and short legs.

Two-year-olds still sleep approximately half the time, about 13 hours, although the range of normal is anywhere from 8 to 17. By now the morning nap is gone but most children will still take an afternoon nap of an hour or two. Even if the child does not actually sleep, the parent or other caregiver should provide a quiet rest time in midafternoon.

Motor skills continue to advance at a uniform pace in this year, but the development will not be quite as dramatic as it was in the first and second years. The advances will be refinements of skills previously exhibited.

At 24 months, toddlers should be able to walk and run quite well, negotiating the house easily and no longer bumping into furniture or knocking over small items at every turn. Unlike one-year-olds, who spend a certain amount of time each day simply practicing motor skills—walking, climbing, or manipulating objects—two-year-olds tend to incorporate the practice of skills into exploration and play. They like to walk by themselves and will resist most attempts to carry them or put them in the stroller. Outside, they are still likely to fall often as they run

exuberantly after playmates or butterflies, explore playground equipment, or climb low walls. Their play tends to be rough-and-tumble and parental supervision is still needed to prevent serious mishaps. It is impossible, and probably unwise, for parents to prevent every minor fall, but it is still necessary that they be there to comfort the child afterward.

Typically, the two-year-old can stack five or more blocks on top of one another and can jump in place with both feet together. Most can take off shoes and socks and will try to dress without help. Their physical grasp is more finely developed and they can easily turn doorknobs, hold crayons or pencils, and manipulate eating utensils, although not yet as an adult would.

INTELLECTUAL DEVELOPMENT

Language

The third year is a critical period for language development. Vocabulary increases markedly while the subjects of communication grow in complexity and sophistication. Words begin to take the place of action. Now not only does the child express thoughts but he or she also begins to express emotions (e.g., "I'm sad"). Whereas younger children typically use language to make observations ("Kitty run") or describe or comment on topics ("Ball bounce"), two-year-olds begin to use speech to communicate needs and desires ("Danny want milk") and to influence the behavior of important adults ("Mommy play ball [with me]").

What makes this great forward leap possible is the convergence of several developmental factors that affect the ability to acquire language. According to child-development pioneer Jean Piaget, two-year-olds leave the sensorimotor stage, in which their primary frame of reference is the present and in which they can only think about or understand something by actually experiencing it. They are now able to remember and recall what is said. Entering the stage of representational intelligence, they are able to think symbolically. They will, for example, develop a mental picture of Mother, so that Mother will exist even when she can't be seen. Or, seeing Daddy's hat, the child may recall last night's playtime with Daddy and imagine what might happen tonight when Daddy returns.

Symbolic thought—and language is one form of symbolism—allows the child to think and talk about things that may have occurred in the past, fitting these events into current concepts, or to conjure up sequences of events or behaviors in the mind, manipulating the outcomes and thus "trying out" ideas, rather than having to act out behavior in order to find out what the consequences are. They may practice sharing, for example.

Also critical to the burgeoning of language skills in the third year is the child's strong desire to communicate. The child wants to share thoughts with and emulate parents and other significant adults. Moreover, there is a strong urge for self-expression. This desire to communicate what they are thinking, feeling and, most of all, experiencing, provides two-year-olds with the motivation to develop their language skills. For them, language serves an egocentric as well as a social function.

The ability to express thoughts, wants, and needs facilitates independence. Thus, even during the peak of negativism, a child is rarely negative about language. For two-year-olds, communication helps deal with emotions and fears. Like an adult, the more a youngster can "talk things out," the better he or she feels. Children who are delayed in their language development often have more problems with behavior. Language gives a greater sense of control over self, instincts, and sudden wants, and this control is needed in the quest for greater independence.

Language Skills

At the start of the third year, the average child has an effective vocabulary of 250 to 300 words or simple phrases, more than double what it was only three months earlier. This represents words that are both understood and spoken. (The number of words a child understands but has not yet added to spoken vocabulary brings this total even higher.) On the other hand, a perfectly normal child may only speak 6 or 20 words, yet be able to comprehend hundreds. Parents should not be concerned. Typically a child like this needs a little longer to put things together, then suddenly starts to speak in paragraphs!

During the third year, vocabulary grows at an average of 50 words a month, so that by age 36 months, the child will be able to use about 900 words. Generally boys are a little slower to acquire language than girls, but they nevertheless progress rapidly this year.

A two-year-old's sentences are usually two or three words long ("Erica go bye-bye") at the beginning of the year, progressing to three to four words during the second six months. For the most part, sentences consist of nouns and verbs. Even in these telegraphic utterances, children show an understanding of basic grammar and syntax. Function words, such as articles, prepositions or conjunctions, begin to appear at two-and-a-half. By then the child understands and may begin to use the plurals, possessives, pronouns (*you* and, especially, *me, my,* and *mine*) and the relative prepositions *on, in,* and *under.* Two-year-olds will also begin to use *I* and *me* in place of their names. By the end of the year, they may be able to describe themselves by age and sex and can give their first and last names when asked.

The child of two is usually able to understand simple commands ("Throw the ball to Mommy") and to identify body parts (nose, hand) and common objects (ball, spoon). By 36 months, he or she can understand three-part commands ("Go to the kitchen, open the cupboard, and bring me a glass") and may be able to describe common objects in detail ("The ball is round and red").

Two-year-olds do not need to be taught to speak; they only need to be developmentally ready to communicate and to have an environment filled with aural stimuli. A two-year-old learns most language by hearing it spoken by family members and peers, or on records, radio, or television. Educational television shows such as "Sesame Street" are helpful, but the best source of language education is the child's own family. Parents should speak freely in the child's presence and should respond to questions. Because two-year-olds understand many more words than they can speak, parents need not hesitate to use fairly sophisticated language and to express interesting and advanced ideas. They should remember, too, that children do not learn appropriate language by hearing them speak baby talk!

Parents can facilitate their child's desire to communicate by speaking to the child as much as possible. For example, they can describe their actions and interactions with the child: "I'm making breakfast for you. I'm pouring milk into your glass. Now the glass is full. Here's your glass of milk. The milk is cold, isn't it?"

At this point, the child's pronunciation should not be of concern. A typical two-year-old will be intelligible to a stranger only about 25 percent of the time. By age three, however, this jumps to 75 percent. Rather than correcting pronunciation or grammar directly, parents should simply repeat the child's word or sentence the correct way. Thus, an appropriate response to the child's observation that "flowers is pwitty" is not "No, Lisa, say flowers are pretty," but "Yes, flowers are pretty, aren't they?"

Language and Cognitive Development

There are many theories about the relationship between language and rational thought. Some developmentalists believe that a child's early use of language is nonrational—in the beginning he or she just wishes for things and they appear, reinforcing the idea that the youngster is the center of the universe. This stage is called "egocentric thinking" and essentially it lasts through the preschool years. The child continues to see things almost exclusively from his or her own perspective, which is why toddlers who hide their eyes with their hands may think that no one else can see them. A child experimenting with the television may think that he or she has produced the picture, unable to imagine that it comes from somewhere else. Language reflects this egocentricity, too. A two-year-old will tell a story without identifying who it involves or where it took place because the child assumes that the listener should know this.

After this stage, thinking is dominated by perception—what is seen and heard and is experienced is now believed to be the truth. Finally, as they begin to think in terms of words instead of pictures, children are able to reason abstractly and to use logic.

Although egocentric and associative, the two-year-old begins to have an understanding of consequences, or cause and effect. The child begins to anticipate events, and understands increasingly complex and abstract thoughts. For example, he or she can anticipate basic elements of the day: naptime always comes after lunch. Or, the youngster realizes that when the string is pulled, the curtain closes. "Why" questions are very common by the end of the year and throughout the following, as the child begins the journey toward perceptual thinking.

The change from egocentric to perceptually dominated to logical thinking is a long process, although progress is made during this year. Piaget named the entire period, lasting from about age two to age six, "preoperational." This he divided into the substages of preconceptual thought (until about age four) and intuitive thought (ages four to six). In preconceptual thinking a child's understanding is midway between that of individual objects and classes of objects—or concepts. Unable to think abstractly or form true concepts, the child may recognize similarities and may assign one word to cover similar objects or persons but not be able to make fine distinctions. For example, all men with gray beards may be "grandpa." Piaget relates that one of his daughters, who were the models for his theories, first saw a garden at Uncle Alfred's and thus, until she was able to make distinctions, all gardens became "Uncle Alfred's garden."

During the preoperational stage, cognitive development is characterized by several recognizable thought processes, among them animism and classification. Animism, in which children ascribe living characteristics to inanimate objects, is common among two-year-olds and exists in one form or another through the preschool years. Piaget described four stages in which the child first believes that all objects are alive and gradually refines that concept to include only things that move (even such things as a clock pendulum), then only things that move of their own accord, such as the sun. Finally the concept is narrowed to plants and animals or just animals. In the meantime, the child may firmly believe that a tree root deliberately tripped him or her or that the door wanted to pinch a little finger.

In classification, a child grows increasingly more sophisticated in the ability to group objects by characteristics. At first this is one-dimensional. The child may, for example, be able to match the two green balls, distinguishing them from the red and the blue balls. As time goes on, the child can identify (chain) two or more objects that have a characteristic in common—two green shapes or two balls of different sizes. Eventually the child will be able to sort a number of objects into different groups and finally to classify them according to their relationship to each other, such as lining up blocks in size order.

The best way for parents to encourage growth in intellect is to be open and receptive to all questions and to expose the child to as many different experiences as possible. But common sense should prevail—there is no point in trying to force learning on a child at this age. First, it is not possible to push a child ahead from one Piagetian stage to another: The child must first have reached the appropriate point of neurological development. Second, it can be counterproductive, as it may make learning a task rather than a joy.

Left to develop at his or her own pace, the two-year-old will find learning terribly exciting because it is another part of becoming independent. It is not important that a child learn the alphabet sooner than the next child (or according to any rigid timetable), but that he or she learn it when ready and enthusiastic about it. It is far better for parents to nourish the natural enthusiasm for learning than to teach specific skills before their time.

SOCIAL AND PSYCHOLOGICAL DEVELOPMENT

Behavior

In the third year, children begin to consolidate a sense of self. By 24 months, most have weathered the rapprochement crisis but they still have trouble separating easily from their parents, especially their mothers. They are more interested in social relationships and activities, such as gaining the attention of adults, engaging in conversation, and playing with peers, but they are still egocentric.

The primary achievement of the third year is the development of self-control. Self-control can be seen as the ultimate goal of a struggle between autonomy and social conformity. As the child develops greater language skills and begins to reason things out, rather than simply reacting physically and emotionally, he or she begins to act in more socially acceptable ways. It is something the child will struggle with throughout the 12 months, making real progress in the second half of the year. In the meantime, it may take all the self-control parents can muster to weather this period, often called "the terrible twos."

Lovable as two-year-olds can be, they can also be maddeningly negative, contrary, and independent. Although they want to please their parents, to acquiesce means to give up their independence, so their first answer is always no. Wise parents learn not to ask questions that allow this to happen ("Do you want your bath now?") but to make matter-of-fact statements ("It's bathtime and your bath toys are waiting for you"). They also learn to limit the answer choices to acceptable alternatives ("Would you rather have cheese or yogurt?" "Do you want to go to bed now or in five minutes?").

Another difficult part of this drive for autonomy is the desire to do everything themselves ("I do it, Mommy"). As long as they are not in danger of hurting themselves or destroying property, it is better to let them try. In dressing themselves, they may put on mismatched socks or stubbornly insist on wearing a wool hat in July. Parents can choose to accept this, understanding that it is not a reflection on their parenting skills. Or, if they find the outfit or the decision totally inappropriate, they can propose a compromise that allows the child a small victory ("Okay. You can wear the wool hat until it's time to leave and then we'll let your teddy bear wear it").

Every situation can't be a showdown. If for no other reason than that they are bigger and stronger, parents will always win, but the win will cost both them and their children dearly. Children who aren't allowed to establish their autonomy now will either do it later in a much more self-destructive way or they will not develop it at all.

By two-and-a-half, many children will have a better measure of control over antisocial behavior, but they can become demanding and rather obnoxious in their inflexibility. And their ambivalence can be maddening. Having insisted on making the decision themselves, they suddenly can't decide. The problem is that they don't have enough experience to know whether they are going to prefer one alternative or the other. Parents can sometimes suggest a way they can have their cake and eat it, too. ("Would you like to wear your red dress today and your blue dress tomorrow?" The child will invariably choose the blue dress for today, but the decision-making process will be hastened.)

At some point during the twos, every child has a temper tantrum. No longer able to control their emotions, two-year-olds will shriek, kick, pound their fists, throw themselves on the floor, and even hold their breath. Some children—generally the more active ones who have definite ideas about what they want—may have one or two tantrums a week. Tantrums usually occur when the child is totally frustrated by not being able to do something, either because of the child's own limitations or because the parent has thwarted him or her. They are more likely to happen when the child is hungry, very tired, or overstimulated by an active and social day. If parents are aware of these triggers, they can try to keep them to a minimum.

Difficult as it may be, the best way to handle a tantrum is to ignore it. By responding to it with threats or bribes, by losing their own temper, or by caving in to the unmet demand that produced the tantrum in the first place, parents only reinforce the behavior by bringing the child the attention he or she craves. The parent should be consistent in ignoring the behavior, but must also realize that the child is not rational and may hurt himself or others. Throwing things out the window or pounding violently on a glass tabletop are potentially dangerous behaviors that cannot be ignored.

Although parents should remind themselves that their child is not the only one who has ever had a temper tantrum, it is difficult to ignore this kind of behavior in a public place, especially while facing disapproving stares from strangers. The best response in this case is simply to leave. Forget the cart full of groceries for a few minutes and take the child outside or even to another part of the store until he or she calms down.

When tantrums happen at home, the child should be removed from the scene without comment, taken to a quiet place to wait it out, or left alone in his or her bedroom. Those children who will allow it can be held close until they calm down, and then distracted with another activity.

For some children, tantrums sometimes result in breath-holding spells. This behavior may begin spontaneously at a very young age and is not meant to be manipulative. However, if it prompts the parent to fuss over the child, it may be repeated until it becomes a way for the child to achieve control over the parents. The breath-holding episodes usually follow a specific sequence: the child is denied something, he or she gets very angry, starts to cry loudly and uncontrollably, then suddenly stops breathing. Understandably this can be very frightening to parents, and some will acquiesce to the child before the crying starts in order to avoid the breath-holding. Although frightening, these episodes are not serious: the child eventually gives up and gasps for air or, in rare cases, becomes momentarily unconscious, at which point breathing starts again automatically. Although it may sound callous, the best approach is to ignore this behavior.

Toward the end of the third year, when the child is better at self-expression, the parent can acknowledge the child's feelings ("I'll bet you were really angry that we had to leave the park") and explain that the child has to use words, not tantrums, to express these feelings. Teaching children to put their feelings into words, rather than actions, helps give them the control that they are seeking. By acknowledging the child's feelings ("Sometimes it must seem like your new brother gets all the attention. It's hard being an older sister at times, isn't it?"), parents are laying the groundwork of verbal expression.

Body and Gender Awareness

Part of the developing sense of self is the child's increased awareness of his or her own body. It is, in fact, the two-year-old's greatest possession. Children this age feel very defensive and protective about themselves. This doesn't mean that toddlers will not put themselves in danger—they have only the dimmest notion of consequences—but it does mean that the smallest cut or injury, which a year before may have gone without notice—will produce loud wailing and much concern. Band-Aids become a favorite for children of this age, and putting one over each and every minor scrape is usually all that is needed.

This desire for self-protection is reflected early in the third year in the fuss many children make about going to the doctor. Not only are they afraid of getting a shot, they also fear being probed, poked, and examined by another person. Fortunately, this changes over the course of the year as the vaccination period ends and as children's understanding of language increases, making it easier to console them with words. They become less difficult to examine and may begin to develop a rapport with the doctor as they approach age three.

At this age the child sees everything in terms of the human body ("Why do trees have arms and no legs?"). It also explains why the first introduction to gender differences can be something of a shock.

Sometime during the third year, if not before, children will discover that those of the opposite sex are different. They may notice an older brother or sister, or a new baby of the other sex may join the family. For an only child, the introduction usually comes through a peer: changing into bathing suits for a swim or "playing doctor." The latter is common and altogether normal at this age. It is really a form of mutual education and not sexual or sensual in an adult way. Parents who are upset when they find children engaging in this game may risk conveying the message that there is something wrong or dirty about genitals. Their best course is to ignore it. Or, if they are not uncomfortable, they can use it as a way to open discussion about bodies and as an opportunity for the children to ask questions. Establishing this willingness to discuss bodily functions and sex early will make discussions easier when children are older. If they know that they can get straight answers without being made to feel guilty about their curiosity, children will be more willing to bring their questions home.

Likewise, parents should take a matter-of-fact attitude if they come upon their child masturbating, which is apt to happen at any time during the third year. In fact, the child has probably been enjoying these pleasurable feelings since infancy. Before age six months, many children discover their genitals and find that touching them or rubbing them against something feels good. If the child is not masturbating to the exclusion of other pleasurable activities, the parents have nothing to worry about and they should simply accept the behavior as normal. As children get a little older, they should be taught that masturbation is a private activity that is best confined to their own rooms.

Gender differences in behavior between boys and girls are already quite apparent at this age. Boys are typically more aggressive than girls, and girls are in general more advanced in language development. The differences become obvious when children are observed in preschool and daycare settings, even those that attempt to expose both sexes equally to the same play materials: The girls will be found in one corner discussing whose turn it is to play the mommy, while the boys will be in another corner wrestling for possession of the same trucks. Some theorists believe that these differences are entirely culturally determined, while others believe that there is some genetic basis for these differences that is then strongly reinforced by culture.

Whatever the genesis of the differences, parents who wish to rear children without the stereotypical sex-role characteristics may find it difficult. Even if they manage to eliminate sexist attitudes within the home (they will have to unplug the television set), they may not be able to keep Grandma from making every present to Nancy a doll, and they still will not be able to control the attitudes of their children's peers, which have a strong influence at this age. They may also find that they have transmitted subconsciously lingering beliefs and cultural norms that are so ingrained they are not aware of them. That is not to say that they shouldn't try, only that they should not be surprised if they find that the workbench they have given Sally is being used as a pretend ironing board.

Another aspect of psychological development in the third year is the child's ability to see things from someone else's perspective. Much of a child's personality, however, is shaped by individual environment. Through the second and third years, as the child develops a stronger sense of self, he or she takes an active role in choosing what to be like. A boy may model his walk after his father or a peer; a little girl may imitate her mother's voice and mannerisms.

Social Relationships

The primary social relationships for a two-year-old remain those that he or she has with parents. They are the child's emotional lodestars, no matter how often their overtures are met with the ubiquitous noes. The two-year-old wants their approval and their love. As strong as the drive for independence is, separation is still difficult for the child.

Children at this age also want to imitate their parents and can sometimes do so with amusing or painful accuracy. They enjoy, especially toward the second half of the year, helping around the house, even though their help often results in more work for the parents. They are beginning to develop some sense of satisfaction in doing things for others and delight in accomplishing simple tasks, such as fetching a diaper from another room for a new sibling. Unfortunately this desire to help around the house disappears over the next few years.

As friendly and affectionate as two-year-olds can be (in their good moments) toward their parents, they can be appallingly selfish and aggressive with one another. In the course of a game, they will not seem to care much if another's feelings are hurt because they still don't entirely understand that other children have feelings. Indeed, much of the play of two-year-olds is selfish. As they develop a stronger sense of self, they become very possessive and eager to point out what's theirs. Before now, the two-year-old did not need to claim an item—he or she simply assumed ownership of everything. But as this illusion is destroyed, the child reacts by grasping for personal possessions.

It takes a great amount of cajoling to convince two-year-olds to share their toys, even those they are not currently playing with. They are able to do it occasionally, and more so toward the end of the year, but mostly they are not ready to give up control or even to understand the concept of sharing. When two or more are together, it is best to provide several play materials at a time to be sure that each child has a choice. If they go for each other's toys anyway, distraction is usually the best solution.

Slowly over the year, children begin to gain a perspective other than their own. They are much better able to share, albeit with periodic breakdowns in their control. In group play, they may appear to empathize with other children to a degree. When one gets hurt and cries, they all get serious. But this may be as much a reflection of their concerns about their own bodies and well-being as about their friend's. They won't develop real empathy for a while yet.

The primary social skill that most parents wish their children to develop is simply "proper behavior." They want their children to shift from the egocentric perspective toward understanding the needs and wants of others so that they can learn to live in harmony. What is considered appropriate behavior is culturally prescribed. This socialization process may be more difficult in our society, where independence and individuality are emphasized, than in cultures where conformity is the goal. We present an inherent conflict to children—we want them to be independent, yet we also want them to follow all the rules.

Play

Play is a very important part of life for two-year-olds. It is the mechanism through which they explore roles, test out ideas, incorporate their observations about the world, and deal with their emotions, all important in the quest for themselves.

The nature of play changes during the third year, growing more complex and sophisticated in its themes and in the involvement of peers. It also becomes more constructive and purposeful. For example, once a child is adept at scaling the sofa, climbing it for its own sake will prove less of a thrill. Now the toddler is ready to pretend it's a mountain, so its entertainment level rises again. No longer will the child be happy simply to watch a ball bounce up and down; now, he or she will construct a rudimentary game: How high can it bounce? How far can it be thrown? Can it hit the toy truck? This type of play signals not only greater mental maturity, but neuromotor development as well. First with a parent and later with peers, the two-year-old will engage in cooperative play with the ball.

As language skills develop, more of the child's play becomes symbolic. This may take the form of pretend play, in which the actions of adults are imitated, or of fantasy play, in which the child's imagination takes him or her farther afield. A toddler might, for example, pretend to be a fireman, wearing a bowl for a hat and carrying a rope for a hose. Later, in fantasy play, the child might become a fire truck, rushing through the house making siren noises. This type of play allows the child to test reality, comparing it and differentiating it from inner fantasy. He or she may scold a teddy bear in the same words and tone Mother uses, or, if toilet training has begun, place a favorite doll on the potty. Much of children's early pretend play is an imitation of their parents, who are still the major force in their lives. Later this imitation is extended to other adults and to their peers.

At 24 months, most children engage only in parallel play with peers. Two children of this age will sit near each other and may even play with similar toys, but will not actually play with each other. They may both be pounding blocks on the floor, or each may be completely unaware of what the other is doing, but they will be aware of each other's presence.

As the year progresses, however, the two-year-old will become very interested in what other children are doing and will begin to imitate them. Eventually, in small groups of children, all will be doing more or less the same thing. If one starts hopping, others will join in, and when one falls, the others will fall, too. But interaction is still peripheral at this age and the similarity in action is more the result of imitation than of any sense of cooperation, which does not develop until later. Because children are still quite aggressive with each other, grabbing and pulling toys away, hitting and shoving, their play must be closely supervised.

Pediatrician/author Dr. T. Berry Brazelton and others have noted that play among groups of children this age follows a distinct and regular pattern. It will build from quiet play into loud play, peak at an excited frenzy, then settle into a recuperative lull before building up again. The wails of pain that erupt occasionally from these encounters usually have more to do with the natural cycle of play—it has reached a climax and needs to "cool down"—than with any serious injury. Often children will engage stoically in tussling far more violent than the event that produces the tears, only to yelp later at the smallest injury once they sense the time has come to stop playing. Parental awareness of this and

other patterns of child play can help in planning meals and naps to take advantage of the "lulls."

Appropriate playthings for two-year-olds are those that are safe, simple, durable, and inexpensive. The most successful toys—ones that children will keep coming back to—are those with multiple uses. Blocks, for example, can be boats one day, trains the next, and doll furniture next week. Toys without a lot of specific detail allow children to use their imagination. They are often more interested in things their parents use than they are in manufactured toys.

Manipulative toys such as balls, puzzles, nesting boxes or eggs, and stacking rings, are appealing to two-year-olds. So are toys and material that allow them to express their creativity—clay, finger paint, large crayons, dress-up clothes. Children at this age also enjoy moving in time to music, especially strongly rhythmic pieces, such as marches.

While parents should try to provide a variety of playthings, what is more important is variety of play: the child should have opportunities to play alone, with others, outside, inside, at a playground or another's home. The healthy child is one who eagerly exploits those opportunities.

COMMON CONCERNS OF PARENTS

Discipline

Discipline is often thought of in negative terms and confused with punishment. Actually, discipline is a positive process, a way in which parents help their children develop self-control and through which they pass on their values. If parents think of discipline as a way of showing love, they may find it less difficult to be firm at times when they are tempted to give in to a temper tantrum or to indulge a child's whims.

Parents can be more effective in their discipline if they understand what they want for their children—and for themselves. What kind of behavior do they value? What would they like to see less of? What are they willing to put up with and where do they draw the line? It may be helpful to make a written list (which will have to be changed every few months as the child develops). Some parents are more concerned than others, for example, with having neatly dressed children or preserving the living room as an adult oasis. Others would rather let the child make a mess (within limits) if it provides some diversion that allows them time to enjoy the newspaper. They might be willing, say, to let their two-year-old play with water on the cellar floor, where there is a floor drain and where splashes won't stain the wallpaper, although they would not allow it on the dining-room rug.

Discipline is basically a matter of setting limits and enforcing them—and the two-year-old very much needs limits. At this age, the child wants self-control, not only to satisfy parents, but also to meet individual needs for greater independence. But it's still out of reach, and the two-year-old can find this very frustrating. By using firm, consistent discipline, parents can ease a child's anxiety over control. Erik Erikson, in his seminal work *Childhood and Society*, has a wonderfully precise description of this concept of parental attitude and behavior: "firmly reassuring."

It is much easier to set limits now than later. Generally it will take three or four consecutive and consistent attempts at enforcing a specific behavior for the child to stop testing and accept the parent's wishes. Even though two-year-olds have strong instincts and urges that they want satisfied, they also have a deep love for their parents that provides the best incentive for doing well. This strong relationship with parents and a sincere desire to please them is what drives the two-year-old toward self-control. Of course, parental love and approval are not the only rewards for being "good"—behaving properly also reinforces a sense of mastery and raises self-esteem.

Unfortunately, a child's good behavior often goes unrecognized because it is expected as a matter of course. It is ignored, while bad behavior usually gets a response. And since children prefer any attention—even scolding—to no attention, they tend to repeat behavior that gets that attention. Rewarding good behavior can be as simple as saying "That was great. I'm proud of you," or even just making eye contact, or giving a squeeze or a pat. It can also be a system of gold stars for certain achievements (getting through a meal without spilling or dropping food), with a treat after a certain number of stars are earned. The treat can be an extra bedtime story or a trip to the park—it does not have to be food or a material reward.

Approval also enhances the child's self-esteem. If it is outweighed by disapproval, the child may either become submissive, following the rules automatically without internalizing them, or may become defiant and lose respect for the rules altogether. A child will respond better to a challenge for success than to punishment for failure. When parents tell a child what they want done and how they expect the child to act, rather than emphasizing what they don't want, they provide something positive to strive for rather than something that must be given up or avoided. For example, if a child stands up in the bathtub and the parent wants the child (for safety reasons) to sit down, the parent should say: "please sit down" rather than "don't stand up." Then the youngster can be praised for doing something positive that pleases the parent.

Any punishment that is meted out should be immediate and appropriate; also it should be brief. After it is over, the child should be shown an alternate way of behaving. (Pulling the cat's tail is not acceptable, but tugging on a security blanket is. Pouring water from the bathtub onto the floor is not acceptable, but pouring water from a plastic cup into the bathtub is.)

Many parents find that time out is a very effective method of discipline because it removes the child from the situation that stimulated the behavior and temporarily isolates him or her from the parent, who is still the main source of love and approval. Time out can mean sending the child to sit in the corner or to go to his or her room for a short period (two or three minutes) to think about the misbehavior. The time out is not a substitute for correct behavior. In other words, if the offense was refusing to put blocks away, they will still have to be put away after the time out, or another time out will be called. (For more information on time out, see chapter 12, Emotional and Intellectual Development.)

Rare is the parent who hasn't contemplated a slap or a spank in a desperate moment for a child whose behavior is particularly obnoxious. Some give in to the impulse; some actually believe it is justified in certain circumstances. Physical punishment may be a temporary outlet for parental pique, but as a means of teaching discipline, it is simply not effective. Physical restraint, denial of privilege, or some other restriction is a more effective way of dealing with the situation. Physical punishment may deter the child from a certain behavior, but it does not help establish self-control, which is the real goal of discipline.

A child's self-control does not develop smoothly. For a time, the two-year-old may compromise by doing things that he or she knows are forbidden and then indulging in self-scolding. Or a fantasy character may be created to take the blame for whatever naughtiness is committed. This is another way of testing the limits. The youngster may even progress to outright lying and denial. Although these sound like negative actions, they are, in fact, positive, showing that the child is aware of wrongdoing and that he or she is simply trying to avoid the consequences. Nevertheless, parents should not accept the fib or the imaginary culprit. By letting the child know that they recognize what is going on, they are teaching that the child must accept responsibility for his or her actions. On the other hand, parents should not fear that their child is headed on the road to crime. Lying and covering up are common in two- and three-year olds and if dealt with directly, are easily handled.

Conflicts will arise between parents and children quite frequently, and parents should choose their battles wisely. By ignoring some of the smaller contests, it's easier to concentrate on those that matter most. It's very easy to become emotionally involved in an encounter with an obstinate child, and that emotion can easily cloud judgment. It's also a good idea to let a child win every now and then to avoid fostering a sense of powerlessness.

A well-disciplined child is neither submissive nor unruly, but self-controlled with a strong sense of self-esteem. By the end of the third year, the youngster should have a good measure of self-control, even though he or she will not have what we consider a conscience. At this stage, actions are not governed by what is "right" or "wrong," but by what is accepted and what is prohibited. A true conscience will not emerge for several more years.

Toilet Training

Because parents will most likely introduce their children to the potty and the idea of controlling their bladder and bowel movements before 24 months, this subject is covered in detail in the previous chapter.

While training may begin toward the end of the second year, the goals are not accomplished until later. The first success is often reported between 24 and 30 months, and daytime toilet training is often completed by 30 months. Nap and night training may closely follow daytime training or may take another year or more. Boys tend to take a few months longer than girls.

The child is the key to efficient and trouble-free toilet training. Brazelton's concept of child-oriented toilet training often means waiting until the heat of the negativism phase subsides, when the child has a greater interest in pleasing parents and being like them. Trying to train a child too early (before 18 months) can be arduous, as the child has insufficient verbal skills and little understanding of what's expected. It may, in fact, take longer at this age than it would if the parents were to wait a few months. The child may also suffer more relapses and loss of control than if trained later. Indeed, parents may not want to begin training until well into the third year, when they sense the child is ready for it. Children who are obviously uncomfortable about being in a wet or dirty diaper and want to be changed, prefer training pants to diapers, show a new interest in dressing neatly, imitate parents' toilet habits, and communicate with gestures or words when their bladder is full or they feel a bowel movement coming are indicating their readiness to begin training.

Child-care and Early Childhood Programs

Much more study is needed before we can be sure of all the consequences—positive and negative—of children being cared for from an early age in daycare or other child-care situations that don't involve the parent. There are some who feel that the best situation for a child is to be reared in the home by the mother for at least the first three years. On the other hand, some studies show that child care outside the home is not only not harmful, but can even produce children who are more peer-oriented and independent than children who remain at home. In the end, it must be an individual decision, made by balancing the needs of the child against the needs of the parents. What is right for one family, or even a particular family at a particular stage in life, may not be right for another family or another time.

The issue is fraught with emotion and clouded by individual perceptions and the vast differences among children. The parents, especially the mother, may feel guilty if daycare is used as a matter of choice, or oppressed and frustrated if it is forced upon them by economic necessity. What matters most in the end is quality care, not who renders it. Good daycare is certainly preferable to having a frustrated and unfulfilled mother in the home. (For more information on daycare, see chapter 16).

There is certainly no need for children to take part in early-education classes, especially before the age of three. Even after that, it is uncertain whether these classes will provide educational advantages. Yet, if carefully chosen, they can be a good opportunity for the child to meet other children, and they can provide a break for the primary caregiver.

Nursery schools or preschools, beginning as early as the third year, do seem to help socialize the child. There children are exposed to the structure of the classroom (however loose it may be at this age) and to following instructions from someone other than the primary caregiver. Having gone through the separation process already, children who have attended preschool may adjust more easily to kindergarten than those who have not.

Bedtime and Sleep Problems

Even a child who has not earlier shown resistance to bedtime may begin to resist in the third year.

Children at this age may take longer to unwind and settle down because they are still stimulated from the learning activities of their days. Also, they are now very social animals and would prefer to be with the family than to go to bed alone. But most of all, they are experiencing separation anxiety anew, and bedtime means separation. And so the ritual starts: calling out to ask for water, another story, a toy, to go to the bathroom, or just to ask a question. Sometimes the need is very real—the child may be wet and uncomfortable, genuinely thirsty, afraid, or ill —but most of the time the requests are merely tactics to accomplish the main mission: to prolong contact with the parent and delay bedtime.

Not all bedtime rituals are bad. Actually, parents can use them to ease the separation and help the transition to sleep. A quiet story time, a lullaby, listening to soft music, being rocked or cuddled, saying prayers, brushing teeth, kissing dolls or favorite stuffed animals good-night, looking for the evening star, making wishes on stars, turning on the nightlight, being tucked in—all can provide some comfort by their familiarity, signify that bedtime is near, and help the child wind down. For many parents, this is a very special time alone with the child and one that they cherish. Most families, often drawing on their own childhood rituals, find that they develop a specific set of activities that are repeated each night in the same order.

It is helpful, too, if parents establish a specific bedtime and hold to it as much as possible. For one thing, they are entitled to have part of the evening to themselves, even if the child is playing quietly in bed or listening to music rather than sleeping. Setting a specific bedtime also allows the parent to monitor the amount of sleep the child actually needs. A child who is put to bed at eight and is always awake before six probably just doesn't need as much sleep as the child who doesn't awaken until half past eight. If the parents in this case would rather sleep until seven, they can try keeping the child up an hour longer at night. There is no rule that two-year-olds must be in bed by eight, as long as they get adequate rest. A child who is active, eating normally, continuing to grow at a regular rate, and usually good-natured is getting enough sleep.

After the bedtime ritual, it is best for the parent to say good-night and then leave the room. Children will invariably call out once or twice with questions or requests, and most parents will allow a few of these calls. If the child wants water or a favorite toy, for example, the parent can get it, but can do so without comment so that the social contact is not reinforced. Also, a limit needs to be set ("Okay, I'll tell you what special things we're going to do tomorrow, but first you'll have to promise me no more

questions, because it's time for you to be asleep") and enforced simply by ceasing to respond.

Some parents will remain in the room until the child falls asleep. This has a potential for problems, because the child then associates the parent's presence with going to sleep and won't sleep unless the parent is there. Further, the child expects the parent to be there if he or she wakes up.

Children who persist in calling out or in crying for the parent to return, or who go to sleep, then wake up and cry, present a dilemma for parents. It is difficult to be dogmatic about bedtime; indeed, experts often disagree about how to handle the situation. But the majority seem to concur that the best way to deal with a child who wakes and cries, or who cries after being put to bed, is to check to be sure that there is no real problem and then to leave. If the child is afraid, the parent can stay for a few minutes to reassure the child but announce that he or she will be leaving soon because it is bedtime. Patience and perseverance are key in this matter.

Most pediatricians advise against allowing the child to come into the parents' room and, especially, their bed. This is an easy habit to establish and a hard one to break. On the other hand, some parents enjoy the togetherness and find that it is all right from time to time. In other societies where it is more common, there is some indication that the children themselves outgrow it in a few years.

Although it may be acceptable when the child is younger, sleeping in the parents' bed intrudes on their privacy. It also inhibits their sexual relations or, if it doesn't, exposes the child to sounds or actions he or she doesn't understand or may misinterpret and become fearful about. If necessary, the parent can lie down with the child in the child's room, but it should be understood that this, too, may become a ritual.

If bedtime delaying tactics really become a problem, parents can try the stoic approach, often much more difficult for them than for the child. This means only going to the child's room if his or her crying is so frantic that they are sure something is wrong. Otherwise they must make it clear that bedtime means no more requests and that they do not intend to respond unless there is a serious problem. The child will surely test them and it may take at least a week or two of diligence, but it will usually work.

Fears

Childhood fears are common and quite predictable. Children will be afraid of different things at different ages, ranging from loud noises in infancy through animals and supernatural beings at school age, and sexuality as teenagers. Two-year-olds are afraid of an astonishing variety of things, from vacuum cleaners and bathtub drains to darkness, animals (real and imaginary), and of course, separation from parents. These fears are usually transitory, lasting a few weeks to a few months. They should not be of concern to parents as long as the fears are appropriate for the child's stage of development, do not persist for many months, and do not grow so overwhelming that they interfere with family life.

The fears should not be ignored, however, nor the child belittled. Putting down even preposterous notions ("Don't be silly, David. You wouldn't *fit* down the bathtub drain") will only make the child more anxious because it amplifies self-doubt while failing to provide a mechanism for dealing with the fear.

The best advice for dealing with fears is "acknowledge, accommodate, but don't avoid." Rather than denying the possibility of monsters under the bed, the parent can help look for them, use magic to ward them off ("Let's close our eyes and clap twice to make them go away") or find another harmless tactic for dealing with them. When the fear involves something that can't be avoided for a time—bathing or vacuuming, for example—the parent can help prepare the child. If the child is afraid of the vacuum cleaner, he or she can be warned beforehand when it is going to be used, so the sudden noise won't be startling. The parent might suggest that the youngster play in another room, put on some music, or hold a comforting object (doll, stuffed animal, or blanket). If the child is primarily afraid of the noise and not the machine itself, the parent could offer to let the child turn the vacuum on and off, so the toddler has some feeling of control over it.

More than 30 years ago, child psychoanalyst Selma Fraiberg wrote *The Magic Years*, a classic of child-development literature that is still a popular guide for parents today, in part because of its wonderfully accurate descriptions of children's behavior and practical suggestions for dealing with it. She relates how one child developed a fear of being sucked down the bathtub drain after she had almost lost the teddy bear she threw down a flushing toilet, then stood in the tub while her mother drained the water. To counter this fear, Fraiberg suggested letting the child play with bathtub toys in the sink, where she could control the water and the drain and play out the bath sequence in an environment she could manipulate. At the same time she would be learning about relative size and would come to realize that the toys would not fit down the drain, just as she wouldn't. In the meantime, her mother could

continue to bathe her, being sure that the drain was not emptied until after, perhaps well after, she had left the tub.

Forcing the child to confront something that is terrifying will only make the fear worse and will have a negative effect on the child's relationship with the parent. Rather than forcing a child to pet the neighbor's dog when the child is afraid of even the friendliest of animals, the parent can pet the dog while the youngster observes from a place where he or she feels safe. Parent and child can pet toy dogs, look at picture books of dogs, talk about different kinds of dogs, and gradually prepare for a time when the child feels more comfortable in a dog's presence.

Eating

Parents are understandably concerned that their two-year-olds get a nutritious diet. But this concern sometimes leads to an overemphasis on eating three perfectly balanced meals a day. As long as the child is getting sufficient calories to continue growing normally, there is no need to adhere to rigid rules about meals. In fact, these rules can be counterproductive.

Rarely do children in families who can provide sufficient food suffer malnutrition. If the amount of junk food in the house is limited and the child is offered a variety of foods—fresh fruits and vegetables; bread, grains, and cereals; and small amounts of protein sources—he or she will select a diet that is reasonably balanced. It may be only bananas, celery, and cheese for a month or so, but ultimately tastes will broaden and it will all balance out. In terms of quantity, children can survive quite well and all of their nutritional needs can be met by only one or two meals a day.

If parents understand and accept this, they will be able to bear with equanimity the eating habits of their two-year-olds. Once they are able to become disinterested parties at the dinner table, never showing that it matters to them what the child eats or whether he or she eats at all, they will find that half the battle is won.

Likewise, parents should not be concerned about table manners at this age. Children should be allowed to feed themselves as much as possible. The sense of mastery that they achieve by making their own choices and eating at their own pace lessens their inclination to reject every new food put in front of them. If the table is a happy, unpressured place, the child eventually will want to eat whatever the parents eat.

(For additional information, see chapter 5, Nutrition for Toddlers and Preschoolers.)

SUMMING UP

THE THIRD YEAR, the epitome of toddlerhood, brings tremendous advances in the child's intellectual, social, and psychological growth. The catalyst for all of this is the burgeoning development of language. Functional vocabulary more than triples during these 12 months, but more important, the child begins to be able to communicate feelings, wants, and needs.

Underpinning the growth of language are several developmental milestones. The child leaves the sensorimotor stage where only the present and the visible are understood and enters a stage of representational thought that allows him or her to remember and repeat events of the past, to anticipate events in the future, and to understand that the people and objects not physically present nevertheless exist. Language becomes not only a means of relating to others but also a device for trying out ideas and working through problems. This symbolic thought is evident in communication and in play.

All of this sets the stage for the development of self-control, the major accomplishment of the third year. The child begins the year at the height of negativism, in the throes of "the terrible twos." As mastery of language helps build self-esteem and establish independence, the child begins to substitute words for actions and is able to deal intellectually with situations that in the previous year provoked only a physical response. Parents play a major role in helping the child to gain self-control by setting limits and enforcing them consistently. Great strides are made when limits are internalized and the child can refrain from acting on every urge and want. This self-control extends from toilet training to behavior restraint, as the desire to please parents and bolster self-esteem grows. As the year ends, the child leaves negativism behind—at least until the teenage years—and becomes a loving and more happily independent three-year-old.

11 The Preschool Years

Carol Ann Brown, R.N., M.S.

INTRODUCTION

DURING THE FOURTH, fifth, and sixth years of life, children leave toddlerhood and enthusiastically pursue the learning tasks of the preschool years. The rapid growth associated with infancy has leveled off; the preschooler develops rapidly in terms of skills rather than gaining noticeable inches and pounds. During this period the child develops even more language, self-care, fine and gross motor skills, as well as the emotional, intellectual, and social skills necessary for the launch into the school years.

Each child develops at an individual pace influenced by genes, diet, general health, the relationship to the primary caretaker, and the family's socioeconomic status. Even with all these variables, most children mature at a similar rate, displaying behavior and mastering skills within a broad range of normal.

NUTRITIONAL NEEDS/ MEALTIMES

PRESCHOOLERS NEED FEWER calories in proportion to their size and body weight than they needed during infancy. Growth is more linear, and the youngster may take on a longer, leaner appearance. This physical change—the lengthening of legs in relation to the trunk—is normal for the preschool years and is often accompanied by a decrease in the child's appetite.

Parents frequently worry when their children begin to be less interested in food, but no normal, healthy child offered a balanced and varied diet will starve. It is useless to force a child to eat more than is wanted, and the power struggle can lead to destructive conflicts acted out at mealtime. Certain practices, however, can encourage good eating habits. Child-size portions are more appealing than a heaped plate (the child can be encouraged to ask for seconds to satisfy a hearty appetite). Assistance can be offered in cutting food, but children at this stage should be encouraged to do as much as possible for themselves. Parents should encourage independence and success—sandwiches cut in quarters are easily managed by small hands, a half-full cup is less likely to spill than one filled to the top. As always, good parenting involves sensitivity in creating a context for a child's involvement and growth. Tolerance and patience are required.

As noted in chapters 5 and 10, a preschooler's attitudes toward food can be quirky. While some children will eat anything, more often three- to six-year-olds will be stubbornly ritualistic about what they will eat, how it must be prepared, and the particular manner in which it must be served—down to such details as in what bowl or on which plate. Within reason, accommodate such requests—they will eventually be outgrown.

New foods should be introduced in a relaxed context. A skeptical child can often be reassured by saying, "Just try it—if you don't want it, leave it on your plate." Children who are included at adult mealtimes will respond more readily to parental attitudes toward food and will eventually express an interest in sampling what the grownups eat. Involvement in food preparation is fun for the children and serves as another way to introduce them to unfamiliar dishes.

The healthy social activity characteristic of mealtimes can sometimes distract a small child from the tasks of self-feeding. A parent can approach this problem in several ways. Mealtime activity can be curtailed somewhat so the child can concentrate on eating, or the child can eat before the family meal, joining the adults for company, tastes, and perhaps dessert.

Regardless of the stimuli, children frequently eat different amounts at various meals; nourishing between-meal snacks are an excellent way to fill in the gaps. (For a more detailed discussion, see chapter 5, Nutrition for Toddlers and Preschoolers.)

BEDTIME

CHILDREN BETWEEN the ages of four and six years need approximately 11 to 12 hours of sleep during each 24-hour period, but anything from 8 to 14 hours falls within the normal range. The precise number varies from child to child and with the particulars of current activities. A child in the midst of an unusually stimulating situation will be likely to sleep less than usual, even though he or she may show signs of fatigue.

An overtired child manifests fatigue in a manner similar to a tired adult, but the child rarely understands the relationship between state of mind and the need for sleep. A tired child responds more slowly than usual—even to favorite foods, people, and activities. When tired, the child may be restless and irritable, unable to say what he or she wants. The youngster also may be "too tired" to sleep.

Generally a child will sleep as much as is needed, but those who do not get adequate rest over a long period of time tend to be more susceptible to infections and other illnesses. The parent can help

by reducing the activity as bedtime approaches or by creating a subdued atmosphere to encourage a nap. (The four- and five-year-old may not take an afternoon nap, but nonetheless a quiet time is useful for both child and parents.)

By the time a child is four, it's likely that the "delay-bedtime-at-all-costs" struggle common to the twos and threes will be resolved. Although parents may no longer have to cajole a child when it's time to retire, bedtime routines will still help make nightly partings go smoothly. A quiet storytelling or picture book sharing is a time-honored ritual that allows a parent, grandparent, or other loved one to share private moments with the child at day's end. A warm bath, putting toys to bed, and other such tactics also may be useful.

Night Fears

Nightmares and waking fears are very common for four- and five-year-olds who can firmly believe that monsters lurk beneath the bed and that dragons are hiding in the closet. A child who is too fearful to fall asleep usually responds more positively to proofs than logic. A look under the bed and inside the closet often provides more reassurance than words. Selma Fraiberg, the noted childhood authority, suggests a bedside cologne atomizer, christened "monster spray," which can serve as the youngster's magic weapon against nighttime monsters. A night-light and slightly open door also can be reassuring.

When a child awakens from a nightmare, a parent should go to the bedside and assure him or her that all is okay. A parent's presence, supplemented by a hug, kiss, and sip of water, is usually enough to erase the scary atmosphere that lingers after a nightmare. Childhood fears of this time are likely to diminish by the sixth birthday, when a child can further distinguish the real from the unreal.

IMPORTANCE OF ROUTINES

THE IMPORTANCE OF consistent eating and sleeping routines goes beyond the concrete concerns of nutrition and restfulness. Routines imply predictability —for the child, an accumulating sense of control over basic elements of the environment. The need for orderliness and stability, considered by many theoreticians to be as basic to human survival as needs for food and shelter, is critical during the four- to six-year-old period, when children are just beginning to learn how their actions affect the world around them.

Specific bedtime, mealtime, and other routine

activities (play, bath, and so forth) help the child organize and predict events. The absence of predictability causes anxiety at the expense of growing curiosity and independence. If a child is anxious about when parents will return home from work, for example, he or she cannot constructively utilize the available time to play and explore. In contrast, being able to count on arrival within a certain time frame gives the child a sense of security and satisfaction.

This is not to say that parents must not ever deviate from schedules and routines. When disruption is necessary, however, advance warning and an explanation of what to expect gives the child a sense of security. The effort to sustain as many of the normal routines as possible under altered circumstances (such as a prolonged visit or a move) will ease the child's anxiety.

The older child, whose language and logic abilities are more highly developed, benefits more from detailed explanations. Younger children may understand the words, but not the meaning. When explanations are offered, it's important for the parent to find out what the child has, indeed, understood.

CHARACTERISTIC BEHAVIOR

THE CHARACTERISTIC BEHAVIOR of children at various ages reflects the behind-the-scenes maturation of the nervous system combined with the skeletal and muscular development of their bodies. The lengthening preschooler not only looks different, but the youngster does different things. It is always miraculous to watch children who could barely stand alone at one year scampering recklessly as three- or four-year-olds. Both actions are examples of gross motor skills. A one-year-old derives pleasure from repeatedly dropping objects into a container; the three-year-old exerts independence by bathing with a parent standing by. These actions are examples of fine motor skills.

The child acquires gross and fine motor skills in a sequence that reflects the maturation of motor pathways. As the pathways continue to mature, the child can refine motor skills further, learning to draw and cut rather than scribble or tear, and graduating from walking to skipping. (Table 11.1 provides examples of age-appropriate fine and gross motor skill development.)

Often the combination of activities characteristic of an age group and the emotional development of children at that age (see What Preschoolers Are Like, next page) form age-typical personalities. The

three-year-old appears reckless and brash; the four-year-old is confident and informative; and the five-year-old appears anxiously aware of more than he or she can manage.

The four-year-old approaches independence in self-care activities because fine motor skill has developed sufficiently by this point. This is a great leap

Table 11.1 **FINE AND GROSS MOTOR SKILLS**

Gross Motor Skills	Fine Motor Skills
3 years Pedals a tricycle; jumps from a low step; can go to toilet unaided; can get undressed in most situations; can go up and down stairs using alternating feet without holding on; throws large ball with one hand; can put on own coat without assistance; catches soft object with both arms.	Begins to use blunt scissors; strings large beads on shoelace; can copy a circle; can help with simple household tasks (dusting, picking up); can wash and dry hands, with some wetting of clothes; can brush teeth, but not adequately; can imitate a bridge made of three blocks; can pull pants up and down for toileting without assistance.
3½ years Skips on one foot; hops forward on both feet; runs well without falling; kicks large ball; twists upper body while holding feet in one place; uses hands to get up from floor; catches soft object with hands; catches large ball with arms.	Can cut straight lines with scissors without tearing paper; manipulates pieces into position for simple puzzles; can weave yarn randomly through a card; places small pegs in pegboard; unbuttons small button; can eat from spoon without spilling.
4 years Jumps well; hops forward on one foot; may catch a large bounced ball with hands; walks backward; catches soft object with one hand; catches small ball with arms.	Cuts around pictures with scissors; can copy a square; can button small buttons; may bathe self, with assistance; folds napkin into a triangle or a rectangle; outlines a picture with yarn.
5 years Can jump rope; runs lightly on toes; alternates feet to skip; gets up without using hands; catches small ball with two hands.	May be able to print own name; copies a triangle; dresses without assistance; may be able to lace shoes; can put toys away neatly; bathes self; threads small beads on a string; eats with fork.

in terms of self-feeding, in dressing and undressing activities, and in toileting—all prerequisites to many nursery school programs. (See Preparation for School, near the end of the chapter.)

WHAT PRESCHOOLERS ARE LIKE

THE EFFORT TO ADAPT to and organize the environment compels preschool children. Their limited experiences and understanding of the world are constantly augmented. Throughout this period, children develop new perceptions of their surroundings that increase in complexity and accuracy.

At three years old, the child does not yet have the power to reason out several ways of looking at a situation. The only way a three-year-old can view any given set of circumstances is "my way," not because the three-year-old is a stubborn breed, but because a child of that age hasn't developed the thought processes required to picture a situation from someone else's viewpoint. The three-year-old's vision is self-centered. Having recently confirmed the meaning of "I," he will hardly give it up easily. By five or six, a child engaged in a verbal argument with a peer actively experiences that two people can see the same situation from different viewpoints.

At three years old, the child has just begun to distinguish between reality and unreality. To three-year-olds, anything's possible. Temperamentally, three-year-olds are expansive and imaginative. The parent seems all powerful and even magical. As a matter of fact, magic plays an important part in the view of three-year-olds, who may actively believe that there are creatures hiding under the bed, that things have feelings, and that wishing can make it so. A child of this age may experience extreme guilt over a wish because he or she cannot always distinguish between having a "bad thought" and doing "something bad."

At three and four, children will often tell white lies. Although untruthfulness should always be corrected by adults (who usually can "magically" see right through the lie), the child's intention is not malicious. Rather, white lies are based on overt fantasies in which the child feels the wishes as if they were true: for example, "I rode on the elephant at the zoo." Lies may also be based on parent-pleasing or wishfulness, in which cases children tell adults what they think will make the adults happiest.

Harsh scolding for "lying" is an overreaction and may have the negative effect of making the child feel ashamed of thoughts or feelings, as opposed to giving the child the confidence to express them. The adult should speak with the child and guide him or her to tell the truth. The parent of a small child who lies often for reasons of self-protection should examine the intensity of his or her own reactions to the child's mishaps or wishes. (See Family Relationships, next page.)

BUILDING BLOCKS FOR THE CHILD'S THINKING

WITH EACH BIRTHDAY, the preschooler accumulates additional building blocks for thought capabilities. In the course of these years, the child exchanges belief in magic and a solely self-centered view for more accurate logical thinking.

At three, concrete perceptions and actions in the immediate environment are the sole contributors to the child's thought and expectations. By the end of the fifth year, the child can construct alternative possibilities out of the information available. For example, at three, when Mommy gets her pocketbook, it means one thing only to the child—that Mommy is going out. Through the development of what Piaget labeled intuitive thinking, the older child can imagine or reconstruct other meanings for this action.

The child's ability to follow multiple directions also evolves during these years. Because the young child can only perceive the environment one element at a time, the meaning of consecutive actions is lost. (Although the child can follow only one direction at a time, he or she still enjoys the results of an adult-supervised series of actions, such as preparing chocolate pudding.) As the attention span lengthens, the child becomes aware of more elements in the surroundings, as well as cause-and-effect relationships; and he or she gains the ability to follow two or more directions in sequence. By five years old, the child is capable of following a three-step direction in the proper order.

The child's work of organizing and mastering the environment is dependent on a growing ability to classify objects and experiences. First the child matches identical objects, then groups similar objects, and finally sorts various objects according to a constant standard. Once the child can grasp more abstract groupings, he or she can order objects by graduating size, color, or shape. The ability to isolate one quality in an otherwise changing group of objects does not commonly emerge until the end of the child's sixth year.

FAMILY RELATIONSHIPS

THE SAME CHILD WHO, as an infant, experiences only "self," and as a toddler falls in love with Mother (or some other primary caregiver), further expands his or her horizons as a preschooler. The preschooler's world includes the whole family unit, where the child learns through experience the lessons of emotional and social development.

The family atmosphere is determined by the parents. Loving, firm, and consistent parents rear children who feel loved, who understand and appreciate existing rules of behavior, and who know what to expect. The child can apply these lessons-by-example to interactions with others in an ever-widening sphere that includes playgroups, nursery and elementary school, and, eventually, the world at large.

There are periods of crisis for the developing child. During these times, responsive parents may observe personality changes in their child. These cycles of behavior occur at predictable ages throughout childhood. Awareness of these tense ages may help parents extend the limits of their patience and reassure themselves. Many parents worry that if their children were "more normal" they would never show signs of nervousness or anxiety. However, anxiety is a normal by-product of growth. The parent who can remain calm and reassuring during the child's tense periods will benefit the child and help ameliorate rather than exaggerate the inevitable tensions of growing up.

SELF-ESTEEM

THE PARENTAL RESPONSE toward children and their moods serves as a model for the child's own response to individual feelings. If Mommy and Daddy are loving, the child feels lovable. If they are proud, the child is proud. The child internalizes parental reactions and makes them his or her own. Positive reactions contribute to a positive self-image for the child. Parents can guide children toward healthy responses to negative emotions. (See Parenting and Discipline, next page.)

The preschool period is a time of mastery for the child during which good feelings about self also are derived from accomplishments. The parental role is to create an environment that keeps up with the child's developing capabilities. At three, four, and five, the child's personality and individual interests begin to emerge. The parent can respond by facilitating activities that both suit the child's interests and will safely challenge the child. The parent

may also encourage the preschool-age child who can be simultaneously attracted to and fearful of the unfamiliar.

A third and significant source of self-esteem also emerges in the fourth and fifth year: the child learns to feel the mother's (or primary caregiver's) love and approval by conjuring a mental image of the loved object. This process eventually helps the child to tolerate separation experiences.

SEPARATION

NO MATTER HOW grown up a child appears to be, and regardless of how well separation is tolerated, the youngster is never too old to need physical affection. Rather than a sign of dependence as some parents fear, coming back for hugs serves to refuel the child for the anxiety-provoking but rewarding challenge of separation.

The preschooler is between two worlds—the known and the unknown—one comforting, the other attractive but possibly threatening. As a result, the child tends to vacillate between grown-up and infantile behavior, feeling independent and dependent and alternating between confidence ("I know how") and frustration ("I can't").

Because the preschool-age child lacks the ability to think abstractly, what is unknown is unknowable except by experience. Locomotor skills have expanded the preschooler's range of experience, and language allows the child to understand and express more thoughts. Sometimes, however, the child wanders too far—physically and imaginatively—and can be frightened with the results of independence.

The continued interest and support of the caregiver eases the anxiety provoked by the child's ever-widening explorations. At younger ages (toddler), eye-contact suffices; as the child's range expands beyond eye-contact, parent-child talks augment the benefits of physical contact. This social time reassures the child of his or her value to the parent, and provides an opportunity for an exchange of warm feelings. The dialogue also provides the parent with an opportunity to "see what's going on" with the child.

One of the rewards of separation for the child is the discovery of meaningful relationships with other members of the family; the father, for example, when the mother has been the primary caregiver. Others outside the immediate family such as nursery-school teachers, babysitters, or a favored aunt or uncle may become the "apple" of the child's eye. The parent occasionally feels a loss, which is best overcome by pride in seeing the child emerge as a social, affectionate, and independent being.

Parent/child separation can illuminate the parents' need for privacy. Children can be helped to understand that parents need to share private time with one another. As the child separates and finds gratification in experiences apart from the parents, he or she perceives that the parents' relationship also exists apart from their relationship to the child. Just as the child's separation rewards the parents with an independent child, a strong relationship between the parents provides the child with a positive model of adult male-female intimacy.

SEX-ROLE IDENTIFICATION

DURING THE THIRD or fourth year, most children have had the opportunity to observe the differences between male and female genitalia. For many children, the immediate reaction is shock, particularly because of age-characteristic fears about body integrity and mutilation. Adjustment to the anatomical differences between the sexes occurs in stages.

Parents must provide information and reassurance to children that nothing has been taken away from girls or will be taken away from boys. In addition, children should be given simple accurate answers to inevitable questions about procreation. Parents should take care to get feedback from children, who often elaborately misconstrue even the most careful explanation. Boys will often express bitter disappointment that they cannot carry a child as can their beloved mother.

At this time, children of both sexes learn about their cultural as well as procreative roles. A positive identification with the parent of the same sex aids the child in accepting his or her gender.

Sexual curiosity is common; once a child has seen another child of the opposite sex naked, the impulse to explore is quite normal. Children discovered in sex play (with other children) should be guided toward another activity. Later, alone with a parent, they should be invited to ask questions to find out what they want to know and told that answers won't become evident by exploration at this life-stage. Although discouraged, the child should not be made to feel ashamed of sex play.

PARENTING AND DISCIPLINE

MUTUAL LOVE is the single most important element of parental authority. Out of that love evolve several mechanisms that allow parents to teach their children self-control, self-discipline, and the appropriate limits to behavior.

Children love their parents and want to be loved by them. This wish to be loved helps younger children aim for the parental approval elicited by "yes" behavior and avoid disapproval associated with "no."
As the child grows up, parental values are internalized. The child feels good if he or she does what the absent parent would want. The internalization of values occurs because parents dispense rewards, both tangible and intangible. By adopting the parent's values, children can be like the all-powerful parent who gives love and provides for basic needs.
Parents are role models for behavior. Through their actions they introduce their children to moral concepts and demonstrate appropriate ways to relate to others.

Constructive use of authority is the ultimate act of parental love. Children cannot succeed in the world at large unless they learn standards for their safety and for social cooperation with others. Nevertheless, the process of imposing the limits can cause anxiety in both parent and child.

The ideal use of authority benefits the child's welfare rather than the parent's convenience. Discipline provides an opportunity for the child to focus on individual choices; therefore, a child should not be punished for doing something that he or she didn't know *not* to do beforehand. The youngster should be informed of the limits rather than threatened with angry foreboding about "next time."

The meaning of disciplinary actions should be clear to the child and related to the misbehavior. For example, being told to sit on a chair for 15 minutes is more appropriate punishment for running out of the house without Mother's permission than a spanking or being deprived of television. The latter two alternatives tell the child nothing about behaving better, but the very act of sitting still for 15 minutes instructs the child to think before acting. The three-, four-, and five-year-old needs to be encouraged to take initiative, and necessary disciplinary measures should not discourage the child's freedom.

A parent who screams, slaps, or spanks out of anger does not teach the child about self-control; the violent, out-of-control parent demonstrates the opposite, providing a bad role model.

From three to five, children learn to substitute language for more primitive physical forms of aggression, and they should be encouraged to express their anger in constructive ways. A parent who says, "You've made me angry; this is why," demonstrates a way to express anger that doesn't hurt others. A five-year-old who wants a new doll may be angry when her mother says, "No, you can't have it now, but you may have it for your birthday." When the child says in response, "I'm very angry at you, Mommy," she safely imitates her mother's past reactions of displeasure yet remains comfortable with her own urgent wish for the doll. The child has demonstrated in a simple way that her wish is not bad in spite of the parental no.

The angry parent, on the other hand, creates a fearful child. The preschooler often responds to forays toward independence with guilt and fear of the unknown. Parental anger justifies the guilt and thus inhibits independence.

TWO-WAY COMMUNICATION

LANGUAGE SKILLS GROW exponentially during a child's third, fourth, and fifth years, and parents should play a central role in this development. The goal of language is communication, and attentive two-way communication with a child is one of parents' most important contributions. Children are most comfortable speaking when they feel they have an adult's full attention. Finishing a child's sentences, correcting grammar and pronunciation, or bombarding the child with a constant stream of quizlike questions takes away from the child's ability to express his or her own thoughts.

Yet children need to improve their language skills. A better way to teach these skills is to first listen and then repeat what they've said using correct vocabulary, grammar, and pronunciation. Children will feel that they have been heard and will begin to absorb correct usage.

Communication is a two-way street. When parents speak to a child, they should determine whether the youngster has correctly interpreted what has been said. Though children frequently *do* understand more than they can express, they often misunderstand what is said because of their limited understanding of the world. If misunderstanding occurs the parent should explain again in simpler terms.

Implications of Language and Speech

Language provides a medium to reach out with words and imagination. A child's increasing use of adverbs and adjectives parallels an increased comprehension of the ideas they express. The child who returns after the first day of elementary school and excitedly says, "Now I understand why they call it the first grade . . . because it's the *first* grade," has learned the meaning of a word that was previously just a reference. The lesson *is* exciting.

Speaking is an act of initiative that, like other expressions of will, requires parental encourage-ment. Parents can teach children by example: speaking clearly, speaking out for their needs and desires. A shy child who has the language skills but lacks the confidence to talk can be gently urged to "speak up" or "speak out." A whispered "Go ahead, say what you said to me" or "You sound so great when you speak loudly" or "You're right! Let them know the answer" may provide the encouragement the child needs.

At times a parent might wish the child would not speak up, particularly when the youngster has learned to insult others with profanities or "bathroom" talk. Although this should not be encouraged, this stage is as normal as the nonverbal stage. Verbal aggression is actually a step forward from less mature expressions of frustration or anger, like biting, hitting, or kicking. A child should be taught more appropriate ways to express angry feelings, rather than being discouraged from their expression altogether.

Stuttering

Most children go through stages when they stutter or mispronounce sounds or words. The repetition of words and phrases characterizes many children's speech, most commonly during the fourth year. Such a child should be provided with opportunities to speak in a relaxed, unpressured environment. A child with ongoing speech problems after the fourth year may need the special assistance of a speech therapist.

Vocabulary and Usage

By the time a child is four years old, his or her speech should be understood by a stranger at least 90 percent of the time, and the vocabulary at that age should be about 1,500 words.

The four-year-old understands and applies many of the regular rules of language, but not the exceptions. In English, he or she can add *s* to make plurals, and *ed* to indicate the past tense, but may make mistakes when these rules don't apply (The sheeps drinked the water). At four and a half to five, the child learns other endings; usually *ing* precedes the comparative *er*. With the help of patient and nonjudgmental parents and teachers, the child will have begun to master even exceptions to grammatical rules by the end of the first year in school.

PLAY

"IT'S JUST CHILD'S PLAY" is taken to mean activity that is easy to do and perhaps insignificant. But play is hardly insignificant; it is a child's lifework. Through play, defined by Webster's as "the spontaneous activity of children," the child not only engages in activity for pure enjoyment (a benefit in itself) but also learns about and tests the environment; discovers, practices, and masters physical and intellectual skills, and learns how to live with others.

Play is active. Through play the child exercises physical and intellectual abilities during all stages of development. The repetitive and ritualistic play of preschoolers is a form of practice that leads to mastery. An increase in the control of fine and gross motor skills (see Table 11.2), contributes to the child's self-esteem ("I can do it!"). Age-appropriate materials provided by the parents can help children to enjoy the full range of their abilities and curiosities, whether they're playing alone or with others. (See box, next page.)

At all ages, physical play is beneficial as an energy release. Toys are increasingly important for preschoolers and serve multiple functions. Exercised muscles grow stronger. The child who is encouraged to learn new skills also develops confidence in physical ability, which will provide enjoyment—through sports, dancing, and physical fitness—throughout childhood and adult life.

Play is explorative. Through play children come to understand the world around them. Play provides direct experience of the concrete environment: Construction sets, hide 'n' seek, and finger painting eventually demonstrate principles of balance and structure, nuances of visibility, and elements of color.

Modeling themselves after adults, children also react to the adult world; in play they can try adult roles on for size. Play is a way for children to "work out" life situations, frustrations, and conflicts. Through play-acting a child may substitute versions of a reality that displeases. Particularly through solitary play, a child can exercise control over objects, say blocks or dolls, to balance experiences in a world that they cannot control.

As the child matures, he or she plays more with others. In nursery school, for example, children play all the time when they aren't eating or sleeping. Social play provides the opportunity for socio-dramatic play. Acting out make-believe situations with other children emerges in play at the age of three and dominates throughout the preschool years. Parents can provide materials—costumes and props to enrich imaginative play for their children.

During the school years, children learn how to play games with rules. Game-playing helps children deal with their frustration in learning and following rules. Younger children, whose desire to win is un-

Table 11.2 **CHARACTERISTIC BEHAVIOR**

Average Age	Expected Behaviors
3 years	Asks many "Why" questions. Talks in sentences using four or more words. May talk about fears. Can give first and last name. May explore environment outside the home if given the chance. "Chains" objects using subjective attribute for categorizing (e.g., red block next to yellow block next to yellow crayon). May retain urine through a night's sleep and wake up dry. May use profane language if older children or adults heard using it. Counts to three.
4 years	Begins many questions with "Where." May talk with imaginary playmate. May threaten to "run away from home." Can count to 5 and is learning number concepts. Can name color of three objects. Can give opposite of up (down), and hot (cold). Can associate familiar holidays with the season in which they occur. Completes 8- to 10-piece puzzle. Understands four to six prepositions. "Magical" power of thought at a peak.
5 years	May begin many questions with "How." Asks the meaning of words. Knows days of the week. Can count to 10. Talks "constantly." Can identify coins correctly. May need to be reminded to eat and to go to bathroom because attention is so externally focused, may not recognize subtle internal cues. Can follow a three-step direction in proper order. Capable of memorizing own address.

bridled yet stronger than their tactical abilities, may become frustrated with difficult games or formidable opponents.

All types of play—solitary, social, with or without materials, physical, and imaginative—are important to the developing child. The parent can help by providing play materials, helpful suggestions when necessary, and a nonfussy play environment where the child can be free. Last, but not least, children need their parents' help to arrange for playmates.

RECOMMENDED TOYS

3- and 4-year-olds

- Manipulative toys
- Trucks
- Trains—nonelectrical
- Puzzles—no more than six large pieces
- Blunt scissors
- Large crayons
- Construction paper
- Clay or Play-Doh
- Finger paints
- Magazines with lots of pictures
- Doll or cardboard figures for practicing buttoning, snapping, zipping, and lacing
- Percussive instruments—drum, xylophone, tambourine, triangle
- Whistles, kazoos
- Large metal or plastic tea set or kitchen set
- Dolls with easy-on-and-off clothing
- Toy telephone
- Blocks
- Magnetic letters and board
- Counting frames with large beads
- Picture books

5- and 6-year-olds

- Puppets (hand and finger)
- Blocks—larger sets with a variety of shapes
- Picture books with some simple words
- Cutout paper dolls
- Clay and Play-Doh
- Watercolors
- Finger paints
- Pail and shovel
- Trucks, trains (simple electrical toys, if provided with supervision)
- Simple board and card games
- Legos
- Activity books
- Chalk and chalkboard
- Dolls/Houses for imaginary play

SCHOOL

AT ONE TIME children were almost universally introduced to school when they began kindergarten. But times have changed; these days the increased number of homes where both parents—or the single parent—work, make it necessary to send the children to preschool. Even where it isn't a necessity, many parents desire to expose their children to a varied, stimulating environment. School helps the child learn about the outside world and gain independence from parents. Whether the process begins at three, four, or five depends upon parental resources, attitudes, and needs as well as the resources available in the community.

Regardless of when the child begins school, all parents want their child to commence formal education with maximum potential. How do parents foster that potential? Studies support what common sense dictates: A child whose questions are answered, whose curiosity is encouraged, who gains exposure to new information through interactive two-way communication with parents, and who as a result masters new skills and concepts, is likely to do well in school.

While educational toys are valuable to the child, continuous quizzes create tension about learning. The need to produce the *right* answer limits the child's curiosity and imagination. And when the parents always ask and the child answers, only one-way communication takes place. Exchanges of conversation between parent and child are better preparation for school because they teach the child that the giving and receiving of information—learning—is useful and enjoyable.

Early Entry

Early entry into the educational system through preschool or nursery school has advantages for children under five. For the three-year-old, the nursery school period comes when the child is feeling a need for independence. Short separations from the parents coupled with daily reunions can help the child master separation anxieties. For four-year-olds filled with curiosity, preschool opens a door to life outside the home and apart from the family. They learn to relate to other children and to adults other than their parents. In a preschool program, the child can expand and satisfy his or her interest in the world, life, and people.

For children who come from learning disadvantaged homes, government-financed preschool programs (Headstart) can help bridge the gap between home and kindergarten. Children who enter kindergarten with solid skills will have an advantage throughout their education.

Preschool or nursery school has advantages over early entry into kindergarten. The child's level of cognitive ability and fine and gross motor skills affects his or her performance in kindergarten. Modern kindergarten curriculums, more challenging than those of the past, may be too difficult for children under the age of five. (See the accompanying box below for a checklist to help evaluate preschool programs.)

Child's Reaction

Initially the child may resist attending school in a variety of ways—crying, being a "slowpoke," clinging to parents, complaining of illness. Separating from the parents for the first time can be difficult, but with coordinated efforts of parents and staff, this can be short lived. Attending school aids in the normal separation process.

Parents should listen to the child's reaction to his or her experience after entry. If the child is not happy, and communication doesn't bring about a solution to the problem, the school may just not be right. The school as a whole has to be evaluated before a change is considered. Parents should talk to staff, other parents, and other children (if appropriate) to clarify and, if possible, solve the problem. On the other hand, sometimes the problem is larger than, for example, a teacher whose style may not be to the child's liking. The philosophy of the school may be too rigid for a child who needs flexibility, too lax for a child who needs structure. Or the size of classes may be too large for a child who needs a lot of individual attention. Ideally, these are factors that should be considered in choosing the school in the first place, but if the wrong choice has been made, it is better to make the change early.

Teacher's Expectations

The prerequisites for school entry vary with the level of the program. Most nursery-school, daycare and Headstart programs suitable for the three- and four-year-old require that the child be toilet-trained. Children are also expected to dress and feed themselves, speak up to express needs, and part easily

---

CHOOSING AND EVALUATING THE LEARNING ENVIRONMENT

Place

The environment should be clean, safe, and designed to be comfortable, fun, and accessible to children.

Types of Learning

Fine motor play, drawing, cutting, pasting, and *gross motor play* to learn about bodies—balance, weight, and gravity, help children hone developing capabilities.

Role-playing releases emotional tension and helps children respond to social roles and experiment with adult roles.

Mastery of fine and gross motor skills, imaginative and social play situations help children feel a sense of accomplishment. The freedom to experiment promotes enjoyment and discovery.

Academic learning (reading, writing, arithmetic, and other educational training) begins in earnest in elementary school, but many nursery schools and preschools introduce children to fundamental concepts.

Material

Colorful books and toys, pens, crayons, scissors, and brushes should be plentiful and in good condition. These materials encourage fine-motor-skill development. Toys such as slides, tricycles, and tumbling mats encourage the development of gross motor skills.

Activities

A combination of fully organized games and songs, and less structured free time encourages children to play and interact with small and large groups. During creative time, children can cut and paste or work with finger paints, concentrating on their own projects with supervision and encouragement from staff.

Staff

The staff sets the tone or feeling in the nursery school. They are responsible for creating an atmosphere that should be relaxed, sharing, loving, and caring. Those who work in the school should be friendly and genuinely interested in children. The ideal ratio between children and adult staff varies depending upon the age of the children in the program. (See chapter 16.)

Selection

Parents should see the school in action before enrolling their child. Several programs should be compared. The school must meet parental needs as well as the child's developmental level. If both parents work, a full-day program is less stressful for them than two half-day programs that require transportation. In any event, the school should be a place the child enjoys going to, whether for six hours a day or for six hours a week.

from parents. To a certain degree, daycare programs help children develop these skills further, to which any parent who has observed an army of children hurling their jackets on the floor to climb into them nursery-school-style can attest.

Admission to kindergarten or elementary school marks the child's official entry into school. The child must be developmentally mature enough to handle the curriculum, and emotionally and socially mature enough to be able to function in the classroom.

The child entering school should be able to part from parents, to share with peers, and to pay attention to, recall, and accurately follow directions. Not only must the kindergartener and first-grader relate well to peers, they must understand the meanings of rules of behavior and have respect for the teacher's authority.

The school-age child should have reached a level of gross motor development at which he or she is able to skip and jump; fine motor development should allow the child to hold a pencil to write, turn pages, and handle scissors.

What academic skills should children master before entering kindergarten or first grade? They should know the alphabet well enough to identify letters and sounds (not *only* the alphabet song). Children who can write their names understand that letters work together to create a word that *means* something, and they are better prepared to learn to read and write.

The child entering kindergarten should know the numbers up to 10. As with letters, rote knowledge is not sufficient. The child should understand concepts, such as less and more, and their significance in numerical terms. Comparatives, such as big and small, should also be familiar to the child. The five-year-old should know colors, the words for simple shapes—circles, squares, triangles, and so forth. Both colors and shapes are often used to direct children to books or assignments, and knowing them is therefore important in following directions. The child also needs to know the difference between left and right.

Preparation for School

Parents can help prepare their children for school in many ways, so that they are ready emotionally, socially, and academically. Children who can not bear to be apart from parents will not learn effectively, regardless of their intelligence or academic preparation. Encouraging separation is therefore fundamental. Typically separation begins early, when the youngster is left occasionally with sitters, grandparents, or friends. Because the fun of playing with other children eases the strain of separation, the child should be introduced to and involved with other children whenever possible.

Educational activities outside the home, like trips to the park or neighborhood sites, begin the process of opening up the world to the child. Keep in mind the child's age and attention span. Children should be exposed to activities—new games, materials, and procedures, and readily encouraged and praised for learning new skills. Children who feel they must do everything perfectly shrink from new endeavors, while those who enjoy freedom to fail can flourish amidst educational opportunities.

Games, rhymes, songs, storytelling, dramatic play, reading aloud, coloring, and dancing to music are all fun ways parents can share learning with their children.

The Meaning of School for Parent and Child

The first day of school is loaded with meanings for parent and child. No longer a baby, and finally "like the big kids," the child begins to spend more time away from home, encounter people and experience responsibilities independently, without the buffer of parental protection. The teacher becomes a significant role model, and peers have an influence. Parents will notice changes in the child's interest, desires, and behavior, especially as the youngster begins to question family rules and regulations and to challenge the absolute authority of the parents.

Parents often respond to these changes with mixed emotions. They don't like to have their authority questioned and they often feel a loss of devotion as the child elevates an outsider—the teacher—to a level of importance once reserved for them alone. They should expect these feelings and consider them the flip side of the child's growing independence. Discussions of school experiences can provide an opportunity to find out how a youngster feels about the outside world. These discussions are also a way of reiterating family rules and regulations by relating them to experiences at school.

Parents may sometimes feel a loss, but they may also feel liberated. Perhaps they have waited for this day with as much anticipation as the child. Whether the new time gained is devoted to work, school, or homemaking, the launching of their child into the world of school entitles them to discovery and the rewards that go with it.

12 Emotional and Intellectual Development

Candace Erickson, M.D.

INTRODUCTION

FROM BIRTH and throughout early childhood, parents and children are involved in an intricate dance, continually adapting to the child's changing capacities as the child masters the physical and emotional challenges of development. During this period, children's needs are affected by both their limitations and their expanding abilities.

In facing the needs of each successive stage of the baby's development, both parents and the family as a whole develop and change. Beginning with conception the new baby's needs affect the relationship between the mother and father, that of the parents and any existing children in the family, and that of the family members to their environment. The resulting pattern of need, reaction and interaction is as fascinating as it is complex.

Each family has its own patterns. Indeed, each child in any given family not only brings a unique personality and set of abilities, but also meets the parents at a point in their own development that is different for each sibling. This results in the wonderful variety of human personality. It also makes it obvious that there can be no single "right" way to manage the many developmental tasks that face a child. The characteristics of the child, the parents, and the family will determine the interaction, and the requirements of this interaction will recommend the most appropriate way to manage issues and problems. However, since the parents are the adults in these interactions, it is incumbent upon them to evaluate the needs of the child and the needs and resources of the rest of the family, and to select the approaches that best fit their family. Most children are very adaptable, and respond well to a wide variety of approaches, developing into happy and successful individuals.

Interactive development exists even in the earliest periods of infancy. When an infant, who has no awareness of time, is hungry, that hunger is experienced as now and forever. No wonder it is signalled by such urgent cries! When the parent responds to the screams with food, warmth, contact, and affection, experience teaches the infant that someone will meet those needs. In this way, the child develops trust. The development of trust is a key emotional task of early infancy, a challenge that is imposed upon the physically helpless child, who must rely upon parents to meet needs. Meanwhile, as the child rewards the parent with contented coo's and smiles, the parent tries even harder to elicit these positive reactions, and the interaction becomes progressively more fine-tuned.

Other emotional developments, such as separation conflicts, also occur in the context of the child's maturing abilities. As children's bodies mature and they develop mobility, they are capable of crawling away from Mother or Father for the first time. As they mature neurologically and cognitively, they can remember the parent is not there. The combination of these developments causes separation anxiety and stranger anxiety.

Many mothers will correctly insist that their child recognized them well before this age, which is approximately nine months; however, there is a difference between recognition and memory. Recognition involves identifying a familiar object on sight; memory involves recall when that object is not within view. Separation anxiety accompanies the child's ability to create a mental picture of a familiar person (usually the mother) who is absent, as the child discovers the emotion of missing that person.

Before, the child was incapable of remembering Mother when she was not there and so was willing to accept a caring substitute. Now, the very presence of someone who is not Mother reminds the child that she is not there. A child who was previously placid and even responsive to strangers and grandparents now will often cry upon seeing them during this phase, called stranger anxiety. Even when Mother is physically present, the infant, who can now hold a mental image of her in mind even while focusing on the other person, will recognize the "stranger" as "not Mother." The infant may then cling to Mother and shun the other person in order to ensure that Mother does not leave.

In play this remembering finds expression in peek-a-boo games. The child remembers the hidden object and delights in looking for it. There is also amusement in covering the eyes and making the world disappear and reappear. The game, in which the infant can control the coming and going, allows him or her to develop confidence that things that go away will come back again. Eventually the child will apply this knowledge to anticipate the parent's return.

Locomotion—first crawling, then walking—further extends the issue of separation. Only now it is the child who is going away and coming back. Mastery of motor skills is intrinsically pleasurable to most children. Moving away brings them into contact with new people, places, and things—all of which present opportunities for the excitement of exploration.

Children who are successful in getting people to give chase as they move away experience the mastery of other people. While this new freedom of locomotion can be exciting and pleasurable, it also can be frightening to children who now find themselves someplace new, out of sight of a parent.

Adjustment to this new phase is an example of the intricate dance between parent and child. The child's new mastery (crawling, for example) may be frightening to the parents as well. They must cope with their anxieties while accommodating the child's ability and need to explore. Parents have the responsibility to allow their child to continue to master the environment. Yet they also must balance the child's needs to explore with their own responsibility to protect the child, setting limits so that he or she can explore in relative safety.

What follows in this chapter is an outline of normal child development and some of the typical problems that arise from changes that the child's development imposes on the family "dance." It should be used as a guide to inform the parents' assessment of their child's and family's development, aided by their own common sense. If they are unsure about a specific problem, they should consult their pediatrician or other professional who knows the child and family well and has a broad knowledge of child development.

DEVELOPMENTAL MODELS

ALL CHILDREN go through the same stages of emotional and intellectual development. The chapter "Eight Ages of Man" in Erik Erikson's book *Childhood and Society* provides the theoretical framework for the stages of psychological development, and Jean Piaget's work provides a framework for cognitive development. These stages are summarized here for easy reference and discussed in more detail in chapters 8 through 11.

Normal Development, Infancy to 18 Months

The first Eriksonian stage of normal development is "trust versus mistrust." Here the child moves from complete dependency upon the environment to locomotion and its accompanying independence. Children must develop trust in their environment, experiencing it as a safe, stable place. They must perceive others as reliable, nurturing, and predictable. This requires consistency so that the child has a stable base from which to move out and explore. Children must also develop trust in themselves, learning that they can delay gratification until their needs are met. For this, they rely upon signals from the environment that provide reassurance.

Piaget's sensorimotor-exploration stage comprises several substages. During the first 4 weeks, inborn reflexes are combined and become more efficient through repetition. Between 4 and 16 weeks, the child repeats rather simple acts just for the pleasure of doing them. Between 4 and 6 months, the child learns to repeat an act to produce a desired effect. Between 7 and 10 months the child develops the ability to remember and begins to repeat past performances from memory. At this age, parents can play hide-a-toy with the child, who now actively searches for a vanished object. The same cognitive skills can be applied to simple problem solving. From 11 to 18 months the child engages in trial-and-error exploration and develops a sense of spatial relationships. Throughout this process the child is using rapidly developing motor abilities to learn patterns of response in the physical environment that will serve as models for intellectual problem solving.

Normal Development in Toddlers, 18 to 36 Months

This is the Eriksonian stage of "autonomy versus shame and doubt." During this stage children learn to master their bodies and such functions and activities as locomotion, feeding, sphincter control, and language. They want to do everything for themselves. This stage incorporates the "terrible twos," when the child's persistent noes are a means of separating from the parent. Every child needs to develop a sense of independence and self-control. Parents must permit the child to take progressively more responsibility without excessive expectations.

In cognitive development, Piaget identifies this as the stage for developing symbolic thought. The child is mastering language and learning that things (such as words) can be symbols for other things. The child uses "magical thinking" rather than cause-and-effect reasoning. At this very egocentric stage, children feel that they are the center of the universe. They feel omnipotent—that they cause everything.

Normal Development in Preschoolers, 3 to 6 Years

This is the Eriksonian stage of "initiative versus guilt." Whereas in earlier stages, children learned to master their own bodies, now they begin to learn to manipulate their environment and the people in it. In the process, they may overstep their bounds and infringe on others. This will lead to restriction, which in turn leads to guilt, but this is also how children begin to incorporate a conscience. Infringement, they learn, is "bad" rather than "acceptable." In this way, they learn social values from family and peers. During this stage children also acquire heightened body awareness; they are becoming aware of the differences between boys and girls and men and women.

In Piagetian terms, children in this stage are "preoperational." They can think about things that are not present. Aware that events have causes, but lacking an understanding of the complex interrelationships of cause and effect, children of this age substitute associative logic. They use perceptual cues as their most powerful determinant: age is determined by who is tallest; sex is determined by the length of hair; the amount of something is determined by its length or height.

TEMPERAMENT

BABIES COME IN many "normal" personalities, with temperaments that range from extremely placid and easygoing to easily startled and very active. That range of normal can be a problem if baby's temperament doesn't match the personality of the parent, or even the parent's expectation.

An infant who is very placid may be viewed as a "happy" or "easy" baby and reinforce the parents' view that they are doing a good job. However, other parents might find such an infant lacking verve and energy. An infant who is slow to warm up to new people or experiences might be seen as rejecting. Yet other parents might view the same behavior as thoughtful caution. An infant with an exaggerated startle reflex (previously labeled as a "difficult baby") has trouble with self-regulation and needs more help from a parent. With sudden, tearful displays of discomfort, this baby may make the parent feel helpless or incompetent. But some parents enjoy this child's intensity and see the child as a youngster who knows what he or she wants, who is alert and curious.

There is no good or bad temperament: it is all in the match between parent and child. Despite this "no fault" viewpoint, it is incumbent upon the *parent*, not the infant, to adapt. That is part of the parental role. Fortunately, we now know enough about different types of temperament that when parents do not find themselves in harmony with their child's personality, specific suggestions from the pediatrician or other child development professional can often help the parents discover ways to enhance their interaction with their child.

WHEN IS A PROBLEM SERIOUS?

EVER-CHANGING CONFLICTS are part of a child's emotional development, and normal parents and children constantly adjust. How do parents determine when their child has a problem that is more serious than the usual? A problem that requires more than the ordinary attention or adjustment?

A clear sign that a problem is serious is when it presents itself as a constellation of changes in several areas that are beginning to coalesce. For example, if the child's behavior toward the parents has been a problem, is it now also difficult with siblings, playmates, and schoolmates? Are sleeping and eating patterns suddenly disturbed? Is the child complaining more about physical problems? Does he or she seem emotionally upset? If there are manifestations in more than one area, the parent should be concerned about an underlying problem that goes beyond normal developmental trials. It is rare that a serious problem exists in isolation.

Another indication that a problem may be more serious than suspected is the observation that the child has remained in a particular developmental phase considerably longer than his or her peers, or has suddenly reverted to behavior no longer appropriate to the child's age group. Sometimes this reversion can be triggered by illness or the arrival of a sibling, but this usually passes in a reasonable amount of time.

If a problem persists, a parent's first course of action should be to consult the pediatrician. When necessary the pediatrician will be able to recommend a mental health professional who can make a thorough assessment of the child and recommend a course of action—sometimes therapy—for the child individually or for the family as a group. (For more information on therapy, see chapter 29, Psychiatric Disorders.)

CHILDREN WITH SPECIAL NEEDS

THE VAST MAJORITY of children develop at more or less the same rate as their peers. Parents are usually able to sense when their child is developing much more rapidly or more slowly than other children the same age. This often becomes more apparent when the child enters preschool.

Parents who sense that their child is developing more slowly than others of the same age or who question whether they are providing adequate stimulation for the child should discuss the issue with their pediatrician or the child's nursery school teacher. Most pediatricians regularly screen their patients for developmental delays. However, since screenings are occasionally inaccurate and since parents know their children better than anyone else, if they have concerns, they should bring them up with the child's doctor. If a developmental problem is suspected, physical causes of delayed development, such as poor vision or hearing, must be ruled out first. If the pediatrician finds nothing wrong physically, he or she may recommend a thorough assessment by a child-development professional. On a more informal basis, preschool teachers have a very good feeling for how a child performs relative to peers and can often inform the parent if there is a problem.

At the other end of the spectrum are children with high cognitive ability. These children tend to be well adjusted if given the opportunity to live a balanced life where they can enjoy the rewards of their intellectual or creative gifts, use play to discharge energy and emotion, and master motor skills and emotional challenges. The most common problem for gifted children is parents who press them too hard to achieve. Kids are supposed to be kids; play is the work of children.

Problems can arise—particularly in the preschool years—when children's cognitive ability outstrips their emotional and motor development. A child who can conceptualize how something should be done, but does not yet have the motor coordination to accomplish it at that level may become quite frustrated. For example, children who understand that a letter or shape looks a specific way may be quite distressed if they do not yet have the fine motor coordination to be able to draw it accurately. Here parents can help by sympathizing with the child's frustration, pointing out some things that the child does well, and reassuring that, as with other things in the child's own experience, getting a little older and having more practice will help the child do it better.

A large disparity between intellectual abilities and emotional development can lead to problems as well. Because of their advanced reasoning skills, gifted children may avoid displaying—or even allowing themselves to recognize—difficult emotions. These young children may see the reasons why they "shouldn't" feel angry or afraid and therefore try to deny the feelings in spite of the fact that the feelings are both real and age-appropriate reactions. Suppressing the feelings robs the child of the opportunity to find ways to resolve them. A gifted two- or three-year-old may understand the reasons for not feeling frightened and be able to recite them, but still may not be able to cope effectively with the fear.

When parents pressure a gifted child to develop his or her cognitive abilities, ignoring emotional growth, the gap gets bigger. And in our culture, where feelings are often denied, parents will frequently find it easier to encourage cognitive development at the expense of emotional or social development. But parents of gifted children must make an equal effort to educate their children emotionally, to help them identify emotions and find appropriate ways of expressing them. When the child is experiencing an emotion, parents should label it, rather than deny it or try to reason it away. They should explore what it means, and explain appropriate outlets; for example, they might suggest that hitting and biting are *not* acceptable ways to let go of anger or frustration, but that punching a pillow or "bop bag" is. This helps the young child identify, express, and resolve often confusing feelings. It also clearly demonstrates that feelings (over which the child has little control) are not bad, but rather it is how we act on them that is either appropriate or not. The child who must "learn" in every spare moment does not have the energy to invest in emotional and social development.

Of course, a child who initiates "learning" activities should be encouraged to pursue that interest, but not to the exclusion of other activities. The key is balance. The child needs physical play for motor development and contact with other adults and children for social development.

Because children try very hard to please, parents must encourage cognitive development without vesting it with their own need to prove that their child is gifted. A primary source of problems in the family of a gifted child is the parents' need to have such a child. Parents who wonder if they are putting too much pressure on their child should ask themselves these questions:

- Am I structuring all my child's time?

- Am I excessively disappointed in my child's failures?

- Am I disappointed if my child's performance is less than perfect?

- Are my child's achievements too important to me?

- Can I enjoy the process of my child's learning or am I only interested in the result?

- Do I appreciate my child as a child or only for his or her accomplishments?

Parents should also be alert to the possibility that the child's self image has become too dependent upon achievement. If the child is *too* good, never showing anger, or if the child is too intent upon perfection when attempting a task, rather than involved just for the enjoyment of it, something may be amiss. These signs need to be evaluated qualitatively, however. There are good-natured children who rarely lose their tempers and there are children who are highly motivated intellectually. The issue is balance. Gifted children need to be encouraged equally in *all* areas of development.

BEHAVIOR MANAGEMENT: A RATIONAL APPROACH TO DISCIPLINE

THE PROCESS of socialization involves instilling in children a sense of what is appropriate behavior and what is not, teaching them to do what we want them to do and not to do what we don't want. The simplest way to do this is to reward the desired behavior and discourage the unwanted behavior, a technique that could be called "behavior management." Although it may be hard for parents of a two-year-old to believe, children would rather behave as their parents wish than misbehave. Unfortunately, parents often inadvertently reinforce problem behavior by taking the child's good behavior for granted. The child whose good behavior is ignored and who only gets parental attention for misbehavior will choose negative attention over none at all.

In order to avoid the "negative feedback is better than none at all" trap, parents need to actively strengthen positive behavior. The reward can be a smile, touch, praise, or special privilege. Positive behavior should be reinforced immediately, consistently, and generously. A sincere effort that produces less than perfect results should also be rewarded. Insincere praise of results should be avoided, however.

Unwanted behavior can be weakened by using a nonreinforcing, unstimulating punishment (such as sitting on a chair or standing in the corner) in combination with reinforcement for appropriate behavior. The parent should intervene early in the case of bad behavior and resist arguing with the child to the point where both the parent and child are out of control. In order to follow through, the parent needs to remain calm; scolding, nagging, and physical punishment give the child attention, thus reinforcing the unwanted behavior and disrupting any progress made on the behavior front. The latter type of punishment also reinforces out-of-control behavior by example.

Whenever possible, punishments should relate directly to the bad behavior. If, for example, a young child writes on the wall with a crayon, it should be explained that the child clearly does not know how to play with the crayon properly and the crayon must be taken away. If an older child dawdles getting ready for school in the morning, the parent should explain that the child must be too tired to get ready on time, and therefore, must go to bed 15 minutes earlier in order to be more awake. Then 15 minutes should be subtracted from bedtime each day until the child responds by being ready on time. Time can be added back again as a reward, with an explanation of the parent's reasoning.

Time out is a useful nonreinforcing punishment. It means the absence of attention and stimulation for the child, which is punishment enough. Before using time out as a punishment, the parent should explain the terms to the child. For example, "You are being told to sit in this chair to give you time to decide to act differently." The child can either be allowed to sit until he or she has decided to complete the task (tidy up toys, apologize for hitting and play nicely) or for a specific short period of time. In either case, the required task must be performed at the end of time out.

Time out is especially good for children with impulsive behavior styles. It gives them a chance to collect themselves and reconsider their behavior. Punishments such as scolding and hitting don't give children that opportunity to evaluate. A young child should never have to sit for more than 5 minutes, but the timing should not begin until the child is quiet. The child who continues to argue and negotiate should be reminded that time out does not begin until talking has stopped. Time out is not a replacement for the desired behavior.

Parents must be very consistent in the use of any technique to teach proper behavior, or the problem will be made worse. If the parent makes a rule, but then succumbs to the child's temper tantrum or whining, the lesson taught is that if the child pushes hard enough the parent will give in. The child will have learned the opposite of what the parent wanted.

Parents must learn to pick their battles and not make every instance of misbehavior an issue. The most important rules to make are those that ensure the child's safety and the parents' sanity. Rules allow the family unit to function smoothly. It is also important to recognize that families are not democracies. Children do not have to agree with or appreciate the value of the rules. Parents must remember that they are in charge for a reason: They are the adults and have more experience and reason. That is why they make the rules. On the other hand, while it is all right for parents to set some rules that are arbitrary ("just because I say so") or not to feel compelled to explain the reason behind every rule, it is not all right to riddle a child's life with too many arbitrary demands.

The behavior-management technique described above works if parents mean it, in other words, if they are consistent. We all know people to whom this technique comes naturally. Children recognize this quality, too. When these people say, "Stop it now," children obey in a flash. A parent whose application of behavior modification does not work should remember that it is not the child who is bad, but the program. It should be modified until it does work.

In applying behavior management, it is important to actually count and record the number of times a behavior occurs each day (or week), both *before* the intervention program begins and episodically during the program. This is particularly important if the behavior to be changed occurs frequently. Suppose, for example, that a child hits other children 20 times a day. After a week of behavior management, the hitting is down to 10 times a day. If the parent did not actually count the instances first, no improvement will be noted because 10 times a day is still a lot. The parent will correctly report that the child is still constantly hitting. Feeling that the program is not working, the parent will probably stop it. In reality, however, the frequency of the hitting has been cut in half. If progress continued at this rate (and if the parents are consistent there is no reason why it should not) in another two or three weeks the child would not be hitting at all.

If behavior management appears not to be working, the parents should check the program for problems. The most common ones are:

1. The punishment is actually reinforcing the problem behavior (e.g., the parents spend more time arguing with the child about time out than praising the child for appropriate behavior).

2. The parents are not consistent in reinforcing good behavior (e.g., they don't notice when the child is being good).

3. The parents are inconsistent in using time out for bad behavior (e.g., they skip it when it is inconvenient or embarrassing).

4. The parents do not insist that the child comply with requirements after time out (e.g., the child sits in the chair for five minutes and then doesn't have to clean his or her room, a trade-off even a parent might find appealing!).

5. The behaviors necessary for a reward are too diffi-cult, so the child never succeeds and never experi-ences positive reinforcement (e.g., a child who is hitting three or four times an hour must go two hours without hitting before being praised, an unreason-able expectation that is inevitably unsuccessful. Five or ten minutes would be more appropriate to start, increasing the length of time required as the fre-quency of hitting decreases.)

6. The "reward" is not rewarding (e.g., the parent praises the child with a snarl or gives a "prize" that the child does not want, so there is no incentive to change the behavior.)

Remember, if the program does not work, it is the program that is bad, not the child.

HABITS

CHILDREN DEVELOP habits that are disturbing to par-ents, despite their attempts to discourage them. Often the parental response reinforces the behavior, although the parent neither understands its moti-vation nor his or her own response. Many so-called habits are responses to transitory emotional or physiological needs.

Thumbsucking

As the infant's oral needs reach a peak, and as the baby begins to teethe, the thumb, fingers, some-times the whole hand, winds up in the baby's mouth. Thumbsucking often increases when the child is weaned from the breast or bottle.

As an emotional response, thumbsucking is just one way babies have of comforting themselves. Hair pulling or hair twisting, presleep rocking, and mas-turbation are all comforting behaviors. In his popu-lar books, pediatrician T. Berry Brazelton applauds thumbsucking and its counterparts as the sign of a resourceful child; he indicates that the behaviors are part of the child's efforts to cope with emotional challenges.

Thumbsucking usually peaks in the second half of the first year, but older children often suck their thumbs in stressful situations. Most children give it up voluntarily by the age of four. Parental interven-tion is most successful with infants if it takes the form of prolonging nursing or encouraging the sub-stitution of a toy or pacifier for the thumb. Wrench-ing the thumb from the child's mouth is a bad idea and creates an unhealthy struggle (which the child will win) over control over the thumb. With older children for whom thumbsucking is more regres-sive, trying to understand the cause of the habit without criticizing the behavior is the best ap-proach.

Many parents have tried to stop thumbsucking by scolding, covering fingers with gloves, and put-ting bitter-tasting compounds on the thumb, all to no avail. Studies indicate that such punitive mea-sures rarely help and often worsen the behavior. In an otherwise normal infant or child, thumbsucking should be regarded as a normal behavior that will likely resolve spontaneously. If thumbsucking per-sists beyond age four, the parents should seek a den-tal evaluation to be sure that the habit has not caused any misalignment of the teeth. If it has, an oral appliance might be necessary to correct the alignment. It will also simultaneously break the sucking habit.

If it is necessary to help a child stop thumbsuck-ing, the most successful methods are behavior man-agement programs that enlist the child's drive toward mastery and reward efforts to discontinue the habit. Thumbsucking is usually a habit and done without thinking. Remembering this, the parent can help the child notice when he or she is sucking and help the child to substitute some other behavior, such as grasping one hand with another or stroking the hand with the thumb. Quiet, gentle signals to help the child notice the behavior are sufficient. Re-minders should never involve nagging, scolding, or embarrassing the child. If the child chooses to con-tinue sucking, the parent should ignore the behavior completely. If the child tries to use the substitute behavior, the parent should praise the child's efforts with both words and physical affection.

If the child catches him- or herself thumb-sucking and uses the substitute behavior without parental reminders, or if the child simply does not suck the thumb at a time when he or she habitually does so, the parent should be even more reinforcing, pointing out and praising the child's increasing mastery over the habit. With this approach, com-bined with support in exploring other, more age-appropriate self-calming strategies, the thumbsuck-ing should diminish over time and disappear.

Nail Biting, Hair Twirling, and Hair Pulling

Nail biting and hair twirling are habits very similar to thumbsucking and can be treated in the same way. Nail biting is an extremely common behavior engaged in by up to 60 percent of school-age chil-dren. However, this habit usually does not begin until four or five years of age. Treatment is very sim-ilar to that for thumbsucking, and should include increasing the child's awareness of behavior and positive reinforcement for mastery. Negative rein-forcement and punitive measures are not successful and can often make the situation worse.

Hair twirling often occurs concomitantly with thumbsucking, but may continue even after the thumbsucking stops. Hair pulling is less common and is thought to affect less than one percent of children. With hair pulling, the child may twist off, pluck, or rub off hair, usually from the scalp, but sometimes from eyebrows or eyelashes. It is usually not recognized and probably not a problem unless the child has pulled enough hair to cause visible areas of hair loss. If hair loss appears to be the result of habitual pulling, the parents should discuss it with the pediatrician, who may make a referral to a mental health professional for evaluation of possible psychological disturbances.

Bed-wetting

This can be a normal stage in the toilet-training process, a response to the stress of toilet training or, with an older, physically ready child, a response to unrelated emotional problems. Even children who can stay dry during the day have a more difficult time controlling their bladders at night (girls develop overnight bladder control sooner than boys). Parents can cope with this in a practical manner by keeping a diaper on the child until he or she consistently wakes up dry in the morning, by limiting liquids in the evening, and by waking the child for a bathroom trip before the parents themselves go to sleep.

The child struggling with bladder control needs to learn at an individual pace and without the shame of failure. Most children should have developed daytime control by 36 months. Nighttime control usually occurs by age five, but it is not unusual for children of six or seven to continue wetting the bed. Beyond that age, bed-wetting may be the result of something other than the child's physiological limitations. Parents should try to identify the problem, and the child should be given positive reinforcement for progress. As with thumbsucking and nail biting, scolding, punishing, and embarrassing the child are rarely successful and often make the problem worse.

On the other hand, engaging the child in an effort to master the developmental task and praising his or her accomplishments are usually successful. Rewards such as special new pajamas, new sheets, or a sleepover after a period (perhaps a week or two) of consecutive dry nights may increase the child's motivation to master this task. Daily verbal rewards should be used as well because young children have a different sense of time, and for them a week or two may be difficult to imagine. A two-week chart with a star or sticker for each dry day can provide daily reinforcement and help the child conceptualize the

two-week period. But a parent's praise and affection are the most powerful rewards available. When the child does wet the bed, it should be treated casually as a normal part of the effort toward mastery. Little attention should be paid to the event. A child who seems upset by the event may be helped by a comment such as "When you are learning something new, sometimes you do things the old way. But each day as you get older and practice more it will get easier and easier until you can be dry every night." Parents should be careful not to overdo the reassurance so that the child gets more attention for the accidents than for dry nights.

FEARS AND ANXIETIES

THE DEVELOPMENT of a child's fears and anxieties parallels cognitive and psychological development. A two-month-old will cry when the mother leaves, indicating that a bond has been formed, but the child can be appeased by a substitute. Later, from five to eight months, the infant accepts a substitute much less readily, having developed the cognitive ability to remember Mother. Sometimes the eight-month-old will even react to Father as if he is a stranger if, for example, the baby's sleep schedule and the father's work schedule have kept them apart.

Parents can cope with stranger and separation anxieties by familiarizing the child gradually with alternative caretakers and limiting the duration of separation from the primary caretaker.

Certain fears are typical of certain ages. At two years, children are often fearful of loud noises; at three and four, they often fear animals, even pets they once accepted; at four and five, they often fear the dark; at six, they may be afraid of getting lost.

In their text *Childhood Behavior*, researchers F. L. Ilg and L. B. Ames delineated the following list of dos and don'ts in dealing with children's fears:

- Don't make fun of the child's fears.

- Don't humiliate the child in front of others because of his fear.

- Don't force the child to confront the fear, for example by forcing his hand to pet a dog when he's afraid.

- Don't call the child a baby because he has a certain fear.

- Do realize that with time the child will outgrow the majority of his fears.

- Do allow the child a respected period of withdrawal from the object or situation that evokes fear before gradual attempts are made to work through the fear. For example, if the child is afraid of the ocean, take him to the edge; then carry him in, then hold him while he floats.

- Do try within reason to avoid situations that scare the child so much that he cannot cope.

FEEDING

FEEDING IS TYPICALLY a problem area, one that parents unintentionally may turn into a battleground. Although nutrition is a subject that can be treated logically, even parents who understand the situation intellectually often have a strong emotional response to whether or not they believe that their child is getting enough to eat. What often begins as an almost fearful concern becomes a power struggle when the child decides not to eat. This is not healthy for child or parent.

Unless he or she is seriously physically or psychologically ill, a child will respond to normal body cues and eat enough to grow appropriately. If the nutritional content of the food available is reasonable, the child will meet the body's nutritional needs. Since many foods children will eat, such as cereals, breads, and milk, are fortified with iron and vitamins, most will get sufficient amounts of these nutrients even if their tastes in food are limited. Parents should learn to trust the child's body cues regarding hunger and satiety and should not invest food with emotional meanings that will become the basis for future eating disorders. There are two simple ways to remain logical about what is adequate:

1. If the child is not losing weight, and over the months is growing along the appropriate growth curve, he or she is getting an adequate amount of food.

2. If the child will only eat a few types of food and the parent is concerned about adequate nutrition, use of vitamin drops or a multiple vitamin pill can be discussed with the child's pediatrician. In this situation, the vitamin supplementation is being used primarily to reassure the parent that the child, despite picky eating habits, is getting adequate nutrition.

Feeding and Development

Certain feeding problems coincide with normal developmental stages. For example, when breastfeeding, a mother often tries to guide the baby to her nipple by placing her fingers on the baby's cheek and trying to turn the baby's face toward the breast. The baby responds by turning his or her face toward the mother's fingers (and thus away from the breast) and trying to suck them. This reflex action, called a rooting reflex, is often interpreted as a rejection of the mother's breast, and therefore of the mother, or as an indication that the child does not want to nurse. Neither is true. Rather, it is a way of helping the baby survive: If it is the nipple that is touching the baby's cheek, the rooting reflex helps the baby find it and get it in the mouth to suckle.

At six to eight months, babies can feed themselves finger foods. Part of this developmental period, which usually ends by twelve months, is dropping or throwing food on the floor. The baby is fascinated by seeing things disappear (as in peek-a-boo) and by the process of taking and releasing. Parents find it difficult to respond positively to this fascination. They may feel the food is being rejected; they may dislike the mess; they may resent constantly picking up the food the baby throws onto the floor. Some parents feel the baby is manipulating them.

Since there is little a parent can do to prevent this behavior, it is better to let the baby enjoy this stage of development. Limits, however, can be set. Parents have to decide how much they can tolerate. Certain practical tips can be helpful.

In any given meal, it is safe to assume that a baby who begins to throw food on the floor is no longer very hungry. If the baby is no longer eating, the parent can end the meal if the food dropping has become untenable. Cleaning up once per meal, rather than constantly, eases the pressure to keep up with the baby's activity, and takes the parent out of the game-playing danger zone. Some parents have learned to place a washable shower curtain under the highchair. Or better yet, they use bags saved from the dry cleaners and just throw them out after each meal. It is up to each parent to decide what is comfortable.

At 18 to 30 months, toddlers want to play more than they want to eat. Their enchantment with the world is so powerful that it is difficult to stop their play to interest them in eating. Even the mastery of utensils intrigues them more than eating itself. Parents play an important role in helping to calm down the toddler so he or she can concentrate on eating. If they want the child to sit through a family meal, they learn that the child has to be entertained.

Toddlers won't eat much, but they will eat what they need. Often several small snacks, the nutritional equivalent of "three squares a day," are more suitable to the toddler's limited appetite attention span.

After 30 months, a child who absolutely refuses to eat is most likely engaged in a power struggle. The parents must be responsible for taking mealtimes out of the emotional arena.

Like battles over sleeping and toilet training, parents cannot win battles over eating. When they invest all their energies into something they cannot win, they are frustrating themselves and setting useless limits for the child. The parent cannot use force to get the child to eat, but most children, even terrible twos, can be coerced with positive attention. Positive reinforcement works with every child (and adult, for that matter) and is extremely important. The parent who cannot tolerate it when the child plays with food (a completely normal activity) *can* set limits. But the parent should be careful to choose which battles are worth fighting and not make everything a "no." (For additional information, see section above on behavior management.)

Food as Comfort and Reward

If the parent interprets each cry from the baby as hunger, or in desperation offers the baby a bottle to comfort every ill, the baby learns that food is a sourse of comfort rather than a means to satisfy a hungry belly. When food is used to satisfy needs other than hunger, it is likely to lead to problems of obesity. Older children often are introduced to this pattern of oral satisfaction with candy and other sweets. This pattern also teaches children to ignore other needs and therefore stunts the development of alternate means of satisfaction.

In a related pattern, parents often use food treats as a reward or an enticement. They should let logic be the guide. If it becomes a question of retaining sanity or rewarding the child with food, they should give the child the food. However, they must be careful not to "train" with food. Positive parental attention is a powerful reward, one that ultimately is more satisfying and beneficial for the child. Parents often dole out more negative than positive attention, scolding their children more often than praising, or simply interacting, with them.

Food Preferences

As noted in chapter 5, children are fickle about food. What they love one day, they are likely to refuse the next. (They are noted for refusing food especially after the parent has bragged about how well they eat!) Parents must learn to live with it. Although they want their child to eat, they need not worry that the child will starve if they do not provide a constantly changing menu. In past generations, when there were genuinely fewer options, children did not starve. Nor will children today. When they are hungry, they will find something to eat. The trick is to make sure that what is available is consistent with good nutrition and sound eating habits. (See chapter 5 for a more detailed discussion.)

13 How Does Your Baby Fit In?

Elizabeth Anisfeld, Ph.D.

INTRODUCTION

EVERY CHILD is born into a unique environment. For each new birth there is a singular set of circumstances that must be considered, a particular constellation of family relationships subtly distinct from all others. This perpetual novelty of environment and interaction intrigues and frustrates social scientists because it defies precise measurement and the development of models. The intimate details of the family environment are difficult to observe and even more difficult to classify.

Beliefs about the role and influence of parents in shaping their children have changed throughout history and vary across cultures. For many years it was assumed that the child was a "tabula rasa" and was shaped by the environment, with no consideration given to the capacity of the child to affect the behavior of others. At other times and places in history, it was believed that the developmental course of the child was predetermined at birth and external influences could do little to change that.

From investigations in recent years, it has become evident that babies are born with certain characteristics that may affect the process of their development. Some of these factors may arise from genetic makeup, some from the intrauterine environment; but whatever the source, the baby's unique combination of characteristics will have an effect on the family into which he or she is born.

Some babies are difficult from the beginning for no apparent reason (for example, babies with colic). Other babies may survive nicely, even thrive, in the most untoward circumstances. Parenting is not the determining factor in such cases. Something in the baby's own self is at work.

Not only are babies different from birth, but so are their parents. Parents come with different relationship histories, different family constellations, such as reconstituted families, and different expectations and hopes for their offspring. The important factor in determining a favorable parenting outcome is the willingness and ability of the parents to adapt to the particular needs of the child they are parenting and to treat that child as a unique individual.

COPING WITH THE STRESS OF A NEW BABY

THE ENVIRONMENT into which a child is born comprises many elements: the parent or parents, the presence or absence of siblings, grandparents, or other household members; the physical surroundings and whether they are part of an urban, suburban, or rural setting; the financial resources available; and the amount of support available to the primary caretaker from spouse, relatives, friends, or household employees. Though it is difficult to document the precise effect of any of these elements on the child's development, it would appear that they are significant.

Every new baby is either a firstborn, a later-born, a twin, or rarely, a triplet or quadruplet or a survivor of a multiple birth. The environment in the first few years is very different for each of these.

The Firstborn

In most instances, the arrival of a firstborn child is one of life's most joyous occasions. Even when the pregnancy has been unwanted or unplanned, there is often a response of wonder at the miracle of birth. The changes that accompany the birth of a first child encompass every aspect of the parents' lives. Such sweeping change inevitably carries with it a certain amount of stress, even under ideal circumstances. When conditions are less than ideal, that stress can be overwhelming.

Because most people become parents, society tends to support the view that parenting is a "natural" function and therefore needs little special attention. The result is that many new parents have unreasonable expectations of the ease with which they "ought" to assume this new role. When the initial excitement dies down, they find themselves with reduced physical resources, varied and confusing emotional states, and the task of adjusting to a totally different life-style; yet they may feel guilty or inadequate if they don't seem to be completely happy, fully capable, and in control.

No one can anticipate all the stresses that will be encountered in a new situation. Prospective parents can be prepared, however, to meet some of the typical problems and to be aware of others that might appear. They can accomplish this in several ways.

First there is information gathering. The local library is apt to have a good selection of books about becoming parents, such as *Ourselves and Our Children* by the Boston Women's Health Book Collective. The most helpful are those containing the actual thoughts and experiences of new parents, that address not only why the decision to have a baby is made, thus helping to sort through personal needs and expectations, but also what feelings and events have surprised, disappointed, or disturbed new parents.

Second, parents can locate during pregnancy the services or support that may be needed after the baby is born. It is much easier to get out and about to ask questions or make exploratory visits before the baby is born. And it is generally more comfort-

able to make decisions when the need is not pressing. Each question answered, each detail handled in advance represents one less possible source of anxiety in the early months when everything is new and wits may seem scattered.

Parents should consider hiring temporary household help after the baby is born if help from relatives is not available or not desirable because of space problems or poor relationships. Although it is possible for a woman to manage without any outside help after a normal birth, it is far better if the regular chores can be handled by someone else while mother and baby get acquainted and begin to develop a routine. It is also important for the mother to get sufficient rest, especially if she is breastfeeding, as her milk supply can be affected by lack of sleep. If she is recovering from a cesarean section while adjusting to a new baby, she has all the more reason to need help.

If the mother will be returning to work, provisions for child care should be investigated and arrangements made far enough in advance to allow for a smooth transition. Both parents-to-be can share in the process of gathering information and making decisions about child care.

If the mother will be staying at home, she may want to investigate parent support groups, neighborhood drop-in centers, or other avenues that provide regular contact among new parents. All new parents can benefit from frequent association with others going through the same experience. Although it may be difficult for working parents to achieve, it is well worth the effort.

Both husband and wife should understand and accept the fact that each will sometimes feel the need for extra attention and nurturing at precisely the time when the other partner may be least able to fill that need. This is a period when fatigue, the lack of private time together, and the adjustment to the demands of being totally responsible for another person can result in increased stress. Clearly communicating to each other any special needs, working together to provide whatever help is possible, and reminding each other that the situation is temporary can go a long way toward alleviating this stress. (See chapter 3, The Role of the Father.)

One approach to keeping stress to a minimum is the development of a healthy attitude toward parenting. While parents can have a major influence on a child's feelings of security and self-esteem and the values that become a part of each child's identity, they need not feel total responsibility for the final outcome.

Infants need and deserve consistent, responsive caretaking, which takes time and motivation. By realizing this from the beginning, parents can plan to reduce temporarily their outside commitments. Time invested during the first months in satisfying an infant's needs pays off later in a more independent child.

There is no great mystery to baby care. It is merely the close observation of another's needs, the development of skills to meet those needs, and the willingness to put in the necessary time and attention. Like all new jobs, caring for a baby involves the establishment of new relationships and the learning of new tasks. As with most jobs, it takes about a year to become fully adjusted and to feel competent. Unlike many jobs, though, there is rarely a dull moment—trying times, fearful times, puzzling times, but not dull times. And the rewards are lifelong.

Laterborns

By the time a second child is born, the job of parenting has become familiar. Husbands and wives have worked out a system for dividing duties. Many of the stresses that accompany the birth of the first child are not present at subsequent births. Even some of the inevitable stresses of fatigue and lack of time are better understood and therefore less frustrating. What cannot be anticipated is how the older child or children will respond to the new arrival. The chief stress becomes how to cope with the demands of a new baby while meeting the needs of each sibling.

It is normal for the arrival of a new baby to precipitate behavior problems in older brothers or sisters, especially in firstborns and in those nearest in age to the new baby. Indeed, a child of any age can feel that a new baby is something of a threat to his or her share of time and attention. It is not unusual for a child to revert to an earlier stage of behavior for a while after the arrival of a new baby. Some children "act out" their jealousy while others (older children in particular) become morose. Some will even become overly solicitous, a behavior that is pleasing at first, but that may be a sign of trouble.

Difficult or erratic behavior in an older child can be trying for the parents, unpleasant for the child, and even dangerous for the baby. Parents can prevent many potential problems by fostering positive feelings of self-worth in the older child. Studies indicate that children tend to accept a new baby more readily when they are included in discussions about what the baby may be like and how the older child can help with the baby's care. Even a very small child should be included in the baby's care whenever possible. When the child is disinclined to help or cannot appropriately participate in caring for the baby, the parent should be prepared to divert the child's attention from the baby. He or she might offer a toy, sing a song with the child, or tell a story. Daily exclusive time with the older child, even for a few minutes, helps resolve much sibling rivalry.

Parents should avoid major changes in the older child's daily life, such as moving or changing schools, for a reasonable period after the baby arrives. It may be worthwhile to enlist the help of grandparents, relatives, or sitters to continue to provide sufficient time for play and special attention. A family conspiracy to accord the older child generous praise while overlooking small transgressions also may ease the way.

Even under the best of circumstances, all children will be somewhat jealous and some children will be truly difficult. For most, the frustrations and conflicts of this period act as catalysts for the development of a sense of self, and the short-term setbacks do not have long-term consequences. Occasionally, however, there will be a significant disturbance. Parents who sense that an older child is truly suffering after a reasonable period of adjustment should seek professional help.

There is nothing to indicate that strong feelings of jealousy toward a newborn are any indication of how the children will get along later in life. Many elements enter into sibling relationships as they grow, such as sex constellation, age difference, temperament, and interpersonal relationships with other family members. Remembering that parents can affect but not control their children's behavior may relieve some of the stress of the adjustment period. A sense of humor and respite from the children are even more effective.

The Special Case of Twins

The birth of twins represents a crisis of about a year's duration in any family. The level of crisis will depend on many factors: the money available for employing extra help; the degree of cooperation by the father; the presence of other children and their ages and temperaments; the experience and disposition of the mother; and the nature of the twins themselves, to name a few. The twins' arrival may be especially hard on any older siblings as not one, but two rivals appear, commanding attention from all corners and demanding most of their parents' time.

Twins are not fundamentally different from single babies. That is, they are not born with peculiar traits. The conditions of twinship produce an environment, however, that is radically different from that of singly born babies. This has ramifications for the way the household is organized, the way the babies are treated, the way in which the twins develop, and often for the way siblings respond. The only situation that approaches twinship in families with singly born children is when two children are born within 10 months or less.

Twins require more than twice as much work as a single baby. Some studies have shown the work required to be up to four times greater. Not only must everything be done twice, but often it must be done while one twin is protesting being second in line. If there are other small children, the logistics may be mind-boggling. The net effect of this is that neither twin gets as much attention as a single baby, and neither twin ever has the experience of having the exclusive attention of a parent. There is competition for the mother's time and attention from the first day of life.

Parents expecting twins will do well to get in touch with an organization such as Mothers-of-Twins—for support, if there is a local chapter, or if there is not, for lists of resources. (A local hospital may know of a chapter; see also the Resources section of the appendix.) If an official organization for parents of twins is not located nearby, other twin parents may be found through friends, a pediatrician, or a hospital. The best information and support comes from those with personal experience. Although many of the works on twins are scholarly rather than practical, Amram Scheinfeld's *Twins and Supertwins* is most readable and informative and is an excellent guide to resources.

It is important to recognize that certain options open to parents of singletons will not be available to parents of twins. Demand feeding, for example, is a practice that appeals to many, but it may be impractical with twins. Likewise, the daily bath may have to be confined to every other day for twins, alternating babies at bathtime. The rewards of this compromising come later on when the twins begin to require far less individual attention than siblings born close together. At about nine months, many things can be done for both at the same time, and later still, the twins begin to entertain each other a great deal.

During the early months it makes no difference whether the twins are identical (monozygotic) or fraternal (dizygotic). They will require the same amount of extra effort and attract the same amount of attention both within the family and without. As they grow older, however, fraternal twins tend to attract less attention and to develop as individuals. Identical twins remain the focus of attention throughout life and are often, if not usually, treated as a pair. The ongoing situation with identicals may be particularly difficult for children near in age and of the same sex.

All twins are affected similarly by having competition for the mother's attention from birth, by being constantly in association with another infant at the same stage of development, and by being treated as a unit. Consequently, all twins may have a greater struggle to achieve individuality.

It is well documented that, on average, twins test slightly lower than singletons in verbal skills throughout childhood and adolescence. Whether this is the result of less verbal stimulation in infancy, the ease of nonverbal communication for two infants developing in company simultaneously, or the effects of low birthweight or premature birth is unclear. However, this modest deficit does not affect overall achievement in life. Indeed, parents of twins often report that twins do many things for themselves earlier than their singleton siblings. When one twin discovers a new skill, the other usually follows suit immediately, perhaps sooner than if left to himself.

The development of an individual identity is a greater struggle for twins than for other children. It may be the nature of this struggle that contributes to the special relationship throughout life that is almost universally observed and is reported by twins themselves. With the exception of a small group of disturbed twins, however, even identicals develop individual characteristics that are easily discernible to family and close friends at a very early age. It is interesting that the personality traits of identical twins often tend to be complementary, so that each has different areas of competence or strength.

For parents, the problem of twin individuality is most apparent in decisions regarding dressing alike or differently, schooling together or in separate classes. Discussions with other parents of twins and consultations with teachers may be helpful. In the end, however, parents will have to rely on their own judgment, especially with identical twins; fraternal twins will automatically go their own way in most cases if permitted. Twins, after all, are individual children born into a special circumstance. As with singly born children, the best approach to their care and teaching will be a highly individual one that evolves out of the particular constellation of personalities and resources of the household.

The difficulties that accompany the early months of caring for twins are usually amply rewarded with the pleasures that accrue as they grow and become independent. There is a special joy in watching two children unfold at the same time with the added stimulation of the mysteries of the twin relationship.

The Only Child

In recent years the myth of the only child has been proved to be a myth indeed. Onlies have been studied from almost every angle. The one way in which they differ significantly from children with siblings is that they tend to achieve a higher level of education. This should come as no surprise since parents with only one child, or those whose second child comes many years later, would naturally be able to devote proportionally more time, effort, and money to his or her education than parents with two or more children.

The extra care and attention that is sometimes accorded an only child can foster independence and self-esteem. On the other hand, it can produce a spoiled and dependent child. Having all the resources of the family available to one child can provide greater advantages, but this can be accompanied by greater expectations and more pressure to perform well.

Because the only child must go outside the home for companionship, there is greater exposure to a variety of social situations. This can produce either a self-reliant or an insecure child. Research, however, indicates that the personality traits traditionally ascribed to only children—such as selfishness, dependence, and rigidity—occur in only children, as they do in other people, for a variety of reasons that have nothing to do with lack of siblings. The traits may be inherited or they may be influenced by relationships outside as well as within the family.

There is apparently neither an advantage nor a disadvantage in being an only child. As it becomes more widely known that having an only child does not have a negative impact on that child in later life, there may be a greater tendency to opt for the single child. Parents who feel they can afford only one child no longer need feel guilty about not having a second child as a companion for the first.

Because only children are also firstborns, there is little to add about special needs or circumstances. The only caveat is that should an only child also be an only grandchild or an only niece or nephew, some agreement among the extended family may be needed to prevent overwhelming the child with possessions.

Birth Order, Family Size, and Development

There are many popular notions regarding the effect of birth order and family size on personality and intelligence. Firstborns are often described as brighter or more responsible, only children have a reputation for being selfish and poor marriage risks, laterborns are thought to be easygoing, and the youngest of the family may be expected to be spoiled. Children from large families are supposed to get along well with others, and twins are considered to have a special and exclusive relationship.

In fact, recent studies show that birth order alone has little, if any, effect on the intelligence of a child, and personality traits attributed to birth order tend to be exhibited largely within the family rather than outside. As methods of investigation have improved and variables have been more carefully controlled, less and less importance is being assigned to the effect of birth order on intelligence, and the ideas about the effects of family size are being revised.

Clearly there are certain biological risks affecting intelligence related to the age and health of the mother. However, in normally healthy women who are neither physically immature nor well past normal childbearing years, there are no indications that intelligence is influenced by biological factors nor that birth order influences the risk of minimal brain dysfunction.

It appears that the development of intelligence is related to the amount of stimulation. While large families *may* be able to provide stimulation for all children, short birth intervals make this very difficult to do. This is especially so when the family size and spacing are related to impoverished conditions where both social and biological factors are not conducive to normal development. In conditions providing adequate nutrition and care, however, the intelligence of the parents is the salient factor.

As far as academic achievement is concerned, size of family or order of birth appear to have no effect. As in the case of IQ, academic performance relates to the prevailing social conditions and parental intellectual capacity rather than to family size directly. Likewise, in later life there appear to be no differences in occupational status related to birth order.

The belief that children reared in large families are better adjusted than others is likewise not supported by recent studies. In fact, it appears that personality problems increase with family size, particularly in lower social classes. This may be due to lack of attention or even to punitive behavior on the part of the parents. Children from lower-class large families tend to have less self-confidence, but it is difficult to ascribe any personality differences to family size as such.

If there are any personality traits associated with birth order, they would appear to be the result of the socialization process rather than any inherent condition. Most single firstborn children receive more attention and verbal stimulation than twins or laterborns. It is not surprising, then, that firstborns often exhibit higher self esteem and report a closer tie to parents than laterborns. Parents, likewise, often feel a difference in their relationship with their firstborn.

In short, the popular notion that being an oldest, middle, or youngest child automatically confers certain personality traits is outdated. Although birth order can certainly have a strong effect on some children, its influences on personality and IQ have been overrated. And whether there is one child or many becomes significant primarily when the physical, emotional, or economic resources are inadequate to provide satisfactory care. In sum, it is the unique environment into which each child is born and the novel way in which the child interacts with that environment that is important.

THE ROLE OF GRANDPARENTS

IN EVERY CULTURE there are probably grandparents who would be considered "ideal." Examples in our culture might be the grandmother who comes to help after the birth of each child and provides babysitting services through the years. Grandparents who offer the children unconditional love, act as their confidants, and provide advice to the parents *when asked* are to be especially cherished.

This is a wonderful picture, all the elements of which can contribute to the security and well-being of a child. For those who live near their parents or have strong family ties that make a close long-distance relationship workable, this is a scenario much to be desired. Children need all the love they can get, and it is good for them to have a defender when parental authority seems harsh. Parents, too, can benefit from the respite offered by obliging grandparents, and their advice is often helpful in times of trouble or uncertainty.

For many reasons, a close relationship with grandparents cannot always be achieved. Grandparents in their forties and fifties may be at the height of their careers with little time for grandparenting. Older grandparents may move away upon retirement, spend considerable amounts of time traveling, or live in a retirement community where small children are not always welcome. Some grandparents are quite willing to lend financial support but want no part of babysitting. Others may be going through a major crisis such as divorce and be seeking a helping hand rather than extending one.

Disturbed relationships can also prevent close grandparent contact. If parents do not get along with grandparents, the grandchildren may be kept away for the parents' sake. Divorce may deprive a child of one set of grandparents, and remarriage may provide another set who have established relationships with other grandchildren. Some grandparents are not ideal people themselves, and their children may minimize the time with the grandchildren because they believe the circumstances are negative. For example, some grandparents play favorites or are unduly harsh in their criticism.

Timing makes a difference as well. A grandmother who still has teenage children at home may not be inclined to add babysitting for a grandchild to an already crowded schedule. An older grandparent who is having health problems may not be as patient with the noise and clutter of later grandchildren as with earlier ones.

These impediments notwithstanding, a close grandparent-grandchild relationship can provide a sense of belonging, a perspective on aging, and an enlargement of interests, as well as that all-important extra measure of unconditional love.

Grandparents can make a useful contribution in every stressful situation that parents are likely to encounter and they can contribute immeasurably to the safe passage of their grandchildren through difficult times. The configurations of family relationships are legion, the obstacles to nurturing relationships many, but the advantages of such relationships are well worth making considerable efforts to achieve.

SUMMING UP

HAVING CHILDREN is a great cooperative venture with kaleidoscopic variations. Regardless of popular notions, scholarly theories, family expectations, and personal preconceptions, the business of bearing and rearing children turns out to be a highly intuitive process, unique to and for each parent and child.

How children turn out depends not only on how they are treated by their parents, but also on personality tendencies present at birth, experiences outside the family environment, the influence of their peers, and their relationships with significant adults other than their parents. This is why children reared in the same family may be very different from each other.

Parents, by providing a nurturing and stimulating environment responsive to the individual needs of each child, can help children develop to their fullest potential.

14 Ensuring Your Child's Safety

Leslie Davidson, M.D.

INTRODUCTION

INJURY, NOT DISEASE, poses the greatest threat to children's life and health. Injury is the leading cause of death in children over one year of age. Although problems at birth and congenital anomalies account for many more deaths than do injuries during the first year of life, the rate of death by injury, 37 per 100,000, is greater in the first year than at any time except the late teens. Injury is also the leading cause of hospitalization in children, and although precise figures are not available, it is certainly a major cause of both long- and short-term disability. According to statistics, being black, of lower socioeconomic status, or male substantially increases a child's risk of death due to injury.

Every year in the United States some 26 million children age sixteen and under are injured, and as many as 11,000 die as a result of those injuries. Nearly 400 children under the age of four die from accidents every month. An accident severe enough to require medical attention or restricted activity befalls one of every two children. Although this chapter concerns injuries to children age six or younger, the statistics cited include older children as well. It is important for parents to develop a perspective on how safety needs will change as their children become independent and take increasing responsibility for their own well-being.

One half of the childhood deaths due to injury are caused by motor-vehicle injuries, either passenger or pedestrian. Other major causes of death and disability in children from birth to age six are suffocation (choking, smothering), drowning, fires and burns, and falls (see table 14.1). Poisoning, although still cause for concern, has decreased greatly in recent years due to improved packaging of medications, the use of lead-free paints, and other safety measures. Child abuse and homicide, although important causes of childhood injury and death, are not addressed in this chapter, which deals with unintentional injury only.

Because the leading cause of death by injury in children is automobile accidents, vehicular safety is discussed in a separate section. All other injuries will be discussed together in order of developmental importance.

Table 14.1 LEADING CAUSES OF ALL DEATHS FOR SELECTED AGE GROUPS (1985)*

Cause	No. of Deaths	Death Rate
	All Ages	**874.0**
All Causes	**2,086,440**	323.0
Heart disease	771,169	193.3
Cancer	461,563	64.1
Stroke (cerebrovascular disease)	153,050	**39.1**
Accidents	**93,457**	19.2
Motor-vehicle	45,901	5.0
Falls	12,001	2.2
Drowning	5,316	2.1
Fires, burns	4,938	1.7
Poison (solid, liquid)	4,091	31.3
Chronic obstructive pulmonary disease	74,662	28.3
Pneumonia	67,615	15.5
Diabetes mellitus	36,969	12.3
Suicide	29,453	11.2
Chronic liver disease, cirrhosis	26,767	10.0
Atherosclerosis	23,926	8.9
Nephritis and nephrosis	21,349	8.3
Homicide	19,893	
	Under 1 Year	**1,071.5**
All Causes	**40,030**	510.4
Certain conditions originating in perinatal period	19,068	229.1
Congenital anomalies	8,561	142.3
Sudden infant death syndrome	5,315	24.6
Heart disease	920	**23.8**
Accidents	**890**	4.8
Motor-vehicle	179	4.6
Mechanical suffocation	171	4.6
Ingestion of food, object	170	3.0
Fires, burns	111	2.4
Drowning	90	18.9
Pneumonia	705	8.1
Septicemia	303	
	1 to 4 Years	**51.4**
All Causes	**7,339**	**20.0**
Accidents	**2,856**	7.1
Motor-vehicle	1,016	4.3
Fires, burns	613	4.2
Drowning	600	0.7
Ingestion of food, object	102	0.6
Falls	80	5.9
Congenital anomalies	840	3.8
Cancer	543	
	5 to 14 Years	**26.3**
All Causes	**8,933**	**12.5**
Accidents	**4,252**	6.8
Motor-vehicle	2,319	1.7
Drowning	570	1.3
Fires, burns	453	0.7
Firearms	235	0.2
Falls	71	3.5
Cancer	1,183	1.4
Congenital anomalies	469	

* Adapted from *Accident Facts*. Chicago: National Safety Council, 1988.

† Per 100,000 population in each age group.

THE SAFE ENVIRONMENT

THE REQUIREMENTS of a safe environment differ according to the developmental level of the child. The risk of injury changes as the child's ability expands. For example, a toddler is at greater risk of choking on a peanut or a pebble than is an infant of three months, and a one-year-old is in greater danger than a five-year-old of drowning in the bath.

Developing a Safety Perspective

Parents' first task is to monitor the various environments in which their child spends time, modifying appropriately whatever elements pose hazards to their child at each stage of development. Some basic safety standards apply to all children, especially in the home and the automobile; others are particular to certain ages. The primary environments of small children are the home (parents', grandparents', sitters'), the daycare center or school, neighborhood play areas, and vehicles.

New parents may need help in determining where hazards may exist for their baby, as they can be numerous and unexpected. In most households, the arrival of a baby requires both a reorganization and the purchase of appropriate equipment. The Home Safety Checklist (see table 14.2) is an excellent tool for home safety evaluation. Some of the items, such as toddler gates or cabinet latches, are only necessary when the child becomes mobile.

Table 14.2 **HOME SAFETY CHECKLIST**

General Safety

Yes	No	
1. ☐	☐	Home has two unobstructed exits.
2. ☐	☐	No loose, chipping, or peeling paint.
3. ☐	☐	Plants out of reach of child.
4. ☐	☐	Basement not accessible to child.
5. ☐	☐	Attractive items/food not stored over stove.
6. ☐	☐	No space heater or electric appliances in bathroom.
7. ☐	☐	Nonaccordion toddler gates at top and bottom of stairs.
8. ☐	☐	No frayed or dangling electric cords.
9. ☐	☐	Extension cords out of reach of child and not overloaded.
10. ☐	☐	Space heater or woodstove in safe condition.

Child Area Safety

Yes	No	
11. ☐	☐	Shock stops in unused electrical outlets.
12. ☐	☐	Toy chest has safe closing mechanism or no top.
13. ☐	☐	Crib not near window or outlet.
14. ☐	☐	Crib slats 2⅜ inches apart or less; mattress fits safely.
15. ☐	☐	Adequate guards on all windows.
16. ☐	☐	Windows in safe repair.

Hazardous Product Storage

Yes	No	
17. ☐	☐	Medicines/vitamins out of reach of child.
18. ☐	☐	Cleaning supplies not stored with food.
19. ☐	☐	Cleaning supplies out of reach of child in kitchen and bathroom.
20. ☐	☐	Shampoos, soaps, cosmetics stored out of reach of child.
21. ☐	☐	Matches, lighters, flammables out of reach of child.
22. ☐	☐	Knives, razors, cutting objects out of reach of child.

Safety Aids in Use

Yes	No	
23. ☐	☐	Syrup of ipecac in home, use understood.
24. ☐	☐	Poison Control Center sticker on phone.
25. ☐	☐	Working smoke detectors properly placed.
26. ☐	☐	Shock stops in all unused electrical outlets.
27. ☐	☐	Cabinet latches in use.
28. ☐	☐	Working fire extinguisher available.

Safety Practices in Use

Yes	No	
29. ☐	☐	Children tested for lead within last 12 months.
30. ☐	☐	Children properly restrained during all auto travel.
31. ☐	☐	Fire escape plan has been developed.
32. ☐	☐	Children always attended in water or on high surface.
33. ☐	☐	Children know "stop, drop, and roll."
34. ☐	☐	Stove safety understood.
35. ☐	☐	Hot water at safe temperature—125 degrees F. or less.

No checklist, however, can cover all potentially hazardous situations. Parents need to develop a safety orientation, to see things from a child's vantage point, both literally and figuratively. They will need to examine habits that may pose no problem in a childless household, but that now can present a danger. Do they, for example, throw things other than paper in wastebaskets? Do they put soap in an unlocked dishwasher, waiting to add a few more dishes before locking and running it? Do they view vitamins as harmless supplements that they keep on the kitchen counter with the condiments and take with morning coffee?

Parents will, as soon as the baby becomes mobile, have to go through the entire house or apartment looking for safety hazards on or near the floor. They may want to consider doing this before the baby is born, while the household routine is a little more relaxed and flexible. In fact, the entire household must be examined periodically to determine what changes or additions are necessary for safety. Potentially poisonous items, unless they are absolutely needed, should be thrown out. Outdated medications should also be thrown out; other medications should be kept in a locked cabinet. Anything sharp, breakable, flammable, or potentially poisonous stored on low shelves or in bottom drawers must be moved. Special locks are available for drawers and cupboards. Books should be packed tightly into bottom bookshelves. Wastebaskets or trash cans that don't have tight-fitting covers should be placed in cabinets with latched doors.

Now is the time, too, to resolve to stick to certain safety rules. There are few absolutes in child rearing, but there are three in the area of safety. Parents must make it a practice to *never leave a baby or young child alone:*

- in the house
- in the bath or near any body of water
- in a high place such as a bed or changing table

These three measures will considerably reduce the risk of almost every major cause of childhood accidents: falls, burns, scalds, poisoning, and drowning. A fourth rule—*Make sure the home is equipped with adequate smoke alarms in working order*—will minimize the risk of injury or death by fire. A fifth rule—*never allow a child to ride in a car without a car seat or shoulder and lap belt*—would reduce auto deaths and injuries considerably. This should begin with the trip home from the hospital or childbirth center. Last, *never drive while under the influence of alcohol.*

Even the most dedicated parent cannot supervise a child every second of every day, and it only takes a few seconds for an enterprising child to experiment with a new and potentially hazardous object. For this reason, parents need to remove as many potential dangers as possible. They should also keep in mind, however, that no matter what they do, their children will fall, cut themselves, sample scraps from the garbage or the dog's dinner. The idea is to minimize the chances of serious harm. Parents should never feel so constrained by safety considerations that they inhibit the learning and independence that come from healthy exploration.

Safe Baby Furniture and Equipment

Parents need to develop a safety orientation about baby furniture and equipment. The Consumer Product Safety Commission has set standards for cribs and the U.S. Department of Transportation has set standards for car seats (see Vehicular Safety, later in this chapter) because inferior products in these categories have caused accidents or failed to protect their occupants. Unfortunately, standards have not been set for other categories of children's furniture. Compounding the problem, many parents use baby furniture borrowed from friends or passed down as family heirlooms. No crib should be used unless it meets these safety requirements:

- Slats no farther than 2⅜ inches apart.
- A minimum of 20 inches from top of mattress to top of side panels when they are in an up position.
- A minimum of 9 inches from top of mattress to top of side panels when they are lowered.
- A double-action side release mechanism (to protect against accidental dropping of the sides when hit).
- No horizontal pieces that would provide a foothold for climbing out of the crib.

If the crib has been painted, be sure that lead-free paint was used. If it hasn't or if a parent can't be sure, the crib should be repainted with at least two coats.

When purchasing other furniture or equipment, parents should check the following:

- *Balance.* Some baby bouncers or walkers may become top-heavy and topple if a baby stands up in them. Highchairs should be broad-based.
- *Hinges.* Hinges should be made so that they cannot close inadvertently or so that children cannot close them. X-type hinges should be covered with a guard.
- *Small parts.* Some baby furniture comes with attached beads or other toys to amuse the baby. They should be sturdy enough not to break or come off.
- *Safety straps.* Changing tables, highchairs, infant seats, carriages, and strollers should all come with straps or harnesses.

Toy boxes can be dangerous for two reasons: they often have a heavy wooden lid and a hinge that

Table 14.3 **TIPS ON TOYS**

Toys can be dangerous if they are not related to the age level of your child. For example, a toy that has many small removable parts is fascinating to the 6-year-old—and to his baby sister too, but that little creeper would very likely swallow so small an object. And there are tools that can be handled skillfully by the 12-year-old that might cause injury to his younger brother. The chart below lists both dangerous and safe toys for children of different ages.

Age and Interests	Hazards	Suggestions
Under 1 Age of Awareness	Avoid toxic, heavy breakable toys . . . sharp edges that might cut or scratch . . . small attachments that might become loose and be put into ears, nose, or mouth.	Brightly colored objects hung in view . . . squeak toys . . . sturdy, non-flammable rattles . . . washable stuffed dolls with embroidered eyes . . . colored balls . . . cups or smooth non-breakable objects to chew on.
1–2 Investigative Age	Avoid small toys that may be swallowed . . . flammable objects . . . toys with small removable parts . . . poisonous paint on any object . . . stuffed animals with glass or button eyes.	Rubber or washable squeak toys and soft stuffed dolls or animals . . . blocks with rounded corners . . . push-and-pull toys with strings or rounded handles . . . nests of blocks.
2–3 Explorative Age	Avoid anything with sharp or rough edges that will cut or scratch . . . objects with small removable parts . . . poisonous paint or decoration . . . marbles . . . beads . . . coins . . . flammable toys.	Sandbox with bucket, shovel and spoon . . . large peg boards . . . wooden animals . . . cars and wagons to push around . . . tip-proof kiddie cars and tricycles . . . large crayons . . . low rocking horse . . . small chair and table. Simple musical instruments.
3–4 Imitative Age	Avoid toys that are too heavy for child's strength . . . poorly made objects which may come apart, break or splinter . . . sharp or cutting toys . . . highly flammable costumes, electrical toys.	Small broom and carpet sweeper . . . toy telephone . . . dolls with simple wrap around clothing . . . doll buggies and furniture . . . dishes . . . miniature garden tools . . . trucks and tractors . . . non-electrical trains . . . drum . . . clothes, building blocks.
4–6 Beginning of Creative Age	Avoid shooting or target toys that will endanger eyes . . . ill-balanced mobile toys that may topple easily . . . poisonous painting sets . . . pinching or cutting objects.	Blackboard and dustless chalk . . . simple construction sets . . . paints and paint books . . . doll house and furniture . . . small sports equipment . . . skipping rope . . . washtub and board . . . paper doll sets with blunt end scissors . . . flame-retardant costumes . . . modeling clay.
6–8 Beginning of Dexterity Age	Avoid non-approved electrical toys . . . anything too large or complicated for child's strength and ability . . . sharp edged tools . . . poorly made skates . . . shooting toys.	Carpenter bench and well-constructed, lightweight usable tools . . . sled . . . construction sets . . . roller skates . . . approved electrical toys . . . kites . . . equipment for playing store, bank, filling station, etc. . . . playground equipment . . . puzzles and games . . . sewing materials . . . dolls and doll equipment.
8–12 Specialization of Tastes and Skills	Avoid air rifles, chemistry sets, dart games, bows and arrows, dangerous tools, and electrical toys UNLESS used under parental supervision.	Hobby materials, arts and crafts, photography, coin and stamp collections, puppet shows . . . musical instruments . . . gym and sports equipment . . . model and construction building sets . . . electrical train with Underwriters Laboratories (UL) approval . . . bicycle.

Reprinted with permission from the National Safety Council.

collapses easily. Children love to hide in the box and may not be able to get the lid open or may crush their fingers in the hinge. Plastic crates or small laundry baskets make better toy storage. If a wooden box is used, the hinge should be a double-action one. (See chapter 1, Before the Baby Is Born, for more information on purchasing furniture and equipment.)

Toy Safety

Toy safety is, again, tied to the developmental stage of the child. What is safe for a four-year-old, who is generally past the stage of exploring everything by mouth, is not safe for a one-year-old. Obviously, toys made of flammable materials or with faulty wiring are unsafe for any child. Table 14.3 adapted from the National Safety Council, gives guidelines on types of toys that are safe and unsafe at various age levels.

The U.S. Consumer Product Safety Commission publishes periodic lists of products that have been banned for safety reasons. Other sources of information on toy safety are listed in the Resources section of the appendix. Parents should be aware that some imported toys, especially low-priced copies of popular American items, may not meet acceptable standards.

Daycare and Babysitters

Safety considerations of daycare centers and nursery schools are as important as the training and philosophy of the staff. In many communities, daycare centers must meet certain safety standards to be licensed, but parents should nevertheless satisfy themselves that the staff and administration are cognizant of safety precautions. This is especially important when parents make less formal arrangements for care of their children, in individual or small group settings which may not fall under state or municipal jurisdiction. The School and Daycare Safety Checklist (table 14.4) provides some key questions for parents to ask when choosing a school or center. (For additional information, see chapter 16, Daycare.)

Parents who might otherwise demand that their children be entrusted to only the most highly qualified teachers sometimes enter into babysitting arrangements more casually, either out of desperation to find a last-minute sitter or because they view the situation as only a temporary one. Nevertheless, they owe it to their child to choose carefully each caregiver, even if employment lasts only a few hours.

Teenage babysitters have traditionally provided

Table 14.4 **SCHOOL AND DAYCARE SAFETY CHECKLIST**

Parents can apply the Home Safety checklist in table 14.2 to schools and daycare centers as well as to their homes. In addition, these questions should be asked:

1. Are there fire extinguishers that work and do staff know how to use them?
2. Are there smoke detectors or a sprinkler system (preferably both)?
3. Are there fixtures or furniture with sharp edges?
4. Have soft surfaces or mats been installed under play equipment?
5. Are the cleaning closets locked?
6. Are the fire exits unobstructed?
7. Is there a plan with drills for evacuation in the event of fire?
8. Are there instructors who have been trained in first aid and resuscitation of children?
9. What is the plan for the care of injured children?
10. What kinds of injuries have occurred at the school or center?
11. Is heating equipment protected?
12. What is the temperature of the water in the taps?
13. Is the kitchen off limits to the children (i.e., locked or separated by a gate)?

an important service at reasonable cost, but the quality of the care they provide and the amount of responsibility they show varies considerably. Children under 13 or 14 should not be given the sole responsibility for looking after younger children. Some high schools, Y's, 4-H Clubs, and similar groups sponsor babysitting courses that cover the rudiments of child care and safety practices. Parents may check with these organizations for a list of their recent graduates or work to encourage establishment of such courses in their community.

Older adults may provide the patience and perspective that teenagers may lack. Senior-citizen centers, retirement communities, and church groups may be a source of names.

Parents should check references when hiring a babysitter who isn't personally known to them and should discuss with any sitter what is expected of him or her. The main points to cover are: not opening the door to anyone and what to do in case of fire, accident, or sudden illness.

A permanent emergency telephone list should be posted near the phone, updated periodically, and pointed out to the sitter. This list should include phone numbers for the fire department, police, and ambulance (if 911 does not cover all services), the child's pediatrician, the local Poison Control Center (see Appendix A for listing) and several close friends, neighbors, or relatives who can help out in an emergency. This list should be supplemented on each occasion with the number where parents can be reached. If parents will be unreachable, they may want to make arrangements with a specific friend or neighbor to cover for the time they will be out.

Building and Renovation

The addition of a room or the renovation of a house or apartment can pose many hazards. In particular, parents should be watchful of paint chips during renovation. Until 1948, indoor paint contained lead, which is toxic to children; it may still be contained in outdoor paint. Paint remover is extremely caustic to the skin and its fumes are toxic. Some types are highly flammable. If major renovation is in progress, parents may want to live elsewhere for the period of paint stripping or chipping.

Travel Safety

When traveling, parents should pack syrup of ipecac and keep medicines, razors, scissors, and other potentially dangerous items in a lockable suitcase. If they will be staying at a private house, they may want to take outlet covers and a safety gate along. If they are planning to fly and then rent a car, they should either bring a car seat along (it can be checked with the luggage and does not need to be boxed) or check to see if the car rental agency has one for rent. (For more information, see chapters 1 and 8.)

a window shade or venetian blind, or an electrical cord from a lamp or other appliance. Toys dangling across the crib on a string can also cause suffocation.

Once crawling has begun, floors and reachable surfaces must be kept free of small objects such as coins, jewelry, plastic packaging materials, and anything else that might go into the mouth or over the face to prevent breathing. Sewing and crafts paraphernalia are dangerous as well, not only as items than can be put into the mouth but because they are often sharp and pose a threat to the eyes as well.

The chief concern about toys for children under age one is that they not provide a means of choking or strangulation. (See figure 14.1.) Toys for infants should not:

- Be small enough to swallow.
- Have small parts that could come off, such as glass or button eyes on stuffed animals.
- Have cords that could wrap around the neck, such as those on toy telephones.
- Be decorated with lead-based paint.

The Heimlich Maneuver, a method of helping older children and adults expel food or foreign objects when choking, is not recommended for infants under one year of age. Backslapping is more effective. It can be used when a baby is choking or to expel water in a drowning situation. Parents should learn this technique so that they will be prepared should their child need it. (For more information, see chapter 34, Medical Emergencies and First Aid Procedures.)

SAFETY RISKS

The First Year

During the first year the greatest dangers are drowning, suffocation or strangulation, falls, and scalds. Prevention is a matter of appropriate equipment, proper arrangement, and constant supervision.

Suffocation and Strangulation. These can occur all too easily, in ways that would not be obvious to many parents, and in ways that may only be a problem at this age and not later. Soft pillows, plastic bags, widely spaced banister or crib slats, venetian blind or drapery cords, infant necklaces and pacifiers on ribbons have all caused infant deaths. Balloons, buttons, pacifiers with two parts, or any other object that a baby might suck on can obstruct the windpipe and cause choking. Care should be taken not to place the crib, carriage, changing table, or playpen in reach of any cords, including those from

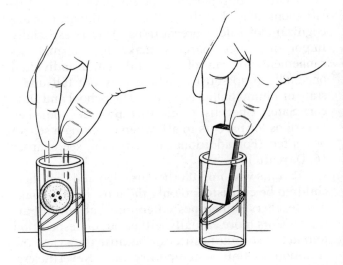

Figure 14.1. **Toy Measure.**
A simple cylinder device, available from some toy companies, allows parents to test whether a toy or part is large enough to be safe.

Falls. The only safe place to leave a baby alone is in a crib or playpen. The tiniest infant can eventually wiggle all the way off a bed, chair, or changing table. The crib mattress must be lowered a little with each new accomplishment to keep the crib a safe enclosure. Especially determined infants have been known to hoist themselves up and over the crib bars, landing on their heads. If this happens, it may be necessary to move the child to the playpen to sleep until he or she is accomplished enough to get out of the crib feet first.

About 40 percent of injuries sustained during the first year of life are head injuries, many of which are the result of falls. Falls that occur before the baby crawls are almost always the result of leaving the baby unattended on a bed or other high surface.

There is no need to have a high changing table. Babies can be changed on a low bed, an upholstered chair, a hassock, or on a blanket on the floor to avoid the possibility of a fall.

Once the process of creeping, pulling up, and walking begins, some falls are inevitable. Here the task is one of minimizing possible damage. As soon as the baby is crawling about, any stairs should be fenced both top and bottom. Expansion gates should not be used because they can contract and pinch tiny fingers, or worse, children are apt to put their heads through the openings.

Furniture with sharp edges should be moved out of the baby's play areas or replaced altogether. If this is not practical, the corners can be covered with foam tape or special plastic adhesive-backed corners that are sold in hardware and baby-supply stores.

Scalds and Burns. It is not unusual for mothers of small infants to hold them while having a cup of tea or coffee. An infant can awaken suddenly with a startle reflex, while older babies can bounce about, jarring the parent's arm, or tug at a place mat or tablecloth, causing a spill that can scald. Trying to manage a baby while drinking a hot beverage is a dangerous practice to be avoided from the very first. Parents must decide either not to hold the baby when drinking hot beverages or resign themselves to drinking lukewarm coffee for a year or two.

Bathtime is fully supervised at this age, and scalding in the tub is less likely than it may be a year or so later when the child may be able to turn on the hot water faucet. Nevertheless, this is the time to adjust the thermostat on the hot water heater to produce water no hotter than 130 degrees F., and preferably 120–125 degrees F. In apartment houses this may be difficult, but an appeal can be made to the landlord or superintendent, pointing out that this safety measure protects the elderly as well as small children. Barring this, a regulating device can be purchased that fits onto an individual tap.

Burns, particularly from contact with a hot object, can best be prevented by childproofing the home. Radiators and hot water pipes, heaters, woodstoves, and fireplaces must be surrounded by guards. Hot irons and electric coffee pots should never be left unattended, nor should the cords hang down within the child's reach.

To prevent electrical burns and shocks, any unused electrical outlets should be covered. Plastic plug-in blanks can be purchased at baby-supply or hardware stores, or outlets can be covered with heavy electrical tape. Because most electrical burns to infants result from sucking or chewing on electrical cords, these should be kept as much out of the way as safe use will permit.

Although ignition of clothing from an open flame is a small risk in the first year, flame-resistant night clothing should be provided from birth. Some fabrics, such as acrylics, may be flame-resistant, meaning they will not burst into flame, but they are capable of melting and causing severe burns. Imported night clothes may not be flame retardant.

Drowning. A baby can drown in only one or two inches of water, making it imperative that a parent never leave a baby or young child alone near water of any depth, not even for a moment. Parents should learn to let the phone or doorbell ring at bathtime or take the baby along if they feel they must answer.

Baths are not the only place a baby can drown. A mop bucket, a foot tub, a toilet, a puddle in the back yard—all perfectly harmless in the childless home—are hazardous for a baby.

The Toddler Period, Ages One to Three

The toddler is into everything: opening doors, emptying drawers, climbing on almost any surface, and exploring every small object by putting it in the mouth. The one-year-old's world is expanding to include the yard, the playground, and other public places. Drowning now tops the list of possible dangers, with fires and burns following close behind. Falls and choking on food or other objects remain major concerns.

Childproofing the Home. Now that the child is more mobile, it is time for another safety assessment of the whole house, concentrating on the kitchen and bath. The same assessment should be made of any home where the child routinely spends time— the babysitter's, daycare center, grandparents', or vacation home.

The kitchen is particularly dangerous for the toddler. Gas stoves, ovens, and hot liquids and food-stuffs on stove or countertops can be lethal. Matches, a source of endless fascination, must be kept locked away. Furniture polish, cleaning agents, pesticides, and lye-containing drain treatments, traditionally kept under the sink or in the broom closet, must be kept out of reach or locked up. Knives and other sharp tools and small electric appliances with attractive cords and engaging knobs and switches cannot be left about. To prevent burns, fires, and poisoning, parents should take the following precautions:

- Teach the meaning of "hot."
- Use back burners of the stove for cooking.
- Turn pot handles toward the back wall.
- Lock up matches and candles.
- Keep small appliances and their cords out of reach.
- Do not allow the child to turn on hot water faucets.
- Put all hazardous cleaning supplies out of reach, under lock and key.
- Put safety latches on all cabinet doors and drawers.
- Keep stepladders, stools, and chairs out of the cooking area.

Bathrooms, too, can be a place where burns, fires, and poisoning are hazards almost equal to that of drowning. The following precautions should be taken:

- Keep space heaters of all types out of the bathroom.
- Adjust maximum water temperature to below 130 degrees F. and secure hot water faucets so that they cannot be turned on by a child.
- Cover the hot water tap in the tub with heavy terry-cloth (such as an old towel) or purchase a special rubber fitting for the tap (some come disguised as a whale) so that the hot metal cannot burn the child.
- If hair dryers, radios, and electric shavers are kept in the bathroom, be sure that they are unplugged and out of the reach of a child standing on the toilet or sink.
- Keep all medications and cleaning agents locked up or well out of children's reach. (When determining out-of-reach locations, keep in mind that many children are skillful climbers.)
- Avoid taking medications in front of children to reduce the chances of their attempting to imitate this behavior.
- Keep cosmetics and safety razors locked or on the top shelf of the medicine cabinet.
- Clean up broken items by vacuuming first, then wiping with a damp paper towel.

A variety of locks and latches are available in hardware and baby-supply stores that make ordinary drawers and doors safe. One type, for example, involves a long, flexible plastic catch that screws to the inside of a cabinet door. The door can be opened with one hand far enough to depress the latch until it clears the plastic catch that is the other half of the set—easy for an adult to use but not a child. Another type, useful for metal kitchen cabinets, is a giant plastic hasp that slips through both handles on the outside and locks them together.

The important thing is to choose a storage method that is not so troublesome that parents find themselves not using it. If a lock can't easily be put on a medicine chest, for example, then perhaps the contents can be transferred to the bathroom linen closet, which can be locked with a simple hook and eye near the top. Dangerous items might also be kept in a file box or fishing tackle box with a lock.

Poisoning. Although poisoning deaths in this country have become relatively rare, dropping from 456 in 1959 to 57 in 1981, poisoning injuries in the one-to-five age group are still common (more than 110,000 in children under five in 1983) and must be guarded against. The major reason for the decrease in poisoning deaths and injuries has been the institution of childproof caps on prescription and over-the-counter drug containers. Parents should be aware, however, that medications—especially aspirin—are available in containers with easy-open caps for arthritis patients and other adults who do not have the strength to open safety caps. Care should be taken to purchase medications with safety packaging, as pharmacists do not always supply them automatically. Parents should also recognize that grandparents and others who live in childless households may routinely purchase drugs in nonsafety containers. If an older relative lives with the family or if the child spends time in a grandparent's home, these containers should be kept safely out of reach.

Potential poisons, including some common house plants, can be found throughout the home. (See table 14.5, Poisons in the Home.) Parents should eliminate any that are not essential and store the rest in locked containers or closets. Never should toxic substances be transferred to another container such as a soda bottle. Not only does this make it easier for a child to confuse the contents, but it eliminates the information about contents, safe use, and poisoning emergency instructions.

Parents should be prepared for a poisoning emergency by having syrup of ipecac (an emetic that induces vomiting) in the medicine chest and the number of the Poison Control Center posted near the phone. Vomiting should not be induced if the child

Table 14.5 **POISONS IN THE HOME**

The following are examples of potential toxins found in various locations throughout the house. Not all of them are commonly considered poisonous, but when taken by a child they can have toxic effects. This list should not be considered all-inclusive.

Bathroom

Prescription drugs and medications such as: acetaminophen, aspirin, cold medications, contraceptives, cough medicine, diet pills, hydrogen peroxide, iodine, laxatives, rubbing alcohol, sleeping pills	Cosmetics, such as: deodorants, depilatories, hair dyes and bleaches, hairspray, makeup, nail polish and remover, perfume, permanent-wave lotions, shampoo

Miscellaneous

Lighter fluid	Liquor
Shoe polish	

Laundry

Bleach	Spot removers
Detergents	Cleaning fluid (carbon
Fabric softener	tetrachloride)

Cleaning Supplies

Ammonia	Metal polish
Disinfectant	Room deodorant
Drain cleaner	Rug cleaner
Floor wax	Wall and window cleaner

Workroom/Garage/Garden Supplies

Antifreeze	Kerosene
Benzene	Motor oil
Car wax	Paint
Charcoal starter	Paint thinners and
Fertilizer	removers
Gasoline	Pesticides
Glue and cement	Rat poison
Hand cleaners	Turpentine
Herbicides (weed killers)	Varnish and shellac

Kitchen

Dishwasher soap	Sodium bicarbonate
Insecticides	Vitamins

Common Poisonous Plants *

Autumn crocus	Dieffenbachia *(also called dumbcane)*	Lantana	Rapeweed
Azalea		Larkspur	Rhododendron
Belladonna	English ivy *(berries and leaves)*	Lily-of-the-valley	Rhubarb *(leaf and roots; only the stalk is edible)*
Bird-of-paradise *(seed pod)*	Foxglove	Manchneel	
Buttercups	Grass peavine	Mistletoe *(berries)*	Skunk cabbage
Cassava	Holly *(berries)*	Monkshood	Sweet pea
Castor bean	Horse chestnuts	Mountain laurel	Tomato plant leaves
Chinaberry	Hyacinth *(bulbs)*	Oleander	Water hemlock
Chinese evergreen	Hydrangea	Philodendron	Wisteria *(seeds)*
Christmas pepper	Iris	Poinsettia	Yew *(needles, bark, seeds, and berries)*
Corncockle	Jack-in-the-pulpit	Poison hemlock	
Daffodil *(bulb)*	Jasmine *(flowers)*	Pokeberry	
Daphne	Jerusalem cherry	Potato *(sprouts, roots, and vines; only the tuber is edible)*	
Deadly nightshade	Jimson weed *(also called thornapple)*		
Delphinium		Purple locoweed	

* From *The Columbia University College of Physicians and Surgeons Complete Home Medical Guide*, © 1985. Used with permission.

has swallowed anything corrosive such as lye or a strong acid or if the child is drowsy, unconscious, or having convulsions. If the child eats or drinks something that may be poisonous, the parent should call the Poison Control Center or local hospital emergency department and describe the substance and the state of the child. Unless instructed otherwise by the pediatrician or Poison Control Center, the parent should take the child and the toxin, if known, to the hospital immediately. A basin should also be taken to preserve anything the child may vomit, as it may assist in diagnosis and treatment.

Drowning. Because toddlers can sit up by themselves, it is more tempting to leave the toddler alone in the bath "for a moment" than it is to leave a baby.

It is equally dangerous, however, as is leaving a tub full of water standing for any reason.

When a youngster graduates from the sink or the baby bath to the tub, a nonskid rubber mat should be placed in the tub (large enough to cover the whole bottom) and a skidproof rug on the floor to ensure safer footing.

Wading pools, swimming pools, culverts, uncovered wells and cesspools in the yard or neighborhood are potential danger areas for toddlers. A parent should check the surrounding blocks for any pools or culverts that might pose a threat and then see that children are kept out of the area. Those living near ponds, lakes, or other large bodies of water will need to be particularly watchful. Parents should work with community officials to see that, where feasible, these attractive nuisances are fenced or attended. Where this is not feasible, children should not be allowed in the area unsupervised. Any child taken out in a boat, even a rowboat in a pond, should wear a life preserver or personal flotation device in the appropriate size.

The best way to protect against a child's wandering into harm's way is to fence his own play area and to choose neighborhood play areas that are properly fenced. In the back yard, the wading pool should be emptied when not being used. If there is an in-ground pool, parents may want to consider installing a special alarm that is triggered if anything heavier than five pounds falls into the pool.

Many parents these days teach their children to swim before age three. Although swimming is a valuable skill, it does not provide a guarantee against drowning. Even parents whose children are quite at home in the water must be as vigilant as those whose children cannot swim at all.

Choking. The highest incidence of fatal choking is in children under two. Fatal choking in children usually involves round objects, more often food than anything else. Pieces of hot dogs are the chief culprit, along with candies, nuts, and grapes. These foods, as well as popcorn, crisp bacon, raw vegetables, chicken or fish with the bones still in, should be avoided until a child is three or four.

Typical objects that cause choking are undersize pacifiers, small balls, pieces of toys, pebbles, marbles, and uninflated or underinflated balloons. Parents need to keep an eye out for any small objects within a child's reach. This is especially difficult when there are older children around who have toys with many small pieces. The older child must be cautioned about carefully putting away such toys, and he or she must have an area in which to play with these toys without interference.

Falls. Tumbles associated with cuts and bruises go along with the toddler phase, but serious falls with head injuries need not occur if proper precautions are taken. This is the time to be sure that stairs are protected and that all entrances to hazardous places (basements, attics, driveways) are secure. Window guards—on all windows, if possible, and certainly on all windows above the first floor—are critically important. Furniture should be checked for sharp edges, stability, and placement to be sure that chairs or tables do not provide access to unsafe objects or locations. Safety glass should be installed in doors and colored decals should be placed on large expanses of glass.

When the child begins to walk, scatter rugs should be removed, tacked in place with double-faced rug tape, or placed on top of a nonskid mat. This is a good general safety practice, especially if there are elderly living in the home as well.

Playgrounds should be chosen for safety rather than convenience. Exposed cement anchors for slides and swings, cement or asphalt surfaces, or areas constructed to accommodate both older and younger children are dangerous for toddlers. Hard surfaces increase the chance of head injuries; uneven surfaces add to the risk of falls, cuts, and gashes; and the presence of older, more accomplished children increases the risk of collisions and may encourage younger children to mimic activities for which they are not ready. (See Safe Playground Checklist, table 14.6.)

Traffic Safety. By the time a child is two, traffic safety will begin to be significant. Firm discipline is required to keep adventuresome two-year-olds out of streets and driveways. Parents can set a good example and begin to explain and practice traffic rules, such as crossing only at lights and looking to the left and right, even though children should also be taught never to cross the street without taking an adult's hand. Tricycles and other riding toys should be ridden only on sidewalks and never across driveways. Children of this age cannot comprehend danger, and though traffic safety "education" should begin, most safety efforts are matters of discipline and supervision at this stage.

Ages Four to Six

During this period children begin to leave their own yards or to go beyond the block, often with older children. They play rough games, explore new territory, and begin to participate more fully in family life by helping around the house and garden. Children will begin to play out of parents' sight for longer and longer periods of time, but frequent

Table 14.6 **SAFE PLAYGROUND CHECKLIST**

The Consumer Product Safety Commission has developed the following Voluntary Product Safety Standards for home and public playgrounds:

1. Equipment should be simple, natural, and inexpensive.
2. Equipment should be safe. Be aware of and try to avoid any sharp edges, protruding parts, and weaknesses or flaws in materials.
3. Make periodic checkups and replace any worn or damaged pieces of equipment.
4. Equipment should be attractive. Some like bright colors. Environmentalists like natural earth-tone colors.
5. Surfaces beneath and around equipment should be absorptive so children will not incur a force greater than 40 to 50 g when they fall. Sand, wood chips, pea gravel, shredded tires, etc., are recommended surface materials.
6. Equipment anchored in the ground should be set in concrete for stability. To avoid a tripping hazard, all types of anchoring devices should be placed below ground level.
7. Open-ended hooks that can catch skin or clothes should be avoided. If **S** hooks are used, pinch the ends in tightly.
8. Moving parts, particularly on gliders and seesaws, can pinch or crush fingers.
9. Hard, heavy swing seats can strike a dangerous blow. Choose light-weight seats or ones with an absorptive surface.
10. Equipment that requires children to climb should not have steps greater than the knee height of those who will use the equipment.
11. The spaces between bars of horizontal climbing equipment should not exceed 14 inches.
12. Rails or runs on any equipment should be cylindrical and about 1 inch in diameter.
13. Equipment should be an appropriate height, never more than 6 feet from the ground.
14. Sliding surfaces should be wide so that more than one child can slide at a time.
15. Equipment should not have radical angles for sliding or climbing.
16. Standing surfaces should have protective rails that can be reached comfortably by children.
17. Crawl spaces should have openings large enough to permit access by adults if necessary.
18. Equipment should be designed to guard against entrapment or situations that may cause strangulation. Swinging exercise rings should be removed from playgrounds used by young children.
19. Inertial effects or rotary motion from equipment should not cause dizziness or spatial disorientation.
20. Preserve all wood materials with a nontoxic substance.
21. Drill holes in the bottom of all tires for adequate drainage.
22. Place metal equipment in the shade when possible or facing a north-south direction to prevent exposure to direct sunlight.
23. Moving equipment (swings, merry-go-rounds, etc.) should be located toward the edge or corner of a play area to prevent injuries to children as they run from one apparatus to another.
24. Equipment should be arranged so that children playing on one piece will not interfere with other children playing on, or running to another piece of equipment.

Reprinted with permission from The United States Consumer Product Safety Commission.

checks on their activities are still vital.

The risks for this age group are similar to those for toddlers, except that the chance of choking and scalding decreases with each year, while the risk of injury by firearms enters the picture. The chance of pedestrian injury also increases markedly. With both firearms and pedestrian injuries, the risk is far greater for boys than for girls.

A more thorough neighborhood check is in order as children begin to play farther afield. It is now time to look for construction sites, deep holes such as abandoned wells, discarded appliances or cars, vacant buildings, bodies of water, etc. Dangerous places should be pointed out to the child and rules laid down about avoiding them.

Traffic and Bicycle Safety. Traffic safety rules can be more thoroughly explained and must be continually enforced. Such rules as "Never run into the street after a ball" and "Never go between parked cars" can now be understood and must be reiterated regularly. Boys are more at risk than girls, and blacks more than whites, of being hit by a car. Five-year-old boys are the most likely to dash into the street and be fatally struck by an automobile. Although children must learn to obey traffic safety rules and need opportunities to practice these rules, they are far safer playing in enclosed areas where there is no chance of being lured into the street by a stray ball.

Bicycle safety should be taught along with general traffic safety. In addition, parents should provide equipment and clothing that promotes safe riding. This includes a hard-shelled helmet with polystyrene liner, reflective belts or bands, as well as a bicycle of proper size equipped with reflectors, bell or whistle, and chain guard. Helmets are regularly worn by serious cyclists and by about 10 percent of college students. Young children, however, are rarely provided with helmets or requested by parents to wear them. As cycling is an almost universal childhood activity and head injuries are the most common result of bicycle accidents, parents should invest in safe and properly fitted helmets for their children.

Drowning. Water safety can be taught children at this age. Children can learn the Lanoue water-survival method of floating even before they learn to swim. For those living in cold areas where ponds and lakes freeze in winter, the dangers of playing on frozen surfaces must be explained and strict rules set forth.

Safety Education. As children begin to help around the house, they should be taught safe ways to handle kitchen equipment, cleaning supplies, and tools. Where garages or basements contain power tools, the dangers must be clearly explained, and children should always be kept away from lawn-mowers.

This is also the time to reinforce teaching about the danger of matches, open flames, hot substances and objects. The possibility of chemical burns should also be explained. Children are now old enough to be taught to "stop, drop, and roll" should their clothing be ignited. Paints, petroleum products, insecticides, and gardening products should be stored in locked cupboards or on high shelves out of reach of any small child. In all matters, parents can teach safe behavior best by practicing safety themselves.

Children should also be taught how to approach a strange dog, even one that acts friendly. The safest way is to make a fist and extend it slowly to allow the dog to sniff it. Only after the dog seems satisfied and reacts positively should the child expose any fingers or attempt to pet the dog.

VEHICULAR SAFETY

BECAUSE HALF of the childhood deaths due to injury are caused by motor vehicle accidents, traffic and automobile safety is the single most important precaution parents can take to ensure the lives and health of their children. Beyond fatalities, a significant number of children in traffic accidents sustain head and spinal cord injuries that result in epilepsy and paraplegia.

Fatal pedestrian injuries are more common than fatal passenger injuries in preschool and school-aged children. Yet this problem has not been studied in a systematic fashion that can identify children particularly at risk, environmental hazards commonly involved, or psychosocial or geographic factors that may be influential. It is clear that boys of all ages are at greater risk than girls, and it may be that children with emotional and behavioral problems are more frequently involved in pedestrian accidents. Children under 10 often do not have the cognitive ability to negotiate traffic safely. At present there is no program or body of facts that can help reduce death and injury to children in pedestrian accidents other than vigilance and constant reinforcement of traffic safety rules.

With regard to fatal passenger injuries, however, the picture is much brighter. It has been clearly demonstrated that for children four years of age and under, use of proper child restraints in automobiles can reduce the probability of both death and serious injury by more than 50 percent. For children over four years of age, the use of lap belts produces similar results. All 50 states have adopted mandatory passenger restraint laws for children. Educational programs have been mounted on television, in schools, and in physicians' offices.

While improvement in the death-and-injury rate of restrained children is evident, large numbers of children still ride unprotected, or restrained by devices that are inadequate or improperly installed. Some 600 to 700 passengers under age five are killed each year and more than 50,000 are injured as a result of vehicle collision and sudden stops and swerves. Perhaps half of these deaths and injuries could be avoided or the injury consequences reduced with proper restraints. It is no wonder that some have labeled failure to provide this protection as child abuse.

Automobiles

People of all ages need to be protected against impact with automobile interiors or being thrown from the vehicle during collisions or sudden stops. When a vehicle going 30 miles an hour suddenly stops, all unrestrained passengers continue to move at that speed until they are stopped by their own collision with another passenger, the vehicle interior, or the ground outside the car. For a young child this is equivalent to the impact of falling from a third-floor window. A child held in the arms of an unrestrained adult is in even greater danger. The child not only suffers the forward impact, but is apt to be crushed by the adult moving with a force equal to 30 times the child's weight.

All children up to 40 pounds should (and in many states, must) ride in a crash-tested safety seat. Children over 40 pounds but under 55 inches in height should use a lap belt with or without a booster seat, and children over 55 inches in height should wear both a lap belt and a shoulder harness.

To be effective, child restraints must be of an

appropriate design and correctly installed. Because some child safety seats cannot be properly installed in certain car models, parents should be sure that the seat they purchase is compatible with their car. Parents who do not have a car but whose child rides regularly in someone else's car should provide a safety seat for the child's use. Those who cannot afford to purchase a safety restraint may be able to get one through a loan or rental program. Pediatricians and hospital social-service personnel are usually knowledgeable about such programs. Safety seats may also be purchased secondhand. This should be done only under the following conditions:

- The seat was manufactured after January 1, 1981.
- The seat is on a list of devices meeting Federal Standard 213-80.
- The manufacturer's instruction booklet is available.
- The seat is in good condition, free of rust, discoloration, or frayed belts.
- The buckle works properly.
- All securing devices are available and in good repair.
- The seat has never been involved in an accident.

Some three- or four-year-olds begin to rebel against car seats and may try to squirm out or unbuckle the straps. Parents should make it a rule to stop the car and not continue until the child is secure again. They can also set a good example by never driving unless they are wearing seatbelts themselves. If possible, the child safety seat should be placed in the middle of the back seat. This is not only the safest place for it, but will allow the child the best vantage point.

Children may also put up resistance when they move from a safety seat to regular seatbelts, because they can no longer see out the window. Parents may want to consider a booster seat which comes with a body harness or can be used with a lap and shoulder belt, and which can be used for children up to 65 pounds.

The only occasion when it might be impossible to provide a child safety seat is while riding in a taxi, when seatbelts should be used. Auto rental companies usually have seats available for rental at a small charge, and airlines, trains, and buses accept safety seats along with regular luggage. A consideration in purchasing a seat for the family car is that it should be easily transferred to another vehicle, making it easy to provide the seat when riding with others.

Further information on automobile safety and child restraint devices that meet Federal standards can be obtained from the sources listed in table 14.7. The box on Auto Safety Guidelines lists practices that always should be followed.

Table 14.7 **INFORMATION SOURCES FOR CHILD CAR SAFETY**

American Academy of Pediatrics
P.O. Box 1034
Evanston, IL 60204

American Association for Automotive Medicine
P.O. Box 222
Morton Grove, IL 60053

Consumers Union, Washington Office
1511 K Street, N.W.
Washington, DC 20005

National Highway Traffic Safety Administration
400 7th Street, S.W.
Washington, DC 20690

National Safety Council
444 N. Michigan Avenue
Chicago, IL 60611

Physicians for Automotive Safety
Communications Department
5 Eve Lane
Rye, NY 10580

Family physician, hospital, county health department, and local auto club.

AUTO SAFETY GUIDELINES

- All passengers, not just children, should use seatbelts.
- Loose objects should not be placed on the dashboard or back window where they may fly off if the car stops suddenly.
- Doors should always be locked when children are riding in the car. Children should not be allowed to play with the locks, open windows, or stick their hands out windows.
- The car should not be left unlocked or running in the garage or driveway.
- Children should not be allowed to play with the steering wheel or any of the buttons in the car, even with a parent present, because they may attempt it when they are alone.
- Children should never be left alone in the car.
- Parents should not attempt to discipline a child while driving. They should stop the car and pull over.
- Because boredom often leads to trouble, parents should be in the habit of bringing toys, games, and books on car trips, even short ones.

Bicycles

Many parents, especially in urban areas, use bicycles both for short errands and recreation. As soon as their children reach the early toddler stage, they buy child bicycle seats and take the child along. A study at Northwestern University found that in a seven-year period there were more than 2,500 injuries to children riding in these seats, and three-quarters of the children were under age three. Most of the injuries were to the head or neck, and 81 percent were considered to be severe or moderate. To make this mode of transporting a child as safe as possible, the following precautions should be taken:

- Be sure the seat is securely mounted.
- Be sure the seatbelt is adequate to firmly secure the child.
- Equip the bicycle with spoke guards.
- Provide the child with a helmet.

Other Vehicles

Mile for mile, airplanes, trains, and buses are much safer means of transport than automobiles, motorcycles, or bicycles. Whenever there is a choice, public transport is the safest place for the traveler of any age.

FIRE SAFETY

CHILDREN FROM BIRTH to four years of age are four times more likely to die in a fire than their parents, and they are less likely to survive serious burns or smoke inhalation than adults. Those who do survive severe burns frequently suffer permanent disfigurement and psychological damage.

The hope is to prevent fires altogether. The second line of defense is early detection. The United States leads all nations in the incidence of death due to fire. Parents cannot afford to be casual in their approach to the subject. The most important tool to reduce the risk of injury or death from house fires is a working smoke alarm. The accompanying guidelines on reducing fire hazards in the home and preparing a family fire-escape plan has been produced by the Ambulatory Pediatric Association.

Reducing Fire Hazards in the Home

Smoking: Careless handling of cigarettes is the most common cause of deaths and injuries in residential fires. If there are smokers in the house, the increased risk of fire can be reduced by:

1. Depositing cigarettes and cigars in large ashtrays, not in wastebaskets.
2. Double-checking the house before going to bed to be sure there are no smoldering cigarettes in chairs or sofas.
3. Keeping matches and lighters in a place inaccessible to children.
4. Not smoking in bed.

Kitchen: The kitchen is the most common origin of house fires. These can be avoided or their danger reduced by:

1. Not leaving anything that is cooking unattended.
2. Keeping curtains, towels, dishcloths, and other flammables away from the cooking area.
3. Mounting a fire extinguisher near the kitchen.

Storage: Fire hazards caused by improper storage methods can be reduced by:

1. Storing combustible and flammable materials in safety containers and away from children and potential sources of heat.
2. Keeping storage areas such as attics and basements free of unnecessary items.
3. Not piling clothes and papers against light fixtures.

Electrical: To reduce fires from electrical sources, avoid:

1. Overloading multiple-outlet plugs.
2. Positioning large appliances in areas where there is poor air circulation.

Fireplaces and wood-burning stoves: Prevent destructive fires in fireplaces and wood-burning stoves by:

1. Using protective fireplace screens.
2. Making sure the fire is out before going to bed or leaving the house.
3. Keeping flammable materials away from the fireplace or stove.

Family Fire-Escape Plan

Before a Fire Occurs

1. Draw a floorplan of the house showing halls, bedrooms, stairs, windows, and doors. Mark the normal exit route from each bedroom with heavy arrows and alternate routes with lighter arrows.
2. Provide a rope or metal ladder for bedroom windows that are too high above the ground for safe exit. The ladder should be securely attached to the windowsill or to a radiator near the window.
3. Install and maintain smoke detectors for each bedroom area.
4. Assign to each family member specific duties, such as calling the fire department from outside the house and assuring the safe exit of children or handicapped members of the family.
5. Sleep with bedroom doors closed if smoke detectors have not yet been installed outside each bedroom area.
6. Agree on a specific meeting place outside the house, and prohibit reentry until the fire department has arrived and given the okay.

7. If you live in a high-rise apartment, plan and practice a fire-escape plan that specifically excludes the use of elevators.

When a Fire Occurs

1. If you suspect there is a fire or if the smoke detector sounds an alarm, leave the house immediately. Do not get dressed, call the fire department, gather valuables, or search for the source of the fire.
2. If you plan to exit through a bedroom door, feel the door before opening it. If it is warm, keep it closed. If it is not, open it slowly, bracing your shoulder against the door to prevent it from being forced inward by pressure on the other side. Check for smoke before exiting.
3. If you can't escape through the doorway, stuff cloth under the door and exit via the window.
4. Try to leave the house through areas where there is no smoke. If this is impossible, get down and crawl; the best air is near the floor.

ADULT BEHAVIOR AND FAMILY SITUATIONS THAT AFFECT CHILD SAFETY

THERE ARE SPECIAL CIRCUMSTANCES and adult behaviors that put children at increased risk. Some cannot be changed; others are subject to modification.

Stress

Times of change and stress in a family increase the risk of childhood injury. Moving, illness, death, or divorce are all circumstances in which adults are apt to be distracted or incapacitated so that supervision is diminished. At moving time, or when staying in another's home, children have more opportunities to find objects they should not, or to get into situations of potential danger. These circumstances cannot usually be altered, so the only recourse is to be aware of the risks and to get additional assistance or exercise greater vigilance.

Alcohol

In one half of the deaths due to motor-vehicle accidents, two-car collisions, or vehicle-pedestrian accidents, at least one person involved has a blood alcohol level above the legal limit. Sometimes this person is the parent who is driving with a child while impaired. Alcohol is also a major factor in child-abuse injuries.

Parents have a particular duty not to expose their children to abuse, either physical or vehicular, by drinking to excess. Parents can support public and private efforts to curtail drunk driving on a broad level and make sure that their children are not entrusted to anyone who might be involved in substance abuse.

Smoking

Careless handling of cigarettes is the most common cause of death and injury in residential fires. Leaving the health aspects of smoking aside, the safety factor is significant. The idea of banning smoking in the home is one worth considering from the standpoint of fire safety as well as that of general health. If smoking is allowed, it should be remembered that cigarettes and alcohol are a particularly dangerous combination, because alcohol consumption may diminish the awareness of cigarette hazards.

Firearms

About half the homes in America contain at least one gun. Although these guns are generally purchased for hunting or sport, about three-quarters of owners also consider them as a form of protection. In addition to the 200 million powder firearms in private possession, there are an unknown number of nonpowder firearms (BB guns and the like) owned by children and young adults. Children under 15 years of age account for over 30 percent of all firearm-related deaths happening in the home, usually as a result of the unintentional discharge of a gun.

The findings of a recent six-year study in the state of Washington of firearm deaths call into question whether the protective function of guns is equal to the risks involved in having them in the home. This study showed that 54 percent of deaths by gun occurred inside the home in which the gun was kept, and of those deaths, 84 percent were suicides, 50 percent were homicides, and 3 percent were accidental gunshot deaths. Only 0.05 percent of the deaths involved an intruder.

Regarding nonpowder firearms, boys ages 5 through 14 are at greatest risk of being killed or injured, but boys in all age groups are involved. Injuries most often occur inside the home and are usually accidental rather than intentional. With injury rates as high as 35 per 100,000, it would seem that these firearms are too dangerous to be considered toys.

Many child development specialists feel that gunplay promotes antisocial behavior. It may also contribute to accidents when a real gun is handled in a hazardous manner because the child is unaware that it is not a toy. Parents should take these facts into consideration as they decide whether to allow their children to play with toy guns or use nonpowder firearms.

Those parents who choose to keep firearms in the home should follow strict safety rules. All guns should be in a locked cabinet, and ammunition, also locked up, should be kept in a separate location.

SUMMING UP

THE CHILD IS a developing being whose safety is closely connected to each stage of development. A child's level of cognitive development may limit his or her ability to avoid potential injuries. While the educational process should begin early with teaching of rote safety rules, it should be remembered that few of these rules can be reliably carried out by most children until they are about eight years old. Consequently, most of the responsibility for the child's safety until this time lies with the parent or other adult supervisor. The key to preventing injuries in early childhood is to provide appropriate supervision and to ensure a safe environment through modification and frequent reassessment as the child develops.

15 The Family in Transition

Rosemary Barber-Madden, Ed. D.

INTRODUCTION

IT HAS BEEN many years since the American family fit the "traditional" pattern: father in the workforce, mother full time at home with two or more children. Although this pattern was heavily predominant in the 1950s, by the early 1970s only a third of all families fit this description; today, less than a fifth do so. And, despite the apparent return to more conservative values in many areas of American life, continuing radical changes in family structure seem likely in the future.

High divorce and remarriage rates are the major social factor shaping new family structures. One marriage in three ends in divorce; one of every five is a remarriage. As a result, there has been a large increase in the number of single-parent families, usually headed by women; an increase in the number of adults living alone, usually men; and an increase in the number and the complexity of stepfamilies. Even within two-parent families, mothers at home are increasingly rare: two-thirds of all women with children under age 18 now work or are looking for work outside the home.

Families, moreover, are smaller than at any time in history. While the smaller family can be seen as part of a long-term trend beginning in the late nineteenth century and broken only by the "baby-boom" families of the 1950s and early 1960s, more recent contributing factors are the tendency toward later marriage and the postponement of pregnancy by women pursuing careers. The extension of adolescent dependence on parents—in large part the result of extra years of education—often results in children remaining at home longer.

Another social factor affecting family patterns is the generally more relaxed attitude toward sexuality. There are increasing numbers of teenage mothers—some married, the majority not—and of older, never-married women raising children alone.

SEPARATION AND DIVORCE

DIVORCE RATES in the United States have been rising steadily since 1860, the first year for which such data are available. Within this steady curve, the lifetime level of divorce for those who married in the decade after World War II is unusually low; for their children, the baby-boom generation, it is predicted to be unusually high. It is projected that half of all recent marriages will end in divorce. About half of all divorces occur within the first seven years of marriage, resulting in large numbers of children experiencing family breakup at a very early age.

The central events of divorce—departure and loss—are psychologically comparable to the event of death and often evoke similar responses. But maintaining a failed marriage "for the sake of the children" places a heavy burden on the children, who are supposedly being protected, and causes more suffering, and in a more prolonged form, to both parents and children than a reasonably amicable breakup.

The most serious risk to children from their parents' divorce is the deprivation of the sustained emotional support that they need to grow into stable adults. When both the custodial and the noncustodial parents make ongoing efforts to provide each other support, the children will be better able to adjust to their changed circumstances. In bitter divorces, children frequently become pawns in their parents' rancorous contest—they may, for example, be offered by one parent to the other in return for a better property settlement. The emotional damage caused by divorce varies, of course, with the circumstances and the children's personalities, but if the conflicts can be resolved quickly, or at least limited to occasional brief flareups of resentment, children may prove to be more resilient than had been expected.

In addition to providing emotional support and trying to limit their hostilities, parents need to help children develop their own resources. Children who gain a sense of mastery in overcoming obstacles usually come away from stressful situations stronger than before—and divorce is no exception to this general rule.

Timing and Announcement of Separation

When parents decide to dissolve their marriage peacefully, questions arise as how to best break the news to the children, and how soon to part. Economic factors are likely to be an important part of the latter decision—for example, the shortage of affordable housing keeps some couples together much longer than they would wish.

The sooner the children are told about the coming divorce, the better. Even if they cannot articulate their awareness of what is going on, children will sense tension and hostility between their parents. Attempts to hide marital discord inevitably lead to anxiety on the children's part.

Child therapists differ as to whether there is a "best age" for a child to undergo the parents' divorce—and, if so, what that age is. Some hold that divorce is the most traumatic to children if it occurs during the oedipal period (age four to five). At this time, children (especially boys) often wish that the same-sex parent were no longer around and may feel directly responsible if that parent does in fact leave the home. Other therapists feel that the younger the child, and the longer the child lacks two parents, the greater the potential for damage.

Both parents should participate in the announcement of the coming divorce. This tends to lessen the insecurity and also carries the implication that both parents will be available for similar conversations in the future. Most therapists advise telling all the children together, even if this means repeating each statement at different levels of comprehension. Separate discussions with each child foster feelings of secretiveness and consequent distrust.

With children of any age, the focus of the initial discussion should be two-fold: the decision to divorce, and the children's worries about the future. Some guidelines:

- Children should be told only when the decision is firm. They should not be subject to the emotional upheaval that accompanies ambivalence. A firm decision does much to relieve the anxiety caused by parental conflict.

- Parents should avoid blaming each other, saying only that they are no longer happy together, that they have tried unsuccessfully to work things out, and that it is best for everyone that they live apart. They should focus on the basic reason for the divorce—the fact that the marriage is no longer workable—rather than on specific problems. The younger children are, the less able they are to understand the idea of a joint contribution to difficulties and the more likely they are to look for a reason to blame one parent.

- Children should be reassured that they are not responsible for the breakup. The problems are between the parents and it is for the parents to deal with them.

- Children should also be reassured that, although the parents no longer love each other, they both continue to love their children. This statement is more convincing when it is made while both adults are still relating lovingly to the children—that is, while both are still at home. It is also important that the children understand that love shown for one parent will not jeopardize their relationship with the other.

- Concrete information should be provided about when the departing parent will leave, where he or she will live, and how often and where the child will be seeing him or her in the future. Such specifics reduce anxiety, especially regarding abandonment.

- Parents should not be afraid to admit that they make mistakes and that the marriage was one of them. Understanding that their parents are not perfect helps children to tolerate the deficiencies in themselves and others.

- Young children should be reassured that the basic necessities of life—food, clothing, shelter—will still be available to them.
- The lines of communication with both parents should be kept open. This is more important than the actual information that is given.

Children's Reactions

Children's reactions to divorce vary with age, as would be expected, and also by sex. For reasons that are not clear, boys have a more difficult time adjusting to a divorce than do girls. Boys tend to be more aggressive and to have poorer social skills and more problems at school than their sisters, who show their distress mainly by becoming quiet and withdrawn.

In the immediate aftermath of a divorce, children usually experience a number of emotions that are hard to handle:

Grief. With divorce, a child suffers the partial or total loss of a parent, the loss of familiar routines and symbols, perhaps the loss of a secure environment. Grief under such circumstances is natural and should not be inhibited by, for example, admonitions to "be brave." As the child faces the daily reality of the loss—and, particularly, as discussions and questions about the breakup are repeated—he or she will gradually become desensitized. Reassurance that the absent parent is still involved with the child, and regular visitation rights scrupulously observed by that parent, help in resolving the grief.

Guilt. More commonly than the parents realize, children hold themselves responsible for the family breakup. They will need to be reassured—perhaps many times—that no "bad" actions or deficiencies on their part had anything to do with the separation. Children may also experience profound guilt over loyalty conflicts. Even if they are not asked to decide which parent they will live with, some "taking sides" is inevitable. And since children are expected to express equal affection for both parents (whether they feel it or not), the situation is fraught with potential for guilt. Guilt may also follow expressions of hostility toward one or both parents. Since children know from experience that being punished usually lessens their feelings of guilt, they often behave in ways that predictably bring punishment.

Anger. The sources for the anger that children commonly feel in the wake of a divorce are legion. Among them: the preoccupation of the parents with their own problems; inability to live with the preferred parent; an unreliable noncustodial parent; the loss of a peaceful household; being different from peers; straitened circumstances, and a drastic change from the accustomed life-style. The very nature of the divorce situation tends to inhibit children in the expression of anger: if they show their feelings they might see less of the visiting parent, and the custodial parent might leave as well. Repressed anger may be channeled into such symptoms as proneness to accidents, stomach aches, or depression. Parents must gently try to bring anger into the open and teach the child to deal with it constructively. Other children release their anger by acting it out. Very young children may throw temper tantrums; older ones may be disruptive at home or at school, or they may bully their friends or persecute animals. Spending more time with the children will reduce their need to gain attention by behaving in a provocative way; giving them more affection will make them more secure and less likely to test parents' loyalty by acting-out behavior.

Fear of Abandonment. Despite reassurances, children tend to persist in the idea that the parent who has left has abandoned them. In light of all this, all relationships seem unstable—they may come to fear that they themselves may be made to leave home, or that the custodial parent will leave. The fear of being abandoned shows itself in sleep problems, poor concentration, separation anxiety, and "school phobia," among other signs. Some children deal with this fear by provoking punishment (punishment proves that the parent is still there), or by anxiously placating whichever parent they are with, at the expense of the other. When parents remain in touch with the child, fears of abandonment usually yield to the experience that they are unwarranted. It is also reassuring to list for a child the near relatives and friends who will be able to look after him or her, if for some reason neither parent can do so.

Preoccupation with Reconciliation. Children almost always react to the news of their parents' divorce with despairing pleas that they stay together. This is one of the most guilt-provoking experiences of divorce and some parents give in rather than suffer it. After separation, children may attempt to get their parents together again by promises of good behavior, threats, bribery, and manipulation. They may fantasize that the divorce has never happened and that the absent parent is still in the home. In time, most children accept the finality of the breakup, but sometimes the preoccupation with reconciliation persists even after both parents have remarried. In such cases, the parents usually have failed to separate psychologically and are in fact still involved with each other—but in anger and continued economic dependency.

Regression. Regressive manifestations are common in any situation where a child's usual sources of satisfaction are missing. Bed-wetting, thumb-sucking, clinging, and other regressive behaviors generally disappear quite rapidly. If they do not, it is usually because the parent is being overprotective as a result of his or her own guilt feelings.

Generally by the second year after the divorce, family relationships become smoother and most children suffer no long-term damage. They seem to make the best recovery when they have a continuing relationship with both parents, when the parents avoid involving them in their disputes, and when the custodial parent can provide an orderly household routine, with structure, discipline, and emotional support.

Custody and Visitation

The decision about which parent will have custody of the children after the divorce should be made by the parents themselves, if at all possible. (When custody must be decided by litigation, parents relinquish their right to many decisions for their children, and the family structure is at the mercy of the court.)

The primary consideration must be the best interest of the children. Parents must realistically assess which of them is better able to meet the children's needs for consistent affection, approval, guidance, discipline, and physical safety and protection. They must also consider who is better able to make a home for the children, realizing that this means the loss of much of their free time and some of their social life.

Traditionally, mothers were always awarded custody unless they were demonstrably "unfit." Today, the mother is still the primary or sole custodial parent in the great majority (89 percent) of cases, though some 60,000 children live with their fathers. A woman who relinquishes custody of her children may suffer the social stigma of "unnatural mother," but neither parent should be concerned about what others think of the custody arrangement, nor should custody be used as a weapon by one parent against the other.

Over the past few years, there has been a trend for parents to share custody. This has been encouraged by the law, which in 33 states permits the courts to order joint custody. In joint physical custody arrangements, the children live part of the year with each parent. But a recent study suggests that, although the children of parents who have divorced amicably do well in joint custody, those of bitter divorces do not. Shuttling back and forth between two parents who are still angry with each other causes significantly more stress than living all the time with one.

In general it would seem that the nature of the custody arrangement is less crucial to the child's development than is the quality of the relationship he or she develops with at least one caring adult after the divorce.

When a divorce is acrimonious, it is important that the decree be very specific about the hours and days (including holidays) for visitation. Vague terms such as "reasonable visitation hours" invite conflict. Where there are disagreements, it is helpful to remember that visitation is the children's right, not a way for parents to satisfy their own needs. To the child, the consistency and dependability of visitation are more important than the actual number of hours.

The noncustodial parent should make the child feel not only welcome, but also needed in his or her home. As far as possible, responsibilities and rewards—as well as rules—should be the same in both households. The temptation to overindulge the child may be great. But being a "good-time parent" encourages a child to look forward to gifts and entertainment rather than the quality of the time spent together.

SINGLE-PARENT FAMILIES

ONE OF EVERY FOUR children in the United States is living with only one parent; three of every five will spend some time in a single-parent household before they leave home. Separation and divorce account for two-thirds of these households, most of them headed by women. In addition, a large number—perhaps as many as two million—are headed by women who have never married. The independence of these households represents a further change in family structures: it was once common for separated and divorced women to move back to their parents' home, and for never-married mothers to remain under the parental roof.

It used to be believed that children in "fatherless families" suffered from a lack of discipline, and that boys in particular had problems stemming from lack of proper role models. Recent studies, however, do not support these generalizations. Less crucial than the number of parents in the household is the ability of the existing parent to cope.

There is no question that raising children alone is stressful. Single parents must make every decision and meet every need without support from a partner. They must always be on call to provide emotional support, even when their own emotional resources are depleted. Their day is never done. Moreover, divorced women are almost always much worse off financially than they were when married, even if they receive alimony and child support payments regularly. Most must work full time, which may mean trying to reenter a competitive job market with rusty skills. For those with preschool children, the lack of quality daycare compounds the difficulties.

Single parents with children in school have to contend with a strong bias toward the "traditional" family. Textbooks seldom reflect changed family patterns. Teachers tend to have lower expectations of children from divorced families, expectations which are self-fulfilling. After-school activities often require that a child be accompanied by a parent of the same sex. At work, single parents may encounter hostility from employers, since they are not free to work late or to travel. Getting credit may be a major hurdle, particularly for women who have never held a full-time job. Nevertheless, despite the difficulties, many divorced women develop an increased sense of self-worth from the independence and greater control of single-parenthood—and both sexes experience a freedom and spontaneity they did not have when they had to please a full-time partner.

Emotionally, a never-married mother may be better off than a woman who has had a bitter divorce—her child, too, has not experienced the pain of separation. Financially, however, she is likely to be far more needy. Although out-of-wedlock children are legally entitled to child-support payments from their fathers, many women hesitate about initiating the necessary paternity suit.

It is important that the child should not discover the facts of his or her birth from others. Finding the right words may not be easy, but the child should be told as soon as he or she begins to ask questions about the father.

STEP-FAMILIES

FIVE OF SIX divorced men and three of four divorced women marry again. When one or both of the new parents has children from a previous marriage, the structure of the family becomes complex. Since the ties between parents and children tend to remain intact even when the ties between the parents themselves are broken, the new family may extend across two or three households. Kinship and quasi-kinship are ramified and the definition of *family* becomes problematic, with no generally accepted rules as to who should or should not be included.

In addition, there are no generally accepted solutions to many of the problems that step-families face in day-to-day living. These range from what to call the stepparent (first name, a nickname, or some variant on "Mother" or "Father"); to defining the financial obligations of a stepfather to the children of previous marriages; to resolving sexual tensions between step-relatives in the absence of a clear incest taboo. Each step-family must work out such problems on its own, adjusting to itself without the benefit of societal guidelines. The process often takes several years.

The lack of social support may account for the fact that families formed by remarriage have more difficulties than would be expected, given that the parents are older and presumably more mature. Disruptive behavior is so common among children living in step-families that it might be said to be normal. Children living with a mother and a stepfather are significantly more likely to need help for emotional, behavioral, or learning problems than are children from two-parent families or families headed by a woman.

Someone marrying a person with children marries a parent. This statement may seem obvious, but in fact its implications are often not fully appreciated. The new spouse must respect the parent's relationship with his or her children, which has a long history and strong protective, biological ties, while at the same time building a primary relationship with the partner. A stepparent cannot expect to be accepted as "Mother" or "Father," yet has parental responsibilities within the household. The parental role itself will be shared by step- and biological parents—and there are no guidelines for such shared parenthood.

Problems with discipline are common in step-families. Conflicting styles of discipline may be carried over from previous marriages. Stepparents may be too lenient with their stepchildren and too severe with their biological children, from fear of seeming to favor their own. Frequently, children challenge the stepparent's right to discipline them at all. However, some therapists believe that a stepparent can "earn" this right. Early in the marriage, a period of time should be defined during which the stepparent nurtures the child without setting any limits on behavior. This creates an approximation (appropriate to the age of the child) of the emotional and physical bonding of parent and newborn, and so gives legitimacy to demands made later by the parent.

In addition to improved behavior, discipline in step-families has the important goal of clarifying the parent-child relationship. The stepparent may hope to eventually "parent" the child, or may aim for a role similar to that of an aunt or uncle (an acknowledged member of the family but at some distance from the parent-child bond), or may wish to become a friend or mentor to the child. The choice of role must always have the support of the spouse.

The birth of a new child ("their" child) changes relationships within a step-family, since siblings now have a biological bond that crosses the other boundaries in the family. The new child also provides a stepmother with an important sense of legitimacy. Statistics suggest that step-families with "new" children make a better adjustment.

The Step-Family and the Emergency Room

Under American law, a stepparent who has not taken legal measures to adopt a stepchild has no guardianship powers over that child. A hospital, therefore, may not accept a stepparent's consent for the child's treatment, in the absence of the natural parent. In circumstances where the child's life is clearly endangered, the hospital can treat without obtaining parental consent. But in less-threatening (and more common) situations, treatment of the child may be delayed while the matter of parental consent is sorted out.

It is up to individual families to take precautions. The natural parent can confer the right to consent upon the stepparent with a simple notarized statement, a "consent to give consent" document. Some urban hospitals have a VIK (Very Important Kid) program, which is particularly helpful when parents are away at work. Under this program, natural parents register their children at school or at the local hospital and name three individuals who have the right to authorize emergency treatment for the children.

TEENAGE PARENTHOOD

BY THE TIME they leave high school, about half of all American teenagers are sexually active, and one girl in every four has a pregnancy. Every year, about 400,000 teenage girls have abortions and about 470,000 become mothers, usually remaining single. It is estimated that, of brides age 17 and under, one in three is pregnant. The cost of teenage pregnancy and parenthood is high, for the teenagers themselves, for their children, and for taxpayers ($1.3 billion a year).

Under the law, schools are required to let pregnant teenagers continue with their studies. However, pregnancy and parenthood are the major causes for girls' dropping out of school. Many of these young mothers turn to welfare for support; lacking education and skills, their future is bleak. Nor is the outlook bright for their children: low birth-weight and infant mortality are disproportionately high among the babies of teenagers.

Better sex education in the schools may be the answer to the rising teenage pregnancy rate and its associated problems. Certainly the teenage birthrate is lower in those countries where sex education has a larger place in the curriculum than it does in the United States. However, some parents oppose such education as implying the consent of parents and teachers to sexual activity, or question its usefulness when adult behavior and values send conflicting messages. If uncritical publicity greets the birth of celebrities' out-of-wedlock children, pregnancy hardly seems reprehensible to impressionable adolescents.

Among other factors that help prevent the issues of teenage pregnancy from being dealt with successfully are:

- The lack of a comprehensive examination on a national scale of the differences in birthrates between certain groups.

- Government's desire for a "cure-all" answer, combined with its reluctance to work on complex solutions.

- The fact that many confuse antipregnancy campaigns with pro-abortion campaigns.

- The tendency to absolve teenage boys from responsibility for the pregnancy and the support of the child.

- The propensity of political leaders to seek dramatic, easily identifiable solutions to problems—and to avoid becoming involved in situations that cannot be readily resolved.

CHILD ABUSE

EACH YEAR in the United States approximately one million cases of child maltreatment are reported, about 80,000 of them involving sexual abuse. Many more thousands of cases of abuse go unreported.

Most instances of sexual abuse involve an individual known to the child. Family members, friends, relatives, and people perceived by the child as being relatives are the usual perpetrators although some well-publicized cases have involved daycare personnel. Occasionally a separated or divorced parent with visitation rights is accused of sexual abuse by the parent with custody. Some of these accusations have proved to be true, others false, and still others mere tactics in legal battles for custody and other rights. In these circumstances, intensive questioning of the child can have harmful psychological effects, whether abuse took place or not. (For detailed information on child abuse and how, when, and where to report it, see chapter 16, Child Care; for a discussion of child abuse in the family, see box near end of chapter.)

DEATH

MOST YOUNG CHILDREN have a healthy curiosity about death. Even if parents are able to shield them from violence and monitor their television-watching, children will be aware of death around them—in the bodies of wild animals on the highways, in lifeless pets, or in withered flowers and falling leaves. It is natural for them to wonder what death is like, and what it means to them and to their families and friends.

The death of a pet, or that of someone not close to the child, gives parents an opportunity to open a discussion, and the opportunity should be taken. Talking about a death that is not close gives children a chance to articulate their fears; the discussion can lay a groundwork that will be helpful when a death is closer and more painful. Similarly, the ceremonial burial of a pet can make a child's first contact with funeral rituals less traumatic.

Parents should answer a child's questions about death simply and clearly and at the child's level of comprehension. They should avoid giving more information than the question requires. If they do not know the answer, they should say so—some parents will wish to phrase their response "No one knows for certain, but I believe . . . " They should not deny the child an answer in order to "protect" him or her: where questions are not answered, children will draw on fantasy for explanations that may be more frightening than reality. It is not unusual for children to repeat the same question over and over, testing the answer while gradually coming to understand it. Parents should not be surprised if some of their children's questions about death are startlingly matter-of-fact.

It must be remembered that young children tend to take words literally. If, for example, a parent tries to explain death by likening it to sleep, a child may assume that a dead person will soon wake up. Similar difficulties may be encountered when a child is faced with the common euphemism "lost," for example, "He has lost his mother," or a parent's description of an afterlife. For instance, if parents assure a child that "Grandpa is in heaven, watching over you," the image that the child receives may be that of a malevolent spy. Parents need to be sensitive

to the child's concerns and level of understanding, while remaining true to their own beliefs and traditions.

Death in the Family

Adult. Even a very young child should be told when an adult in the family dies. It is understandable that the parents may want to shield a child from painful emotions, but this is a mistaken "kindness." Children will inevitably sense the sadness in the household and pick up on the disruption of ordinary routine. If they are suddenly sent away to stay with a friend or neighbor, it will be clear to them that the visit is due to some unexplained occurrence at home, from which they are being excluded, and they are likely to feel both rejected and anxious.

Young children can benefit by sharing in some of the rituals that surround death. While parents are the best judges of what their children can handle, generally children should be encouraged to attend the funeral or memorial service. However, they should not be forced to do so if they express strong antipathy. A child who is old enough might participate in the ceremony, perhaps by reading a poem or a selection from scripture. Viewing the body is also helpful, as this tends to discourage the development of unrealistic fantasies. Parents should prepare their children for a religious ceremony or a visit to the funeral home by explaining clearly what will happen and what is to be expected.

The grief span of children is different from that of adults: most children move quickly into and out of grief. They find it hard to tolerate a long exposure to grieving and may run out to play with apparent lack of concern. Generally, there are three phases to a child's grief for a loved person:

- Protest and denial.

- Pain, despair, and disorientation as the child begins to accept the loss.

- Acceptance, with the child gradually returning to usual routines, interests, and pleasures.

As much as two years may elapse before a child completely absorbs the loss. Parents should not be reluctant to grieve openly in front of their children: if adults' sadness is not expressed, children may doubt the appropriateness of their own grief. Tears are therapeutic and grieving together gives adults and children the chance to comfort one another. But adults should never lean on children for support or make a child an emotional replacement for a dead person.

Grief may affect a child's performance at school, or result in the emergence of depression or anxiety

CHILD ABUSE IN THE FAMILY
Arthur H. Green, M.D.

There is evidence that child abuse has existed for many centuries, but it was not addressed as a social issue in the United States until the nineteenth century, which saw the establishment of asylums for maltreated children, humane societies for child protection and, at the turn of the century, separate juvenile courts. Child abuse was not considered a medical issue until after World War II; it gained wider attention in the early 1960s when the most severe form of physical abuse, later to be called the "battered child syndrome," was recognized.

Today, laws in virtually every state require health care providers, child welfare workers (and in some cases, teachers) to report suspected cases of abuse and neglect, but define the two terms very broadly. Thus, it is often left to the reporter and sometimes ultimately to the state child-protective system or the court to determine when a child has been abused or neglected.

It is not surprising that the laws are vague, given our cultural belief in the sanctity of the family and the right of parents to raise their children as they see fit. At the extreme, few would argue against the conclusion that incest or multiple cigarette burns constitute abuse. The problem comes in determining when, for example, malnutrition or emotional deprivation represent true neglect or are merely the unfortunate outcome of poverty or parental ignorance or inadequacy, and in determining when neglect moves into the category of abuse. Regardless, children would be better served if attention were focused on identifying and helping troubled families rather than on trying to categorize maltreatment or determine authority or culpability.

Generally speaking, abuse is repeated physical or sexual violence against a child and may, in extreme cases, include emotional abuse as well. Neglect could be considered the failure of parents to provide adequate care, thereby jeopardizing the emotional or physical development or well-being of the child. Care can include such diverse factors as food, shelter, clothing, education, intellectual stimulation, affection and emotional support, medical attention, and adequate concern with safety.

It is very difficult to determine how large the problem of child maltreatment is, because figures are based only on reported cases. The number of recognized cases has grown substantially in recent years, but there is no strong indication that this is the result of an actual increase in incidence rather than greater awareness and the institution of reporting requirements. Nevertheless, reported cases are probably only a fraction of actual cases, and abuse is far less common than neglect.

Cultural factors influence the frequency of child abuse, with some societies more punitively oriented than others. In some cultures where aggression is otherwise freely expressed, children are rarely struck.

The possibility of abuse should be considered in every child who is seriously hurt, or who sustains frequent and inexplicable injuries. Injuries—at least those that are visible—range from black-and-blue marks to fractures and burns.

Abusive Parents

Abusing parents share common characteristics. Frequently, parents who abuse their children were abused or neglected themselves as children. Without intervention and counseling to break the cycle, abuse tends to recur in each generation. Although both sexes demonstrate this cyclical pattern, the abusive mother and the abusive father tend to have a distinct set of characteristics.

Compared to a nonabusive parent-child relationship, the abusive relationship has a joyless, strained quality. The abusive parents are out of sync with their children. Consumed by their own feelings of rage, insecurity, and inadequacy, they cannot perceive the needs of the child.

Mothers. The abusing mother often continues to have a destructive relationship with her parents who, more often than not, abused her in childhood. Often this maltreatment took the form of exploitation or sexual or emotional abuse. Because she is unable to depend upon them or upon siblings (usually abused as well) for help, she lacks much-needed emotional and practical support. Such a mother is prone to immature, impulsive behavior because she never learned the controls demonstrated by an effective parent. Yet, simply by virtue of the fact that she is female, she is expected to take primary responsibility for child care and to be a nurturing and effective parent, and the social sanctions against her when she fails are stronger than they are against abusing fathers.

Abusive mothers are often dependent upon abusive men and may have few, if any, friends. They are lonely and isolated and may resort to drugs or alcohol to relieve their depression. The combination of a lack of support and emotional immaturity often contributes to another phenomenon of child abuse: role reversal. The abusing mother is abnormally dependent upon her children. She needs her child's approval and constant acquiescence to bolster her own self-esteem. This role reversal places an extraordinary burden on a child, who needs to become independent from the parent without risking the loss of love or violent reprisal. At the same time, the abusing mother talks less to her child than the nonabusing mother, and abused children ignore their mothers.

Children who, because of their own needs, cannot respond to the mother's childlike needs are targets for abuse. This in no way places blame for child abuse upon the victim, but it does introduce a factor that might trigger an abuse-prone mother.

Children who are demanding—physically or emotionally—are most likely to be victims of child abuse. Often there is one "target" or "scapegoat" among several children in a family. A child who is physically ill, with chronic or disabling medical problems, or one who is either hyperactive or underresponsive, may pose problems to the abuse-prone mother. A premature baby, often poorly bonded with the mother and difficult because of its slower development, is more likely to strain an immature mother's low threshold and trigger an abusive or neglectful response.

In the delicate emotional balance between mother and child—especially in the case of a mother who was abused herself—increased stress or a loss of support can push her close to or over the edge and send the family into chaos. For example, if the spouse leaves, or if a grandmother or even a trusted babysitter is no longer available for child care, the mother is forced to deal with the child's increased demand for care, and abuse may result.

A stressful environment is often linked to a lack of money. Child abuse is statistically higher among the poor, whose limited resources stress existing relationships, and for whom financial solutions to child-care stresses are unavailable. The presence and availability of paid caretakers among the well-off, from full-time nannies to the occasional babysitter, reduces the demand for a mother's attention and alleviates the stress on the abuse-prone parent. It is possible that abuse is underreported among the affluent, who often live farther from one another's scrutiny, in larger houses with greater privacy. The same money that buys space can also provide discrete professional support in child-care responsibilities.

Fathers. Fathers who are abuse-prone react to a child as they would to siblings: they compete rather than adopt the supportive paternal role. Often their relationship with the mother is stable until the child is born. The birth of the child evokes feelings of loss in the father, whose response is to strike out at both mother and child.

In half the cases of abuse by fathers, alcohol is involved. Under the influence of alcohol or other drugs, abusing fathers often beat their spouse as well as their children. Abuse-prone men also were frequently emotionally deprived and beaten during their own childhoods.

Most sexual abuse of children of either sex tends to be by adult males, and frequently this takes the form of a father or stepfather abusing a daughter. The father in such a case may have great feelings of inadequacy, may also be abusing the mother, and may use the daughter as a surrogate wife, especially if physical, mental, or emotional illness prevents the wife from fulfilling her role as a sexual partner. Unfortunately this behavior is often chronic and may involve one or more children for long periods of time before it is discovered and stopped.

Treatment

The treatment for child abuse involves counseling and providing support. To be effective, it must be multidisciplinary, addressing the variety of contributing factors: the emotional immaturity of the mother or father or both, alcoholism, environmental stress factors, and the extraordinary needs of the child.

The mother may be depressed, beaten, ineffective, totally disorganized, isolated, and without support. Psychological counseling, which may include marriage counseling, can help the parents deal with emotional difficulties. Environmental stress can be alleviated with social-service support through the welfare system and child-rearing services. Someone can enter the home on a regular basis to help the mother organize the household; in addition, outside homemakers can help identify other available support resources—neighbors, friends, family.

Treatment must also target other factors that contribute to child abuse. The abused child should be evaluated, and hyperactive or chronically ill children should be treated. The psychological and emotional treatment of the abused child in therapeutic programs may take quite some time. Younger children can be placed in a nursery program; older children, five and up, might benefit from individual treatment, such as play therapy.

In play therapy, the child engages in spontaneous play with materials such as dolls, puppets, clay, and crayons in the presence of a therapist. The therapist guides and encourages the child to express reactions to and reenactments of traumatic experiences in the abusive household. Play therapy helps the therapist pinpoint the dynamics of the child's home life and inner life. Verbalization, in the context of a safe, abuse-free relationship, helps a child to master his or her response to the trauma.

Most children feel they are responsible for their own victimization. The therapist's benign and supportive stance demonstrates that an adult can be caring and nonabusive, providing an alternative experience. The therapist can also explain to the child that he or she is not responsible for provoking the parent's anger. Play therapy helps to bolster and restore the child's self-esteem. A more secure child has an increased opportunity to mature into a secure adult. The rehabilitation of the abused child (combined with stopping the abuse within the family) is the most compassionate and effective way to prevent the perpetuation of child abuse, generation after generation.

In sexual abuse cases, the prognosis is good if the child can be helped to believe in his or her own innocence. This almost always requires complete separation from the abusive parent, as effective treatment for pedophilia has not yet been developed.

or problems such as insomnia or headaches. Parents can best help children by keeping all lines of communication open. Some children will want to talk—not just be talked to. Others may work out their feelings through play, or telling a story, or painting a picture. A child who is angry about the death should be given physical outlets for the anger and helped to understand that such feelings are normal. Acting-out behavior is a not infrequent response of grieving children.

Looking at photographs and souvenirs of pleasant times, observing birthdays and anniversaries, or retelling favorite stories can help adults and children share their loss through the sharing of memories. Such memories also reaffirm the statement that those whom we have loved continue to live on in our minds. Visiting the grave can help remove some of the mystery of death and provide a sense of an ongoing family.

Children. It is very important that a young child who is dying continue to feel a member of the family. If the child is hospitalized, this may not be easy. Frequent parental visits are, of course, essential to keeping the child in the family fold, but siblings also should visit regularly, if there is no risk to them. (Such visits may require special permission from the hospital authorities.) Siblings are often even closer to one another than they are to their parents, and the benefits of their visits to the dying child will be evident.

Should fatally ill children be told the truth about their condition? Much, of course, depends on the age of the child and the nature of the illness, but many dying children—like adults who are close to death—know the truth without being "told." Parents should share with the child—at his or her level of comprehension—whatever support their religious or philosophical beliefs provides them.

When a child is not expected to recover, parents should prepare other children in the family by openly discussing with them the illness and eventual death of their brother or sister. If a child's death occurs without forewarning, parents should speak to siblings as soon thereafter as possible and give as much information about the circumstances of death

as the children's ages and understanding allow. In either case, parents should encourage children to express their grief or fears about the death. It is important to allay any sense of guilt or responsibility that children may feel regarding a sibling's death. At the same time their sense of loss should not be overlooked or minimized. Parents should bear in mind that it may take months for full adjustment.

If bereavement counseling is available it may be wise for the family to take advantage of it, especially in cases where signs of depression are exhibited.

Infants. Parents' grief at the death of an infant only a few days or weeks old may be intense. The brevity of the child's life and the relative lack of memories often sharpen the sense of loss.

If possible, the parents should be with the infant at the time of death. A special room may be available at the hospital where they can be alone with their child. The baby, no matter how brief the life expectancy, should be given a name. The name confers a firm identity and aids the parents in their memories of the child. A simple funeral or memorial service is a comfort to many families. (For more information see chapter 6, If Things Go Wrong.)

If parents are concerned that their genetic makeup may have had a bearing on the infant's death, they should consider an autopsy.

TRANSCENDING TRANSITION

Separation, divorce, remarriage, or death can have a major impact on a family; for some, it is devastating. But it is rarely permanent. Social scientists have found that families do manage to cope. These reconstituted families, made smaller by death or divorce, larger by remarriage and sometimes by more children, not only survive but become stronger.

No longer is there one model for the ideal family. Families come in many constellations, and family members, given time, transcend the turmoil and succeed at building a nurturing environment.

16 Child Care

Rosemary Barber-Madden, Ed.D.

INTRODUCTION

ABOUT HALF the American mothers of children under age three work, most of them full time. Some of these women rely on relatives or in-the-home baby-sitters to care for their infants and toddlers, but an estimated 40 percent of young children whose mothers work are now cared for out of the home by non-relatives. This rapidly growing social phenomenon has received only reluctant attention from the federal government. In fact, the United States is often cited as the only developed country without an official policy to assist working parents in the care of their very young children.

Despite repeated studies and surveys demonstrating an acute shortage of adequate and affordable daycare, federal funding of daycare centers has actually declined during the 1980s. At the same time, the problems of child abuse, infectious diseases, accidents, and neglect at various daycare facilities have received wide media attention.

Contrary to popular belief that daycare is a recent phenomenon, it actually has a long history in this and other countries. Formal programs began in the United States in the nineteenth century with kindergartens and day nurseries for the custodial care of children from the lower economic classes. During the Depression, daycare centers for workers' children were publicly funded, and shortly afterward licensing of centers became more widespread. In World War II, child-care centers were established near factories and hospitals so that women could contribute to the war effort by working. In the 1950s, privately run centers were established, and the 1960s witnessed the funding of a number of programs, including Head Start.

Despite the long history of outside-the-home care for preschool children, the concept of daycare for very young children has been controversial. Fears have been expressed about the "Sovietizing" of the American family and it has been speculated that the toddlers might be unduly influenced by the bureaucrats in government-run daycare facilities. Some have felt that essential links between mother and child might be irretrievably lost through separation for so many hours on the five working days of the week. Care by "strangers" at the centers has been blamed for producing ill effects in very young children.

While these are difficult charges to disprove absolutely, a growing body of research indicates that neither maternal employment nor out-of-home care, per se, is harmful to young children. (However, individual care situations may indeed be detrimental, if they fail to meet basic standards of quality and safety.)

Expert opinion is most split over what effects infant group care may have during the first few months. Infants need a great deal of physical care and individual attention, which may not be forthcoming unless the group is limited in size and the caretaker dedicated and loving. Nevertheless, there is no evidence that infants in quality care situations suffer negative effects. Still, the debate over daycare's long-term impact may not be decided until a generation or two of closely monitored youngsters mature into adulthood (if even then). Meanwhile, the reality is that for a great many American families, out-of-home care is not a life-style option, but an economic necessity. Single-parent and dual-income families now outnumber the traditional model of a working father and an at-home mother. The nuclear family has also tended toward diffusion; fewer households today can call on resident grandparents or other relatives for regular babysitting.

Clearly, then, daycare is here to stay. The dominant issues are no longer theoretical pros and cons, but practical concerns about adequacy and accessibility of care. This chapter will describe different types of child-care arrangements that may be available and will provide basic information that may help parents in making choices.

TYPES OF CHILD CARE

CHILD CARE ARRANGEMENTS for the children of working mothers may be divided into several categories:

- home care and care by relatives
- family daycare (in the home of a nonrelative)
- daycare centers
- public and private nursery schools, preschools, prekindergartens, kindergartens, and Head Start programs
- regular all-day, part-day, and after-school care

Because information is not collected on a systematic basis for very young and preschool children, no complete account can be given of the number of children involved in various care options. Out-of-home care for infants and toddlers (that is, for children under the age of three) is rapidly expanding, but it is still not meeting the demand from working women with children in this age range. Children in family daycare situations outnumber those in formal or licensed daycare centers about two to one. In 1986, an estimated nine million preschoolers, toddlers, and infants spent their days with someone other than their mothers.

Home Care and Care by Relatives

Because of family privacy, not much is known about this category of care. Home care is often less costly than other types of daycare; however, the caregiver is usually an untrained relative or neighbor and rarely are there controls over the environment.

At one time, it was relatively easy to employ someone to come into the home to care for children. But as the American workforce becomes more educated and seeks higher paying jobs, it becomes harder to find American citizens who are willing to be employed as child-care workers in the home. In border states and large metropolitan areas, the demand for persons hired for in-home care has often been filled by au pairs or nannies from other countries. Until recently, many of these have been illegal aliens, but new immigration laws restricting the hiring of these "illegals" is expected to sharply reduce this source of child care.

Au Pairs and Nannies

Au pairs have traditionally been young, middle-class European women taking a year or two before continuing their education to experience life in the United States by living as a quasi-family member who is paid a small amount to care for the family's children. In more recent years, au pairs have been not necessarily middle class, not always female, and not always short-term. Many speak little English and may have little in the way of references or experience. They usually earn about $100 a week, plus room and board. New immigration laws restrict the number of visas available and limit the stay to one year.

Nannies may or may not have child-related training, and may or may not have a work permit; they may cost as much as $300 or more per week. Some have been trained at special nanny schools in Great Britain or at the few recently established in this country, and these generally can command a high salary and fringe benefits.

The hiring of au pairs and nannies has been affected by the 1987 immigration law, which makes employers of illegal aliens liable to fines up to $10,000. While strict enforcement of the law for au pairs is not expected, few parents will be sanguine about the prospect of having to break the law to find care for their children. As of 1988, the government allows 3,100 legal au pairs per year, through the auspices of the American Institute for Foreign Study and the Experiment in International Living.

Family Daycare

This is the most popular out-of-home child care option, largely because it is often the only option available to working parents. Typically, family daycare is an informal arrangement between parents and a neighborhood person who agrees to take in and care for one or more children during the day. The caregiver may be a parent who chooses to stay at home with his or her young child and wishes to make some money on the side; it may be a trained child-care professional who operates an unofficial little center out of his or her home; or it may simply be an individual who likes working with small children. The range in quality among family-care settings is very wide, as most (more than 75 percent) of these arrangements are not licensed, and therefore are not monitored by state regulatory agencies. Referrals are usually made by word of mouth (though there are also some referral agencies, see Resources section at the end of this chapter), and it is up to the parent to check out the caregiver and the premises carefully before making a commitment. Of course, this advice holds for *any* child-care situation, but in a licensed center, there is at least the promise that basic standards of care and safety will be met.

With the right caregiver, family daycare can be an excellent opportunity for the child to receive loving, homelike attention. On the other hand, some family-care situations have provoked parents to complain about inadequate sanitation, safety, and play equipment, marathon television watching, and overreliance on snack foods for meals. Parents may be charged for family care on an hourly, weekly, or flat-fee basis; typical costs range from $50 to $125 per week, depending on the area and the hours of service.

Center Care

There are at present approximately 60,000 licensed daycare centers in the United States, about half of them nonprofit. Although their number is expanding, the supply in no way is keeping pace with the demand, and an overall shortage of center care prevails. Moreover, aside from meeting the basic qualifications for licensure—which in themselves vary greatly from state to state—no two daycare centers necessarily have much in common. Nonprofit church-run centers and government-funded Head Start programs, for example, may have operating principles and facilities very different from those of for-profit centers run by private individuals or by proprietary chains (such as Kinder-Care, Inc., which operates more than 1,100 centers nationwide). By the same token, a child-care cooperative administered by parents may have a different philosophy and meet different needs than a Montessori program or one of the private preschools that are becoming increasingly popular for the early education of three- and four-year-olds (whose families can afford the tuition payments).

Yet all of these possibilities are lumped together under the term "licensed center care," which suggests far more uniformity in quality and services than actually exists. In 1971, a bill to create a national daycare network with federally mandated standards was vetoed by President Nixon. Since then, most efforts to link and organize daycare providers have been on a local, grass-roots level. Now in the late 1980s, some lawmakers have begun to catch on to the changing needs of their constituent families, and a number of new daycare-center proposals are being considered at various levels of the legislative process.

Workplace-Related Care

The child-care needs of working families is not exclusively a governmental problem. During the 1980s, many corporations began to realize that mothers with children under age six are the fastest growing segment of the workforce, and that these workers' productivity may be affected by their parental responsibilities. Some companies have concluded that it makes economic sense to assist in establishing child-care facilities for their employees, because the increase in working parents' productivity would offset the cost of operating a child-care program.

Many other firms, however, object to this approach on the grounds that the corporation should not interfere in family private life (and vice versa), or that the cost of providing daycare would be difficult to justify in a hard-nosed budget.

Even in companies with a commitment to daycare, the actual facility is usually located away from the workplace. Many companies choose to subsidize existing daycare facilities rather than found new ones. Out of six million American employers, only about 150 provide a child-care facility at or very near the workplace.

Altogether about 3,000 companies are involved

in some way in helping their employees with day-care. Procter & Gamble, IBM, AT & T, Campbell's Soup, Southland, CBS, Merck, and Polaroid are some of the better-known companies that have taken an active role in providing facilities for the children of employees. Nevertheless, the U.S. Armed Forces actually operates more daycare services for its employees (both in this country and stationed overseas) than any other American employer.

School Systems

Several city school systems run pre- and after-school care programs for children ages five and older, and some urban centers are now extending this care to infants and toddlers. For example, the Hewlett-Woodmere school system in New York puts its pre-kindergarten and kindergarten children into one building; 300 children attend the center, which is open from 7:30 A.M. to 6:00 P.M. An attempt by the Boulder, Colorado, school system to open a similar program was abandoned because of opposition from private daycare-center operators.

CONSIDERATIONS IN CHOOSING DAYCARE

Cost

Many women, especially single mothers, have no economic choice but to work and to use whatever kind of daycare is available or affordable. Cutbacks in federal spending have caused the closing of some daycare centers dependent on public funds. Non-profit church-sponsored services are on the increase, as are for-profit private services. The cost for day-care centers varies from $40 to $120 per child per week. For quality care, the cost is often $100 and up.

As a general rule, church and community day-care centers tend to be less costly than private operations, or at least more amenable to sliding-scale fees based on what a family can afford. On the other hand, some private centers and preschools offer scholarships to selected youngsters who otherwise would be unable to enrol. In many instances, the only way to find out for sure if there is any flexibility in the fee structure is to speak openly and directly about cost considerations with a center's director.

Quality

In 1979, the Day Care Division of the U.S. Department of Health and Human Services published a national study entitled *Children at the Center*. This report acknowledged that "young children reach out to capture all the 'raw resources' (including adults) that are available to them. Using whatever is there, they move forward each week, sometimes each day, to improve some new skill, to add some new understanding to their universe."

The study attempted to assess the major quality-of-care issues that affect a child's social and learning experience in daycare. It concluded that the three most important elements are group size, the caregiver-to-child ratio, and the quality and training of the caregivers. The report recommended, for example, that the ideal size of a group for infants and toddlers under two is no more than six children, with at least two adult caregivers. For children in the two-year range, no more than eight to a group with at least two caregivers was recommended.

Not every center approaches the ideal, however. As a general rule, there should be a staff member for every four (or fewer) babies; one for every six to eight toddlers (mid-twos to three-year-olds); one for every ten to twelve preschoolers (three and four years); and one for every twelve to fifteen five-year-olds. Group size should also remain fairly small, with no more than eight to ten babies, ten to fifteen toddlers, and fifteen to twenty preschoolers.

Nevertheless, most parents of children in day-care agree that the single most important component of quality care is the individual teacher. And, unfortunately, the economics of the situation undermine the likelihood of finding high-quality, professional caregivers for our children's crucial formative years. Early child care is an extremely low-paying line of work—many caregivers earn the minimum wage—and the individuals who are successful at it and who have invested in their own training and education tend to move on to more financially rewarding teaching positions. One of the reasons child-care wages are so low, of course, is that the parents who are ultimately footing the caregivers' salaries are often themselves strapped to meet the cost of care.

The national daycare study found that for infants and toddlers, staff qualifications such as formal education and specialized training was not quite as important for the delivery of personalized, quality care as it was for older, preschool children. Even so, the study noted that caregivers with formal education usually had more social interaction with the children and gave the youngsters more verbal stimulation. Children in their care also tended to show less apathy and were less often exposed to potential harm. Moreover, children cared for by adults with training in child development evidenced higher levels of cognitive and social skills than youngsters cared for by adults without specialized training. (The accompanying box, Judging the Quality of Care, outlines some of the criteria parents should use.)

Home vs. School Atmosphere

While many parents of very young children are limited in the child-care options available to them, those who have a choice of different types of arrangements may face an interesting question. Should they put their youngster into a less structured, "child-centered" atmosphere or into one with a more organized schoolroom program?

Experts disagree on the age at which formal schooling should start. Five-year-olds attend kindergarten in nearly every school system. It is now known, however, that children three and younger can perceive, organize thoughts, and respond on a much higher level than was previously recognized. Are their precocious intellectual gifts being wasted by traditional, undemanding child care?

Some educators hold that basic learning patterns become irreversibly set before age three, and that encouraging the child's learning development during this early stage can have lifelong benefits. And, certainly, few people would argue with the notion of feeding a child's curiosity and boosting his or her learning skills through a stimulating environment and creative play. Yet the methods sometimes employed to promote early learning are the subject of considerable controversy, especially the use of flashcards and other techniques to teach children to read, speak foreign languages, do mathematics, play musical instruments, and so on.

It is true that some youngsters may thrive on such methods. Most child-development specialists agree, however, that toddlers and preschoolers should be allowed to develop at their own natural paces and should not be pressured into very early achievement. There's no evidence that enforced learning in the first few years of life has any lasting carryover into later school or career performance. Moreover, intense and structured schooling at a very early age may produce the opposite effect, causing children to burn out and turn off to the educational process.

There is also some question about how much useful learning a child actually derives from a results-oriented teaching approach. A toddler, for example, may please his or her parents and caregivers by learning to count to 40, but without any understanding of the concept of 40 separate items. His or her basic logic skills may be better served by games or toys that emphasize the similarities among various shapes, colors, and textures. In other words, for very young children stimulating learning may just

JUDGING THE QUALITY OF CARE

Quality of care can be measured by observing children and staff and by administering standardized tests to the children. Three principles underlie this approach to judging the quality of care:

1. The child's well-being comes first and foremost.
2. As well as shielding the child from harm, quality daycare must also promote social, emotional, and learning development.
3. The child's actual experience, not the center's stated goals, must be used to judge the quality of care.

The following are among the factors that observers should consider:

- How much time does the staff spend in close interaction with the children? In maintaining order? In detached observation or administrative tasks?
- How much of the children's time is spent in a group activity? In independent, reflective play, wandering aimlessly?
- How much verbal initiative do the children show?

Staff Qualifications
- Years of formal education.
- Diplomas and degrees.
- Education or training in young-child-related fields.
- Years of previous daycare employment experience.
- Tenure in current center.

The following points were also made in the federal daycare study:

- Parent participation can be important when access to the center's staff is provided without making unrealistic time demands on working parents.
- Additional space beyond that required by state regulations does not seem to make a difference.
- Supplemental services at centers need to be organized.
- Although children at centers specializing in school readiness score higher in standardized tests, no standardized federal curriculum for daycare centers is justified.

as easily take place in an informal, homelike setting as in a structured classroom.

Safety Considerations

The safety of children in out-of-home care situations is a source of anxiety for both parents and caregivers. Accidents and injuries are the main cause of death to American children from age one through five years. Tragically, one-third of early childhood deaths from injury could have been avoided through adequate precautions.

Many daycare workers have no training in how to deal with injuries, and an even greater number have not been instructed in their prevention. One study found that two-thirds of the injuries in daycare settings occurred on the playground. The objects most frequently involved in accidents were, in order of importance, climbers, slides, hand toys and blocks, other playground equipment, doors, indoor floor surfaces, motor vehicles, swings, pebbles and rocks, and pencils. (For more information see chapter 14, Ensuring Your Child's Safety.)

Health Considerations

Placing a number of very young children in close proximity for several hours a day is bound to raise the risk of communicable diseases. In addition to the ubiquitous runny nose, sore throat, and other respiratory complaints, daycare children are vulnerable to outbreaks of diarrheal illnesses, chicken pox, conjunctivitis, head lice, and other distressing but not truly threatening ailments. More serious infections, such as hepatitis and meningitis, are also reported with some frequency in daycare settings. Measles outbreaks have also become more common in recent years, indicating that immunization efforts have not been as successful in reaching young children as public health officials may have thought.

Health codes in virtually every state require immunization against measles, mumps, rubella (German measles), polio, tetanus, pertussis (whooping cough), and diphtheria as prerequisites for elementary-school registration. Unfortunately, some parents wait until their children are of school age to have them vaccinated, which leaves daycare youngsters at increased risk. For this reason, most licensed centers (and well-run unregulated programs, as well) insist on a medical exam and certificate of vaccination before enrolling children. Within the last few years, a new vaccine against *haemophilus influenzae* type B, the organism responsible for most cases of meningitis in children, has become available. This development is only a partial solution to the infectious meningitis threat, however, because it is recommended for youngsters at least 18 to 24 months old and the peak incidence of the disease is among children less than a year old.

While immunization is an essential first step toward the prevention and spread of dangerous diseases, attention to basic hygiene can also reduce the rate of many daycare-related illnesses. Health care professionals point out that simple measures taken in daycare facilities such as proper food handling and refrigeration, prompt disposal of soiled diapers and used toilet tissues, handwashing before meals and after trips to the bathroom, and adequate and sanitary toilet facilities could go a long way toward preventing many common contaminations.

To ensure basic health and safety standards at daycare centers, staff should be specifically trained in the fundamentals of first aid and sanitation, as well as in the management of mildly ill youngsters who remain in the group.

Nutrition

Many centers offering full daycare provide lunch for children, and some serve breakfast as well. Even half-day programs usually offer a midmorning or midafternoon snack of some kind. (See box on Assessing Nutritional Standards.)

ASSESSING NUTRITIONAL STANDARDS

1. Are the number of meals and snacks sufficient and are they well spaced?
2. Do the meals and snacks meet nutritional standards?
3. Are food preparation and serving sanitary?
4. Is the type of food likable and easy to handle for children?
5. Is the food served without delay?
6. Does a caregiver sit with the children during mealtimes?
7. Are tables, chairs, and utensils suitable to the age group?
8. Is the atmosphere relaxed, without the threat of punishment?
9. Are menus prepared at least a week in advance and accessible to parents?
10. Does the food have sufficient variety in color, flavor, shape, and temperature?
11. If a child is on a special diet, are the parents' instructions posted where they will be seen?
12. Are special diet foods supplied by parents stored and served properly?

CHOOSING A DAYCARE PROGRAM

Identifying Possibilities

In addition to the referral services mentioned in the Resources section at the end of this chapter, parents can get the names of daycare providers and facilities from many sources—the telephone book, pediatricians, teacher (especially of kindergarten and lower grades), fellow employees, church groups, friends and neighbors with young children.

If a center passes the initial telephone screening, the next step is setting up an appointment to visit the center. Visiting parents should allow themselves ample time to talk with the director, stroll through the premises, and observe classroom and playground activities. A return visit—or perhaps even a series of visits—may be warranted, as a thorough investigation of a program at this stage may pay off in time and worry saved later on.

Meeting the Director

Because the director of the center is the person ultimately responsible for the child's well-being, parents have to judge whether this individual has the temperament and qualifications appropriate to the position. The director should be able to give straightforward answers to just about any question a parent may have. Parents should also observe how the director interacts with the staff and with children in the program. (For example, does the director appear to know the names of the youngsters encountered as he or she leads a tour of the center?) Other basic issues to cover in the meeting with the director include his or her own credentials and experience in child care; his or her concept of quality care (Is the emphasis on the program, or on the needs of the individual child?); who would actually care for the child and what the room would look like; and what happens if the child needs special attention, is injured, or becomes ill. (Also see box on Questions Parents Should Ask.)

Looking over the Premises

In a licensed facility, the parents can expect that some effort has been made to meet minimum fire, sanitation, and health requirements. But, as stated above, licensing itself is not a guarantee of quality and safety, and visiting parents should keep an eye out for things like nonfunctional fire exits, worn-out or unsafe playground equipment, carelessness in food handling and bathroom hygiene, inadequate enclosure or protection from the street and from passersby. The first priority is that both the parents and the child must feel secure and comfortable with the environment, and it is up to the family to make that determination for themselves. The box on What to Look for During Your Visit outlines specific aspects that should be observed. Also see the boxes on Health and Safety, and on Resources, and see table 16.1, next page.

CHILD ABUSE

UNFORTUNATELY no type of child care is guaranteed free from child abuse; abuse and neglect cases are just as likely to involve in-home or family care as public centers. In fact there are two aspects of child abuse directly relevant to daycare: abuse or neglect by members of the daycare program staff, and abuse

---

QUESTIONS PARENTS SHOULD ASK

Initial Screening

Much time and energy can be saved by asking the center's director or admissions officer the following questions over the telephone:

- What age groups are served? (If toddlers are accepted, do they have to be toilet trained?)
- What are the hours of care?
- What are the fees?
- Is the program licensed?
- Is some particular educational system (such as Montessori) followed?
- How much parent participation is expected?

WHAT TO LOOK FOR DURING YOUR VISIT

Physical Aspects

- Playground: Are there large structures for climbing and sufficient room to run freely?
- Classroom: Are there manipulative toys, puzzles, and construction sets? Art materials? Picture books? Musical instruments?
- Classroom walls: How much of the work displayed in the room is done by children? Is only the "best" work displayed, or does there seem to be an effort to include every child, regardless of skill?
- From the artwork displayed, is individuality or uniformity emphasized?
- What part do the children have in the upkeep of the room?
- Are there plants and animals in the room for nature study?
- Is the overall environment friendly, cheerful, and comfortable?
- If you were a child, would you want to spend your day there?

(continued next page)

WHAT TO LOOK FOR DURING YOUR VISIT (continued)

Program

- Are activities outdoor as well as indoor?
- How much choice do children have in what they do?
- Can children work on their own as well as in groups?
- Are children encouraged to be independent in dressing, eating, toileting, and washing?
- Is work given so children can help each other, or do they do their work individually?
- What kind of learning is stressed? Social skills, accumulation of data, academic skills, motor skills, dramatic skills, verbal skills?
- Is the emphasis on children's being taught or on children's discovering?
- What kind of learning experiences take place outside of the school building (class trips, etc.), and how often?
- In what ways are parents included in the school process? How often do parents come in and what do they do?
- How are the children divided for different activities —by sex, age, skill, etc.?

Staff and Staff/Children Interactions

- Do the caregivers seem to enjoy their job? (Is there life in the classroom, or does the teacher seem to be "cranking it out"?)
- Are staff members rigid or flexible in their dealings with children?
- Do staff members cooperate with one another?
- Do staff members really listen to the children?
- Are the children responsive to the caregivers? Do they look fearful when spoken to?
- How do caregivers resolve conflicts between children?
- What kind of emotional support is provided to distressed or upset children?
- Do staff members talk with the children, contributing to their verbal skills?
- In what ways are the children trusted or not trusted?
- Do staff members help the children feel positive about themselves?

Table 16.1 **CHECKLIST FOR DAYCARE CENTER SELECTION**

Name of center: _____ **Date visited:** _____

Screening Questions	Yes	No	Program	Yes	No
Infants and toddlers accepted?	☐	☐	Balanced daily schedule?	☐	☐
Hours suitable?	☐	☐	Activities age-related and varied?	☐	☐
Fees affordable?	☐	☐	Daily outdoor activities?	☐	☐
Program licensed?	☐	☐	Girls and boys equally encouraged?	☐	☐
Conveniently located?	☐	☐			
Learning system followed?	☐	☐			
Parent participation?	☐	☐			

Environment	Yes	No	Play Materials	Yes	No
Warm and cheerful?	☐	☐	Manipulative toys?	☐	☐
Safe and well maintained?	☐	☐	Picture books?	☐	☐
Children lively and happy?	☐	☐	Blocks?	☐	☐
			Art supplies?	☐	☐
			Musical instruments?	☐	☐
			Water, sand, clay, and dough?	☐	☐

Care Workers	Yes	No	Parent Participation	Yes	No
Enough staff to give children individual attention?	☐	☐	Scheduled parent meetings?	☐	☐
When children need help, do staff respond quickly?	☐	☐	Regular parent/caregiver conferences?	☐	☐
Do staff have good communication with children and parents?	☐	☐	Parents welcome at center?	☐	☐
Do staff participate in children's activities?	☐	☐	**Notes**		
Are staff aware of health and safety factors?	☐	☐			
Director accessible and responsive?	☐	☐			

HEALTH AND SAFETY

Following are some of the factors considered by daycare licensing agencies in New York and Connecticut. Parents can use this checklist in assessing a center.

- Each child gets an annual physical checkup.
- Appropriate immunizations are given, with later booster shots.
- Health records of children and staff are reviewed.
- Menus are monitored for their nutritional content.
- Staff and children are instructed in hygiene.
- Vision, hearing, and disability screening is provided.
- Outbreaks of infectious disease are quickly treated.
- Staff are instructed on communicable diseases.
- Assistance is given in the care of children with special needs.

Sanitation and Environmental Hazards

- Water supplies are tested for purity.
- Food-handling techniques are checked for contamination risk.
- The environment is checked for hazards such as asbestos and lead.

- An overall inspection is carried out for dangerous conditions such as broken playground equipment, uncovered electrical outlets, and the presence of toxic substances.

Child Growth and Development

- Training and instruction in growth and development are given to the staff.
- The children's program is reviewed for content and quality.
- Staff qualifications are examined.
- The child/staff ratio is fixed according to the children's age group.
- Group size is controlled according to age group.
- Links with community resources are encouraged.

Child Abuse

- Complaints are investigated.
- Staff qualifications and child/staff ratios are screened.
- State police check staff for criminal records and previous abuse.
- Cooperation is offered to other authorities in this area.

RESOURCES

The following information was adapted from the April 1988 issue of *Working Mother* magazine, which contained a useful and extensive "special report" on child care.

The *State Child Care Fact Book,* published by the Children's Defense Fund, contains a state-by-state listing of daycare regulatory agencies and of childcare advocates. It is available in some public libraries or can be obtained by sending a check for $7.45 to CDF Publications, 122 C Street NW, Washington, DC 20001.

The Child Care Action Campaign, 99 Hudson Street, Suite 1233, New York, NY 10013, will provide lists of child care resources and referral services and fact sheets on other aspects of child care free of charge.

The Children's Foundation, 815 15th Street NW, Washington, DC 20005, will supply the name, address, and phone number needed to obtain information on licensed family daycare in your state. Send 50 cents and a stamped, self-addressed business envelope along with a note that you would like your state's fact sheet from the *Family Day Care Licensing Study*.

For referrals and/or information about nannies, contact the International Nanny Association, 976 West Foothill Blvd., Suite 591, Claremont, CA 91711; and the American Council of Nanny Schools Delta College, University Center, MI 48710, which publishes the *Nanny School Directory*.

To find out more about au pairs, write to Aupair Homestay USA, 14TI K Street NW, Suite T100, Washington, DC 20005; and Au Pair in America, 102 Greenwich Avenue, Greenwich, CT 06830 Tel.: (203) 863-6123.

A Little Bit Under the Weather is a guide to sick-child care, available for $20 (check or money order) from Work/Family Directions, Inc., Nine Galen Street, Suite 230, Watertown, MA 02172.

or neglect detected by the staff (presumably parental abuse).

In cases where the caregiver is responsible, cooperation between the state agency regulating daycare and law-enforcement authorities is crucial to bringing charges. Such cooperation may also be useful in prevention, as in New Hampshire, where state bureaus and state policy jointly check the criminal records of all individuals who work in licensed care facilities. No facility in New Hampshire is issued a license until all workers are cleared, and each facility must report data for each new staff member hired.

Parents may also play a role in preventing or detecting abusive situations by being attentive to their child's behavior, especially if there are any marked changes that persist for more than a few weeks, or if the child says anything to suggest that unusual punishment or discipline methods may be employed. Some parents' first reactions may be to deny or downplay their fears; nevertheless, it may be helpful to drop by the center unannounced or to pick the child up extra early one day to see for oneself. Parents *should* have access to visit a center at any time, and any attempt by the staff or director to discourage visiting should be grounds for suspicion.

Parents who suspect that their child has been abused should make a careful effort to find out what really happened. The best way to do this is to have the child relate the simple facts exactly as he or she sees them. Parents should then stick with these facts, rather than elaborate on them with or without further assistance from the child. Discussing suspicions with other parents is a natural impulse and in some instances may prove helpful, but if the suspicions turn out to be groundless, spreading damaging rumors can lead to a libel suit. Suspicious *facts*, however, can and should be reported to the state authorities without danger of libel action.

Talking with the Child

Young children may not have the words to describe precisely what has occurred. Parents must first find out if the child has been injured, if the injury still hurts, and if the child is still in a state of fear. Patience and understanding are essential; the child should be made as comfortable as possible and assured that he or she is now safe. Parents must convey to the child that they believe what he or she tells them and that they intend to take action to prevent it from ever happening again.

When talking with the child, *do not:*

- Indicate that he or she is in any way to blame for what has occurred or has brought shame or trouble upon the family.

- Point out the child's inability to render a clearcut, concise version of events.

- Suggest answers to the child; his or her own version is the one that will count.

- Pressure the child into giving information he or she may be unwilling or unable to give.

- Show surprise, shock, or disapproval at what he or she has to say.

- Demand to see the injuries. Allow the child to show them when he or she is ready.

- Bring in an outsider as a witness in the parent-child talk.

- Expect the child to repeat what he or she has told the parents to a third party in the parents' absence.

What to Report

States differ in their definition of child abuse and neglect, but most include some form of nonaccidental physical injury, neglect, sexual abuse, and emotional maltreatment (also known as mental injury or emotional neglect). No state requires the parents to *prove* that an incident of child abuse occurred; it is sufficient for parents or other reporters to "have reason to believe" that abuse has occurred; the occurrence may be described as a "suspected incident." Bear in mind that the child's testimony may be inadmissible evidence in court. For these reasons, the local authority's trained personnel may be able to do more than the parents to make a legal case against the offender.

When to Report

Reports of a suspected incident should be made as soon as possible, certainly no later than 48 hours after discovery. Waiting for proof further endangers the child, and conclusive evidence may never be forthcoming. Some states require an immediate oral report, followed by a written report within 48 hours. A toll-free 24-hour telephone hotline facilitates reporting in some states.

Where to Report

The agencies to which child abuse should be reported differ from state to state. The department of human resources, social services or public welfare, is usually the responsible agency. Other participating agencies may include the police department, county or district attorney's office, juvenile or district court, and the health department. The local authority may or may not have a special unit, often known as Child Protective Services (CPS), to deal with suspected child abuse cases. Parents should make sure they report to the appropriate agency and that their statement will be kept confidential.

DAYCARE FOR CHILDREN WITH SPECIAL NEEDS

IN YEARS PAST, when a child differed physically or emotionally from other children, adults were apt to shake their heads and say that the youngster would probably "outgrow it." It was also taken for granted that some children just grew up "different" or "strange." Today a great deal more is known about child development, and these attitudes are somewhat less widespread—but they do persist, even among some pediatricians, who may tell parents not to concern themselves about an apparent cognitive or emotional problem and that everything will work itself out in the end.

In fact, if ignored, a child's problem may not go away. And, unless proper attention is paid, a social situation like a daycare center may actually make matters worse.

Other children are quick to notice a classmate who is "different," and young children are not noted for their compassion. Alerted by the reactions of other youngsters, caregivers are often the first to bring a problem to the parents' attention. Before selecting a program, parents need to consider whether their child is physically and emotionally resilient enough to thrive in the environment of a daycare facility.

Parents of children with problems will find the interview with the facility director to be particularly important. (See box on Special Considerations.)

SPECIAL CONSIDERATIONS

- What exactly is the nature of the child's problem?
- To what extent will the problem affect his or her relations with other children?
- Would this child be better off in the more protective environment of the home, or in a specialized center for children with similar problems?
- How can parents and caregivers best work together to ease or solve the child's problem?
- How do the director and staff feel about caring for a child with special needs?
- Has the director or a member of the staff any qualifications or experience in caring for children with special needs?
- Will the caregiver be able to spare the time and energy for the child with special needs without neglecting the other children?

17 Adoption and Foster Care

Charmaine Fitzig, R.N., Dr. P.H.

INTRODUCTION

BECOMING A PARENT, whether through adoption, foster care, or by conceiving and bearing a child, is a major decision for a couple. But the decision to adopt a child or provide foster care is significantly different from and more complex than a decision to have children by achieving pregnancy.

It is essential for adults considering adoption or foster care to understand the emotional challenge involved. The process can be long and it often follows what has already been a prolonged, unsuccessful attempt to conceive. But it also brings special rewards. While the challenge cannot be ignored, it is not insurmountable—millions of couples have created happy and loving families through adoption and foster care.

In addition to the emotional issues involved are the intricacies of the process itself, which has changed dramatically in recent years and which varies from state to state. Social concern for the protection and well-being of children, as well as for their natural and adoptive parents, has greatly affected both the law and social-agency practice.

The adoption process has also been greatly affected by the decline in the number of infants and young children available for adoption in this country. The wide use of contraceptives, social acceptance of unwed mothers who keep their babies, and easy access to abortion have all had a dramatic impact on the number of infants available. According to the federal government's National Child Welfare Indicator Survey, 50,000 children were available for adoption in 1982, as compared to 102,000 in 1977.

ADOPTION

ADOPTION IS AT LEAST as old as the Bible, if not older. The Pharaoh adopted Moses and, according to those who believe in the principles of "adoptionism," Jesus Christ became the son of God through adoption, and was not born as such.

Through the centuries, the desire to have heirs and to carry on the family name and tradition has resulted in adoption becoming a socially acceptable —and even desirable—form of creating a family. While this is still true, the focus today has changed from the adoptive parent to the adopted child.

The value that society places on a child also has changed during the last century. In the 1870s, the child was useful and productive, valued for potential and actual economic contributions to the family. The perception of children was essentially, although not exclusively, utilitarian and instrumental. Two generations later the child was economically useless, but emotionally priceless. The child was, and continues to be, valued almost exclusively for sentimental, affectionate, emotional contributions—companionship, love, and pleasure.

Adoption today is a process involving a variety of individuals and institutions: the natural parents, the adopted child, the adoptive parents, private and not-for-profit social welfare agencies, independent law firms, the legislature, the courts, and the health care industry. The interests of all these individuals and organizations have to be satisfied before an adult can bring home an adopted child.

Meanwhile the federal government has set policy that will, through family-planning objectives, continue to reduce the number of infants available for adoption. For example, the United States Public Health Service has set objectives on family planning intended by 1990 to:

- Reduce unintended births among single American women aged 15 to 44 years to 18 per 1,000, from the 1978 level of 26.2 births per 1,000 unmarried women of the same age.

- Reduce the fertility rate for 17-year-old girls to 45 per 1,000, from the 1978 level of 52.1 births per 1,000.

- Reduce the fertility rate for 16-year-old girls to 25 per 1,000, from the 1978 level of 31.8 births per 1,000.

It has been predicted that the likely candidate for adoption, at least from the foster-care population, will be older (age 10 to 12 or over), will be from a minority group, and may have some disability.

Experts agree that data on children available for adoption in this country are scanty and somewhat unreliable; data on adults seeking to adopt are equally unreliable. An often repeated estimate is that about 8.5 million Americans cannot have children by birth. That figure, however, only refers to *infertile* individuals. Some number of *fertile* couples and individuals also must be added to derive a total number of prospective parents seeking to adopt.

The field of adoption changes each year, as the adoption process evolves through new legislation, court decisions, changes in social values, and the changes in the numbers of both children available for adoption and adults interested in adopting them.

That is the status of adoption today—a complex social and legal process. The fact that adoption has evolved into a quagmire of government and social-welfare concerns should not deter adults from adopting a child. It is crucial, however, to understand that adoption is a process. The word *adopted* is not merely an adjective to describe a child. Rather it refers to a process by which a child becomes a part of a family. Adoptive parents should not make any effort to conceal the fact that a child has become a part of their family through the adoption process; society is primarily concerned about the love and affection that exists between parents and children, not whether the family is created by adoption or biology.

The Adoptive Parents

All individuals or couples who are recognized by the law as adults and who are deemed to be stable, both financially and emotionally, are capable of adopting a child. The universe of adoptive individuals can be broken down to four broad categories:

- Infertile couples, with or without a living child.

- Fertile couples who are at risk of producing a genetically impaired infant.

- Fertile couples who elect not to bear additional children.

- Single adults, both male and female.

The Infertile Couple

It is ironic that the events that lead to the joyous occasion of bringing a child home through the adoption process often begin with the realization that a couple will not be able to bear children of their own. After all the tests have been performed, various attempts at pregnancy have failed, and the biological alternatives such as artificial insemination are rejected for personal or medical reasons, the couple is then faced with the emotional trauma of infertility.

What is infertility in the context of its initial emotional impact? For many childless couples, infertility brings a feeling of loss, grief over the death of an unspecific person, and grief over the death of a dream.

A Feeling of Loss. A couple trying to achieve pregnancy wants more than to have a child. The nine months of pregnancy are an important intermediate event and it is normal for a couple to anticipate the joy of those nine months of gestation. The excitement of telling friends and relatives about the pregnancy, the buying of maternity clothes, feeling the baby move, guessing the baby's sex, and baby showers, are all events that a pregnant couple anticipates and enjoys.

The infertile couple has not only lost the ultimate result of pregnancy—their own baby—but has also lost the intermediate events. The feeling of loss begins with the feeling of not being able to enjoy pregnancy itself.

Other feelings of loss have to do with losing a part of oneself. The ability to bring children into the world by choice is an inherent part of life. When infertility takes that choice away, it may seem to the couple as if they have lost a part of their own lives.

Grief over the Death of an Unspecific Person. Part of the excitement of pregnancy lies in its largely unpredictable outcome: What sex will the baby be? Will the baby favor the mother or father in appearance and disposition? What will the baby's personality be like? Even though a couple may think of a baby as their own, the baby itself is an unspecific person. A pregnant couple finds joy in anticipating this unspecific person. An infertile couple experiences the death of this unspecific person, who, in fact, has not even been conceived. Such couples often grieve over the loss of what their child would have been.

The Death of a Dream. The dream of having a family, of having, loving, and raising children, is a powerful motivator for couples to have babies. For infertile couples that dream is lost. Its place is taken by the anxiety-ridden reality of infertility. Each time the couple faces a family, they are reminded of their own infertility, and the loss of the dream can be intensified, at least in the early stages.

The heartbreak can be overwhelming. When the final medical verdict of infertility has been delivered, many couples have difficulty in coping with it. The first step in dealing with infertility is to make a concerted effort to resume a normal life. It takes a substantial effort at first, for the sight of every pregnant woman, and every baby, serves as a reminder of the couple's loss. In many cases, infertility counseling is required.

Considering Alternatives

The process of adjusting to the potential reality of infertility should begin while the couple is still pursuing medical remedies. Reviewing options should begin at the same time. In looking back on their experiences, a majority of couples have one regret in common: not acting sooner to face reality and, subsequently, not acting sooner to review options. This does not imply that potentially infertile couples should not devote their time and energy to medical options. The first option should always be to achieve pregnancy, but there comes a point when that option should not exclude all others.

Alternatives may include a decision not to have children at all, pregnancy through insemination with donor semen, in vitro fertilization, embryo transfer, surrogate parenting, and adoption and foster care.

The first option, not to have children, does not reflect an escapist attitude. For some individuals, the desire to have children is a strong personal need. If that need cannot be fulfilled through the usual means, some couples find it emotionally easier not to have a family.

An infertile couple interested in pursuing artificial insemination, in vitro fertilization, embryo transfer, or surrogate parenting should consult with medical and legal experts in the field before proceeding. (For more information about these alternatives, see the chapter on Infertility in *The Columbia University College of Physicians and Surgeons Complete Guide to Pregnancy*.)

Other Candidates for Adoption

Fertile Couple Advised Against Pregnancy. Adoption and foster care are also options for couples advised against having children because the mother has a serious medical condition that would be adversely affected by pregnancy or because one or both have genetic traits for disorders that might be passed on to offspring. Some couples in these circumstances suffer the same painful emotional experiences as infertile couples unable to have biological children.

Single Adoptive Parent. The traditional view among social workers assumed that married couples represented the ideal, if not the only, source for placing children available for adoption. More recently, however, child-care professionals are widening their search for adoptive parents by considering singles. With the growing number of children being raised by single parents as a result of divorce, social-welfare institutions have accepted the fact that an unmarried responsible adult is capable of providing the care and attention needed to raise a child. The norm, however, is for adoption agencies to place children with a single person only when a two-parent home cannot be found.

Although there is no research to support the assertion, some adoption experts believe that the motivation to become a parent may be stronger in some single parents than in some married people. Because these individuals are not expected by society to become parents, their decision can be viewed as an assertive effort to undertake that role.

One of the first reported single-parent adoption programs began in Los Angeles in the mid-1960s when the County Department of Adoptions could not find two-parent families for all children needing a home. Since then, several other adoption institutions have begun placing children in single-parent homes.

In considering single applicants for adoption, social-service agencies look beyond the usual considerations such as ability to provide a stable and loving atmosphere to factors that are unique to a single parent. Because there is no second parent to rely on, the health of the prospective single parent may be of greater concern than it would in a two-parent adoptive family. Because it will probably be necessary for the single parent to also be the sole wage earner, the availability and quality of child care is an issue. The adoption agency will also want some assurance that the applicant has an extended family who can supply emotional support, substitute short-term care in case of illness, and provide role models of the opposite sex. Fairly or unfairly, there may be careful scrutiny of the individual's sexual identification and contacts. In other words, why isn't the applicant married? And, as in any prospective adoption, the motivation of the applicant will be questioned.

A single person considering adoption could well ask these questions of him- or herself. Each consideration has a corresponding responsibility, and unless the prospective parent is willing to accept that responsibility, it is unlikely that adoption would be in the best interest of either the child or the adult.

Singles wishing to adopt should be aware of one major hurdle: the concerns of the child's natural parents. The natural parents must be convinced that a single parent can be a better source of love, affection, and growth for their child than they themselves can be. An unmarried mother, perhaps already dealing with guilt feelings for placing her child for adoption, may well feel more guilt once she becomes aware that the child will be raised by another single parent.

The Decision to Adopt

The process through which a couple arrives at the decision to adopt a child is purely a function of the spouses' relationship with each other. Questions that a couple should consider are: What is the motivation for wanting to adopt a child? Is it to satisfy the need to carry on the family name and tradition? Or is it to satisfy the desire to love, care for, and provide for a child? Are both partners committed to the creation of a family through adoption? Do the partners see adoption as a way of "saving" a marriage? Is their decision based on a good samaritan attitude of wanting to "rescue" a child?

The desire to love, care for, and raise a child should be the supreme motivation behind adoption. Other motives may doom the decision to failure, and

an adept adoption counselor will be able to recognize when the decision is being made for the wrong reasons.

Before going to an adoption agency and getting caught in the emotional whirlwind of the process, prospective adoptive parents may want to discuss their decision with family and friends, and with other parents who have adopted a child. The value of openly discussing the subject with family lies in assessing how the adopted child will be accepted by siblings, cousins, nephews, and the child's grandparents. While any disapproval from relatives should not dissuade a couple with a strong desire for children, the process may be smoother if they know ahead of time what to expect. It is not unreasonable to consider how the adopted child's acceptance by the family will affect the child's adjustment and emotional growth. On the other hand, many relatives who are initially against the decision come to love and accept the child once it becomes clear that the adoption is final.

A number of community agencies offer free counseling on adoption, and parents should take advantage of these opportunities. These counseling sessions or seminars not only help the parents in shaping their own beliefs and attitudes about adoption, but they also serve to explain general family life with an adopted child.

The Adoption Process

Once the decision to adopt is firmly accepted by both spouses or by the single parent, the next step is to find an agency, either public or private. Most adoptions—except for those by stepparents and other relatives—take place through agencies.

Public agencies, which are tax-supported, usually do not charge for their services. Private agencies, which are often affiliated with a religious group, usually have a sliding-scale fee based on the parents' income. The fee can be very low or it can be as high as 7 to 10 percent of one year's gross income. The charges for adoption are not for the child, but for the services provided by the agency—the counseling, the home study, and postplacement visits. Legal fees are usually extra.

If the fee from a private agency is excessively high, there is reason to question the agency's purpose. If money, rather than placing homeless children in families, is the primary interest of the private agency, then the social responsibility for the child's interests may be sacrificed.

Most states regulate adoption agencies by establishing minimum standards for licensing. Licensed agencies that are also accredited meet a more rigorous set of standards set by professional organizations, such as the Council on Accreditation of Services to Families and Children. Working with a licensed agency is generally an assurance that standards of professional conduct will be met and that the parents will receive proper psychological support and guidance.

In some areas, there are referral agencies that do not handle adoptions directly but will help prospective parents locate the most appropriate agency for them. For example, some agencies specialize in children of a certain racial or religious background.

Some agencies conduct group orientation meetings for prospective parents. The purpose of the first meeting is to inform the parents of the types of children available through the agency, perhaps through pictures and slides; to explain the agency's policies; and to outline the entire adoption process. Other agencies accomplish this through an individual interview with an adoption counselor.

Prospective parents who are interested in entering the process are then asked to fill out an extensive application, giving information about their family, personal, financial, employment, and medical background.

The next step is the home study. The social worker assigned to the case will meet with both parents together and individually. If other individuals or children share the home, it is likely that the worker will also want to discuss with each of them their feelings about adoption.

The home study is an investigative process during which parents are often asked to reveal many details about their private lives. The social worker is not snooping; he or she needs to understand the quality of home life in the search for the best home possible for each child. The agency needs to know, for example, that there is no critical illness in the family, especially any illness that will jeopardize the child's sense of stability. The home study serves an important purpose in that it can help point to attitudes or problems that need to be dealt with before adoption.

Assessing income is also a part of the investigative process. A large income does not necessarily give applicants an advantage; a stable income does. If there are two parents and both work outside the home, reliable arrangements must be made for the child's care. If the child has special needs and the income necessary to provide for those needs is not available to the parents, the child may be eligible for a medical subsidy. Almost all states provide such subsidies.

During the entire process, applicants must realize that the agency has the authority to disapprove an adoption. The rejected applicants may not find out why they were not accepted, but most agencies today will talk with rejected applicants about why adoption doesn't seem possible at a given time. Rejection by an agency does not preclude the applicants from reapplying or working with another agency.

After the home study is completed and the prospective parents are accepted, the agency worker will discuss specific children who are available and may provide pictures of them. While the agency can recommend a certain child for the parents, the decision to accept or reject that recommendation lies with the parents. The parents can express specific preferences for the type of child they want.

Children available for adoption, as well as the prospective parents, can be categorized by the following characteristics: age; race; ethnic, cultural and social background; religion; education; and physical, mental, and personality characteristics.

The social worker generally relies on the following guiding principles as they relate to each of the characteristics listed above. Parents should also consider each of the characteristics as they proceed in their decision to adopt.

Age. Age is a factor for both the parents and the child. As a general rule, the parents selected for a child should reflect the normal age for natural parents of a child of that age. Older parents, however, are not automatically disqualified. If the parents show the ability to take care of the changing needs of a child, then their age is not a source of discrimination.

On the other hand, older children—10-, 12-, or 14-year olds, for example—are often a more demanding challenge for the parents. Typically, such children may have been abused or may have spent years in one or more foster homes. As a result, they may have developed a distrust for adults. Other older children may have spent most of their young lives in institutions. Their problems in adjusting to family life are even more difficult.

Developing a relationship with an older child requires skill and patience. These children are "growing people," and they have already formed habits, beliefs, and behavior patterns. Adopting an older child means having to work hard to make the adoption work. It requires flexibility on the part of the parents and a willingness by any children who may already be a part of the family to accept the new sibling.

Personality characteristics, too, play a significant role in the adoption of older children. Similarities in personality traits may aid in the assimilation of the child into the family, especially if other children are already a part of that family. In any case, prospective parents must be willing to face a host of emotional challenges that the child will bring into the family.

Prospective parents who want to adopt an older child should be aware that the eventual success of such adoptions is yet to be demonstrated by research. One study indicates that adoption disruptions increase with the age at adoption. The disruption rate varies from as low as 7 percent for children between birth and age five, to as high as 47 percent for children between the ages of 12 and 17.

A 1986 study by the Child Welfare League of America (CWLA), however, reached a different conclusion. The CWLA study found that 73 percent of parents interviewed indicated that adopting an older child was a "good" or "excellent" experience. The vast majority of the parents said that they would adopt the child if they had to do it over again and that the adoption had added meaning to family members' lives.

Given the inconclusive results of this research, adoptive parents should not let age deter them from adopting an otherwise desirable child. With proper pre- and postadoption counseling, the adoption can be successful.

Race. Adoption counselors will often attempt to place children with parents of the same race, but a child is rarely, if ever, denied an adoption by parents of another race when parents of the same race are unavailable.

Adoption counselors believe that children placed in adoptive families with similar characteristics, such as color, race, or ethnic background, can become more easily integrated into the family and community. But, as in any adoption, the interests of the child are paramount. Parents considering interracial adoption should seek community resources to help themselves and the child with issues of cultural heritage and identity. Helping the child feel loved and wanted can help overcome any preoccupation the child may have with not looking like his or her parents.

Opponents of transracial adoptions argue that children do not develop a strong sense of identity unless they grow up with a family of their own race. But parents who elect to adopt across racial lines disagree; giving the child a positive self-image can overcome the race issue. A desire to adopt a minority child should not, however, be based on the fantasy of rescuing a child.

Ethnic, Cultural, and Social Background. These are often not considered important factors in the intracountry adoption process, except if the child is older or if the parents have shown an obvious interest in adopting a child of a background similar to their own. Cultural and social behavior are not en-tirely inherited traits; they can be acquired.

International adoptions, however, make ethnic, cultural, and social backgrounds major issues. As they grow up, children from other countries may feel, for example, "American on the inside, Korean on the outside." Again, the development of a positive self-image can help the international adoptee overcome the sense of not belonging to any one place.

Parents considering international adoptions have more to worry about than just ethnic background. International adoptions are governed by several state and federal laws, as well as the laws of the child's home country. Federal requirements for an intercountry adoption vary, depending on whether the child is brought here for adoption or is being adopted in the country of origin.

Adopting a child from another country also puts a responsibility on the parents to make sure that the social-welfare agency arranging the adoption is a reputable one, and not engaged in child profiteering.

The advantage of an international adoption is that the waiting period for adopting an infant or toddler is often not as long as it would be to adopt a child within the United States. Adopting transnationally, however, involves additional expenses, such as air fares, legal fees in both countries, fees for the orphanage in the child's country, special medical attention to guarantee that the child is healthy and properly immunized, and language training for older children. Parents should also recognize that adoption does not automatically grant the child from another country American citizenship. The law does allow for the parents to file for naturalization of the child as soon as the adoption is final in the United States.

Religion. Religion can be a basis for creating the adoptive family, but it is usually not the sole determinant for the selection of a child.

Social-welfare agencies that are under the auspices of a religious order, however, are free to stipulate requirements consistent with their faith. Parents who have a strong religious faith are encouraged to contact their clergyman or other appropriate religious leader for an evaluation of factors that may affect the child's religious upbringing.

Education. To some adoptive parents, the education level of the child's natural parents is an important factor. They believe that a child from a well-educated family is likely to inherit a predisposition to value education. There is no empirical evidence to support this. From the adoption counselor's viewpoint, the educational status of the child's natural parents is not a reliable index of the potential development of a child. On the other hand, the adoptive family should offer an environment in which the child can develop his or her own capacities, and not be expected to fulfill any unrealistic goals of the adoptive parents.

Physical, Mental, and Personality Characteristics.

Just as race is not a determining factor, mere physical resemblance is not considered important in the placement of a child. It is not practical or advisable to match all blue-eyed blond parents with blue-eyed blond children. The shortage of children available for adoption precludes the social-welfare system from putting any emphasis on physical appearances.

The mental development of a child, although important, can be facilitated by the adoptive parents.

Children with physical or mental disabilities are often described as "hard to place," posing a challenge to social-welfare agencies and adoptive parents alike. Such children are often older and may have experienced the trauma of rejection from both foster-care parents and adoptive parents.

It is important for the adoptive parents to realize that hard-to-place adoptees are children first of all, with the same emotional and physical needs and wants as all children.

Although a child's disability can complicate the day-to-day life of the adoptive family, many parents who have adopted a child with special needs have learned to face things one at a time and seek out help when needed.

The decision to adopt a child with a disability requires a special commitment from the parents. It means getting accustomed to awkward moments, stares, and comments when in the company of friends or strangers. It means having to learn that the child may be avoided by other children of similar age. It may mean modifying the household routine or even the physical arrangement of the household to accomodate the child.

The first step in adopting a disabled child is to get a complete medical evaluation of the disability. The child may not have received good general medical care, the condition may have been misdiagnosed, and the child may not have received appropriate treatment. Correcting such mistakes often reduces the severity of the disability.

Adoption counselors will not deny that the job of parenting a child with special needs is strenuous in many ways. But, as with any child, the rewards are also great.

Placement

Once a single parent or couple has narrowed the decision to a specific child, the adoption agency then provides more detailed information on the child's developmental history, including birth history, weight and height, eating and sleeping habits. The parents also receive information on the child's personality and temperament, along with medical data, known hereditary conditions, and nonidentifying information about the natural parents.

Information about the natural parents is critical for the adoptive parents to know and share with the child as he or she matures. Adoptive parents are also told why the child was placed for adoption.

When a particular child has been selected for adoption, and the social agency approves the parents' selection, both the parents and the child are then "prepared" for placement. The preparatory work depends on the child's age and the particular needs of the adoptive family. The older child is always given an opportunity to become gradually acquainted with the new parents, with the social worker acting as liaison and providing continuity of contact during the transition phase.

The entire process can take several months to several years before a child actually joins a family. That is followed by a "probationary" period when the agency worker will visit the adoptive home several times. The first visit is often within a week. The frequency of subsequent visits will vary, depending on the parents' need to talk with the worker, the age of the child, and any substantial changes in the parents' life-style.

In most cases, after the probationary period is over and the agency is satisfied with the placement, the parents, the child, a representative of the agency, and the parents' lawyer have to appear in court for a final adoption decree. Most states require consent from children above a certain age—generally over age 10—and all states require consent by birth parents, unless parental rights have been terminated by a court.

Until the 1970s, the unmarried birth father's consent was rarely taken into consideration. But as a result of a U.S. Supreme Court ruling that the birth father, too, has rights to the child, the rights of both parents must be terminated, either voluntarily or through court action, before a child is "free" for adoption.

Independent Adoptions

Not all adoptions are arranged through agencies. Some children are placed through private or independent adoptions, usually arranged by an attorney, doctor, clergyman, or relative. Sometimes prospective parents will place ads in community newspapers stating their desire to adopt an infant and offering to pay the medical expenses of a pregnant woman who intends to release her baby for adoption.

Although these adoptions can be successful, there may be risks involved. Prospective parents wishing to pursue independent adoption should satisfy themselves that they are dealing with a reputable attorney, one who is willing to furnish references of other couples he or she has helped. Fees should be reasonable to cover expenses of the birth mother and the attorney, but not out of line with agency fees.

One of the drawbacks of independent adoption is that there is no agency to provide counseling to the family in adjusting to their new situation. Parents who feel this would be helpful can seek the services of an independent social worker. Sometimes social workers who are certified to perform home studies are available to provide counseling.

Current Issues in Adoption

The current state of the field of adoption is often described as a "time of experimentation." Although most experts consider recent developments to be positive, the changes have raised questions about generally accepted customs and practices. The three most prominent changes are in the areas of adoption laws, open adoptions, and alternatives to adoption.

Adoption Law. While there are some federal laws that affect adoption, most regulation is at the state level. The primary purpose of adoption regulations has been to ensure professional placement services, but more recently some state legislatures have been concerned with the confidentiality of the adoption process. Starting in the late 1970s, some states moved to open adoption records to adult adoptees, while others moved toward limiting the access.

Bills have been introduced or passed in almost every state concerning access by adult adoptees to information about their genetic heritage and birth records. On the question of information identifying birth parents, there have been three basic approaches: proposals allowing unrestricted access by adult adoptees to records containing identifying information; proposals allowing adult adoptees contact with a birth parent through an intermediary who would secure the birth parent's consent to such contact; and a registry to match names of birth parents with adult adoptees, when both are willing to have contact. (See list of resources at the end of this chapter.)

Open Adoptions. "Open adoption" is a term used to mean either that the birth mother or both birth parents are involved in choosing the adoptive parents for the child or that ongoing contact is arranged beween birth parents and the adopted child.

Such practices are fairly rare, but growing.

Because older children often know their birth families, it is unrealistic for the adoptive parents to expect the child to forget them. Unless the birth parents have abandoned their rights to the child or the rights have been terminated by a court, it is difficult to prevent an older child from wanting to maintain some contact with natural parents.

In many open adoptions, birth parents meet the adoptive parents and participate in the placement and separation process. Although they relinquish all legal, moral, and nurturing rights to the child, they retain the right to continued contact and to knowledge of the child's whereabouts and progress in life.

There is little evidence about whether open adoptions work. Some children remain in foster care because their birth parents cannot accept the idea of never seeing them again and therefore do not terminate their parental rights. For these parents and children, open adoption may be a positive step toward providing a permanent home.

Alternatives to Adoption. Several alternatives are available for people who want to provide love and nurturing to a child but who are not qualified to adopt or who do not feel prepared to accept the responsibilities of adoption. They can fulfill that desire through work as a volunteer in a school, daycare or child-care center; by joining the Big Brother or Big Sister movement; or by volunteering as a tutor in a community center. They can also become foster parents.

FOSTER CARE

FOSTER PARENTS play a vital role in the process of finding permanency for children. Foster care provides children with a temporary residence, daily care, understanding, and affection that is aimed at promoting healthy physical and emotional growth and family life until they can be returned home or adopted.

For foster care to succeed, foster parents have to accept the fact that they are a part of a team of professionals working together to provide the best possible care for their children. Others on the team are the caseworker, teacher, doctor, school social worker, and public health nurse. Few people possess the qualities that enable them to open their homes and their love to an unknown child on a temporary basis, provide a loving and caring atmosphere, and become attached to the child, yet be able to let go when the placement is terminated.

Becoming a Foster Parent

Volunteering a home and a family as a foster parent is quite different from adopting a child. As an adoptive parent, an individual takes on the responsibility of acting in the child's interest permanently. Once the adoption is finalized, there is limited interaction between the social-welfare agency and the adoptive family, unless a disruption occurs. Foster parents, however, are in continuous contact with the social worker.

The foster-care training and placement process generally follows these steps:

Orientation. This is an educational process in which prospective parents learn the kinds of social, family, and personal problems that lead to family breakdown, creating the need for children to be placed in foster care. It prepares the foster parent to anticipate problems and to deal with them through an understanding of the principles of child development. The foster parents learn what their own rights and responsibilities will be, as well as those of the agency staff and the child's natural parents.

Certification. This signifies that the adult has met the necessary legal and agency requirements to become a foster parent. Following formal approval, the agency issues a certificate that contains the name, address, and religion of the family, along with the age and sex of the children who may be available for placement.

Training. Once a foster home has been licensed or certified by the agency, the prospective foster parents receive further training in helping the children who will be in their care to cope with the separation and feeling of loss; in discipline and developmental issues; and in crisis intervention. To help ensure a secure and stable placement, most agencies will provide parents with basic information about agency policy on removal of a child from the foster family, and an explanation of how parents can request an administrative review of agency decisions.

Supervision of Children in Foster Care. After a child is selected and placed in the foster home, the agency is required to supervise the placement. The agency will provide an estimate on how long the child will need care, facts about the child's health, handicaps, school and educational experiences, and relationships of the child with its biological parents.

Recertification. Every year an agency caseworker reviews the parents' license or certificate and prepares a written evaluation of the home and family life, describing care given by the parents to the children and the parents' working relationship with the agency. A physician's written statement about the family's health is also needed for recertification.

Effect of Foster Placement on Children

Being placed in foster care is a traumatic event for most children, causing them to experience a wide range of emotions. Children entering placement for the first time are likely to experience fear, loneliness, hurt, anger, guilt, shame, and powerlessness. The foster parent has a major responsibility to allay the fears of the child, help him or her to feel secure and hopeful about the future, and to help the child cope with powerful negative emotions.

Some children keep their feelings bottled up because it is less painful than sharing them with someone else. Others can't find the words to express their feelings, and parents should watch for opportunities to make the child comfortable enough to vent his or her emotions.

Foster children often wonder why their parents did not keep them. They may feel hurt that "no one wants them," not even their own parents, or anger at their parents for "giving them away."

Younger children will transfer their attachments to other "parent figures" more easily than will older children. Children who have a strong reliance on their natural parents will have strong feelings about foster parents. They may have been neglected or abused, leaving them confused; yet many will retain their love and affection for their natural parents.

Critical Issues in Foster Care

Adults considering foster care must be sensitive to the personal and legal ramifications of accepting a child. (See Guidelines for Foster Parents.)

Even though the foster child is often a minor, the child has rights, a personal history (such as a name, religion), and privileges. These legal and personal needs are the responsibility of the foster parents. The most important of these are confidentiality, family name and religion, Social Security and other income, and education.

Confidentiality. Information regarding children in foster care and their families must be held in confidence by all concerned. The caseworker or the natural parents of the child may share important information about the child and the child's family life with the foster parents. Foster parents should never discuss the child's personal history or other details with relatives, neighbors, or friends. Children in foster care often become upset or lose faith in their foster parents if confidentiality is violated.

GUIDELINES FOR FOSTER PARENTS

The following guidelines for foster parents are based on recommendations from the New York State Department of Social Services:

- Work with the child's caseworker to arrange preplacement visits that are gradually increased in length and frequency. Keep in mind that in most cases, a child can only cope with one stress at a time.
- Make certain that the child's caseworker tells the child as clearly and directly as possible the reason for coming into the care of the agency and the reason for being placed in a foster family home.
- Recognize that the child will have fears about the foster family that can be allayed by an adequate number of preplacement visits that are satisfying and reassuring.
- Be aware of the child's special need to be helped with feelings about separation. Actively encourage the child to express any feelings about being separated from the biological parents.
- Recognize that a child's tempestuous expression of anger in the early stages of placement is necessary and helpful in resolving loss.
- Encourage and promote visits with the biological parents according to the agency plan.
- If there is serious doubt about the placement based on preplacement information, do not accept the placement. A placement that breaks down is traumatic for everyone concerned, but much more so for the foster child.
- Offer food to the child during visits and at the time of placement. Show the child the private living space allocated in the home.
- Allow the child to select the name by which he or she will call the foster parents. If the child cannot decide on a name, offer suggestions.
- Encourage the child to bring along some favorite object.

Any questions regarding the child should be referred to the agency caseworker. Medical information about the child and natural parents is also considered confidential.

The right to confidentiality also extends to situations involving the mass media. Foster parents should obtain permission from the agency before granting interviews or pictures to television, radio, newspaper, or magazine reporters.

Foster children are also entitled to personal confidentiality, which allows them to receive or send mail; receive, refuse, or make telephone calls during reasonable hours; and contact an attorney or a clergyman.

Family Name and Religion. Children in foster care have to use their legal names in all situations. Neither the agency nor the foster parents have the right to change a child's name while the child is in their custody.

Like the family name, the religion of all children must be preserved and protected during foster care, and most states have laws to this effect. The natural parents of the child have a right to determine a child's religion and to request that the child be placed in a foster home of the same faith. Foster parents who accept children of another faith must make arrangements for the children to participate in the religious events of their faith. Similarly, foster parents cannot impose their own religious beliefs or practices on the child.

Social Security and Other Income. Many states require that children in foster care have a Social Security number; it is the responsibility of the agency to obtain it. Children under 18 may receive Social Security income in certain situations, and this income is applied against the cost of foster care. At 18, foster children who are still attending school are entitled to receive Social Security benefits directly until one month after their nineteenth birthday. Those classified as handicapped may be eligible to receive benefits indefinitely, subject to evaluation and approval by the Social Security Administration. Foster parents have the responsibility to report such income to the agency in order to make adjustments to the allowance paid to the foster parents.

Some children may have guardianship accounts, trust funds, or other sources of income that they are entitled to at age 18. The caseworker informs parents of such benefits, and arrangements are made to pay the benefits directly to the child.

Education. A child in foster care has to be registered in the local school under his or her legal name. The foster parents act, however, as if they were the child's natural parents by signing report cards and attending school functions. It is important for the foster parents to be involved in the child's academic progress and activities, to show that they are interested and that they care about the child. The agency should also be kept informed of the child's progress in school.

Laws Relating to Foster Care. Foster care involves several legal relationships: between the

DEFINING RIGHTS AND RESPONSIBILITIES

Foster parents have the right to:
- Be given pertinent information on any child to be placed in their home.
- Receive an explanation of all agency policies and procedures regarding foster parenting; receive training and ongoing supervision and assistance from an assigned caseworker.
- Have complaints and disagreements heard and responded to by the agency.
- Receive preference over all applicants interested in adopting the child, provided the child has been in foster care with the family for a specified time, usually 18 continuous months.
- Intervene as an interested party in any court proceeding involving the custody of a child who has been in the foster parents' home for 18 continuous months or longer.
- Be given notice and a right to participate in any family court review hearing on a child placed voluntarily who has been in the parents' care continuously for 18 months or longer.

Foster parents have the responsibility to:
- Provide temporary care for foster children with the same love given to natural children.
- Provide guidance, discipline, a good example, and as many positive life experiences as possible.
- Encourage and supervise school attendance, participate in teacher conferences, and keep the caseworker updated regarding any special educational needs.
- Attend to the regular and special medical and dental needs of the child.
- Facilitate visits between the child and biological parents.
- Help children adjust emotionally to the problems in their lives.
- Tell the caseworker promptly about any problems that arise or help that is needed.

Biological parents have the right to:
- Help make the plans for their children in placement.
- Be notified as soon as possible of any serious medical emergency or major treatment given without parental consent.
- Visit their children and develop a visiting plan with the caseworker.
- Be notified about and attend any court action concerning the custody arrangement.
- Be represented by a lawyer in any court action concerning their children or affecting their parental rights.
- Give consent for medical care, hospitalization, marriage, release of information, driver's permits.

Biological parents have the responsibility to:
- Work with the caseworker to develop a plan for the children's future.
- Work to solve the problems that prevent their children from living at home.
- Visit their children regularly, at a time and place agreed upon with the caseworker.

Agency or governmental caseworker has the right to:
- Assist the child in managing any transitional role status as a result of replacement, transfer, or discharge.
- Support the child's development (physical, mental, and emotional).
- Maintain or improve the child's relationship with the biological family.
- Represent the agency in developing a permanent home for the child.

The caseworker has the responsibility:
To the foster family to:

- Supervise the placement of children in the home by supplying parents with information and services that facilitate foster parenting.
- Act as the parents' link to the agency, interpreting policy and procedures to help the parents to use the foster-care system.
- Act as a resource for any problems or crises that may arise.

To the biological parents to:

- Help assess problems in the family that affect their ability and willingness to provide for their children.
- Help decide on the child's best interests in terms of a permanent home.
- Help develop and execute service plans that demonstrate their commitment to care for their children.
- Keep them informed of a child's development, progress and health.

To the agency and/or court to:

- Carry out the responsibilities to the family and to report to the appropriate authorities at specified intervals about each child's progress.
- Demonstrate that effort has been made to reunite a family within specific time frames.
- Report on the efforts or lack of efforts of the parents.
- Pursue termination of parental rights when the parents are either unwilling or unable to care for their children.

agency and the natural parents, between the agency and the foster parents, between the agency and the child, and between the foster parents and the child. Most legal matters involving foster parenting are settled through administrative proceedings, although in extreme situations, such as criminal abuse and neglect, the matter may go to court, typically family court.

If a court is involved in a foster-care matter, a legal guardian is often appointed for the child. The foster parents can and should seek legal counsel, but expenses for such counsel are not covered. The agency is represented by its own attorney.

The rights of various parties involved are summarized in the box on Defining Rights and Responsibilities.

SUMMING UP

ADOPTION AND FOSTER CARE are community responsibilities carried out by committed adults in the interest of children.

All children—including those born through unintended pregnancies, those with special needs, and those abandoned by their parents—are entitled to placement in a family that can love and nurture them and guide them toward becoming responsible adults who will ultimately make their own contribution to community welfare.

Sharing responsibility for providing these children with homes are the government, social-welfare agencies, individual communities, and all adults. The professional services provided by adoption and foster-care programs play a pivotal role in assuring permanency for children who would otherwise grow to adulthood without an understanding of family relationships. Ultimately, the responsibility for providing proper adoption and foster-care services lies with individual communities and the individuals in those communities.

Society's attitudes about adoption and foster care are changing. There is growing recognition that the focus needs to be on the child's future, not on the child's history or that of his or her parents.

The growth in child-welfare programs, both private and public, is a clear indication that children continue to be recognized as a valuable resource, both for the present and the future. Adults interested in taking advantage of such programs should contact a local agency or one of the national information or referral organizations listed at the end of this chapter. County and state social-welfare agencies are also an excellent resource for information about adoption and foster care.

ADOPTION AND FOSTER CARE RESOURCES

Adoptees Liberty Movement Association
P. O. Box 154
Washington Bridge Station
New York, NY 10033

Child Welfare League of America
440 First Street, NW, Suite 310
Washington, DC 20001

Committee for Single Adoptive Parents
P. O. Box 4074
Washington, DC 20015

Latin American Parents Association
P. O. Box 72
Seaford, NY 11783

National Committee for Adoption, Inc.
1346 Connecticut Avenue, NW, Suite 326
Washington, DC 20036

North American Center on Adoption
67 Irving Place
New York, NY 10003

18 Getting Off to a Healthy Start; Instilling Good Habits

Stephen J. Atwood, M.D.

INTRODUCTION

ALL PARENTS WANT to give their children a headstart on a healthy life-style, but only recently have we started to reevaluate the positive effects of fostering good habits in exercise and nutrition at an early age. There is mounting evidence that cardiovascular diseases, obesity, and other serious disorders actually begin in early childhood, and many experts think that early health promotion may prevent or delay these diseases. More research is needed to determine whether this is true, but almost everyone agrees that being physically fit and adopting a healthy life-style certainly adds considerably to general well-being. In this chapter we will offer suggestions on how parents can help their children to be more physically fit and attuned to a healthy life-style, particularly by emphasizing functional exercise, such as walking or hiking instead of riding in a car, that can and should be a part of everyday life. It is also about what parents can do to set a good example for their children.

EXERCISE

DESPITE INCREASED EMPHASIS on adult physical fitness, studies of American children indicate that the average youngster is woefully "out of shape." The recent National Children and Youth Fitness Study found that more than 40 percent of American children do not participate in even minimal appropriate physical activity year-round. Up to a fourth of all elementary-school-age children have too much body fat, and less than half of our children participate in physical activities that can be carried on into adulthood. Increasingly, experts urge that even very young children be encouraged to participate in regular aerobic exercise, with emphasis on family-oriented activities.

We know that vigorous physical activity is the key to fitness. Most babies and toddlers are naturally bundles of activity—they are constantly kicking, waving their arms and legs, crawling, climbing, walking, and running. These normal activities build strong muscles and develop good coordination. At an early age, parents should foster and protect the baby's natural activity by providing a safe environment for the child to move about as much as possible. Keeping a baby confined to a playpen may ensure safety, but it is usually for the parents', not the baby's, well-being and does little to encourage the youngster to explore and really move about. Baby walkers and jumpers partially meet the parents' and baby's needs—the baby is more protected but can still move around. But neither is completely safe and should not be used as a substitute for parental observation and interaction.

Functional exercise begins even in the first few months. Parents can support a baby's normal physical activity by engaging in certain types of play. There are a number of postpregnancy exercises designed to help both mother and baby "get in shape" and, at the same time, have fun. For example, most babies love to be lifted up high and allowed to stretch out—a maneuver that can be done when the baby is about eight weeks old. The mother lies with her back flat on the floor or a firm bed with knees bent and the baby lying face down on her chest and upper abdomen. With both hands, she lifts the baby up until her arms are fully extended. The baby will naturally stretch out, holding his or her head up and kicking while being held aloft. Doing this helps the baby develop the strong neck and back muscles needed for head control, while it strengthens the mother's back, shoulder, and abdominal muscles.

In recent years, there has been a move to teach babies how to swim almost before they can walk. Many babies do love to splash around in water, and this can help strengthen muscles and avoid later fear of water. They don't have to learn to swim to exercise. If parents just hold them (in water that is not too cold) in such a way that they don't get too much water in their eyes and mouths, they will kick and splash and get plenty of exercise. It isn't necessary to go to the swimming pool or beach—the baby can splash around in a bathtub full of lukewarm water. Of course, any child—even one who can swim —should *never* be left unattended, even for two or three minutes, in a pool or bathtub. Each year a number of child drownings result from youngsters' being left alone in tubs or pools.

Parents should take advantage of a young child's natural tendencies—encourage his or her love of climbing, for instance, by providing a safe place to climb. A back yard or playground jungle gym installed over a sandbox or a well-padded surface provides an ideal environment for active group play. Old tires can be arranged into a safe, imaginative, and inexpensive climbing and swinging area.

In a city, parents can walk (not drive) with their children to school playgrounds or parks and turn the kids loose. Children always find something to do given a chance. With an only child, parents can invite a friend or two to come along. Two or three children don't need any equipment at all to exercise!

Many youth or community centers and exercise facilities offer special parent-child classes in aerobic dancing and other physical activities. These can be fun and beneficial to both parents and children. But dancing doesn't have to be done at a special facility —it can be done at home in the living room. Parents who turn off the TV and turn on the radio find that dancing is fun, and their children love doing it with them.

It is not necessary to limit exercise to the home or to aerobic exercise classes. In many countries, exercise is a part of everyday life. People walk or bicycle to work. When they go shopping they take their shopping bags with them to carry their purchases home.

(People who must carry their own groceries may find themselves cutting down on the quantity they purchase!) Escalators and elevators are also a bit less common than they are in this country, or they are reserved for invalids and the elderly so that everyone else uses the stairs.

Obesity tends to be less common in countries where sedentary activity is frequently interspersed with physical exercise. Long hours of sitting—particularly in front of a television—are uncommon. When mothers or fathers go for a walk they take the baby with them in a soft baby carrier, a backpack, wrapped in a shawl on their backs, or in their arms. If the children are old enough, they walk too—strollers are rarely seen.

As children grow older, they copy their parents' lifestyle, another reason why parents should continue to encourage and practice active living. All children should be encouraged to engage in active play, preferably in activities that they can pursue for life and parents or other family members can join in on. Walking, hiking, stair climbing, bicycling, jogging or running, swimming, aerobic dancing, ping pong, tennis, Frisbee throwing, and roller skating are among the many activities that can be learned at an early age and pursued for life. What's more, they can all be done by the family together. Simply walking or bicycling when going on short errands, such as trips to a neighborhood grocery, provides exercise and teaches a youngster that it's not necessary to travel everywhere by car. Children can also be invited to go along when walking the dog. Indeed, any number of everyday activities offer an opportunity for family-oriented functional exercise.

Unfortunately, many parents equate physical activity with organized competitive sports, such as Little League baseball, junior hockey, football, and other such sports. Although these sports have much to offer to the older child if they are properly organized and supervised, they should be kept in their proper perspective. If a child enjoys baseball and his or her father likes coaching a team, this can foster healthy adult-child companionship and promote building sports skills. But if the youngster, encouraged more often than not by parents/coaches, becomes overly competitive and pushes or is pushed too hard to achieve, or if the parents show disappointment in the child's performance, the stage is set for emotional turmoil as well as possible physical harm. All too often, a child is expected to fulfill a parent's unaccomplished goals, or alternatively, to live up to a parent's past sports stardom. It is important to remember that sports should be fun for all participants. Rather than pushing a youngster who does not relish organized competitive sports to participate anyway, parents would do better to find an alternative physical activity that he or she enjoys. Again, bicycling, jogging, swimming, skating, hiking, or gymnastics are examples of physical activities that can be enjoyed by parents, relatives, friends, and children, and will provide a good basis for healthy, lifelong exercise programs.

A HEALTHY DIET

ADULT EATING HABITS (and problems) also are formed in early childhood. Increasingly, experts think that proper childhood nutrition can be an important factor in preventing heart attacks, high blood pressure, obesity, diabetes, and other nutrition-related diseases.

Unwittingly, some parents actually encourage poor eating habits. Many worry that their children are not eating enough or are "bad eaters." To encourage eating, these parents will resort to everything from threats to bribes: "You cannot go out to play until your plate is clean," or, "Show Mommy how much you love her by eating all your peas," or, "Eat two more bites of broccoli and you can have some ice cream." Others will try to get a child to eat more by offering snacks throughout the day; as a result, the youngster never feels really hungry and his or her appetite is understandably sluggish. Eating is not a virtue, nor should food be a reward or pacifier.

As noted in chapters 4 and 5, the large majority of children will eat as much as they need for normal, healthy growth. If a youngster is growing normally, and is neither losing weight nor getting fat, it is safe to assume that he or she is consuming adequate calories. Children will consume more food during growth spurts and less in between.

The important thing is to offer a variety of nutritious foods and to instill a regular eating pattern. And, even at an early age, a child can learn the basics of sound nutrition, namely, eating moderate amounts of a variety of foods. Although likes and dislikes should be respected, young children should be encouraged to try at least a little of every food

that is served. If dislike is so pronounced that the child actually gags when attempting to eat a certain food, parents should avoid it for a time and come back to it later. They should offer choices but make sure that the choices are between nutritionally similar alternatives, such as squash or carrots; broccoli or peas.

Sweets

Some babies are born with a natural preference for sweet-tasting foods. Studies have found that even before birth, a fetus will turn toward glucose (blood sugar) that is infused into the amniotic sac. There is nothing wrong with sweets as long as they are consumed in moderation. But a diet that is high in cookies, cakes, candies, and other sweets is also likely to be high in fats (especially the saturated fats that are used in commercial pastries and baked goods), and thus high in calories. And it is well known that sweets promote the growth of cavity-causing bacteria in the mouth. Thus it is wise to limit sweets to mealtimes, and to emphasize fruits and low-fat sweets over pastries, baked goods, and candies. Also, whole fruits are better than juices or "fruit drinks" and are less likely to be abused than sodas and other soft drinks.

Dietary Restrictions

In recent years, the association between diet and disease, especially cardiovascular disorders, has been emphasized. The American Heart Association and others concerned about lowering the toll from heart attacks and high blood pressure have advocated a prudent low-salt, low-fat, high-carbohydrate diet. Although many nutritionists advocate a prudent diet for the whole family, some of the restrictions should not be extended to very young children. For example, babies and young children need a bit more fat than adults; skim or low-fat milk may be fine for the parents and older children, but it is not recommended for children under the age of two. In contrast, some restrictions should be extended to children. If there is a family tendency to develop high blood pressure, restricting a child's salt intake may well help prevent hypertension later in life. Similarly, obesity tends to run in families. If there is a familial tendency to gain excessive weight, an early common-sense approach—a balanced diet that is low in processed sweets and that encourages normal eating habits—can help prevent later weight problems. Parents should make sure the child eats enough for proper growth and development, but not so much that he or she gains excessive weight. In this respect, encouraging physical activity will also help ensure normal weight. (For a more detailed discussion of specific dietary recommendations, see the chapters on Nutrition in the First Year, and Nutrition for Toddlers and Preschoolers.)

TELEVISION

SURVEYS HAVE FOUND that the average American child will spend more waking hours watching TV than playing, going to school, or engaged in any other activity. Some watch as much as eight or nine hours a day, which obviously leaves little time for anything else. Not uncommonly, youngsters become avid television viewers during infancy, especially if their mothers are in the habit of watching television while nursing, feeding, or otherwise tending their babies. By the time they start school, they are "TV addicts" with little interest in or appreciation for other activities.

In recent years, there has been growing concern about the possible negative influences of television on a child's social, intellectual, and even physical development. No one questions the strengths of the television medium or its ability to alter behavior, at least temporarily. Although definitive data have not been gathered on the social impact of television, there have been some reports linking violent or antisocial behavior and even childhood suicides to TV viewing. All too often, a child will prefer television viewing to engaging in physical activity. If TV watching becomes a substitute for active play and exercise, physical fitness is bound to suffer.

In addition to inhibiting physical activity, excessive TV viewing is often at the expense of social interaction such as playing with peers, talking with parents, and developing hobbies. A child may find retreating into a world of solitary TV more comfortable and less demanding than forming friendships with other children or even interacting with family members. If the programs viewed offer a skewed view of the world, it may be difficult for the youngster to cope with everyday reality. In real life, for example, the high-speed car chases or feats of daring are not likely to have the happy outcome that they do in so many television shows.

The social values fostered by many television programs also can have a negative effect on a child. Program sponsors and story themes often encourage excessive materialism. The overemphasis on physical attractiveness, athletic ability, or the seeming effortlessness with which goals are achieved do little to encourage the effort and hard work required for success in almost any venture. And excessive

television viewing does not foster creativity and independent thinking as much as does reading or imaginative play.

Of course, not all television has a negative effect. Educational programs like "Sesame Street" encourage early learning, provide attractive role models, and foster sound social values. They also can be highly entertaining and funny. Balance and discriminate viewing are what is important. Parents should firmly limit television viewing, preferably to no more than an hour or two a day. Television should not encroach on family time. Having it on during meals or at other times that should be set aside for conversation and social interaction can interfere with those activities.

Parents should make it a point to know what programs are being watched. If possible, they should try to join the child while watching a program, especially if they are not familiar with its content. Obviously, programs that are filled with violence, and other subject matter inappropriate for young viewers should be banned. Watching with a child gives a parent an opportunity to teach critical viewing by discussing the message in commercials and teaching the child to separate real life from what is on the screen. In this setting, programs with objectionable content, such as the use of drugs or violence, can help open the way for a healthy family discussion. In fact, many educational TV programs are designed to foster parent-child communication about difficult subjects.

Watching television is a passive, "lazy" habit, requiring less effort than reading, playing outdoors, getting together with friends, and so forth. All too often, we turn on the TV out of boredom or loneliness, rather than a real desire to see a specific program. Parents who find this is happening in their household should make a special effort to break the TV habit. Parents and children can become immersed in a project; for example, baking cookies, going for a walk, or water-color painting. Instead of having a TV on for "background" noise (if a set is on, chances are a child will watch it) they can listen to the radio or music. Again, setting a good parental example is one of the best ways to ensure that television is not abused or overused.

SAFETY AND ACCIDENT PREVENTION

OBVIOUSLY ALL CHILDREN should be provided a safe environment in which to grow, explore, and expand their personal experiences and horizons. Even young children can be taught safety habits. For example, all babies and young children should be securely buckled into a car safety seat, even if the trip is only a block or two. (See chapter 14, Ensuring Your Child's Safety.) In this regard, a toddler or older child will be much more accepting of a seatbelt or car restraint if the parents also use their seatbelts. Similarly, if parents always wait for a green light before crossing a street and practice other basic safety habits, their children are more likely to follow their good examples.

In teaching a young child the basics of safety and accident prevention, it is important to instill a healthy respect for potential dangers without making a youngster overly fearful or timid. Obviously, parents do not want to add to a child's natural fears of the world, but at the same time it is important to foster caution where it is necessary. For example, a child should be taught not to approach dogs, cats, and other unknown animals, but it should be done in such a way that he or she will not develop an irrational fear of animals. Many children who grow up with a household pet naturally assume that all such animals are friendly. Unfortunately, animal bites are extremely common, and young children are the most frequent victims. But bites can be avoided by teaching a child that it is all right to play with pets he or she knows, but always to ask before trying to pet a strange dog, cat, or other animal.

Similarly, children should be taught what is and what is not safe to eat or taste. Young children naturally tend to put almost anything they can pick up into their mouths. At an early age, children should be taught that it is safe to eat anything on their plates or any other food that is given to them by their parents or other people they know. But candy, gum, and other food or objects found on the floor, around the house, or in the street, or offered by strangers should be shown to a parent before they are tasted. All medicines should be kept locked in a cabinet out of any toddler's reach.

SETTING A GOOD EXAMPLE

CHILDREN ARE great imitators, and the people they imitate most are their parents. If parents smoke, abuse alcohol and other substances, overeat, or spend hours staring at TV, chances are their children will follow their example. Indeed, it makes little sense to expect a child to avoid a particular bad habit, such as smoking, if the parents smoke. So if parents have undesirable health habits, the best time to break them is before the first baby is born. Still, it is never too late to change, and making the effort to change a bad habit or begin a new good one, such as stopping smoking or embarking on a regular exercise program, will have a positive effect on a youngster.

Having children offers couples a unique opportunity. It provides parents with the motivation to improve their own life-style as they help their children get off to a healthy start. The whole family benefits when good habits rule.

19 How to Find a Specialist

Fred Agre, M.D.

INTRODUCTION

VIRTUALLY EVERY field of specialized medical care that is available to adults is also available to infants and children. In addition, children have their own specialists—pediatricians. These physicians have had at least three years of additional training beyond medical school, making them "board-eligible." If they are board-certified, they have passed a qualifying exam as well. There are also several sub-specialties of pediatrics, such as cardiology, endocrinology, and neonatal-perinatal medicine, which deals with problems of the newborn.

Most children are fortunate enough never to need a specialist other than a general pediatrician. A pediatrician can handle most medical problems that a child may encounter. There are times, however, when either the pediatrician or the parent feels that the young patient should be examined by another specialist. Parents should not hesitate to seek the advice of a specialist, either one recommended by the child's pediatrician or one that they find through one of the avenues discussed in this chapter.

WHY A SPECIALIST?

REASONS A CHILD should see a specialist include:

- A problem that a pediatrician is unable to diagnose within a reasonable length of time.

- A problem for which surgery is suggested.

- A problem that has been diagnosed as a chronic, potentially fatal, or extremely rare disease.

- A physical illness that the pediatrician believes has an emotional basis and that the parent believes has a physical basis.

- An illness or condition that the pediatrician feels is beyond his area of competence.

- Loss of confidence by the parents in the pediatrician.

Illnesses or conditions that may require a visit to a specialist range from recurring middle ear infections (otitis media); to crossed eyes (strabismus), to asthma or unusually short stature. The pediatrician is usually the one to suggest that his young patient see a specialist. Although the pediatrician will have had some training in whatever medical problem afflicts the child, he or she may feel that it would benefit the child's health to see someone who has greater experience in that particular field (see section, later in this chapter, titled What Is a Specialist?).

Sometimes, though, it is the parent who believes that the child should be seeing a specialist, in spite of the pediatrician's assurances that there is no need. It is best for the mother or father to handle this situation as tactfully and honestly as possible. The parent should tell the pediatrician that he or she would like to take the child to a specialist, rather than going without the pediatrician's knowledge. It is best to say simply, "I am concerned about this problem and I would feel better if I had a second opinion." This will usually elicit an understanding response from the doctor.

FINDING A SPECIALIST

WHETHER THE PEDIATRICIAN suggests a specialist or the parent brings up the issue with the pediatrician, the pediatrician will probably be the one to give the name of a specialist he thinks his patient should see. The benefits of seeing a specialist recommended by or at least known to the patient's pediatrician are many. A parent who has faith in the pediatrician will most likely also have faith in his choice of a specialist. Also, the lines of communication are open between the two doctors working on the child's case, and the sharing of information ultimately benefits the patient.

Of course, it is possible that the pediatrician does not know a specialist to recommend. Or the parent may not feel comfortable with the pediatrician's choice. (Parents who are not at ease with the pediatrician's original diagnosis may want a second opinion from a specialist not personally known by their pediatrician. The parents may feel that the pe-

diatrician will choose a specialist whose diagnosis will likely be the same as his or her own.)

In situations like these, how can a parent locate a qualified and trustworthy specialist? There is no way to guarantee finding the perfect doctor on the first try, but the guidelines listed in How and Where to Look should make the hunt more productive.

WHAT IS A SPECIALIST?

A SPECIALIST IS a doctor who has not only completed the usual four years of medical school and received an M.D. degree, but who also has had two to six years of additional training in a specific field. Board-certified physicians have, in addition to training, also passed an examination given by the appropriate American specialty board. Board-eligible physicians are those who have completed training but who have not taken the qualifying exam.

HOW AND WHERE TO LOOK

1. The parent can ask other people in the community for their recommendations. This method, however, has its drawbacks, as the average person is not always a good judge of a doctor's skills. He or she can tell, though, whether or not a doctor is pleasant, available, or expensive. A friend or neighbor's recommendation is based on a single experience, which may not be the same for someone else.

2. The parent may contact a major medical center, such as a medical university or university-affiliated hospital. Teaching hospitals like these usually have the finest reputations and are at the forefront of medical advances. If the hospital does not have its own doctor referral service, the parent can call the department of pediatrics and ask for the name of a specialist in the area needed. Although the disadvantage of this method is that it is a blind one, the parent can rest assured that he or she has contacted a group of well-trained doctors who have been recognized by the hospital for their expertise.

3. The parent might contact the County Medical Society (listed in the white pages of the phone book). The society can give the names of board-certified physicians with a specialty or subspecialty in the area desired. Again the method is blind, but the doctors listed are qualified.

4. The parent can contact another family physician. If the child's pediatrician does not come up with a name, the parent may wish to call another family

doctor, such as the father's internist or even the mother's gynecologist, to ask for a recommendation for the child. Often these doctors will know of other doctors with specialties in the area in question.

5. The parent may wish to contact organizations that were founded to combat or research the particular medical problem from which the child suffers. Often these groups can provide educational materials, pamphlets, or referrals to local specialists. (See the section on Health and Medical Organizations at the end of this book for a list of voluntary health agencies and associations.)

6. A parent could check the Directory of Medical Specialists, published by the American Board of Medical Specialists. The volume is usually available at the reference desk in the library or at the County Medical Society's office. A geographical listing under each specialty makes it easy to find a physician according to city and state. All doctors listed are board-certified physicians. Next to each name is a brief personal biography, including medical school attended, degrees awarded, teaching positions, honors, and medical and scientific organizations of which the doctor is a member. Parents should be aware that listing in this directory is voluntary. The absence of a particular physician's name does not necessarily mean that he or she is not board-certified, or that a listed physician is superior to an unlisted one.

SPECIALISTS A CHILD MAY NEED

Allergist: A specialist in exaggerated reactions to everyday substances (reactions include sneezing, itching, skin rashes, or asthma).

Cardiologist: A physician with special knowledge of the heart and circulatory system who deals with such problems as congenital and acquired heart disease.

Dermatologist: A skin specialist.

Endocrinologist: A specialist in the working of the endocrine glands (hormone-secreting glands such as the pituitary, thyroid, and adrenal) who can deal with such problems as abnormally short stature or delayed sexual development.

Gastroenterologist: A physician who deals with diseases of the stomach and intestines.

Hematologist: A specialist of diseases of the blood-forming organs and of the blood, including the leukemias.

Neonatologist: A pediatrician who specializes in problems of the newborn encountered in the first months of life, including prematurity and congenital defects.

Neurologist: A physician trained in the treatment of nervous-system diseases and disorders.

Nephrologist: A specialist in diseases and problems of the kidney.

Ophthalmologist: A specialist in the anatomy, diseases, and problems of the eye, who can also perform surgery.

Orthopedist: A specialist in bones, joints, and the skeletal system.

Otolaryngologist: A specialist in diseases of the ear, nose, and throat, more commonly known as an ENT. These doctors also perform surgery.

Psychiatrist: A physician trained in the diagnosis and treatment of mental disorders. (Other mental-health professionals are discussed in chapter 29, Psychiatric Disorders.)

Pediatric Surgeon: A surgeon who limits his or her practice to children and performs such procedures as hernia repair and appendectomies.

Plastic Surgeon: A physician who specializes in cosmetic and reconstructive surgery.

Rheumatologist: A specialist in joint structure problems, such as arthritis, or in a connective tissue/autoimmune disease, such as lupus.

Urologist: A surgeon who specializes in the diagnosis and treatment of problems of the genitals and urinary tract.

Pediatric subspecialists are physicians who limit their practice to specific health problems of children. Generally they have received certification in general pediatrics from the American Board of Pediatrics as well as from one of its subspecialty boards. Currently, subspecialty certification is available in allergy-immunology, cardiology, endocrinology, gastroenterology, hematology-oncology, neonatal-perinatal medicine, nephrology, neurology, psychiatry, rheumatology, and surgery.

Parents may take their child to a pediatric specialist or to a specialist who usually treats adults. The accompanying box lists some of the specialists a child may come to need. Appendix B at the end of this book lists useful organizations and agencies.

20 Infectious Diseases

Anne A. Gershon, M.D.

INTRODUCTION

YEARS AGO, infection was a major cause of death in children in the United States, but fortunately this is no longer true. Many illnesses such as measles, mumps, rubella, polio, whooping cough, tetanus, and diptheria can now be prevented by immunization. Smallpox, which is caused by the variola virus, has been virtually eradicated worldwide as a result of immunization and quarantine measures. When a vaccine is not available to prevent disease, there is usually an antibiotic that will help cure the illness. Many viral diseases that once were considered untreatable now can be diagnosed rapidly and accurately, and treated successfully.

The effects of infection vary with the site, the type of organism, and the age and immune status of the child. The following is a guide to the most common infectious diseases that affect children. It is arranged in alphabetical order by organ systems.

BONE AND JOINT INFECTIONS

PUNCTURE WOUNDS and skin infections that allow bacteria to enter the bloodstream can cause osteomyelitis, an infection of the bone, and bacterial arthritis, which inflames the joints.

Osteomyelitis

Staphylococcus bacteria are the main cause of osteomyelitis, although streptococcus and other bacteria also can cause this disease. The infection begins when bacteria enter an open sore on the skin, or it can follow trauma. Osteomyelitis (which is not contagious) tends to occur in children, primarily boys. The inflammation usually is secondary to an infection that is present in another part of the body. Fever, swelling, severe tenderness, and pain in the bone are among the symptoms. This blood-borne infection spreads rapidly and can damage the bone if left untreated.

Diagnosis of osteomyelitis usually consists of a blood test and an X ray of the infected bone, and may include surgical biopsy of the bone as well. Antibiotics are administered for four to six weeks, often intravenously for the first two to three weeks, and then orally, as the symptoms begin to subside. If the child does not respond to treatment initially, surgical drainage of any pus may be necessary.

Children with sickle-cell anemia are at risk of developing osteomyelitis from salmonella bacteria. A diagnostic drainage procedure is extremely important for such patients to make certain that the correct antibiotic is given. Drainage may also be part of the treatment.

Bacterial Arthritis

Various bacteria can cause bacterial arthritis, although staphylococcus and streptococcus are mainly responsible for this inflammation of a joint. The hip, knee, elbow, and shoulder are the most common sites of infection.

The organisms invade the joints after gaining entry into the blood through a skin infection or by a penetrating wound. Acute joint pain and swelling occur, often accompanied by fever and malaise; range of motion is severely limited.

Early diagnosis and treatment are essential to prevent permanent damage to the cartilage. A small amount of the synovial fluid that surrounds the joint is removed and cultured to determine which organism is causing the infection, so that the proper antibiotic can be prescribed. Drainage of the affected joint also may be necessary.

If antibiotic therapy to halt the infection is delayed, there is a greater risk of joint damage. This can result in a secondary condition that can cause the joint to degenerate.

Lyme Disease

A relatively newly described cause of joint swelling in children is Lyme disease. This form of arthritis is spread by tiny ticks that live on dogs and cats and in the wild on white-tailed deer and white-footed field mice. It is seen primarily in the Northeast, Midwest, and Far West, particularly during the warmer months. The disease is associated with a rash, usually in the form of a striking red blotch or circle. The joint swelling (especially in the knees) may occur weeks or years after the rash. A variety of other symptoms such as headache, malaise, and fever may accompany the disease, which is usually successfully treated with penicillin or erythromycin. The earlier the antibiotics are given, the more effective they are.

CARDIOVASCULAR INFECTIONS*

Endocarditis

When bacteria enter the bloodstream, they can latch onto the endocardium, a thin, smooth membrane

---

* See also chapter 21, Childhood Cardiovascular Disease.

that lines the inner surfaces of the heart. There they can grow and produce an inflammation of the tissue, known as infectious endocarditis. If the infection is not controlled with antibiotics, it can lead to abscesses, heart failure, or death. Children most likely to develop infectious endocarditis are those with congenital heart disease, although this infection also can occur, albeit rarely, in a child without a heart defect. Some children develop endocarditis several years after undergoing heart valve repair or after suffering rheumatic fever. Staphylococcus and streptococcus bacteria are the most common causes of infectious endocarditis.

Endocarditis can have an insidious course. Weeks of fever, malaise, night sweats, and loss of appetite and weight may pass before a diagnosis is made. A blood culture is needed to determine the cause of the infection. Treatment involves the administration of antibiotics for four to six weeks while the patient is hospitalized.

Children who are at high risk of developing infectious endocarditis—those who have had rheumatic fever or heart surgery and who are about to have dental care or minor surgery—should be given antibiotics as a preventive measure before they undergo any procedures that could allow bacteria to enter the bloodstream.

Myocarditis

The myocardium, or muscle wall of the heart, can become infected by such agents as the Coxsackie B and ECHO viruses, which are prevalent in warm weather. Such infections, known as myocarditis, are rare, but severe cases can result in permanent damage to the heart muscle.

The symptoms accompanying myocarditis are fever, shortness of breath, weakness, and abnormal heart sounds. Diagnosis is made by an electrocardiogram, chest X ray, and throat culture to check for the virus. Treatment consists of bed rest under a doctor's supervision.

EAR INFECTIONS

EAR INFECTIONS are common in children, particularly otitis media, an infection of the middle ear, and otitis externa, which affects the outer ear canal.

Otitis Media

Children under age six often develop this acute childhood disorder. Many have recurrent attacks. Those who develop it initially during their first year are more prone to recurrent episodes throughout early childhood. Otitis media occurs year-round, but is most prevalent during the winter. It is usually caused by bacteria such as pneumococci or hemophilus. Allergies and congenital abnormalities also can play a role in causing this disorder.

Infection results when the eustachian tube is blocked and secretions cannot drain from the middle ear into the nose and throat. As fluid accumulates, the area becomes inflamed. Left untreated, the infection can cause permanent hearing loss. Irritability, ear pain, and fever are the main symptoms of otitis media. On examination by a physician, the eardrum may appear red and swollen, and show decreased mobility with pressure change. Infants and small children may tug on their ears when such an infection is present.

Antibiotics are routinely prescribed to relieve the pain and inflammation. If the child does not recover after a 10-day course of antibiotic treatment, he or she may require an additional course of treatment. A sample of the fluid in the middle ear may be cultured to identify the exact organism that is causing the infection. Fluid in the middle ear may persist once the infection is cleared. (See chapter 8, The First Year.)

A follow-up examination should take place after an otitis media infection. Children who suffer up to six ear infections a year may receive preventive antibiotic therapy. It is also recommended that they undergo hearing tests.

While not all middle ear disease is infectious, infections require treatment. If the symptoms do not improve within two days after therapy is begun, the practitioner will want to check for complications such as pneumonia or meningitis. (For more information, see chapter 26, Eyes, Ears, Nose, and Throat.)

Otitis Externa

This bacterial infection of the outer ear canal often is associated with swimming, hence its name "swimmer's ear." Repeated wetting of the skin from bathing and trauma of the ear canal from a cotton-tipped swab or other foreign body are the common causes of infection. The pain and discharge that accompany the infection can be relieved by treatment with topical antibiotics.

Malignant external otitis, also a bacterial infection of the external canal, is characterized by severe pain and tenderness. This rather unusual infection spreads into tissue surrounding the ear and can damage the facial nerve alongside the affected ear if left unattended. In rare cases it can cause brain abscesses and lead to death. Systemic as well as topical antibiotics are used to treat this infection; surgical drainage of the area also may be necessary. (For more information, see chapter 26, Eyes, Ears, Nose, and Throat.)

EYE INFECTIONS

WHEN BACTERIA enter the eye or the area around it, they may cause such infections as conjunctivitis, sties, and orbital cellulitis.

Conjunctivitis

Also called pink eye, conjunctivitis is an inflammation of the outer covering of the eye. The part that normally is white becomes red or pink and the eye may discharge pus. Pink eye is contagious and easily spreads from one child to another at home and at school. Pink eye may be caused by bacteria and some viruses. If it lasts more than several days, is extremely painful, or is accompanied by pus drainage from the eye, a doctor should be consulted.

Sty

A sty is a painful swelling of the skin around the edge of the eye, usually due to an infection in a hair follicle at the base of an eyelash. Sties are caused by bacteria, especially staphylococcus. Placing a warm compress against the eye for 20 minutes, four times a day, will hasten drainage of the sty. The physician may also prescribe an antibiotic ointment.

Orbital Cellulitis

Orbital cellulitis is a severe eye and skin infection caused by *staphylococci, streptococci,* or *Hemophilus influenzae* bacteria. It produces redness, pain, and swelling around the entire eye. Sometimes the eye may protrude and may be difficult to open. A physician should always be consulted for treatment, which consists of antibiotics (given by injection) to prevent complications.

Some eye infections are caused by viruses, particularly the herpes simplex virus. When the eye is infected with herpes, the virus can produce conjunctivitis that does not respond to antibiotics. An eye doctor (ophthalmologist) should be consulted promptly, since antiviral medication is crucial in order to preserve good vision. Herpes eye infections are a leading cause of blindness in the United States. (For more information, see chapter 26, Eyes, Ears, Nose, and Throat.)

FUNGAL INFECTIONS

FUNGAL INFECTIONS occasionally occur in healthy children and cause a wide variety of infections of the skin, mouth, nails, lungs, and other organs. Infants and children with an underlying immune deficiency may suffer from severe fungal infections.

The fungi that cause infection are microorganisms that are larger than bacteria. Infection can occur at any age or any season of the year. Some fungal infections are more common in certain geographic areas. For instance, *histoplasmosis*—a flu-like illness primarily affecting the lungs that is acquired by inhaling airborne spores of contaminated droppings from chickens, birds, bats, or other animals—is common in Tennessee, Kentucky, and some midwestern states. *Coccidioidomycosis,* which resembles influenza and also affects the lungs with cough, fever, and chest pain, is contracted by breathing in dustborne spores or by contact with infected soil in the Southwest. It is also called desert fever, San Joaquin Valley fever, or simply valley fever.

Ringworm, with its ringlike shape, is a common and highly contagious fungal infection that children often catch from one another by common use of towels or combs. (See chapter 32, Childhood Skin Disorders.) *Candida,* a yeastlike fungus that commonly causes thrush, is often acquired by infants as they pass through the vaginal canal at birth. When thrush is present, the tongue is coated with a white discharge and the infant usually has a diaper rash, also caused by candida. Pediatricians treat candida with Mycostatin, an oral antifungal that can also be applied topically to the diaper rash. Candida is commonly seen in babies under three months old. Older infants and children with severe, persistent oral thrush should be evaluated by a physician for a possible immune system deficiency.

A child with a fungal infection who has an underlying disease, such as cancer, may need treatment with amphotericin B, a potent antifungal drug that must be administered in the hospital under a physician's supervision.

GASTROINTESTINAL INFECTIONS

INFECTIONS OF THE intestinal tract, which affect infants and children as well as adults, are caused by a wide variety of microbes—primarily bacteria and viruses, although fungi and parasites also are responsible for some. Whatever the cause, the main symptoms are diarrhea and vomiting. Worldwide, diarrheal disease is responsible for the deaths of about five million children a year. Diarrhea is rarely fatal in developed countries such as the United States, where good treatment is readily available. Babies in the developing countries are at greatest risk.

Bacteria—including *salmonella*, *shigella*, and *Escherichia coli*—and viruses, especially rotavirus, are responsible for most gastrointestinal infections. Poor hygiene and improper handling of food and water cause some, but not all, gastrointestinal illness.

The doctor should be consulted for infants under one year of age if there are more than eight stools in 24 hours, especially if the child also has been vomiting.

Rotavirus

Human rotavirus, which takes its name from its wheel-like appearance, is the most common cause of diarrhea in infants and children, especially those under five. Rotavirus infection can occur year-round, although more outbreaks have been reported during the winter than in other seasons.

Symptoms appear 24 to 72 hours after infection, with diarrhea often accompanied by vomiting. The virus injures the villi, the tiny, hairlike structures in the intestine's mucous membrane that help absorb nutrients. Treatment consists of giving fluids to restore those lost and to prevent dehydration and electrolyte imbalance. Oral rehydration solutions (O.R.S.) provide the proper amount of electrolytes. The infection can be severe in some infants, requiring hospitalization and intravenous administration of fluids.

Salmonella

When salmonella bacteria enter the body, they can produce a number of infections. The most common is gastroenteritis, also known as food poisoning or stomach flu.

The bacteria may be present in water or in food that has been contaminated by an infected food handler. The microorganism also may be transmitted through the meat and eggs of infected fowl. Family members who have direct contact with the contaminated hands or clothing of an infected child may spread the infection. Careful hand washing after using the bathroom can help prevent the spread of gastroenteritis.

Symptoms may develop within a few hours or a few days after ingesting the salmonella bacteria. Nausea, vomiting, abdominal pain, and, in some cases, fever, occur and spontaneously disappear within one or two days. Premature infants and children under one year may become seriously dehydrated and require hospitalization for the replacement of fluids. In young babies, the bacterial infection may spread to the bloodstream, for which antibiotics need to be given.

Salmonella infections can be prevented by ensuring good water sanitation and food hygiene, proper handling and cooking of potentially contaminated foods, and strict handwashing practices to limit the fecal-oral spread of the infection.

Typhoid Fever

When water or food is contaminated with *Salmonella typhi*, it can result in typhoid fever in those who ingest these contaminated materials. Epidemics from this microorganism tend to occur in developing countries, although rare, small-scale outbreaks have been reported in this country. The organism is sometimes spread by someone who has recently traveled to a developing country.

Headache, lethargy, loss of appetite, a slowly increasing fever, abdominal pain, and malaise are the first signals. Diarrhea is unusual, although this can be caused by other types of salmonella. In some children, small rose-colored spots are present on the skin of the abdominal area.

To diagnose the disease, cultures of the stool and blood are taken. Treatment with antibiotics is effective against typhoid fever but hospitalization is required since this is potentially a very serious illness. Stool cultures are taken for three to six months after the illness has disappeared to determine if the microbe remains in the intestinal tract. If the bacterium continues to show up, the patient may be a carrier of the disease. There is no risk that the carrier will develop typhoid fever again, but for public health reasons it is important to know whether this problem has developed. Antibiotic therapy will not usually eliminate the carrier state.

Shigellosis

Dysentery, an infectious disease that affects the colon, is transmitted by the *shigella bacterium*. The infection, also known as shigellosis, is spread via contaminated hands, foods, and excrement. House flies also have been linked with the disease.

Shigellosis can strike any age group, but more than half of all cases occur in children ages one to nine. Most cases are reported during the summer months, although the disease can occur any time of the year.

The incubation period is usually three days, but may be as long as seven. Fevers are common, often before the onset of the diarrhea. During this time, the mucosal lining of the intestine becomes inflamed and swollen, there is increased mucus secretion, and diarrhea develops.

Mild cases may resemble a simple case of diarrhea in that the child hardly seems to be ill. If the diarrhea is more persistent, the stool may contain mucus and streaks of blood. In such cases there is danger of dehydration from the loss of fluid and electrolytes. Severe dehydration is characterized by sunken eyes, dryness of the mucous membranes, little urination, and failure to produce tears when crying. Such a condition requires immediate hospitalization.

Treatment includes the restoration of lost fluids, and antibiotics may be prescribed. Patients should get sufficient rest and nourishment while they regain their weight and strength. Drugs such as Kaolin-Pectate to stop the diarrhea are *not* recommended because they actually may prolong excretion of the organism.

E. Coli Infections

The *Escherichia coli* bacterium, which occurs in a variety of forms, normally inhabits the human intestinal tract without incident. It is only when a child comes into contact with a foreign strain of E. coli that infection resulting in diarrhea can occur. E. coli is the main cause of so-called traveler's diarrhea, or tourista. When the bacterium enters the gastrointestinal tract, it causes the intestinal cells to slow down digestion and to secrete an increased amount of fluid and electrolytes, resulting in diarrhea. E. coli infections may also develop in hospitalized babies.

Symptoms are apparent within a few days after exposure to E. coli. Diarrhea appears first, sometimes accompanied by abdominal cramps, fever, and vomiting. The stools are watery, without any sign of blood or mucus. Severe dehydration and accompanying weight loss can result.

Treatment consists of fluid replacement to prevent dehydration. A bismuth preparation (such as Pepto Bismol) may be helpful but should be avoided in young children. Antibiotic therapy usually is not necessary, but may be prescribed for severe cases.

E. coli infections can be spread by contact with contaminated hands or clothing in a nursery. Attention to hygiene can help prevent spread of E. coli bacteria.

HEPATITIS

SOME VIRUSES primarily infect the liver and may cause hepatitis, a liver infection with jaundice. These viruses include hepatitis A, hepatitis B, and a group of agents called non-A, non-B hepatitis.

Hepatitis A

Formerly known as infectious hepatitis, hepatitis A occurs most often among children and adolescents. It is transmitted through saliva or stool (a method known as fecal-oral spread).

Children in daycare centers and those who live in institutions are at the highest risk for acquiring this form of hepatitis. In daycare centers, children often crowd together and share playthings. Young ones may not be able to carry out good hygienic habits.

Children with hepatitis may not show jaundice or other symptoms, often transmitting the disease to unsuspecting family members. The illness in an adult, in contrast, is accompanied by fever and jaundice. In rare cases it may be fatal.

Hepatitis A can occur at any time of the year. When symptoms appear, they first resemble those of the flu: weakness, muscle aches, fever, headache, and severe appetite loss. After about a week, diarrhea, itchy skin, nausea, vomiting, and jaundice appear. Full recovery usually takes up to six weeks. There is no specific treatment for hepatitis A other than bed rest and a nutritious diet high in carbohydrates. When hepatitis A exposure is recognized, e.g., in a daycare center, a gamma globulin injection can prevent the illness. For this and other reasons a physician should always be consulted when jaundice develops in anyone.

Hepatitis B

Hepatitis B, formerly called serum hepatitis, affects adults more than children. This disease is transmitted through direct contact with infected blood. In general the disease poses a risk to health care workers, drug addicts, the newborn children of infected women (including hepatitis carriers), and anyone who has close personal contact with someone who is infected with or a carrier of hepatitis B. It can be sexually transmitted.

Unlike hepatitis A, hepatitis B can reside in a carrier state in people who are otherwise healthy, but who are capable of transmitting the disease to others. Only a blood test can determine whether a person is a hepatitis B carrier. It is unusual for people in this country to be carriers. In the Far East and in some African countries, however, as many as 20 percent of the population may be carriers of the virus.

The infant of a pregnant woman who is a hepatitis B virus carrier should be given hyperimmune gamma globulin and hepatitis B vaccine immediately after birth to prevent the baby from becoming a carrier or developing hepatitis. The hepatitis B vaccine also is used to protect other infants and children at high risk of exposure to hepatitis B.

Treatment is similar to that prescribed for infectious hepatitis—bed rest, a high-protein, high-carbohydrate diet, and regular evaluation of liver function tests.

Non-A, Non-B Hepatitis (Hepatitis C)

The third type of hepatitis, non-A, non-B, which recently has been referred to as hepatitis C, presents symptoms similar to the other forms. Injections with gamma globulin may be used to protect those who are exposed to the virus. However, no screening test is available for persons who might be infected with non-A, non-B hepatitis, nor has a vaccine been developed.

HERPES INFECTIONS

A NUMBER OF CLOSELY related viruses, all belonging to the herpes family, are responsible for a wide range of infections—from chicken pox to shingles, cytomegalovirus, cold sores, and genital herpes. Infections caused by the herpes simplex virus are often referred to as herpes infections. There are two types of herpes simplex viruses: type 1 and type 2. A large number of people with *herpes simplex virus Type 1 (HSV-1)* acquire the infection during infancy and early childhood. HSV-1 commonly infects the upper body, primarily the mouth, lips, and face, although the infection can occur on any part of the body. The virus produces blisters or ulcers, or both, of the skin and mucous membranes.

Genital Herpes

Usually called *herpes simplex Type 2 (HSV-2)*, genital herpes often affects the genital and anal area, where it can cause clusters of blisters. There are no strict anatomical barriers however; herpes simplex 1 and 2 both can infect the oral and the genital region. Most herpes simplex infections are self-limiting and, although they are annoying until they run their course, they are not life-threatening. There are two exceptions: herpes of the newborn infant and herpes encephalitis.

Neonatal herpes can occur in newborns who acquire the disease as they pass through the birth canal if the mother has genital herpes. Infection at birth can cause skin blisters, brain damage, mental retardation, blindness, and death. When a woman near term to deliver a baby develops an active HSV-2 infection, obstetricians prefer to perform a cesarean section. This will reduce the risk of the mother transmitting the virus to the infant.

Herpes encephalitis is the most common form of nonepidemic encephalitis in the United States. Children and adults can acquire this form of the infection, although it is not understood why some people develop herpes encephalitis and others do not. Among its symptoms are fever, headache, change in personality, and seizures. If left untreated, this disease has a very poor prognosis—it claims the lives of 80 percent of those it afflicts and leaves its survivors with severe brain damage. Treatment with the drug acyclovir, if given early in the illness, is effective in curing this disease.

Both oral and genital herpes can be spread by direct personal contact with an infected area of another person or from one area of the body to another by self-contact. The mucous membranes of the mouth and genitals or a cut on the skin are particularly vulnerable areas. Children with oral herpes can give themselves a genital infection by touching a cold sore on the mouth and then touching their genitals. The eyes also can become infected if they are touched or rubbed after an open lesion has been touched.

Herpes acquired after the newborn period is characterized by clusters of blisters, which may be painful. The skin turns red, swells, and develops fluid-filled blisters that eventually pop open. Scabs form over the area and healing takes place within five days to two weeks. Children may also develop dramatic mouth sores, swollen and bleeding gums, and tonsillitis.

Once the area heals, the skin returns to normal. The virus, however, remains in the body in a dormant state in the nervous system. From the original skin lesion the virus travels along the course of a nerve to deep nerve centers, or ganglia. Oral herpes infections reside in the ganglia in the neck, while genital herpes lies dormant in nerves at the base of the spine.

When an infection first occurs, there may be flu-like symptoms, including low-grade fever, aching muscles, headache, and tender, swollen lymph nodes, in addition to the skin or mucous membrane blisters.

In some people, the virus is quiescent—never to become active again; others are more prone to suffer recurrences or reactivation of infections. These flare-ups or reactivations of the latent virus are due to such diverse factors as sunlight, stress, menstruation, pregnancy, or trauma. In reactivation infections, a tingling and burning sensation may be noticed in the area before any sores appear. Commonly, reactivation of Type 1 herpes causes fever sores at the corners of the mouth. Primary or first-time infections in infants can affect the gums and mucous membranes of the mouth and throat, a condition known as gingivostomatitis. These infants have fever and difficulty in eating and drinking because of their mouth pain. Hospitalization may be necessary for intravenous feedings until the infection clears up.

Diagnosis of herpes is made by swabbing a section of the sore with a cotton-tipped swab and culturing this specimen. When a herpes infection of the brain is suspected, a CT scan may be used to make a diagnosis. A surgical biopsy of the brain may also be required if the situation appears life-threatening.

While there is no cure for herpes, the antiviral drug acyclovir is helpful in treating herpes infections. It is usually given orally and it can relieve the pain, reduce the severity of blisters, and help them to heal. Sometimes when the acyclovir is stopped, the virus flares up a bit again. Acyclovir given by intravenous injection has also been helpful when used against such serious herpes infections as herpes encephalitis and neonatal herpes.

Herpes can be prevented by avoiding contact with active sores. Infants under one month of age should not receive care from anyone with an obvious herpes lesion: their immature immune systems are not well enough equipped to cope with the infection. Men with active herpetic sores on the penis or testicles should avoid sexual intercourse with women, especially those who are pregnant. While use of a condom may prevent spread of the infection, it is not 100 percent effective.

While it is an unusual means for transmission of the infection, child abuse should be suspected in young children who develop genital herpes.

Chicken Pox (Varicella)

Children between ages one and ten are very susceptible to chicken pox, a highly contagious disease caused by the varicella-zoster virus. Virtually all children get chicken pox. If a child is exposed to varicella, he most likely will infect others in the family or classroom who are also susceptible.

Most cases occur in the late winter to early spring. A low-grade fever, malaise, and headache often precede the visible symptom of chicken pox— a rash that begins as red bumps that develop into blisters slightly larger than the head of a pin. The rash occurs mainly on the face, scalp, back, chest, and abdomen. The legs and arms usually are not affected as much. Chicken pox is contagious from one to two days before the rash appears until all of the red bumps turn into blisters, break open, and form scabs.

The normal course of chicken pox runs five to seven days. By the end of the first week, and in some children, by the end of the second week, the encrusted scabs will fall away. A child with chicken pox should be isolated from friends who are susceptible to the infection until scabs form over all of the lesions.

As a rule, chicken pox requires no special treatment. The child's nails should be trimmed to prevent the spread of infection if the pox are scratched. Daily baths and change of clothes are also important for comfort and to prevent a bacterial infection. Calamine lotion can be used to soothe any itching, but creams containing hydrocortisone should be avoided.

Severe cases should be seen by a doctor: if there is a cough or chest pain, pneumonia may be present. If the skin becomes superinfected with bacteria, there may be large painful bumps. In rare cases, the central nervous system is affected. Although it is more likely in teenagers and adults, encephalitis may occur and is characterized by disturbances in the child's gait and by abnormal behavior such as extreme sleepiness or seizures.

A child with chicken pox who develops a fever should *not* be given aspirin because of its association with Reye's syndrome. Acetaminophen (such as Tylenol or Datril) should be used instead.

In children who have various forms of cancer, or who are receiving steroid hormone therapy, chicken pox can be very severe or even fatal. They should be treated with varicella-zoster immune globulin (VZIG) as soon as possible after the exposure, *before* they develop chicken pox.

Women who have never had chicken pox should be tested for antibodies to varicella-zoster before they become pregnant. Most women who believe they are susceptible to varicella actually may be immune and their blood will show a positive reaction when tested.

Pregnant women who contract varicella should consult their physician. Babies born to women with active chicken pox at the time of delivery should receive VZIG as soon as possible after birth. Such a baby is at risk to develop severe or fatal varicella.

At this writing, a vaccine against chicken pox is awaiting approval and should be available within one or two years. This vaccine is known to be safe and effective in high-risk children with leukemia and ultimately may be licensed for routine use in healthy children.

Herpes Zoster

Like varicella, herpes zoster (commonly called shingles) belongs to the family of herpes viruses. Unlike varicella, herpes zoster can develop at any time of the year and is characterized by an eruption in a single area of the skin, usually along the course of one or two sensory nerves.

Although shingles is painful in adults, in children it is a much milder illness, lasting two weeks or less. Fever and listlessness usually occur at the beginning. Shingles is as contagious as chicken pox.

Cytomegalovirus

Cytomegalovirus (CMV) is among the family of herpes viruses. Like the other forms of herpes, CMV can remain latent in the body and reactivate later. The infection is common in young children, especially those who attend daycare centers. A healthy child who is infected with CMV rarely shows any symptoms, but may unknowingly transmit the virus to other family members. If the child's mother is pregnant and was never infected with CMV, she can become infected and, even without symptoms, she may transmit the virus to her fetus. A baby born to a mother who experiences a first-time CMV infection during pregnancy is at very high risk of suffering complications and brain damage before delivery. At birth, the infant may have a rash and an enlarged liver and spleen; later, mental retardation and deafness may develop.

On the other hand, a mother who has been previously infected with CMV will confer some immunity to CMV to her fetus. This child is unlikely to suffer any damage from the virus, even if the mother is once again exposed to the virus.

When CMV is acquired during infancy and childhood, it usually is benign and asymptomatic. It is diagnosed by taking a culture of the virus from urine and by testing for antibodies in the blood. Occasionally, CMV results in a febrile illness called CMV mononucleosis, which resembles classic infectious mononucleosis (caused by Epstein-Barr virus, another type of herpes virus). The child usually recovers from CMV mononucleosis without complications or treatment.

IMMUNODEFICIENCY DISEASES

Immunodeficiency diseases result when the immune system is virtually helpless against even the mildest infection. These diseases may be inherited; for example, agammaglobulinemia, in which the body is unable to make antibodies properly, yet still has some immunity because white blood cells are present. Children born with this disorder have an increased likelihood of developing recurring infections, such as pneumonia. Another inherited disease is severe combined immunodeficiency disease (SCID), an often fatal condition in which an infant

is without antibodies, or without the ability to produce infection-fighting white blood cells. Such infants require a bone marrow transplant in order to survive.

A child born to a mother who is infected with the virus that causes AIDS (acquired immune deficiency syndrome) may contract the disease at some point before or during birth. (See section on AIDS below.)

Parents often become alarmed when their child seems to develop frequent infections, and they may wonder whether there is an immune deficiency. Yet immunodeficiency is rare in our population. It is important to remember that the average child will get six upper respiratory infections (colds) a year. Determining whether a child truly has an immune deficiency requires a detailed medical history and physical examination in addition to laboratory testing. Symptoms of an immune deficiency usually include frequent and severe infections. For instance, a child might have more than two episodes of pneumonia that require hospitalization over a one-year period, or a persistent, severe case of mouth and esophageal thrush (candida); frequent viral infections, such as herpes, CMV, infectious mononucleosis, or severe chicken pox; or protozoan infections, such as toxoplasmosis and pneumocystis carinii pneumonia (PCP). (PCP is an exceedingly rare lung infection in the normal population.)

AIDS

AIDS, a fatal disease that cripples the body's defenses against infection, is commanding wide attention from the scientific community as doctors search for a treatment and a vaccine.

AIDS can develop in children whose mothers either have AIDS or who are infected with the human immunodeficiency virus (HIV) that causes the disease, but have not yet become ill themselves. The AIDS virus can be transmitted from a pregnant woman to her fetus either before or during birth. It should be stressed that the virus is not spread by day-to-day contact, such as in schools or daycare centers.

If AIDS is suspected, the blood can be tested for the presence of antibodies to the AIDS virus and even for the virus itself. If HIV antibodies are present, it indicates only that the person has been infected with the virus—it does not necessarily mean that the person has AIDS. It is currently believed, however, that most, but not all HIV-infected persons will develop AIDS.

The Centers for Disease Control suggests that women may want to consider testing for AIDS infection if they are considering pregnancy and:

- Have any symptoms of HIV infection, such as swollen lymph glands, weight loss, or frequent infections.

- Have used intravenous drugs for nonmedical reasons.

- Are or have been sexual partners of IV drug users, bisexual men, men with hemophilia, or men who show any evidence of HIV infection.

- Received a blood transfusion between 1977 and 1985.

- Have been rejected as a blood donor because of a positive HIV screening test.

The symptoms of AIDS vary, but usually the disease begins with frequent fevers; a heavy, dry cough; swollen lymph nodes; fatigue; weight loss; and chronic diarrhea. Neurological symptoms also occur, including loss of memory, sudden mood changes, blurred vision, and difficulty in maintaining balance. Babies may lose their ability to walk and talk.

AIDS is caused by a retrovirus that contains an enzyme called reverse transcriptase, which reverses the normal flow of genetic information during its replication. Once the virus invades the body, it infects certain white blood cells and kills them. This weakens the immune system so extensively that it can no longer normally resist viruses, parasites, fungi, protozoa, and some forms of cancer. Thus these infections and cancer move in and slowly debilitate the AIDS victim. Among these are *Kaposi's sarcoma*, a form of skin cancer, and Pneumocystis carinii, a protozoan that causes a persistent, severe form of pneumonia. Other infections may be present, such as those caused by the herpes viruses, or by fungi, such as the yeast infection candida. Various forms of tuberculosis are common as well. A parasite called cryptosporidium can also enter the body and infect the intestines, causing the chronic diarrhea that accompanies AIDS.

While treatment is available for many of the infections that affect AIDS patients, some infections are resistant to therapy, such as cryptosporidiosis. Once AIDS has been diagnosed, the victim usually grows progressively weaker, suffers recurring infections, and dies within two years of the diagnosis.

An experimental drug called azidothymidine, or AZT, has been shown to be effective in some AIDS patients on a short-term basis. Other new drugs are also undergoing extensive testing for safety and effectiveness. AZT does not cure AIDS, but it does interfere with multiplication of the AIDS virus, and it is helpful to patients.

Kawasaki Disease

Kawasaki disease is an acute illness of the mucous membranes and lymph nodes that occurs in children under ten, primarily those under four. Although there have been outbreaks of Kawasaki disease, it is not known to be contagious. The exact cause is not yet known, but the incidence of the disease seems to be increasing. Children of Japanese origin seem to be the most susceptible, followed by those of black, Hispanic, mixed racial, Chinese, and Korean origin. Caucasian children are least susceptible.

The first sign is a fever that develops suddenly, is typically high, and lasts more than five days and as long as several weeks. Children with Kawasaki disease are usually extremely irritable and may have wide mood swings. In three to five days after the fever starts, other symptoms appear: cracked, red lips; strawberry tongue; and, in 50 percent of cases, swelling of the lymph glands on one side of the neck. A deep red rash may be present and the skin may peel off in scales, especially around the fingernails and toes and, ultimately, the palms and soles. The joints and such organs as the liver, kidneys, heart, or brain may be involved. There is also internal damage to the blood vessel walls in some children with Kawasaki disease.

Because doctors do not know what causes the disease, there are no specific tests to make a diagnosis. The child's symptoms are treated and, usually, aspirin is prescribed to help prevent damage to the blood vessel walls. About 20 percent of patients develop aneurysms, or abnormal outpouchings of the coronary arteries, which supply blood to the heart, a very serious complication. Fortunately most of them recover or become asymptomatic. A small number of cases (0.2 percent) develop fatal cardiac complications. (See chapter 21, Childhood Cardiovascular Disease, for more information.)

MEASLES

MEASLES, once one of the most common communicable diseases of childhood, is now unusual because of the widespread use of measles vaccine, which was licensed for general use in 1963. Recently when outbreaks occur, they usually take place in the late winter and early spring, affecting children who have not yet been vaccinated (younger than 15 months) and college students who may have missed being vaccinated as children.

Measles, or rubeola, often is confused with rubella (also called German measles). They are different diseases, and it is important that children receive vaccination against each. (See section on Rubella below.)

The rubeola virus, an RNA (ribonucleic acid)

virus of the paramyxovirus group, causes measles. The disease is highly contagious, especially during the first few days of the illness before the characteristic rash develops. A low-grade fever, cough, and watery eyes and nose are the first symptoms to appear. White spots (known as *Koplik spots*) on the inside of the mouth may appear next, followed by a rash that begins on the face and moves down the entire body. After the rash begins, the temperature rises sharply over the next few days. The child is usually sick for a total of 10 to 14 days.

Complications may occur during the acute stage of measles. In some cases, bacteria may invade the respiratory tract, causing pneumonia and otitis media. Encephalitis (inflammation of the brain) is fortunately rare, but if it occurs, the disease may result in brain damage or be fatal.

Diagnosis is based on the early symptoms, the observation of Koplik spots, and the development of fever and rash. A blood test is usually performed as well, to check for development of measles antibodies. There is no specific treatment for measles other than bed rest, plenty of fluids, avoidance of bright light if it is bothersome, and a cough suppressant if coughing is a problem.

Measles can be prevented by vaccination. All children should receive the vaccine at 12 to 15 months of age. A second dose of vaccine is now being recommended for older children. Young unimmunized infants who have been exposed to someone with measles can be protected if either gamma globulin or measles vaccine is administered soon after exposure. (The gamma globulin must be given within six days of exposure and the measles vaccine given within 72 hours.) The child then should still receive the MMR (measles-mumps-rubella) vaccine at 15 months. When a measles outbreak presents a possible risk to infants under six months old, gamma globulin may be given. Also, MMR may be given at 12 months instead of 15. Measles vaccine should not be given to children below six months of age.

MENINGITIS

MENINGITIS IS AN inflammation of the meninges, the membranes that cover the brain and spinal cord. The membranes can become infected when bacteria or viruses invade the bloodstream. Immediate diagnosis and treatment are necessary to prevent death or disability, especially from bacterial infection.

Bacterial meningitis tends to be much more serious than viral meningitis. The three main bacteria that produce the disease include: *Hemophilus influenzae*, type B; *Streptococcus pneumonie*, or pneumococcus, and *Neisseria meningiditis* (or meningococcus). Meningitis also can occur after a skull fracture, or following neurological surgery, especially in babies with hydrocephalus. In the latter case, the meningitis is usually caused by staphylococci. Newborns may develop meningitis from group B streptococcal infection.

The winter and spring months are the primary seasons for outbreaks of bacterial meningitis. Children under age five are at the greatest risk of contracting the disease. Those who attend daycare centers are at increased risk. (Children have a tendency to crowd together and it is easy for infection to spread from one toddler to another.) Pediatricians now recommend that at the age of 18 months children should be inoculated with the HiB (Hemophilus b polysaccharide) vaccine, which is effective in preventing many serious hemophilus infections.

The doctor should be consulted when a child under age four years has been in close contact with someone with meningitis or epiglottitis. In some cases, the antibiotic rifampin will be prescribed to prevent the disease from developing. This prophylactic medication also is given to exposed children who have been vaccinated, because they still may carry the bacterium and spread it to others.

Early recognition and treatment of meningitis is crucial. Older children commonly complain of headache and a painful sensitivity of their eyes to light. Fever, vomiting, a stiff neck, and irritability are among the other symptoms of meningitis. In young infants, signs of infection may not be apparent. Often the only indication of meningitis may be irritability and an anterior fontanel that bulges because of an increase in intracranial pressure.

A spinal tap for examination of cerebrospinal fluid is necessary to make a diagnosis of meningitis. After this fluid is removed, it is examined for typical signs of bacterial meningitis: the presence of abnormal white blood cells, low glucose levels, and a high concentration of protein.

Antibiotics and sometimes steroids are used to treat bacterial meningitis. Once it is determined which bacterium caused the disease, the appropriate antibiotic can be administered.

There is no specific therapy for viral meningitis, which may be caused by several different viruses that can enter the respiratory or digestive tract. Viral meningitis tends to occur in the warmer months and is contagious. Usually, it is a self-limiting disease, and the patient requires only supportive therapy such as proper nourishment and rest. Rarely, meningitis is caused by fungi.

IMMUNIZATIONS

Healthy infants born in the United States are routinely immunized against many serious infectious diseases.

Vaccines are made of inactivated viruses or bacteria (or their products) or from live viruses that are specially cultivated so that they will not cause disease. When a vaccine is given, it causes the immune system to react to the infectious organism and creates a long-term memory of this invader so that the body will be protected if it encounters that germ again. Immunization often confers lifetime protection against a disease.

When infants reach two months of age, pediatricians begin the first of a series of immunizations: DPT to protect against diptheria, pertussis (whooping cough), and tetanus (DPT); oral polio vaccine (OPV), to protect against polio; and MMR follows at 12 to 15 months, to protect against measles, mumps and rubella (German measles). (For more information, see chapter 8, The First Year.)

While no vaccine is either 100 percent safe or effective, the vast majority of children who are vaccinated show no adverse reaction. Vaccinated children are at far less risk than those who are not. Therefore it is now a federal law that all children be immunized. On rare occasions, children react adversely to vaccine. Children who develop convulsions or scream inconsolably for several hours after receiving the first DPT vaccine ordinarily should not receive this vaccine again. The pediatrician should be notified and will then usually administer a diptheria-tetanus (DT) inoculation in place of DPT when it is time for the second injection.

Vaccinations against measles, mumps, and rubella (MMR) are given to children at 12 to 15 months. Although serious reactions to MMR are rare, about 5 percent of children receiving the vaccine develop a mild fever following immunization.

The widespread use of MMR, which is required for entry into school, has resulted in a dramatic decrease in the annual incidence of measles by a factor of over 99 percent. Because there has been a recent upsurge in measles, however, a second dose of MMR is often administered. Congenital rubella, once the most common congenital viral infection, now is a rare disease as a result of required immunization. Rubella is not a serious disease if it develops after birth. Rubella vaccine primarily is given to children to ensure that they will not infect others, especially pregnant women, and that young women will be protected from the disease when they reach childbearing age.

The Centers for Disease Control and the American Academy of Pediatrics both recommend that children 18 months old receive one injection of a vaccine against Hemophilus influenza type B (HiB) disease. This disease is highly contagious and is a leading cause of bacterial meningitis. HiB infection also can result in septic arthritis, orbital cellulitis, pneumonia, and epiglottitis, a life-threatening infection of the throat.

A child suspected of having an immunodeficiency disease or in close contact (living in the same household) with a person with an immunological abnormality should not be given a vaccine containing a live virus, such as the live attenuated oral polio (Sabin) vaccine. Instead, the child should receive the inactivated polio (Salk) vaccine.

MONONUCLEOSIS

CHILDREN AND TEENAGERS often become infected with the Epstein-Barr virus, a member of the herpes virus family that causes mononucleosis. This disease is contagious, but usually requires close personal contact to spread, hence the lay description, "the kissing disease." Some infections are very mild or asymptomatic; therefore, some who have been exposed to mononucleosis never develop any symptoms, although they may have been infected.

Mononucleosis often begins with malaise, headache, nausea, and abdominal pain. Additional symptoms are fever, sore throat, and swollen lymph glands. Some patients develop a rash. In younger children, the disease may be a vague illness accompanied by fever.

Often the sore throat is mistaken for a strep throat, but the physician will rule this out when the soreness fails to respond to treatment with penicillin.

To make the diagnosis, the physician examines the white blood cells for the presence of antibodies to the EBV. The test most frequently used is called the "monospot" test, which yields an answer within a few minutes.

Mononucleosis is a self-limited illness and no specific treatment is necessary. Rest is recommended. Some patients may develop an enlarged spleen, which could rupture if they attempt too much activity, such as participation in sports. Jaundice may be present as a result of hepatitis. If so, rest is necessary until liver function returns to normal. Rare chronic forms of mononucleosis have been described in individuals with abnormal immunity. Usually, however, mononucleosis does not recur.

MUMPS

Now THAT children are routinely vaccinated against mumps at 15 months of age, this contagious disease has been very much on the decline. Mumps is often characterized by a swelling of the salivary glands in the neck. Direct contact and infection through the respiratory system are responsible for the spread of the disease. Although mumps can occur at any time of the year, winter and spring are the prime seasons for its spread.

Mumps may be a painful disease, especially if it is contracted as an adult. Young adult males who catch mumps may suffer swelling of the testicles, but despite popular beliefs, mumps rarely causes sterility.

The disease is characterized by fever, headache, malaise, and pain in the neck. The salivary, or parotid, glands in the front of and below the ear rapidly swell for one to three days and return to normal within a week to 10 days. Some patients with mumps may suffer a permanent loss of hearing.

NEONATAL INFECTIONS

NEWBORN INFANTS DO NOT HAVE fully developed immune systems and their infection-fighting white blood cells may not be able to destroy organisms that invade their tissues and bloodstream. Because of this, infection in the first two months of life may be extremely dangerous. Parents should be alert to this possibility and should not hesitate to call the pediatrician if the child suddenly seems fussy or cranky, stops feeding, or just does not look right. Early diagnosis, especially during these two months, is very important.

Some infants become infected congenitally—before birth. If the mother contracted cytomegalovirus, rubella, or toxoplasmosis during her pregnancy, she could transmit the infection to her child in this manner. Other infections, including those caused by hepatitis B and the herpes simplex viruses, may be transmitted to the infant during or shortly after birth.

Among the most serious neonatal infections is neonatal sepsis, an infection in the infant's bloodstream that develops as the result of bacteria present in the mother's intestinal and genital tracts, primarily the group B streptococcus bacterium. Pneumonia often accompanies the sepsis.

Infants with neonatal sepsis usually have a fever or an abnormally low body temperature. They also are irritable, lethargic, have difficulty feeding, and tend to vomit. When neonatal sepsis is suspected, blood cultures are taken to make a diagnosis. Antibiotics are administered, but they aren't always entirely effective. There is no certain way to prevent sepsis, although when it is known that a pregnant woman is heavily infected with the group B streptococcus bacterium, antibiotics may be administered to her intravenously during delivery.

Neonatal conjunctivitis, or an inflammation of the eyes with a watery discharge, usually is caused by the bacteria responsible for the sexually transmitted maternal infections chlamydia and gonorrhea. Infants are infected by their mothers during the delivery. Staphylococcus bacterium is another potential cause. Routine administration at birth of eye drops containing silver nitrate or antibiotics prevents neonatal conjunctivitis in most cases. Antibiotics usually cure neonatal conjunctivitis if it is not prevented. If conjunctivitis due to chlamydia goes untreated, it can lead to pneumonia.

RABIES

RABIES IS A DISEASE that must be avoided or prevented. If prevention fails and rabies goes untreated, it is usually fatal. This disease is transmitted via the bite of infected dogs, cats, bats, raccoons, and skunks. Fortunately, in the United States rabies in humans is exceedingly rare, although the disease does occur in animals.

Headaches, fever, extreme anxiety, and paralysis occur with rabies. The closer to the head that the bite is located, the more quickly rabies may follow, because the virus travels from the skin via the nerves to the brain. Rabies produces encephalitis, an inflammation of the brain that is usually fatal. In some cases the incubation period may be as long as a year. For this reason, it is important that a child who is bitten, whether by a pet, a stray, or a wild animal, be taken to a doctor immediately. The animal that bit the child should be captured if possible and taken to public health authorities. If it is found that the animal has rabies, then antirabies prophylaxis will be prescribed. Prophylaxis includes five rabies vaccine injections and one antiserum injection.

Children should be taught to beware strange animals; rabid wild animals often lose their natural fear of people before showing other signs of rabies. They sometimes act unafraid and may wander into playgrounds and campsites where children may try to pet them. Rabid dogs are unusual in the United States because most pet dogs are immunized against rabies.

RESPIRATORY INFECTIONS

RESPIRATORY SYSTEM INFECTIONS are the most common disorder affecting the pediatric age group. Most upper respiratory infections, such as colds, are self-limited illnesses. But these infections are not always benign; complications can arise and lead to more serious illnesses in the lower respiratory tract, such as pneumonia, bronchiolitis, and epiglottitis. Acute respiratory infections are one of the leading causes of death among infants and children worldwide.

Any part of the breathing apparatus can be involved in a respiratory infection—pharynx, larynx, trachea, and the sinuses (upper respiratory tract), as well as the bronchi and lungs (lower respiratory tract). Involvement of certain parts of the system can lead to serious problems that require immediate medical attention. When a viral infection spreads into the lungs, it causes pneumonia that may be severe. An inflammation of the small airways (bronchioles)—structures that transmit air into the tiny air sacs of the lungs—results in bronchiolitis, a condition with characteristics similar to a severe asthma attack. An infected larynx or epiglottis can produce croup, which leads to marked difficulty in breathing. In young infants, these infections are serious and usually require hospitalization.

All respiratory infections occur more frequently during the winter and early spring months. They are quite contagious and are spread by sneezing and coughing, as well as by rubbing the nose or eyes with fingers that have been contaminated with the virus. Infectious organisms can remain active on surfaces, including the skin and handkerchiefs, for many hours. It is difficult to prevent contact with respiratory viruses, but transmission can be minimized by washing hands frequently and avoiding hand contact with the face, especially the eyes and nose, as much as possible. Used tissues should be discarded promptly.

If an infection is caused by bacteria, it can be treated with antibiotics, whereas viral infections so far cannot. A child with a viral infection should not receive antibiotics—such misuse of medication is not only expensive but is potentially dangerous because it tends to encourage the growth of bacteria that are resistant to antibiotics.

Colds

The common cold, or upper respiratory infection, with its symptoms of nasal congestion, fever, headache, and runny nose, results from an invasion of viruses into the respiratory tract. A whole battery of viral agents are responsible for colds—rhinoviruses, respiratory syncytial virus (RSV), adenoviruses, and parainfluenzaviruses, among others.

A cold usually is self-limiting and lasts five to seven days. Treatment consists of rest and acetaminophen to relieve fever and headache. Decongestants can provide temporary relief from nasal congestion. If a cold persists for two or more weeks, it may involve a secondary infection with bacteria, and a physician should be consulted.

Influenza

Influenza, or the flu, also is an upper respiratory infection caused by a virus. The flu is more severe than a cold, causing high fever, muscle pain, sore throat, cough and, sometimes, nausea and vomiting. The infection lasts a week to 10 days and may leave its victim feeling tired for weeks after the other symptoms have disappeared.

New strains of influenza virus are constantly developing, making prevention difficult. A fairly effective flu vaccine is available, however. This vaccine should be administered every year to children considered to be at high risk for developing complications from an attack of influenza. It is not recommended for healthy children or for those who are allergic to eggs.

Antibiotics are of no use against the flu. Treatment consists of rest, acetaminophen to relieve muscle aches, and the consumption of fluids. Aspirin should not be given, as it may precipitate Reye's syndrome (see preceding section on chicken pox).

Pneumonia

Pneumonia is an infection of the lungs that may be caused by a virus, a bacterium, a fungus, or a parasite. Viruses and bacteria are the most common causes. The infectious microorganisms enter the tiny air sacs of the lungs (alveoli) and cause them to become inflamed and filled with fluid, making breathing difficult.

Symptoms of the disease vary, depending on the type of pneumonia. Those caused by viruses, such as bronchopneumonia, with its patchy inflammation in the lower part of the lungs, usually begin with a brief cold. A fever follows, then a dry cough, and rapid breathing. Bacterial pneumonia (lobar pneumonia) starts abruptly with chills and a quickly rising temperature. The child breathes rapidly and may cough up phlegm that contains streaks of blood.

If these symptoms occur, the physician should be called. In most cases, a child with pneumonia can be treated at home. If the infection is severe, or the child is under a year old, hospitalization may be necessary. Rest and consumption of fluids help relieve the symptoms. If a bacterium is suspected as the cause of the infection, antibiotics are prescribed. With proper treatment, a healthy child will recover from pneumonia in about one to two weeks.

Bronchiolitis

Bronchiolitis occurs most often in infants and young children during the winter and spring. The disease is usually caused by the respiratory syncytial virus (RSV), which infects the bronchioles, the small airways that lead into the lungs. The mucosal linings of the airways swell, thus partially blocking the passage of air. As the child breathes, he or she also wheezes, and may cough fitfully. Most children will recover at home without treatment, in three to five days.

In severe cases, as the child tries harder to draw in air to breathe, he or she may turn blue. A physician should be contacted immediately if this occurs. A child whose skin is blue (cyanotic) must be taken to a hospital and given immediate treatment with oxygen. Healthy children usually recover from bronchiolitis after a few days of treatment. A new medication called ribavirin can be administered in the hospital by an aerosol apparatus to babies with bronchiolitis. This therapy is well tolerated and speeds recovery.

Croup

The viral infection that causes inflammation and swelling of the larynx and windpipe (trachea) is known as croup. This disorder creates harsh, noisy breathing, or stridor, in the child. It is especially heard when the child inhales. Children between six months and three years of age are most commonly affected by croup.

The infection begins with a cold and spreads to the lower respiratory tract. The early symptoms may be mild, with the child hardly appearing ill. The course of the infection can change suddenly, however, and may require emergency treatment. The doctor should be consulted for any child with difficulty breathing.

Some croup attacks may occur at night, awakening the child and frightening him. This is called spasmodic croup and it is due to an allergy, not a viral infection. It is often a recurrent problem. Parents can help relieve the symptoms by exposing the child to steam, which can be created by running hot water in the shower in a closed bathroom. If the child continues to suffer impaired breathing and especially if the lips develop a bluish tinge, a physician should be contacted.

Sinusitis

Sinusitis, or infection of the sinus passages, is often caused by the pneumococci and *Hemophilus influenzae* bacteria. When bacteria enter mucous-lined sinus passages, the infection can obstruct the flow of air and mucus into the nose and create pus. Fever, nasal and postnasal discharge, headache, and tenderness over the sinus cavities are the symptoms of this infection.

Antibiotics are usually prescribed for sinusitis. In some cases, a nasal decongestant may be administered to help the passages drain. If the blockage is severe, the physician may want to bring about drainage by irrigating the area. This is done by puncturing the wall of the nose or the wall of the sinus near the upper lip, injecting fluid, and allowing it to drain through the nose.

When sinusitis is chronic, it usually is due to some cause other than bacterial infection. A child with a deviated nasal septum, nasal polyps, or an allergy is likely to suffer recurring infections of the nose and sinuses. Surgical correction may be necessary in some patients.

Epiglottitis

Inflammation of the larynx, with involvement and rapid swelling of the epiglottis, can obstruct the airway and cause a child to suffocate. The epiglottis is a rubbery structure that helps to close off the trachea (windpipe) during swallowing, thus preventing food and liquid from entering the lungs, directing them instead to the stomach. Epiglottitis, a life-threatening infection of the epiglottis, is usually caused by the *Hemophilus influenzae* bacterium.

Epiglottitis is characterized by its dramatic and sudden onset—a severe sore throat, fever, hoarseness, and an inability to swallow that leads to drooling. The child often refuses to lie down. The airway can become obstructed within hours after the symptoms begin. For this reason, a child with epiglottitis requires emergency hospitalization. An X ray is taken of the neck to determine whether the epiglottis is swollen. Antibiotics are administered and a breathing tube is inserted in the windpipe to help the child to breathe. The child usually improves within a few days after treatment.

Tuberculosis

Until recently, tuberculosis had declined to the point where it was becoming a rare disease in the United States. In areas where poverty forces close living conditions and poor hygiene, however, the disease is on the rise.

Tuberculosis is caused by the bacterium *Mycobacterium tuberculosis*, which is transmitted through airborne droplets produced by coughing or sneezing, especially in confined living spaces. Tuberculosis can occur at any time of the year. Although it is highly contagious if there is direct contact, infection usually occurs after prolonged exposure. Susceptible children usually contract the illness from infected, untreated adults and adolescents. Exposed infants and children with underlying immune deficiencies are at the highest risk.

Symptoms tend to vary, but usually include fever, cough, fatigue, weight loss, lessened appetite, and pneumonialike symptoms that fail to respond to the usual antibiotics. Many children, however, have no symptoms at all.

When the central nervous system is involved the disease is called tuberculomeningitis, and is characterized by fever, headache, lethargy, and a change in personality. If it goes undiagnosed and untreated, it can lead to coma and death. With prompt treatment, the outcome can be good.

Diagnosis is made by a tuberculin skin test. One such test involves injecting the tuberculosis antigen PPD (purified protein derivative of tuberculin) under the skin. If the skin becomes red and swollen 48 hours after the injection, it indicates infection, meaning that active tuberculosis may be present. The Tine test operates under the same principle, but instead of an injection, it employs a device with four small prongs that are coated with the tuberculin antigen.

Some children receive a Tine test before they get their measles-mumps-rubella (MMR) vaccine. This test is performed to make certain that they do not have a mild form of tuberculosis that has been undiagnosed but requires treatment before the MMR vaccine can be given.

Children with positive tuberculin tests require a chest X ray to determine the extent of infection. Swollen lymph glands in the chest, cavities in the lungs, and pneumonia are often seen on X ray in children with TB. Even if the chest X ray is normal, a child with a positive skin test will receive medication.

If a child tests positive for TB, all members of the family must be tested in order to determine how the child was infected. Infected family members also require therapy. Prevention with a vaccine (called BCG) is used in some developing countries where TB is common. Because the disease is rare in most parts of the United States, it is preferable to treat it rather than to try to prevent it with a vaccine.

Whooping Cough (Pertussis)

Whooping cough is a highly contagious disease of the respiratory tract that is characterized by fits of violent coughing. The bacterium *Bordetella pertussis* causes coldlike symptoms for about two weeks, followed by the development of a severe cough with coughing spells that often end in vomiting. Small babies may not vomit, but rather stop breathing.

The disease's first symptoms—a runny nose, cough, and fever—soon worsen, giving way to a copious nasal discharge that severely congests the child. As the child coughs to clear the lungs of mucus, the face may turn deep red or blue and the eyes bulge while the child is gasping for breath. At the end of each bout of coughing, the child makes a whooping sound. This stage of the disease, known as the paroxysmal phase, lasts two weeks or longer.

Malnutrition may occur in infants with whooping cough. The prolonged coughing leaves them exhausted and often unable to eat. Among the other complications of the disease are pneumonia and brain damage from the severe coughing spells. It is an especially severe disease in babies less than one year old, in whom it may be fatal. Older children who develop the disease almost always recover, but are usually ill for some time.

There is no specific therapy for whooping cough. Most children can be treated at home with supportive measures, such as bed rest and administration of fluids to prevent dehydration and malnutrition.

Since there is no therapy, prevention is especially important. Whooping cough is an unusual disease in the United States because of the widespread use of vaccine, which is given as part of the DPT series beginning at two months of age.

The disease occurs mostly in children who were not immunized or who did not receive a full series of immunizations. When such a child develops whooping cough, antibiotics are given to keep the disease from spreading to others. The medication, however, has no effect on the child's own disease.

REYE'S SYNDROME

REYE'S SYNDROME is a serious brain disorder that occasionally follows a viral illness such as influenza or chicken pox. The illness is rare, attacking about

3,000 children a year in the United States, most of them between the ages of 5 and 15.

The cause of Reye's syndrome has not been established, although the use of aspirin has been linked with the illness. Since public health officials have recommended that aspirin not be given to children with influenza or chicken pox, the incidence of Reye's syndrome has decreased dramatically.

Reye's syndrome is difficult to diagnose because its symptoms are similar to other, less serious illnesses. A child with this disease usually becomes lethargic, cranky, confused, and agitated. As these symptoms grow more pronounced, the child begins to vomit persistently. Eventually the child may fall into a coma, which a parent may mistake for much-needed sleep.

Treatment includes intravenous administration of fluids to replace those lost from the constant vomiting and to correct an abnormally low blood sugar. Doctors also monitor the pressure inside the skull, because the condition produces severe swelling of the brain. A spinal tap may be performed to rule out meningitis and encephalitis.

ROCKY MOUNTAIN SPOTTED FEVER

RICKETTSIAE ARE MICROORGANISMS that are larger than viruses but smaller than bacteria. They live in the cells of ticks and other insects, which transmit them to humans via bites. The major rickettsial infection seen in the United States is Rocky Mountain spotted fever, which is transmitted by ticks, especially the dog tick. Despite its name, the disease occurs mostly not in the Rocky Mountain states but rather in the Piedmont Plateau region (primarily the Carolinas), the South-Central states, such as Oklahoma and Texas, and in the islands off Massachusetts.

Because ticks populate wooded areas during the warm spring and summer months, most cases occur during the summer vacation months. Ticks often crawl onto the arms, wrists, legs, and scalps of children who venture into tick-infested areas. After the tick attaches itself to its victim, it burrows its snout into the skin. As it feeds on the blood, it deposits infectious organisms.

Symptoms begin about seven days after a tick bite. They include high fever, chills, headache, muscle aches, and a rash that begins on the extremities and moves inward toward the rest of the body. Treatment with antibiotics, usually tetracycline, is successful if begun early in the illness.

The disease can be prevented by covering exposed areas and using a tick repellent when walking through areas inhabited by ticks. Instead of biting immediately, ticks usually crawl upward, latching onto areas around the waist and at the top of socks. If children have walked through a wooded area, parents should inspect the skin for ticks and remove them promptly. The longer a tick remains on the skin, the greater the chance of infection. If a tick has become imbedded, it should not be pulled or twisted from the skin. The best method of removal is to apply petroleum jelly to the tick, wait about 30 minutes, and gently remove the tick with tweezers. Once the tick has been removed, wash the affected area and your hands with soap and water.

ROSEOLA

CHILDREN BETWEEN six months and two years old commonly develop roseola (exantheum subitum), a febrile illness that is caused by a newly discovered herpesvirus. The illness begins with a high fever that lasts three to five days and is followed by a rash when the temperature falls. In a child under two years, the appearance of rash as the fever is falling, or within a day after it has disappeared, is a pattern typical of roseola.

When roseola occurs, children appear to have no symptoms other than fever, although they may be irritable during this period. There is no specific treatment for roseola, which is a very benign disease and does not recur.

RUBELLA

RUBELLA, OR GERMAN MEASLES, is a viral infection that produces a mild illness in children but poses a great danger to the fetus of a woman who becomes infected during pregnancy. A fetus who contracts rubella is likely to suffer severe birth defects, such as blindness, deafness, cataracts, congenital heart disease, and mental retardation.

A blood test for rubella antibodies is used to determine whether a rubella infection is present. Infants in whom congenital rubella is suspected may require repeat tests up to six months of age to determine if the antibodies to the virus are being produced by the baby and were not passed on by the mother. If the baby is producing its own antibodies, congenital rubella is a likely possibility.

PRECAUTIONS WHILE TRAVELING WITH CHILDREN

Special precautions are needed to protect children when traveling to countries in which infectious diseases that are not ordinarily encountered at home are endemic. Traveler's diarrhea is one of the best known examples, but other more serious diseases, such as malaria, cholera, typhoid fever, giardia, and certain parasitic infections also may be encountered in many countries.

Before embarking on a trip with children, check with your pediatrician or the Centers for Disease Control in Atlanta regarding infectious diseases that may be encountered at your destination. Preventive immunization or medication may be indicated against some, while for others special precautions, such as not drinking local water or eating certain foods, may be advised.

Despite routine immunization of children rubella mini-epidemics still occur in the United States among the unimmunized population, often consisting of young women who did not receive the vaccine after it came into widespread use in 1969 or who were not born here.

The vaccine is given not only to induce immunity in the child but also to reduce the risk of that child transmitting the disease to others, especially to pregnant women. Young women who have not been immunized against rubella should receive the vaccine before becoming pregnant. It is safe to vaccinate a toddler even if the mother is pregnant. If she is susceptible, and her child has been immunized, she will not contract the disease from her child. Pregnant women themselves should not be immunized, however.

When a child is infected with rubella, symptoms will include a low-grade fever, a mild pink rash on the abdomen and chest that lasts a few days and does not itch, and swollen lymph glands. The illness is mild and all symptoms disappear in four or five days.

SCARLET FEVER/STREP THROAT

SCARLET FEVER and strep throat are caused by the same bacteria—group A beta hemolytic streptococcus. Both infections are highly contagious and can lead to serious complications if left untreated.

Scarlet Fever

Scarlet fever actually is a strep throat accompanied by a rash. The infecting bacteria produce a toxic substance that causes a skin rash that begins around the neck and then spreads down the trunk to the rest of the body. The rash makes the skin feel rough, like sandpaper. The tongue takes on a strawberrylike appearance.

The rash tends to appear one to two days after the first symptoms of high fever, vomiting, headache, sore throat, and chills. Within a week, the rash disappears, although the skin may continue to peel for several weeks. Treatment of scarlet fever consists of a 10-day regimen of penicillin (or erythromycin, if the child is allergic to penicillin). Alternatively, an injection of long-acting penicillin may be given.

Strep Throat

When a sore throat begins abruptly and is accompanied by pain, fever, swollen glands in the neck, muscle aches, and a stiff neck, strep throat should be suspected. A throat culture is necessary to verify the presence of streptococcus bacteria. Some doctors use a rapid test that identifies streptococcal antigens in a throat swab for diagnosis. A blood test may also be performed to determine whether the symptoms are due to streptococcal illness or whether the child is just a carrier of the bacterium. Children who carry the organism may have symptoms due to another infection. For instance, a child who actually has mononucleosis may first be diagnosed as having a strep throat because there are streptococci in the throat culture. Yet in this case, the symptoms are a result of infection with the Epstein-Barr virus, which causes mononucleosis.

A patient with a strep infection is usually treated with penicillin (or erythromycin if the child is allergic to penicillin). It takes 10 days of antibiotic therapy to eradicate the strep infection and to prevent the possibility of the body's immune reaction to the bacteria damaging the heart (acute rheumatic fever) or kidneys (glomerulonephritis). Parents must take care to administer the treatment for the full 10 days if the doctor has prescribed oral medication, even if the child no longer appears to be ill. Otherwise, the bacterium will remain in the body. For this reason some physicians prefer to administer penicillin by injection, as one shot is curative. Unfortunately, erythromycin cannot be given this way and must be taken orally for 10 days.

Streptococcal infections can cause rheumatic heart disease in some children. Acute rheumatic fever is due to an abnormal immune reaction to streptococci that causes damage to the heart muscle. Prophylaxis is given daily by mouth or once a month by injection to prevent future strep throats in children who have had one bout of rheumatic fever. This protects the heart from further damage and is usually continued for years.

SEXUALLY TRANSMITTED DISEASES

FORMERLY CALLED venereal diseases, sexually transmitted diseases (STDs) are seen in young children who have been sexually abused and in newborns who become infected as they pass through a diseased birth canal at the time of their delivery. The most common diseases are gonococcal infection, herpes, and chlamydia. Other STDs, including syphilis, hepatitis B, and AIDS, also affect children, although they are less common.

Symptoms vary, depending on the infecting organism. The general signs in postpubertal males include a discharge, an ulcer or vesicle on the penis, fever, painful urination, and swollen lymph glands in the groin. Some infections, such as gonorrhea, herpes, chlamydia, and hepatitis B, may occur without symptoms. Gonococci and chlamydia bacteria can lead to pelvic inflammatory disease, an infection of the upper genital tract that causes inflammation of the lining of the fallopian tubes. Pelvic inflammatory disease (PID) can scar these tubes that lead from the ovaries to the uterus and cause sterility.

Syphilis begins as a painless sore, or chancre, on the genitals. This is referred to as primary syphilis. Skin lesions resembling a rash may appear in the second stage (secondary syphilis), about six weeks later. When the disease enters its third stage (tertiary syphilis), it damages and scars the skin tissue, affects the nervous system, and produces cardiovascular abnormalities. Syphilis is also acquired before birth if the mother has undiagnosed or untreated syphilis. Thus, babies born to mothers who have not had prenatal care should be tested for syphilis at birth.

Infants born with congenital syphilis may have a variety of symptoms. There may be a rash that is most prominent on the face, palms, and soles. Infants often have a persistent, severe runny nose (snuffles). The skeleton also may be affected, with lesions (visible in X rays) occurring in the bones. Some babies have no symptoms initially, even though they are infected.

Diagnosis of these diseases is made by identifying the symptoms and by demonstrating the presence of the offending organism. A blood test to detect antibody titers (VDRL) is also very helpful for diagnosis. It is necessary to test the mother as well as the infant.

Pregnant women are required by law to have their blood tested for syphilis. If the test is positive, they are given antibiotics to prevent the disease from infecting their fetus and to protect themselves.

Silver nitrate solution (or tetracycline or erythromycin eye ointment) is given to all newborns to prevent gonococcal ophthalmia, an eye infection. Newborn infants who are suspected of acquiring gonococcal or chlamydial infections despite prophylactic measures are treated with an antibiotic. If these infections are treated early, complications are unusual. Syphilis and chlamydia usually respond well to antibiotics.

When young children develop STDs, child abuse cannot be discounted and further investigation of the family is imperative.

SKIN AND LYMPH NODE INFECTIONS *

BACTERIAL INFECTIONS of the skin are common in children. Staphylococcus, streptococcus and, more rarely, *Hemophilus influenzae* are the main causes of skin and lymph node infections.

Impetigo

Impetigo appears as round open sores on the skin, usually on the arms, legs, or face. The area is often itchy. When a blister is present, it opens and oozes, leaving a honey-colored crust. If left untreated, the infection can spread to other areas of the skin. Impetigo, commonly seen in the summer, is caused by either streptococci or staphylococci. It is highly contagious, especially to small children.

Impetigo requires antibiotic therapy, which is usually given both topically and orally. Glomerulonephritis (see chapter 25) is a complication of impetigo caused by streptococci in about 3 percent of cases. Some physicians believe that prompt treatment can prevent at least some cases of glomerulonephritis.

---

* (See also chapter 32, Childhood Skin Disorders.)

Boils

A boil, or furuncle, is a localized staphylococcal infection of the skin that usually begins in a hair follicle. As a boil evolves, its diameter often occupies about half an inch and it becomes painful and red. The area comes to a head, from which pus may drain. Older children with boils should be cautioned to avoid picking at them, for this only serves to spread the bacteria further.

Moist heat may be applied intermittently to allow the boil to come to a head so that the pus can drain. In some cases, antibiotics are prescribed for recurrent boils. Large boils may need to be incised by a physician so that drainage can occur. Once drained, they clear up quickly.

Cellulitis

Staphylococcus and occasionally streptococcus and *Hemophilus* bacteria, cause cellulitis, a skin infection that travels from the skin into the underlying soft tissues. The area of skin involved becomes red, hard, warm, and painful. The infected area may be large or small; when cellulitis covers a larger area, it often produces fever, chills, and a general malaise.

The bacteria enter the skin via a cut or sore, and infect the cells and lymph nodes. Cellulitis can be spread to other parts of the body and requires prompt treatment with antibiotics. It is particularly dangerous around the eyes and face.

Cervical Adenitis

Cervical adenitis, caused by streptococcal and staphylococcal bacteria, is a local infection of the skin and lymph nodes, especially those of the neck. The neck or a portion of it becomes warm, red, swollen, and painful, and fever is common. The infection responds quickly to antibiotics, although hospitalization may be necessary.

Cervical adenitis also may be caused by an organism known as mycobacterium, which is similar to the microbe that causes tuberculosis. It is diagnosed by a tuberculin skin test and often by a biopsy of the swollen lymph node. Such an infection is treated with the drugs isoniazid and rifampin. It usually responds well to treatment, although medication is required for several months.

Erysipelas

Erysipelas, a streptococcal infection that affects the deeper layers of the skin and the connective tissue below, is now rare in children. The infection produces fever, swollen, bright red and tender skin, and sores whose borders are irregular and slightly elevated. Erysipelas is caused by streptococci and is treated with penicillin or erythromycin.

TOXIC SHOCK SYNDROME

Toxins produced by the staphylococcus bacteria cause toxic shock syndrome (TSS), an unusual disease but one that can develop suddenly. The rapid onset of fever is one of the first signs of toxic shock. Other symptoms include headache, diarrhea, vomiting, abdominal pain, dizziness, faintness, and confusion. A skin rash resembling sunburn also appears, often on the palms. Toxic shock produces a marked drop in blood pressure, requiring prompt emergency treatment.

Most cases of toxic shock have occurred in women, especially those using highly absorbent tampons during menstruation. Although teenage girls and young women who are menstruating are at greatest risk, toxic shock also can occur in children and in older adults. It is due to lack of antibodies to certain staphylococci.

Toxic shock is treated by giving antibiotics to cure the bacterial infection and other medications to maintain blood pressure and fluid balance in the body until the toxin has been eliminated from the system.

TOXOPLASMOSIS

The parasitic disease toxoplasmosis often produces no symptoms when it infects most children and adults. However, it can be dangerous to the unborn child if the mother acquires the disease during pregnancy, for it can result in mental retardation or in birth defects such as eye abnormalities that can cause blindness. Toxoplasmosis also can result in miscarriage, stillbirth, or death of the baby shortly after birth. A baby who is infected before birth but who does not show symptoms at delivery may show the destructive effects of the disease years later. Patients who suffer from AIDS or whose immune systems are suppressed by disease or treatment are at high risk of developing severe infections of the central nervous system from toxoplasmosis.

The parasite *Toxoplasma gondii*, which is present in raw or undercooked meat and in animal feces, is the source of infection. Cats are the primary host for this parasite, which reproduces in the cat's intestines and excretes fertilized eggs called oocysts in the feces. The oocysts must undergo a maturation period of about 24 hours outside the cat's body before they become contagious. When an animal or human inadvertently ingests a mature oocyst, parasites then invade the body's muscles and organs. Each parasite multiplies, producing cysts containing hundreds more parasites.

To prevent infection, pregnant women should not eat raw or undercooked meat, should wear gloves when gardening, and should avoid contact with cat litter boxes. It is helpful for women of child-bearing age to know whether they have antibodies to toxoplasmosis in their blood. Those with antibodies are already immune and are not at risk to be infected again; therefore their future infants will not be at risk.

A healthy child who develops toxoplasmosis usually shows no symptoms. When symptoms occur, the illness may resemble infectious mononucleosis with swollen lymph nodes in the neck and under the arms, fatigue, malaise, muscle pain, fever, and an enlarged spleen. In rare cases, there is a rash, high fever, pneumonia, hepatitis, and cardiac abnormalities.

When toxoplasmosis develops before birth, symptoms may not appear immediately after birth. Cysts containing parasites may have traveled to the brain, the retina, and the muscles surrounding the heart and the skeleton. When the cysts rupture, they can cause severe organ destruction.

Toxoplasmosis is diagnosed by antibody tests of the blood or by a biopsy of infected tissues. Once cysts enter the body, they cannot be eradicated. If an infant has congenital toxoplasmosis, sulfa antibiotics may help relieve the symptoms and improve the prognosis. Babies who appear normal at birth, but whose mothers had toxoplasmosis during pregnancy, require close follow-up in the event that treatment is necessary. Medications help to prevent blindness and brain damage.

WORMS

A LARGE VARIETY of parasites cause infectious diseases, which in some cases can be debilitating or even fatal. Parasitic infections occur mostly in tropical and subtropical parts of the world, but with changing immigration trends and tourism, some of these organisms have found new breeding grounds in more temperate areas, such as the United States.

Children are easy prey for parasites because they frequently place their fingers or other items that may be contaminated into their mouths.

Ascariasis (Roundworms)

Ascariasis, or roundworm, is the most common intestinal parasite. Worldwide, it infects more than 600 million people a year, including an estimated 4 million in the United States.

Adult worms live in the small intestine and produce eggs that are excreted in the stool. If the stool is deposited in soil, the eggs become infectious after the larvae cast off their outer layer. The eggs remain infectious for a long period of time.

Children who handle the soil and fail to wash their hands may inadvertently ingest the infectious eggs. Once the eggs are inside the body, the worms develop in the small intestine.

Roundworm infections often begin without symptoms. As the worms develop, they occasionally migrate to the lungs, where they can cause pulmonary damage. Cough, fever, and a rash may appear after the larvae invade the lungs. An allergic type of pneumonia or bronchial asthma can persist until the infection is eliminated. A serious infection can produce an intestinal obstruction, which may require surgical correction.

Roundworms are diagnosed by examining the stool for eggs. Many times the worms themselves are excreted during a bowel movement. Treatment consists of oral administration of the drug mebendezole for three days.

Hookworms

Two types of hookworm infect an estimated 25 percent of the world's population. With the exception of the *Necator americanus* (American hookworm), which is common in the southern part of the United States, hookworm infections are rare in this country. The other type of hookworm prevails in the Mediterranean, parts of the Orient, and parts of South America.

The hookworm infects humans by penetrating through the skin of the feet and then migrating to the small intestine. This worm attaches itself to the intestinal wall and lays thousands of eggs daily. These eggs are passed through the stool and when they are deposited in warm, moist soil, they begin to hatch. As the larvae rise to the top of the contaminated soil, they penetrate the skin of barefoot walkers. The larvae pass into capillaries just below the outer layer of the skin on the feet and are carried to the lungs via the bloodstream. After leaving the respiratory system, they migrate to the intestines, where they mature fully.

Because hookworms feed on the blood of their host, anemia may result. Symptoms vary with hookworm infections. If the child is in good health and has an adequate diet, there may be no symptoms. As the number of worms increases, weakness, dizziness, and weight loss may accompany the anemia. This silent form of anemia can retard the child's normal pattern of growth.

Hookworm is diagnosed by examination of the stool for the presence of eggs, developing larvae, and adult hookworms. Treatment with the drug pyrantel pamoate is highly effective in eradicating the worms.

Hookworm infections can be prevented by sanitary disposal of feces and by wearing shoes to avoid contact with egg-infested soil.

Pinworms

The pinworm, *Enterobious vermicularis*, is an extremely common parasite in children. The infection is easy to transmit, especially among young children who share the same bed and children grouped together in nursery school and the lower elementary grades. Infestation can occur at any time of the year and in any climate.

After pinworms enter the body, they set up residence in the intestine. At night, the worm crawls out of the anus and leaves her eggs along the perianal region. Some of the eggs fall onto the bedclothes, where they can be transmitted to another child sleeping on the same bedding. Others fall onto floors and other surfaces where they can be stirred up into dust and into the air and then be inhaled. When a child scratches the egg-infested anal area, some of the eggs will become embedded under the fingernails. When the fingers are placed into the mouth, reinfection can occur.

Anal itching is the major symptom of this disorder. When the child is awakened by itching, small, cream-colored worms may be observed in the perianal region. A physican needs to see the worms or the eggs in order to make a diagnosis. To facilitate this, parents are often asked to apply a piece of transparent tape to the child's anus in the early morning and bring the tape to the physician. The tape then will be examined for eggs under a microscope.

Treatment consists of taking one mebendezole tablet by mouth, with one follow-up treatment a few weeks later. Because pinworms often infect more than one member of a family, it is usually necessary to treat the entire household to ensure complete eradication of the parasite.

Handwashing is the best way to prevent a pinworm infection. When a family member develops an infection, his or her bedclothes and linen should not be shaken, because the infective eggs can become airborne. Frequent laundering can help control the eggs.

Toxocara

Children from one to four years of age often are accidental hosts of this roundworm of dogs and cats. Infection occurs when children accidentally ingest eggs from hands that have touched soil where dogs or cats have deposited their feces.

Some children have a tendency to eat sand from a sandbox and thus have an increased risk of developing toxocariasis, also called *visceral larva migrans*. Children who play with puppies and don't wash their hands before eating or carelessly place their fingers in their mouths also have a higher risk of developing this infection.

Fever, cough, and anemia are among the symptoms of *visceral larva migrans*, which is difficult to diagnose. The disease is self-limiting and treatment usually is unnecessary. Steroids may be prescribed for severe cases.

To prevent this infection, it is recommended that dogs and cats be dewormed routinely. These pets should not be allowed in a child's sandbox.

Tapeworm

Beef and pork tapeworms are acquired by eating raw or undercooked meat. Many times there are no symptoms. However, beef tapeworm may produce gas pains, diarrhea, and weight loss. Pork tapeworm may cause muscle pain, fever, and weakness. When there are a large number of larvae, the pork tapeworms can penetrate the intestinal wall and enter muscle and nerve tissue, causing cysts in the muscle and brain.

To diagnose both forms of tapeworm, the stool is examined for worms or eggs. Praziquantel or niclosamide are prescribed to eradicate beef or pork tapeworms.

21 Childhood Cardiovascular Disease

Welton M. Gersony, M.D.

INTRODUCTION

SOME YOUNG CHILDREN are beset by the same forms of heart disease that affect adults—high blood pressure and elevated cholesterol levels (hyperlipidemia), for example. Others are subject to infectious diseases that may result in heart damage. The most common heart disease in children, however, is congenital.

Congenital heart disease—the general term for a number of conditions present at birth—constitutes serious illness that can often impair quality of life and sometimes lead to premature death. However, most individuals born with congenital heart defects enjoy relatively normal lives, thanks in large measure to constantly improving medical intervention.

These defects are malformations of the heart that take place during the fetal period. They are commonly manifested as "holes" in the partitions separating the cardiac chambers, as malformed heart valves, as the persistence of short-circuit vessels between major arteries that are meant to disappear shortly after birth, or as combinations of these defects. Generally, the result is either an obstruction of the blood flow or a rerouting of the flow.

In all but about 3 percent of these cases, the cause is not known or fully understood. A few causes, however, have been well documented. For example, if the mother has systemic lupus erythematosus or diabetes mellitus or if she contracts rubella (German measles) during the first trimester of pregnancy, the development of the baby's eyes, brain, and heart may be severely affected. Other viral infections, excess alcohol consumption, and occupational exposure to certain toxins during pregnancy may also result in congenital defects.

Heredity plays some role, although it is unusual to have more than one such child in any family. For example, a relatively rare condition called Marfan's syndrome is an inherited genetic disorder that affects the connective tissues of the body, including the blood vessel walls and heart valves. Certain chromosomal abnormalities, such as the one that causes Down's syndrome, are also associated with congenital heart disease.

In the United States approximately one of every 100 infants, or an estimated 25,000–30,000 each year, is born with a heart defect. Precise data are difficult to come by, and these figures are considered to be conservative because many defects go undetected through childhood. In adult years they may prove the basis for conditions such as endocarditis and aortic stenosis.

Some knowledge of the development and function of the heart itself is helpful in understanding congenital heart disease.

THE HUMAN HEART

IN ADULTS, the heart is roughly the size of a human fist, and it is proportionately so in infants. The heart is a hollow, muscular organ with four chambers. (See figure 21.1.) The two upper chambers receive blood and are called *atria*. The lower two pump blood and are called *ventricles*. A thick wall divides

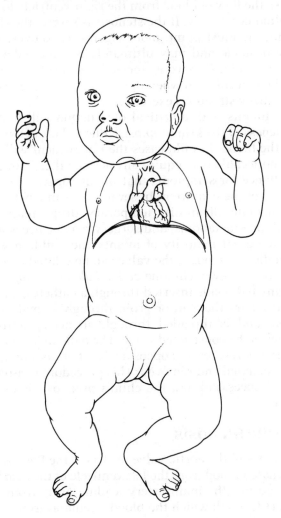

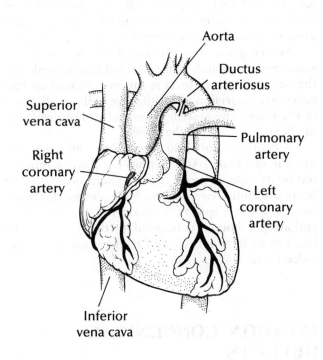

Figure 21.1. **The Heart.**

The drawing at the left shows the placement of the heart and lungs in the baby's chest cavity. At the right is the heart, its major vessels, and ductus arteriosus.

the right side from the left. Although these chambers are separated, they beat simultaneously. Blood flows from the atria through valves into the ventricles, which pump the blood through another set of valves into the arteries, and thus blood is carried to the lungs and the rest of the body.

The blood that travels through the lungs gives up its waste carbon dioxide and gains more oxygen from inhaled air. This oxygenated blood returns to the left atrium of the heart by way of the pulmonary veins. Oxygen-rich blood then flows from the lungs into the left atrium to fill the left ventricle, which in turn pumps the blood into the *aorta*—the main artery to the body. From the aorta, the blood courses into smaller arteries, which carry it to all of the body organs and tissues and then into the *arterioles*, the smallest arterial branches within the body. After it reaches the arterioles, the blood makes its way through very thin-walled vessels called *capillaries*.

The oxygen and nutrients that are in the blood pass easily through the capillary walls to the cells. Conversely, carbon dioxide and other cellular waste products pass back through the walls into the blood to be carried away. From the smallest veins into larger and larger veins, the blood makes its way back toward the heart, enters the superior vena cava or the inferior vena cava, and empties into the right atrium—and the process continues to repeat itself.

Working together, the heart, lungs, and thousands and thousands of blood-filled vessels make up the circulatory system. It is this system that carries necessary nourishment to the live cells in all parts of the body. The system is central to life itself and the heart is central to the system.

A healthy adult heart beats 70 to 80 times per minute, or about 100,000 times per day. In infants, the heart rate is more rapid, generally 90 to 130 beats a minute. Even as the body sleeps, the heart pumps about 5 quarts of blood per minute, or 75 gallons per hour. To respond to this demand the heart must be a durable and resilient organ . . . and indeed it is.

COMMON CONGENITAL DEFECTS

THE CONGENITAL heart defects that can affect the heart's durability and resilience begin to form as this organ develops. In the beginning, the heart is a simple looped and bent tube. Once the walls form that divide the heart into what will become the left and right chambers, the heart starts to beat. Then the valves form that will direct the flow of blood through the heart into the major arteries. From simple tube to complex organ, the heart undergoes critical alignments of structure and formation of tissues. All of this development takes place in the first eight weeks after conception. From then on, the heart continues to grow in size until birth, when other changes take place.

When this complex process goes awry, any of the following malformations can occur. They may result in obstruction or rerouting of the flow of blood, or in a combination of effects. The ones described first, below, are among the most common.

Pulmonary Stenosis

Stenosis simply means a narrowing of an opening. Although any of the four heart valves (mitral, tricuspid, pulmonary, or aortic) may be involved, the latter two are the most commonly affected.

Pulmonary stenosis is a narrowing of the valve or path leading from the right side of the heart to the lungs. When opened, the pulmonary valve allows the flow of blood from the right ventricle to the pulmonary artery. If the stenosis is severe, the right ventricle must pump more vigorously to overcome the obstacle and may ultimately become enlarged *(hypertrophied)*. Severe stenosis can result in rapid fatigue in children when they exert themselves, such as during strenuous exercise.

Infants with a critical obstruction will have a blueness of the skin *(cyanosis)*, due to lack of oxygen in the blood. In mild cases the impairment will not be noticeable nor require any action other than surveillance for symptoms that might suggest a worsening of the condition. In severe cases in newborns, immediate diagnosis, temporary drug treatment with prostaglandins, and surgery may be necessary. In the great majority of infants and children with significant stenosis, the valve can be dilated using a relatively new technique called *balloon angioplasty*. A tiny balloon is inserted through a catheter, a tube that enters the arm or groin through a small incision, and is threaded through an artery until it reaches the constricted valve. The balloon is inflated until it stretches and opens up the stenosis, and then it is deflated and removed. This procedure is usually quite successful and the child's prognosis is excellent.

Aortic Stenosis

Stenosis of the aortic valve obstructs the flow of oxygenated blood from the left ventricle of the heart to the aorta—the main artery leading away from the heart through which the blood circulates to the rest of the body. To overcome the obstruction resulting from aortic stenosis, the left ventricle must pump harder. There usually are no symptoms and the only sign may be a heart murmur. In mild cases there may be no need for surgery to correct the condition, but surveillance and some restriction of activity may be warranted. In severe cases, surgery or balloon angioplasty may be necessary to enlarge the valve opening. If left untreated, children with this condition may show severe symptoms, such as dizziness, fainting, chest pain, and sudden disturbances in heart rhythm.

Coarctation of the Aorta

This condition is manifested by a narrowing of the aorta (the major artery from the heart) and results in restriction of the blood's flow from the heart to the body. Coarctation causes the main pumping chamber of the heart to work harder. In turn, blood pressure increases in the head and arms, and there is less pressure in the legs. In small infants, coarctation is often accompanied by ventricular septal defect (see section next page).

Although there may be no symptoms at birth, an infant with a severe defect may develop heart failure as early as one week of age and may require medication, breathing support, and surgery. A patient severely afflicted by this condition may tire easily, appear pale, and be slow to develop. If the condition is mild, there will usually be no symptoms. Coarctation may go unrecognized for years if arm and leg blood pressures are not taken.

Surgical repair for uncomplicated coarctation is recommended before age four in order to prevent complications, primarily high blood pressure. The surgery may consist of removing the narrowed portion of the aorta or patching it with a portion of an artery taken from the arm or with a synthetic material. The procedure does not involve opening the heart. The results are usually excellent, but the child should be regularly monitored. In rare cases (among infants) the aorta may become constricted again and require repeat surgery. As with most forms of congenital heart disease, the child will be at higher risk of infection (endocarditis) of the heart valves or walls and should be given antibiotics before dental work and before certain surgical procedures.

Atrial Septal Defect

Both atrial and ventricular septal defects are the result of holes in the wall, or septum, which divides the left side of the heart from the right. An atrial septal defect involves an opening in the wall dividing the two upper chambers (the atria) that allows a large amount of blood from the left atrium to flow directly into the right atrium instead of flowing through the left ventricle and out the aorta to the

rest of the body. (See figure 21.3.) This means that oxygenated blood—blood that has already been to the lungs—is returned to the lungs along with blood from the body. Atrial septal defect (often referred to as ASD) results in a greater than normal amount of blood in the right atrium, which may cause its enlargement along with that of the right ventricle.

In many cases, children with atrial septal defect have few, if any, symptoms. There may be a heart

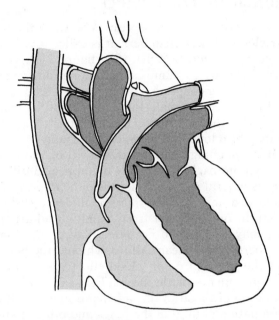

Figure 21.2. **Normal Heart.**

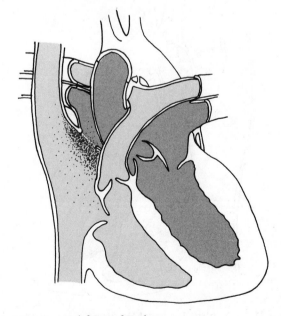

Figure 21.3. **Atrial Septal Defect.**

An opening in the wall separating the left and right atria results in increased blood on the right side of the heart, leading to enlargement of the right chambers and pulmonary artery.

murmur, which usually does not become obvious until after the child is one year old, by which time the volume of blood flowing to the lungs increases. The child's condition should be monitored regularly. If the shunt, or opening in the wall, is significant, surgery may be recommended in early childhood in order to prevent serious complications later on.

Ventricular Septal Defect

When the opening in the septum is between the two ventricles, or lower chambers, it is called a ventricular septal defect, or VSD. (See figure 21.4.) This forces the heart to pump an additional amount of blood, and lung congestion often results.

If the defect is small, the damage will be insignificant and the hole may even close itself. The only sign may be a loud, but harmless, murmur.

If the opening is larger, there will be more obvious symptoms, but they may not appear until the infant is several weeks or months old. Growth may be retarded and the baby may be undernourished. The strain on the heart from pumping additional blood may cause it to become enlarged. In some cases there may be heart failure, which is the inability of the heart to pump blood effectively to meet the requirements of the body. This can lead to a backing up of blood in the veins and may result in accumulation of fluid in the lungs and other tissues

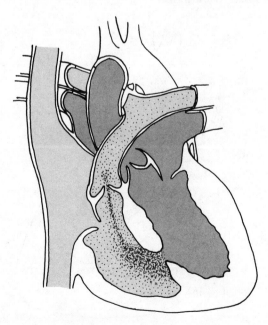

Figure 21.4. **Ventricular Septal Defect.**

Opening between the right and left ventricles results in some blood flowing from the left to the right ventricle and then out the pulmonary artery.

in the body. The large amount of blood pumped to the lungs may result in damage to the pulmonary blood vessels.

To prevent complications later in life, large defects are repaired through open heart surgery in childhood. A Dacron patch is used to cover the hole. Eventually, the tissue that normally lines the heart will grow over the patch and it will become a permanent part of the organ. With this procedure, normal circulation is restored and the long-term prognosis is positive.

As with several other types of heart disease, there is a risk that the child will develop an infection of the heart wall or valves. Infective endocarditis (also called bacterial endocarditis) may be prevented if the child is given penicillin or another antibiotic before any dental work or certain surgical procedures that might leave him or her at increased risk of infection.

Patent Ductus Arteriosus

Normally, blood travels via the pulmonary artery from the right side of the heart to the lungs, where it is filled with oxygen. The oxygenated blood is returned to the left side of the heart and then leaves the heart through the aorta to be transported throughout the body.

In the fetal stage, there is an opening between these two major blood vessels, the pulmonary artery and the aorta. The opening, called the ductus arteriosus, usually closes within hours after birth. In some babies (particularly premature ones), however, the ductus remains open, or patent. (See figure 21.5.)

In premature infants, a bounding pulse is an early and common sign. There may also be a heart murmur. In full-term infants, the murmur may not be obvious until four to eight weeks of age. A child with a large patent ductus arteriosus, or PDA, may breathe rapidly, become easily fatigued, have delayed development, and have an increased risk of lung infections such as pneumonia.

For the premature baby with patent ductus, fluid restriction may be prescribed, as well as diuretics and other drugs, such as indomethacin. Indomethacin may close the ductus, but if this treatment is not successful, surgical closure may be necessary. Surgery usually involves simply tying the ductus off. For full-term babies, if there is heart failure, surgery is done immediately. In asymptomatic patients, surgery may be delayed. Repair of the ductus arteriosus does not require cardiopulmonary bypass. Closure reduces the risk of developing infective endocarditis later on.

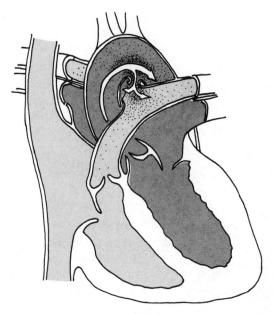

Figure 21.5. **Patent Ductus Arteriosus.**

The duct between the aorta and pulmonary artery in the fetal heart fails to close after birth.

Atrioventricular Canal Defect

This complex defect, also called endocardial cushion defect or atrioventricular septal defect, involves all four chambers of the heart. The main aspect of the defect is a large hole in the center of the heart where the atrial septum—the wall that separates the upper chambers of the heart—joins the ventricular septum—the wall that separates the lower chambers. The second aspect is an absence of separate tricuspid and mitral valves, which normally separate the upper and lower chambers. Instead, there is essentially one valve that spans both sides of the defect. This valve may not close adequately, allowing some backflow (called regurgitation) of blood from the lower to the upper chamber on one side or the other or both.

The result of this defect is that blood that has already traveled to the lungs and become oxygenated flows into the right side of the heart, where it mixes with unoxygenated blood and returns to the lungs. Thus the heart has to do extra work, which may cause its enlargement. The additional flow to the lungs may cause high pulmonary blood pressure, leading to damage to blood vessel walls.

Atrioventricular canal defect is seen frequently in children with Down's syndrome. The first symptoms are most often rapid respirations, poor feeding, and fatigue. There may be a blue appearance to the skin, most noticeably in the lips and fingernails.

Growth and development will be slow and the baby may become undernourished.

If the symptoms are severe and particularly if there is high blood pressure in the lungs, early surgery may be necessary to create normal blood circulation. Generally a Teflon patch is sewn over the hole, the single valve is divided, and two new valves are fashioned to separate the upper and lower chambers. The tissue that normally lines the heart will eventually grow over the patch.

If the necessary surgery is very complex and the child very young, a temporary band may be placed around the pulmonary artery to constrict the flow of blood to the lungs and help control the pulmonary blood pressure. Later the band can be removed and the reconstructive surgery performed. Surgery is generally performed before age one and sometimes as early as two or three weeks of age.

Tetralogy of Fallot

Tetralogy of Fallot represents four related malformations. (See figure 21.6, next page.) A large hole (ventricular septal defect) exists between the two ventricles. There is also a stenosis, or narrowing, of the opening into the pulmonary artery from the right ventricle, which inhibits the flow of unoxygenated blood to the lungs. The third malformation—an enlargement (increased muscularization) of the right ventricle—is a direct consequence of the first two. The fourth is that the aorta lies directly over the ventricular septal defect and thus receives blood from both ventricles. The result of these combined malformations is that venous (unoxygenated) blood leaving the heart bypasses the lung in part and is shunted into the arterial system without oxygenation. This causes blueness, or cyanosis, of the lips and fingernails. It may be evident soon after birth and prompts the reference to "blue babies." A child with this condition may tire easily and may turn somewhat blue (cyanosis), or even faint, as a result of day-to-day activities.

Open heart surgical repair of tetralogy of Fallot is usually recommended in infancy. This procedure involves opening the pulmonary valve, removing the obstructing muscle, and patching the ventricular septal defect. Although the repair can be complex, the risk is low, and the vast majority of patients are then able to lead normal or nearly normal lives.

Transposition of the Great Arteries

In the case of this defect, the pulmonary artery and the aorta are reversed. Normally, the pulmonary artery carries blood from the right side of the heart to the lungs for oxygenation, and the aorta transports

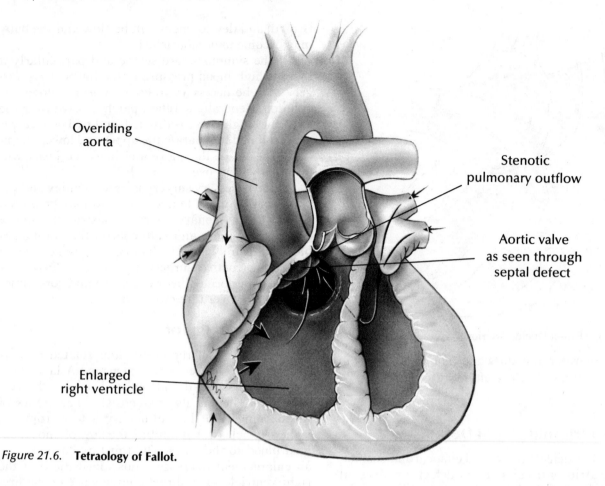

Overiding
aorta

Stenotic
pulmonary outflow

Aortic valve
as seen through
septal defect

Enlarged
right ventricle

Figure 21.6. **Tetraology of Fallot.**

oxygenated blood from the left side of the heart to the body. With transposition of the great arteries, the venous blood does not pass through the lungs for oxygenation but travels directly to the aorta and on to the body. The pulmonary artery receives blood that has been oxygenated and returns it to the lungs for needless reoxygenation.

The transposition defect is a very serious one that becomes apparent shortly after birth because the child appears extremely cyanotic (blue). Ironically, the infant can only survive this condition if there is another defect—atrial septal, ventricular septal, or patent ductus arteriosus—that allows mixing of oxygenated blood with venous blood so that some oxygen circulates to the body.

As an immediate palliative measure, a special technique known as *balloon atrial septostomy* may be used to improve the supply of oxygen to the body. In this procedure, a tiny balloon is inserted through a catheter, a flexible tube that is introduced into the body though a small incision in the groin and then threaded through a vein to the right atrium and across the atrial septum to the left atrium. The balloon is inflated and pulled until it opens the constriction between the ataria, and then it is deflated and removed.

The septostomy temporarily alleviates the cyanosis. Permanent repair of the defect may be performed in the first few weeks or later on, depending on the degree of cyanosis and whether there are other cardiac defects present. Repair may take the form of a *venous switch* (also called an intra-atrial baffle or a Mustard or Senning procedure), in which a tunnel is created inside the atria so that the oxygenated blood can flow through the right ventricle and out through the aorta while venous (nonoxygenated) blood can flow through the left ventricle and out through the pulmonary artery. However, more recently a newer surgical technique has been used to switch the two major arteries with the coronary arteries so that the blood flow is returned to its normal route.

Truncus Arteriosus

In truncus arteriosus, a relatively rare defect, the aorta and the pulmonary artery arise from a single blood vessel and there is a large hole in the wall separating the ventricles. Early surgery is necessary to close this ventricular septal defect and to separate the pulmonary artery from the common artery and attach it via a conduit (tube) to the right ventricle.

Hypoplastic Left Heart Syndrome

An infant with a hypoplastic, or underdeveloped, left ventricle appears normal at birth but becomes severely ill within two or three days. On testing, it becomes clear that the aortic or mitral valve or both are missing and blood has only been able to reach the body from the right heart through the ductus arteriosus, a passageway that is normally open in the fetus but closes shortly after birth. In most cases, the prognosis for infants with this syndrome is very poor. Palliative surgery or heart transplantation are offered at some medical centers.

Tricuspid Atresia

Atresia is a general term for the absence of a structure. In one form, the tricuspid valve, which normally allows flow of blood from the right atrium into the right ventricle, is missing and the right ventricle consequently is underdeveloped. Additional anomalies—specifically a hole in the wall separating the two atria (atrial septal defect) and usually another between the two ventricles (ventricular septal defect)—allow enough blood flow to the lungs and body to enable the child to survive until the defect or defects can be surgically treated. In the interim, however, the infant will appear blue (cyanotic) because unoxygenated blood passes through the hole in the atrial septum instead of traveling to the lungs to become oxygenated. Some blood flows through the ventricular septal defect and finds its way to the lungs, but not enough to prevent cyanosis. The left ventricle provides the entire circulation—pulmonary and systemic.

In some infants, surgery is performed to create a shunt that allows more blood to flow to the lungs and reduces the cyanosis. Later, a repair known as a *Fontan procedure* is made to create an opening from the right atrium into the pulmonary artery, and the hole in the atrial wall is closed. This relieves the cyanosis and allows the left ventricle to perform the normal amount of work. The right ventricle is left out of the circulation.

Pulmonary Atresia

In this condition, the right ventricle is a blind pouch. There is no pulmonary valve to allow blood to flow from the right ventricle into the pulmonary artery so that it can reach the lungs to pick up oxygen. Some blood leaves the right atrium via an atrial septal defect. This hole in the wall of the atrium allows unoxygenated blood to mix with oxygenated blood and this mixture is pumped out through the aorta to the body. Because the resulting mixture is poor in oxygen, the baby is cyanotic. In the mean-

time, the only blood flow to the lungs is through a passageway called the ductus arteriosus, left from the fetal period. This ductus normally closes within hours to days of birth. When it does close, the cyanosis becomes severe. The ductus can be kept open temporarily with drug treatment (prostaglandin) until surgery is performed to create a shunt, or passageway, connecting the aorta and the pulmonary artery.

The type and success of permanent repair depends on how well the right ventricle develops. If it is very small, effective long-term surgical repair may not be possible. If it is not large enough to act as a pump, the Fontan procedure may be used to connect the right atrium directly to the pulmonary artery. A larger right ventricle can be successfully incorporated into the circulation.

Total Anomalous Pulmonary Venous Return

In this congenital condition, the left and right pulmonary veins that normally return oxygenated blood from the lungs to the heart do not connect to the left atrium. Rather, an anomalous vein branches off the pulmonary veins, bypasses the left atrium, and connects indirectly to the right atrium. Oxygenated blood flowing through this abnormal vein mixes with unoxygenated blood in the right atrium. Some of this oxygen-poor mixture then flows through a hole in the atrium wall (atrial septal defect) and eventually out the aorta to the body. The rest of the mixed blood flows into the right ventricle and then is transported to the lungs via the pulmonary artery.

Surgery is required very early on to repair the atrial septal defect with a patch and to connect the pulmonary vein to the left atrium. Prognosis for infants who have this surgery promptly is generally very good.

DETECTION AND DIAGNOSIS

AS IS THE case with many diseases, early detection and diagnosis of congenital heart disease are vital to effective medical and surgical treatment. The diagnostic process includes careful physical examination to detect cardiac enlargement, murmurs, or arrhythmias (irregularities of the heart rhythm). Laboratory tests may also be required, as well as noninvasive diagnostic tests such as an electrocardiogram, X rays, and echocardiography, or invasive procedures such as cardiac catheterization and angiography.

Signs and Symptoms

The presence of obvious symptoms will vary according to the type and the severity of the defect. Severe defects that result in right-to-left shunting of blood (tetralogy of Fallot, complete transposition of the great arteries, and hypoplastic left heart syndrome) produce almost immediate cyanosis and/or respiratory distress, an obvious clue that something is wrong. Another classic sign is a heart murmur, which is simply the sound of blood flow through the heart and which may be normal or abnormal. Not all defects result in murmurs and not all murmurs indicate a problem (some are meaningless and thus called "innocent"). Shortness of breath, enlargement of the liver, and edema (swelling of various parts of the body due to fluid accumulation) are early signs of severe congenital heart disease. A defect may be suspected if the child is slow to develop. Occasionally abnormalities are not detected until adulthood.

If the parent or the pediatrician suspects a problem, the child may be referred to a pediatric cardiologist—a pediatrician with additional training, experience, and board certification in the subspecialty of cardiology.

The Diagnostic Evaluation

The diagnostic evaluation will begin with a history taking, in which the physician will ask about such things as any incidence of heart disease in the mother's and father's family, details of the pregnancy, and what symptoms led to the visit. This will be followed by a thorough physical examination. The doctor will look at the child's skin color, take the pulse and blood pressure, use his or her hands to feel (palpate) the contour of the chest and abdomen, and listen to the child's heart sounds (*auscultation*) through a stethoscope. Palpation helps determine whether the heart is in its normal position and whether there is enlargement of any part of the heart or of other organs such as the liver and spleen.

The doctor will search for the presence of edema in areas where it is typically found: the ankles, abdomen, and eyelids, for example. A blood test may be ordered to measure, among other things, the red blood cell level. Because red blood cells carry oxygen to the tissues, an elevated level may indicate that the body is trying to compensate for decreased oxygen in the circulation.

In older children, another sign that may indicate long-standing insufficient oxygen in the blood is clubbing of the fingers and toes, a condition in which the tips of the extremities become bulbous and the nails curve.

Next the doctor will use any of a number of diagnostic tests to get a more detailed picture of the congenital defect. The following are the most common diagnostic procedures, which may be done either in the doctor's office or in the hospital.

Electrocardiogram (ECG, EKG). This is a painless procedure in which electrodes are attached to the body to measure the electrical impulses generated by the heart as it beats. By studying the pattern of the line recorded by the ECG, the doctor can obtain information about possible heart defects, the condition of the heart muscle, and whether a rhythm irregularity is present. (This test does not introduce any electrical impulses into the body; rather it measures those that the heart produces.) An exercise electrocardiogram, also called a stress test, is simply an ECG performed during exercise, usually on a treadmill or stationary bicycle. It sometimes reveals abnormalities only apparent when the heart is being stressed, not when it is at rest. The test cannot be done on infants, but may be used for some children age four and older.

Chest X ray. Another painless procedure, this test uses an insignificant amount of radiation to produce pictures that allow the doctor to see from different angles the size, shape, and location of the heart, lungs, major veins and arteries.

Echocardiography (Ultrasonography, Ultrasound). In this test, a device called a transducer is passed over the chest and emits harmless high-frequency sound waves. As the waves bounce off structures in the chest they provide a picture that reveals an image of the heart, showing the size, shape, and motion of the heart chambers, valves, and arteries. The technology is similar to that used to detect fish or submarines in the ocean.

Doppler Echocardiography. Using a device similar to that used in a regular echocardiograph, this test is done simultaneously with echocardiography and measures blood flow.

Cardiac Catheterization (Angiography). This procedure directly measures flows and pressures within the heart and allows for visualization of the heart and coronary arteries. It is more complex than the noninvasive ones described above and is carried out in the hospital.

The child is sedated and may sleep through the procedure. After a local anesthetic is administered, a thin, flexible plastic tube (catheter) is inserted through a small incision in the arm or groin and carefully threaded, while the cardiologist watches its progress on a fluoroscope, through a vein into the right side of the heart or an artery into the left side. Venous catheterization is used to assess the functioning of the pulmonary and tricuspid valves and to determine blood pressure and flow in the right atrium and the pulmonary artery. Arterial catheterization may be used to assess the coronary arteries and the functioning of the mitral and aortic valves and the left ventricle.

A dye or contrast material is then injected through the catheter into a blood vessel or the heart itself so that a special X-ray movie can record and define the exact structure of heart chambers, valves, and blood vessels.

The child may experience a hot flush and nausea during or after the experience, but the symptoms do not last long. The child may also be sleepy for several hours and will be returned to his or her room to rest. If no further tests are needed, discharge may be later that day or early the next.

Catheters are also used to treat certain types of defects with balloon angioplasty. (See Pulmonary Stenosis, and Aortic Stenosis.)

MEDICAL TREATMENT

MEDICAL TREATMENT of a congenital heart defect may be all that is needed, or it may be an adjunct to surgery. The following are common symptoms that are sometimes treated medically:

Irregular Heart Rhythms.   The general term for irregular heart rate or rhythm is *arrhythmia* or *dysrhythmia*. *Tachycardia* is a very rapid heart rate, while *bradycardia* is an unusually slow heart rate. Both of them may decrease the efficiency of the heart's pumping action. Arrythmias occur in other forms of heart disease besides congenital and sometimes they occur after corrective surgery. Often no structural heart disease is present and they can be controlled with medication. Rarely, bradycardia may require the implantation of a pacemaker to speed and regulate the heart rate.

Congestive Heart Failure.   When the heart is not pumping sufficient blood for the body to function normally, the condition is known as congestive heart failure. (The heart does not fail to function entirely.) Eventually fluid begins to accumulate in the lungs, which causes rapid or labored breathing and leads to rapid fatigue following even mild exertion. Fluid can also accumulate in other parts of the body (edema), notably the ankles, eyelids, and abdomen.

Drugs such as digoxin or digitalis can be given to stimulate the heart, strengthening its contractions so that it is able to pump more blood with each beat. Diuretics, which promote fluid loss, can be given to help lessen the edema. A low sodium (salt) diet may also be prescribed. Other agents are used to decrease the work that the heart must accomplish.

SURGICAL TREATMENT

IF THE RESULTS of the diagnostic evaluation indicate that surgery is necessary to ameliorate or repair a congenital heart defect, the pediatric cardiologist and pediatric nurse specialists will explain the procedure to the parent and answer any questions. A child old enough to understand will also be given a simple explanation of what to expect.

The Hospital Stay

In order to make the hospital stay as easy as possible on the child, the parent should consider:

- Staying overnight in the child's room whenever possible.
- Encouraging the child to take along favorite toys and other familiar articles.
- Arranging to meet prior to admission the doctors and nurses who will care for the child.
- Discussing with a counselor or the physician possible emotional problems of the sick youngster or the impact of those problems on the family.
- Helping the child to face his or her fears about forthcoming procedures through thorough discussions and explanations and assurances of continuing support from the family.
- Emphasizing to the child the positive aspects of the surgery, i.e., correction of the defects resulting in a more normal life.

(For additional information, see chapter 7, When a Child Goes to the Hospital.)

The Surgery

Heart surgery is among the most complex of operations and requires a highly skilled team headed by a cardiovascular surgeon and his or her assistants. Others on the team include an anesthesiologist, nurses, and technicians, who use sophisticated equipment to administer anesthesia and monitor the patient's respiration and circulation.

If open heart surgery is involved, a heart-lung machine is used to circulate blood through the body, ensuring that it receives oxygen, while bypassing the heart and lungs. On occasion, deep hypothermia is used on infants up to the first year of age. In this procedure, the infant's temperature is dramatically lowered, which permits cessation or limitation of blood flow while repairs to the heart are made.

Following surgery the patient is transported to an intensive care unit (ICU) and carefully monitored on a 24-hour basis by a team of nurses and doctors. The ICU is supplied with an array of equipment that might seem frightening but is quite routine: ventilators (breathing machines), oxygen tents or masks, chest tubes for blood drainage, endotracheal tubes (breathing tubes inserted into the windpipe), intravenous lines for introduction of medicines, fluids, and blood. This type of special care is required as the heart recovers and its function improves.

Visiting hours in ICUs may be brief and restricted during the first few hours after surgery. Once the child's condition is stabilized, he or she will be moved to a regular pediatric unit where parents may stay. Physical and respiratory therapy programs are instituted to begin preparing the child for release. Additional testing may be required before discharge.

Posthospital Recovery

After discharge from the hospital the child will require further convalescence. The parents will be given instructions about amount and frequency of activities and exercise, medication, and diet.

While the cardiovascular surgeon and cardiologist will wish to continue monitoring a child's postsurgical progress, the patient will be returned to the pediatrician or family physician for routine care. Various agencies can also prove helpful in offering home education, vocational counseling, physical or psychological therapy. Among these are the local school district and health department, voluntary health agencies, and others recommended by the medical team.

After heart surgery children usually feel renewed energy and a sense of well-being. Resumption of normal activities is dependent upon the type of defect and surgery, as well as previous physical and emotional health. Most children can return to school within six weeks after a heart operation.

SPECIAL NEEDS

Feeding the Infant with Congenital Heart Disease

A baby's failure to increase in weight as quickly as in height or to develop in other ways is sometimes the first clue that there may be an underlying heart defect. Slow weight gain is commonly seen in infants with congestive heart failure and sometimes in those with cyanotic heart disease.

Rapid breathing, frequent respiratory infections, increased caloric needs (because the heart must work harder), poor appetite, poor absorption of nutrients, and a decrease in oxygen in the blood may all be related to congenital heart disease and may play a role in the infant's inability to gain weight normally.

Pediatricians recommend that babies be breastfed when possible. Supplementary bottles may be necessary if the baby is not getting enough calories with breastmilk alone, or the mother may have to increase the number of feedings. If the baby must for any reason be fed intravenously the mother may express milk in order to keep an adequate supply for later when the baby is able to nurse.

The pediatrician or pediatric cardiologist can advise the parents about how many calories are necessary for the baby's growth and how to ensure that the baby receives them.

Because breathing may be difficult for babies with congenital defects, sucking—on bottle or breast—may also be harder. It may help to hold the baby in a semiupright position during feeding to get the benefit of gravity.

Blue infants may need extra iron, which is available in certain formulas or may be given as drops. The physician can advise about this and other feeding needs.

Exercise and Activity

Except in the case of severe defects, children with congenital heart disease do not need to restrict their activities. Competitive sports may be curtailed in children with certain conditions, but aerobic activities such as bicycling and swimming are generally recommended. Coaches, camp counselors, school nurses, and others who supervise the youngster's physical activities should be aware of any restrictions.

Bacterial (Infective) Endocarditis

Endocarditis is an infection of the tissue in the heart wall, valves, or blood vessels to which people with heart defects are more susceptible than others. Because the bacteria enter the heart through the bloodstream, any procedure that increases the chance of this (such as certain types of surgery or even dental work) increases the chance of infection —although it remains a rare complication. Parents should be sure that any doctor or dentist who treats the child is aware of the child's condition. A prophylactic (preventive) dose of antibiotics is administered before and after surgical procedures. If bacterial endocarditis does occur, it is treated with antibiotics administered intravenously during what is usually a lengthy hospital stay. Prevention is the much better course.

Parents should discuss the appropriate preventive measures with the pediatrician or pediatric cardiologist. A wallet card giving the recommended type and dose of antibiotics is available from local chapters of the American Heart Association or from the pediatric cardiologist.

SUPPORT SERVICES

HAVING A CHILD with a congenital heart defect can impose a financial strain on the family. Some states offer financial aid through various agencies to families who can demonstrate eligibility. These programs may cover initial diagnostic services, hospitalization in an approved medical center, transportation costs, and other pressing financial needs. Social workers, both community- and hospital-based, can assist the family in finding the appropriate federal, state, and local agencies.

Programs of special education can help physically handicapped children (into which category some children with congenital heart disease will fall). These services are provided at no cost to the child's family. However, each state has its own set of rules about provision of these services, and families must contact local school districts for precise information.

OTHER FORMS OF HEART DISEASE IN EARLY CHILDHOOD

High Blood Pressure

High blood pressure, also called hypertension, affects more than 59 million Americans. Children, even infants, can have elevated blood pressure.

Blood pressure refers to the amount of force exerted by blood on the walls of arteries. Each time the heart contracts, arterial pressure rises, and when the heart relaxes, blood pressure goes down. The higher, or upper, pressure is termed systolic blood pressure, and the lower is called diastolic. For example, the doctor may refer to a blood pressure reading of 120 (the systolic) over 70 (diastolic).

Blood pressure is controlled by the arterioles, or smallest arteries in the body. If the arterioles are narrowed, blood cannot flow easily through them and the heart must pump harder to force the flow, causing blood pressure to rise. Blood volume also affects blood pressure.

In about 10 percent of cases, high blood pressure is the result of a specific condition, such as a kidney abnormality or a congenital defect of the main artery supplying blood from the heart to the body (see section on coarctation of the aorta). When this is the case, the condition is known as secondary hypertension. In the great majority of people, however, the cause of elevated blood pressure is unknown and the condition is called primary, or essential, hypertension.

Certain factors predispose children and adults to develop high blood pressure. These include age (adults are more prone than children, and advancing age increases the risk); race (it is more common among blacks than whites); heredity; and obesity.

High blood pressure rarely provokes symptoms, in either children or adults, and can go undetected for years. The main route of discovery is a simple blood pressure test. All children should have a blood pressure check as part of an annual physical, but especially those whose parents have high blood pressure. High blood pressure in adults is defined as a reading equal to or greater than 140 millimeters (mm) of mercury (Hg) over 90 mm Hg (140/90). For children, it is lower, although it increases with age. The doctor should take the blood pressure on several occasions to be certain that the elevation is significant. He or she should be sure that the blood pressure is similar in the arms and legs. If hypertension is present, urine and blood tests may be ordered to see if it is caused by some other disease. Only when no specific causes are found will the diagnosis of primary (or essential) hypertension be made.

If the primary hypertension is mild, with only a slight elevation of blood pressure, it will sometimes respond to simple treatment without drugs. Diet modification is the first choice. If the child is overweight, for example, losing as few as 10 pounds may have a positive effect. Restricting sodium, specifically table salt, also may be important. The pediatrician or family physician can provide a list of high-sodium foods that should be avoided. High on the list are some of the snack items, such as potato chips, that many children like.

It is generally easier on children if the whole family participates in diet modification. Since a varied, balanced diet low in cholesterol and fats (especially saturated fats) and high in carbohydrates, particularly complex ones (starches), is recommended for the entire family, this change will benefit everyone. (See chapter 18, Getting Off to a Healthy Start.)

Exercise can also have a positive effect on high blood pressure directly, as well as indirectly as a method of weight control. Children with high blood pressure can participate in a wide variety of physical activities and generally do not need to be restricted.

If diet modification and exercise are not able to bring the blood pressure under control, the physician may prescribe antihypertensive medications.

Hyperlipidemia (High Cholesterol Levels)

Atherosclerosis, a vascular disease in which the inner layers of the artery walls become thick, irregular, and narrowed, is a major cause of coronary heart disease. This dangerous clogging of the blood vessels is mainly due to deposits of plaque, a hardened form of the fatlike substance cholesterol. A diet high in fat (the typical American diet) can be a major contributor to atherosclerosis.

Some people have a genetic tendency toward accumulating cholesterol in their blood. It is estimated that 1 to 2 percent of American children have this abnormality. Even more are at risk for other reasons, including race (hyperlipidemia is higher in blacks than whites) and diet. In all, approximately 15 percent have elevated levels.

Whether all children should have a blood test to determine cholesterol levels by the time they enter school remains controversial. Certainly children whose parents have an elevated cholesterol level (defined in adults as more than 240 milliliters per deciliter of blood—240 ml/dl) should be tested. Early development of heart disease (before age 55 for men, 60 for women) in the child's parents or grandparents is another clue that there may be hyperlipidemia in the family. Children who are at risk because of family history of hyperlipidemia or coronary heart disease should be retested every few years, even if the original test was negative. In children, the ideal level is about 150 ml/dl.

The American Heart Association recommends that all children age two and over follow the same low-cholesterol, low-fat diet recommended for adults (see chapter 18, Getting Off to a Healthy Start). If a child is found to have elevated cholesterol, changing the diet is usually the first treatment. The American Heart Association recommends that no more than 30 percent of calories come from fat, with saturated fat (found primarily in meats and dairy products) accounting for no more than 10 percent of total calories. Cholesterol (found only in an-

imal products, including dairy foods) should be limited to 300 milligrams (mg) a day. The pediatrician or pediatric cardiologist may recommend that fat and cholesterol be restricted even further in children with hereditary, extremely high blood cholesterol, to 7 percent saturated fat and 200 mg of cholesterol.

Exercise is also helpful in increasing the level of high-density lipoproteins (HDL—the "good" form of cholesterol) and in controlling weight, if this is a problem. Obesity, in and of itself, may increase the risk of heart disease.

Diet changes are successful in lowering cholesterol in about 25 percent of children. If the level is extremely elevated or doesn't respond to diet, cholesterol-lowering drugs may be recommended, but there is not a great deal of experience using these drugs in children.

Rheumatic Heart Disease

Rheumatic heart disease is a residual effect of rheumatic fever, an acute and generalized inflammatory disorder that sometimes occurs after a streptococcal infection of the upper respiratory tract. Two weeks or more following such an infection, commonly known as strep throat, a small number of children (usually less than 1 percent) develop acute symptoms. These may include: fever, skin rash, swelling of the joints, involuntary twitching of muscles (St. Vitus' dance), and inflammation of the heart tissue and valves.

The disease may be due to an overresponse of the immune system: in fighting the streptococcal infection, the body may produce toxins that inadvertently harm its own tissues.

The tendency to develop rheumatic fever seems to run in families, but it is not clear whether this is due to genetics or environment. Although the original streptococcal infection is contagious, the rheumatic fever response is not. Adults occasionally are infected, but most commonly it affects children between ages 5 and 15.

Rheumatic fever has declined dramatically during the last generation, but in some areas it has increased again recently. Traditionally rates have been higher among children of lower socioeconomic status living in a crowded urban environment. The most recent outbreaks, however, have been among primarily middle-class surburban and rural children.

The first step in the prevention of rheumatic fever is to be sure that a throat culture is taken any time a child has an acute sore throat, particularly one that comes on suddenly and is accompanied by fever as high as 104 degrees F., headache, nausea, vomiting, and abdominal pain. Sore throats can be caused by any number of viruses and bacteria (both streptococcal and nonstreptococcal), and only a culture can determine the exact cause. Only one strain of streptococcus—group A hemolytic—can lead to rheumatic fever. There is no effective treatment for a viral sore throat, but those caused by bacteria respond readily to penicillin or other antibiotics, which should be taken for 10 days. Alternatively, penicillin can be given in a single long-lasting injection.

Even without treatment, a child with strep throat will usually recover in a few days. Rheumatic fever may develop anywhere from days to several months after the apparent recovery. The symptoms may be severe or they may be so vague (fatigue, poor appetite, paleness) that they go undiagnosed. In about one-third of cases there will be damage to the heart. This, too, may go undetected, sometimes until adulthood, when valve damage may lead to congestive heart failure.

The two major symptoms that give rheumatic fever its name are a high fever that lasts from 10 to 14 days and arthritic (rheumatic) pain in the joints. The soreness may move from one joint to another and, in severe cases, the joints will swell and redden.

A lacy or wavy skin rash (erythema marginatum) may come and go spontaneously. Neuromuscular involvement may take the form of rapid, involuntary twitching and jerking of the muscles, sometimes known as *St. Vitus' dance* or Sydenham's chorea.

Shortness of breath may indicate that the heart has been affected; the child may become easily fatigued, have a poor appetite, and appear pale. On examination by a physician, the heart may be found to be enlarged and there may be an abnormal murmur. If the doctor suspects rheumatic heart disease, chest X rays and an electrocardiogram may be ordered. Other tests may be used to confirm damage to the heart valves (see preceding section on The Diagnostic Evaluation), but the most important diagnostic information comes from the doctor's physical examination.

Treatment of rheumatic fever primarily involves treating the symptoms. In addition to initial bed rest, aspirin is prescribed for joint pain and inflammation. Steroids (prednisone) may also be used for heart inflammation (carditis). If there is heart failure (a condition in which the heart cannot pump sufficient blood and excess fluids accumulate in the body), digitalis (digoxin) may be prescribed to stimulate and strengthen the pumping action. Diuretics or a sodium-restricted diet may be recommended to decrease fluid retention. If the child has chorea, sedatives or tranquilizers may be used.

Recovered rheumatic fever patients are at risk of recurrent attacks; therefore, they are usually given preventive doses of antibiotics, often in the form of a monthly injection of a long-lasting penicillin or daily sulfonamide or penicillin in pill form. Those who have rheumatic heart disease are most likely to have recurrence, risking further damage to the heart valves; therefore they may be required to take prophylactic antibiotics throughout life. In addition, they are at higher risk of developing endocarditis, a bacterial infection of the heart valves or heart lining. They should have extra antibiotic protection before any surgery or dental procedure that may allow bacteria to enter the bloodstream.

Kawasaki Disease

Also known as mucocutaneous lymph node syndrome, Kawasaki disease is an acute infection of the mucous membranes and lymph glands that has been recognized as a separate entity only in the last 20 or so years. The disease seems to be on the rise, but it is difficult to know whether the increased reporting is due to better recognition or a real rise in incidence. The incidence is highest in Japan, but children of Asian background living in the United States (particularly Hawaii) and other countries are at increased risk as well. However, Kawasaki disease can affect children of any race or ethnic background.

Kawasaki disease primarily affects children under ten, and most patients are under age four. Boys are more likely to develop it than girls. The cause of the disease is unknown. Although outbreaks have been reported, there is no evidence of direct person-to-person transmission or spread by common attendance at social or recreational events. It is very rare that more than one child in a family will develop it.

Because the cause of Kawasaki disease has not been identified, there is no specific diagnostic test for it. Blood and urine tests can give some indication of infection. Beyond that, the doctor will examine the child, look for specific symptoms, and rule out other conditions.

In about 20 percent of cases, Kawasaki disease affects the heart. For the remainder of patients, it is simply an infectious disease that passes within a few weeks.

Typically, Kawasaki disease begins with a suddenly elevated temperature, usually over 102 degrees F. and spiking to 104–105 degrees F. several times daily. The child is often extremely irritable. Other symptoms begin to appear within three to five days after the onset of fever. These include red, cracked lips; strawberry-colored tongue and marked redness of the throat; deep red rash that can appear similar to hives, measles, or scarlet fever; swelling of hands and feet, with dark red or purple discoloration of palms and soles. Swelling of lymph glands on the side of the neck is frequently seen. Some children will have arthritic pain, abdominal discomfort, and/or diarrhea.

As the fever begins to subside, the other symptoms will usually disappear. About the second or third week the skin around the fingertips and toes and, eventually, the palms and soles, will peel, a painless process.

Some 40 percent of children with Kawasaki disease suffer arthritis or swelling of joints, particularly the knees, hips, and ankles. Although this is painful and may persist after the other symptoms have disappeared, it is not permanent.

Only the cardiac complications may become permanent. Approximately 20 percent of Kawasaki patients develop *aneurysms*, or balloonlike swellings, of the coronary arteries. Of that number, a very small proportion will be subject to heart attacks due to spontaneous clotting within dilated arteries. Other cardiac symptoms include pericarditis, cardiac muscle dysfunction or cardiac valve disease, manifested as congestive heart failure, rhythm disturbances, or new heart murmurs.

Aneurysms can be detected by echocardiogram, or ultrasound tests, which reveal the swollen arteries. Most children recover from this swelling. But angina pectoris, or chest pain, and recurrent heart attacks can evolve as a result of coronary clots, and chronic insufficiency of narrowing coronary arteries may result from this disease.

Early therapy for Kawasaki disease includes treating the individual symptoms and making the child as comfortable as possible. Hospitalization is required. The primary medication is aspirin to reduce fever, relieve joint pain, and prevent blood clotting, and intravenous gamma globulin, which is used to reduce the risk of developing cardiac complications.

SUMMING UP

WHILE CONGENITAL heart defects and other childhood heart-related illnesses can be serious, constantly improving medical and surgical intervention allow normal lives for the great majority of infants and youngsters afflicted by them.

Congenital heart defects take form as the heart develops in utero. Some of the more common defects are pulmonary and aortic stenoses, coarctation of the artery, atrial and ventricular septal defects, tetralogy of Fallot, and transposition of the great arteries. Early detection and diagnosis are vital to effective medical intervention.

Signs and symptoms that can occur in children with major heart defects include failure to thrive, tachycardia (abnormally rapid heartbeat), arrhythmia or dysrhythmia (irregular heartbeat), bradycardia (excessively slow heartbeat), congestive heart failure (failure of the heart to pump sufficient blood for normal bodily functions), edema (fluid accumulation), blueness (cyanosis), and endocarditis (infection of the heart wall, valves, or blood vessels).

Heart surgery to correct cardiac defects is common but complex and requires a highly skilled team of cardiovascular surgeons, cardiologists, anesthesiologists, nurses, and technologists, as well as sophisticated machines. The child will require further convalescence after discharge from the hospital. The pediatric cardiologist will continue monitoring the child's progress and the patient will be returned to the ongoing care of the pediatrician or family physician. Various agencies can be helpful in offering necessary services, such as home education and vocational counseling.

While many congenital heart patients will require continuing medical counsel and attention through adulthood, they can usually be expected to live active and normal lives.

Other early childhood heart-related diseases are high blood pressure, which can be controlled by medical treatment; hyperlipidemia, an excess of fats in the blood, which can cause heart disease in later years and which is treated by diet and, rarely, medication; rheumatic fever, which can occur after a streptococcal infection and can result in heart damage, but which can be prevented by treating streptococcal infections promptly; and Kawasaki disease, an acute infection of the mucous membranes and lymph nodes that sometimes has cardiac complications.

22 Childhood Respiratory Disorders

Robert B. Mellins, M.D.

INTRODUCTION

MOST OF THE energy that drives the metabolic process of the body, carrying out vital building and repair functions in each of its cells, is derived from oxygen. A major by-product of this body metabolism is carbon dioxide. Aided by the central nervous system and the circulatory system, the respiratory system is designed to direct the traffic of these two important molecules of life—oxygen and carbon dioxide. The lungs, which are contained in the chest bellows, play a central role in the respiratory process because they are the site at which oxygen from the air enters the body and from which carbon dioxide exits. The circulating blood is the major transport system, moving these important molecules of metabolism between the lungs and the cells of the body.

Breathing is controlled by the central nervous system and is both voluntary and involuntary: we can consciously regulate our breathing or we can breathe without thinking about it, as the central nervous system knows by sensing chemically when the body requires more oxygen or when it needs to blow off more carbon dioxide.

Then mechanisms of breathing (see figure 22.1, next page) begin with the *diaphragm*—a large flexible muscle below the lungs—and the muscles of the chest wall and abdomen. Breathing in *(inspiration)* is accomplished by the contraction of the diaphragm and chest wall muscles, which enlarges the volume of the *thorax* (chest), creating a partial vacuum, and draws air into the lungs.

Air is drawn into the airways through the nose or mouth or both. It travels first through the upper airway, which comprises the nose and mouth; the

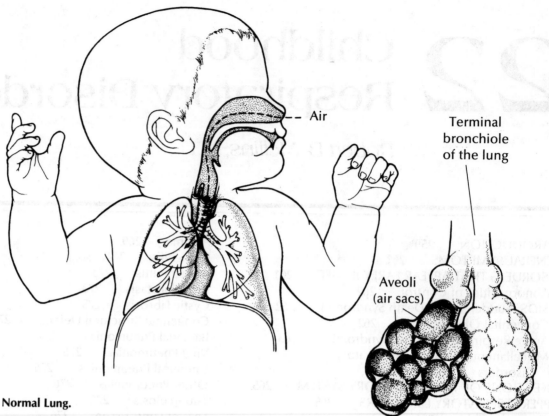

Figure 22.1. **The Normal Lung.**

throat, or *pharynx*, which extends from the back of the nose and mouth to the *larynx*; the larynx, which is the organ of speech located just below the base of the tongue at the top of the trachea; and the upper part of the trachea (before it descends into the protective cavity of the chest). From there the air continues into the lower airway, which comprises the remainder of the trachea, the two bronchi that fork off from the bottom of the trachea and feed into the two lungs, and the numerous subdivisions of the bronchi, including the smallest of the airways, the tiny bronchioles.

The bronchioles deliver the air to the *parenchyma* of the respiratory system. Parenchyma are those parts of any organ that are directly related to the function of the organ and are not just supportive or connective. In the case of the lungs, the parenchyma are the *alveoli*, tiny sacs that fill with air. There are millions of alveoli in the lungs and it is through them that the blood receives its oxygen and expels its carbon dioxide—the gas exchange that is the primary function of the respiratory system. This exchange is conducted through thin capillary walls that allow oxygen to diffuse into the blood and carbon dioxide to diffuse out while keeping the air separated from the blood.

When the gas exchange is complete, the now stale, carbon-dioxide-heavy air is expelled from the alveoli and the lungs by breathing out *(expiration)*. This is accomplished by relaxation of the diaphragm and chest wall, which then allows the natural tendency of the lungs to collapse much like an inflated balloon when the air has free access to escape. As the air escapes from the airways, the volume of the thorax and hence the lungs is reduced. When breathing needs to be very rapid or forceful, the abdominal muscle may help by contracting during expiration.

While the gas exchange is the primary function of the respiratory system, the lungs and airways perform other duties as well. As mentioned, the larynx is the organ of speech. Within it is the *glottis*—folds of tissue that we call vocal cords—that vibrates when air passes over it to produce sound. Above the glottis is the *epiglottis*, a sort of trapdoor that snaps shut over the larynx and glottis every time we swallow, channeling food and drink down the esophagus into the stomach, and keeping it from entering the trachea and lower part of the respiratory system.

The airways and lungs are also the body's first line of defense against infection and contaminants. The nose is lined with tiny hairs that filter the air and snare many infinitesimally small particles before they go any farther. If they do make it farther, the walls of all the airways, from the pharynx to the bronchioles, are lined with mucus that will also trap foreign material. The mucus, containing whatever contaminants it may have captured, is propelled continuously up, toward the pharynx, by means of tiny moving hairs called *cilia*. Once the mucus reaches the pharynx, it is either coughed out or swallowed (most often the latter case with children).

The other main role of the airways is temperature and moisture control. The alveoli in the lungs function best with warm, moist air. The airways will moisten dry air, heat up cool air, and cool down hot air, so that no matter what the air is like outside, by the time it reaches the lungs it is body temperature and moist.

The respiratory system, with its exposure to the outside world through the lungs, is the easiest point of entry for airborne bacteria and viruses. The special characteristics of newborn infants and young children can further complicate the potential for infection and trouble in the respiratory system. For one thing, while infants initially require more oxygen per pound of body weight than do adults, for some time after birth, their respiratory system is not as advanced as an adult's: in the lungs the alveoli are still not fully mature; the central nervous system's control of breathing is still being perfected, and the airways are smaller and easier to obstruct.

This chapter will outline the various respiratory disorders that children face, beginning with the specific problems of the newborn and continuing with a look at each of the major areas of the respiratory system and their related problems.

GENERAL SYMPTOMS

OVERALL there are some general, basic signs and symptoms of a respiratory disorder in children. Any one or combination of the following merits further attention: anxiety or restlessness (often a sign of too little oxygen), dyspnea (shortness of breath), tachypnea (rapid breathing), extra respiratory sounds (most commonly stridor, a high-pitched, harsh, almost musical tone, produced in the larynx during inspiration), cough, fever, chest pain, and cyanosis (a bluish tinge to lips and fingernail beds, caused by the blood's not getting enough oxygen).

The basic treatment for mild respiratory disorders in children is rest and adequate liquids. No one has ever proved that rest is important—and in children, bed rest is impossible—though most doctors feel that keeping children relatively quiet is a good idea. Activity, however, can increase depth of breathing, which may help dislodge mucus and thus be good chest physical therapy. There is no evidence that forcing fluids is beneficial and may in fact be counterproductive in asthma. However, it is important to provide sufficient fluids to prevent dehydration.

Most commonly, airways are obstructed by mucus, and the child's coughing will often be enough to clear it out. Postural positioning—angling the child so that gravity aids the expulsion of mucus—can also be helpful. Acetaminophen should only be given if the child has a fever. Some cases may warrant drugs that dilate the bronchial airways to allow air through, reduce inflammation and swelling (usually corticosteroids and more recently sodium cromoglycate), or combat specific infections (penicillin for bacterial pneumonia is the most well known). Some respiratory disorders require the inhalation of oxygen.

If the disorder is more acute and obstruction of the airways is severe, it may be necessary to insert a tube down the nose or throat into the trachea to provide an open air passage. In very severe cases, the doctor may find it necessary to perform a tracheostomy, surgically creating a passage for air directly through the skin in the neck into the trachea. Respiration may be assisted using mechanical ventilators connected to nasotracheal or tracheostomy tubes.

While respiratory disorders are among the most common ailments a child will face, and while the vast majority of children will never suffer anything worse than the usual cold or flu, any respiratory infection can be potentially serious and must be closely monitored.

DISORDERS THAT APPEAR EARLY IN LIFE

THE RESPIRATORY SYSTEM is not fully mature at birth. While the main division of the bronchi will be completed in the fetus during the first 16 weeks, the alveoli—vital to the gas exchange process—are the last part of the lung to develop and continue to develop well after birth. Therefore, the respiratory system may be vulnerable during the neonatal period (defined as extending from the time of birth to one month of age).

Before birth, the oxygen and carbon dioxide exchange is performed for the fetus by the placenta. During this period, the lungs are filled with liquid. During birth, most of this liquid is expelled when the baby's chest is squeezed as he or she passes through the birth canal, and some is absorbed by the lymphatic and blood vessels. With the baby's first breath, the chest expands and sucks in air.

The first breath is difficult, but inflation of the lungs should be complete within a few breaths and most of the alveoli should be expanded within the first hour. The baby will begin taking deep breaths within about 30 seconds of birth, and after 90 minutes or so should be taking 30 to 60 breaths per minute.

About 10 percent of live births, however, can't make the transition from womb to outside world so smoothly or so quickly. Sometimes they do not breathe fully and are just mildly asphyxiated (cyanosis—bluing of the extremities—is a key sign). Contrary to common belief, the baby is not slapped, but rather, is dried vigorously with a towel and oxygen may be blown over the nose and mouth. Babies that are asphyxiated usually respond to oxygen from a bag and mask, although occasionally a tracheal tube will be necessary. Rarely, a catheter will be inserted into the blood vessels of the umbilical cord to test the baby's blood and administer drugs and more blood if necessary. The progress of infants who have suffered severe respiratory problems at birth is usually followed for several years to see if there has been any long-term damage. In general the recuperative power of the young lung, including compensatory lung growth, is striking.

Abnormalities of Control

The central nervous system controls breathing, triggering another breath when chemical sensors tell it that the blood needs more oxygen. This mechanism, however, may not function completely smoothly in the neonatal period.

Apnea. This is the term for occasional respiratory pauses or cessation of breathing. It is especially common in infants born preterm. It has many causes: infection; respiratory distress; disorders of the metabolic, cardiovascular, or central nervous systems; or the mother's use of, or withdrawal from, drugs. Although apnea early in life, especially of the preterm infant, may disappear spontaneously, it can be a sign of a serious underlying condition and should be brought to the attention of the pediatrician, especially if the infant also suffers from *periodic breathing*—repetitive episodes of waxing and waning of breathing separated by brief respiratory pauses. Periodic breathing often stops if the infant is given oxygen to breathe.

SIDS (Sudden Infant Death Syndrome)

Every year, 10,000 infants between the age of one week and a year are the victims of this unpredictable and fatal disorder. It is the single largest killer of young children after the newborn period and takes the lives of roughly one in every 300 to 400 infants. Characteristically, a baby is put to bed at night apparently healthy and found dead in the morning (hence the colloquial term for the disorder: crib death). At some point during the intervening hours, the baby, for some unknown reason, stops breathing.

While more and more is being discovered about SIDS each year, its cause (or causes) is still not completely understood. There has been no firm evidence that it is caused by any sort of infection. While a popular current hypothesis focuses on abnormalities in cardiorespiratory control, the chain of events leading to death remains elusive. Other theories cite an undiscovered mild to moderate congenital airway obstruction, dedicated nose breathing (many babies do not know to breathe through their mouths for some time) or long periods of REM sleep. Sometimes a baby is found not breathing and can be resuscitated. However, the relationship between these cases of apnea, sometimes referred to as near-SIDS cases (or ALTE—an apparently life-threatening event), and SIDS has not been determined. Furthermore, the majority of children who die of SIDS do not have a history of prior apneic episodes.

Statistically it is known that more boys die of SIDS than girls; that low birthweight and mother's smoking are two predisposing factors; and although no genetic link has been found for SIDS, it is more likely to occur in a family where there has already been a SIDS death. While it can happen at any time and to any family, it arises more often in colder months and in families of lower socioeconomic status. As there is no known cause of the disorder, there is no known treatment. There are devices that can monitor sleeping babies and sound an alarm if there is any cessation of breathing or slowing of the heart rate. These have been found to be useful for the preterm infant with frequent episodes of prolonged apnea and slowing of the heartbeat. Their efficacy in preventing SIDS remains uncertain.

Congenital Obstructions

Congenital obstructions can occur anywhere along the respiratory tract and in most cases they are serious. *Choanal atresia* is blockage at the back of the nose that occurs in twice as many female infants as male. The obstructions are usually bony (90 percent), although occasionally membranous. Both nostrils must be blocked for it to pose a serious problem. The problem is relieved by converting the baby from a nose breather to a mouth breather, then surgically removing the obstruction and keeping it from growing over. Once corrected, it should have no impact on the infant's normal development.

With the *Pierre-Robin anomaly*, the newborn infant's jawbone is too small for the tongue, allowing it to fall back and obstruct the pharynx, potentially causing asphyxiation. In most cases the solution is to modify how the baby is positioned, held, and fed, as the jaw will usually grow to normal size within two to four years. Occasionally, in more severe cases, surgery is required.

Laryngeal Obstructions. These obstructions can take many forms. Complete obstruction, or birth without a larynx, is incompatible with life. Partial obstruction will cause stridor, a high-pitched noise synchronous with inspirations. The obstruction may be caused by *laryngeal webs* (portions of false vocal cords that remain fused and must be surgically removed), cysts (rare, also requiring surgery), paralysis of the vocal cords (one side or both), or even by clogging of an endotracheal tube that may have been put in place to aid breathing shortly after birth. *Tracheal* and *bronchial obstructions* are also possible, and may take the form of cysts or congenital narrowings. These sometimes can be successfully corrected through surgery.

When there is severe narrowing of a long segment of the trachea or bronchi, surgery may not be possible for technical reasons. Finally, some children are born with a relatively soft trachea that is prone to collapse, especially in the area of the larynx, leading to prominent stridor and chest retractions. When there are no other abnormalities, they may gradually improve over the first year of life as the trachea becomes stiffer and less likely to collapse.

Acute Respiratory Distress Syndromes

Hyaline Membrane Disease. This is the most common cause of acute respiratory distress in the newborn, occurring within the first few days after birth, affecting 1 percent of newborn infants. Until 1970, it was the leading cause of neonatal death, taking more than 25,000 lives a year. At that time more than 50 percent of infants with the disease died. Now, with the incredible advances in neonatal care that have been achieved over the past two decades, 80 to 90 percent of infants with the disease survive.

Hyaline membrane disease usually attacks infants born prematurely with immature lungs. Their lungs are often low in surfactant, a soaplike substance that lines the alveoli and reduces the surface tension, thus keeping them from collapsing, especially at low lung volume (as at the end of expira-

tion). Without this surfactant, the alveoli will collapse and not retain air long enough for the oxygen/carbon dioxide gas exchange to take place completely.

Infants with the disease will often exhibit symptoms in the first few hours after birth. Breathing will be increasingly labored as parts of the lungs cease functioning. Cyanosis will develop. For most mild to moderate cases, breathing will continue to be increasingly difficult for 48 hours. After 72 hours of intensive neonatal care, however, the trouble should begin to ease and there should be rapid improvement. The lungs are usually normal within a month, although infants who were more severely affected by the disease and who required mechanical respiration and high levels of supplemental oxygen may take longer to recover (more because of problems associated with mechanical respiration and oxygen than because of the disease itself) and may suffer some long-term effects.

There are predisposing factors for hyaline membrane disease other than premature birth. It occurs in males twice as often as females. The children of diabetic mothers are five times more likely to contract it than the children of nondiabetic mothers. And, infants born through cesarean section, especially if performed before labor sets in, are more likely candidates than babies delivered vaginally.

Two major developments in neonatal care have resulted in decreased mortality and morbidity: the use of constant positive airway pressure during the entire breathing cycle to minimize lung collapse and the use of surfactants administered through the trachea to supplement inadequate or replace defective supplies.

Delayed Absorption of Fetal Lung Fluid. Most of the fetal lung fluid is usually expelled when the infant's chest is compressed while passing through the birth canal. The rest is then usually absorbed into the body within minutes. If it is not, it can block normal respiration, leading to grunting and mild cyanosis. It is most prevalent in males, and those with histories of premature births, cesarean section deliveries, and breech births. Unless the child's lungs are immature and hyaline membrane disease develops, there is usually no long-term problem (oxygen may be required for a short while), as the fluid is absorbed within 24 hours and the symptoms disappear.

Meconium Aspiration. This occurs in 6 percent of live births and accounts for 1.8 percent of all perinatal deaths. Meconium, which accumulates in the fetal intestine, is the breakdown product of swallowed amniotic fluid, fetal hair, gastrointestinal secretions, and mucus. It can be expelled into the amniotic fluid and aspirated during birth; it is especially irritating to the lungs, leading to obstruction of the respiratory tract. If during delivery doctors notice that the amniotic fluid is stained with meconium, they will withdraw or suction out any meconium they find in the nose, mouth, throat, and trachea, and then gently expand the lungs. In more serious cases of meconium aspiration, mechanical respiration may be required.

Miscellaneous Neonatal Respiratory Disorders

Pulmonary Hemorrhage. This occurs 1 to 4 times in every 1,000 live births and accounts for 9 percent of newborn deaths, usually within the first 48 hours. Bleeding in and around the alveoli can fill up to one-third of the lung and severely impair respiration. It often occurs concurrently with bleeding elsewhere. Most infants with pulmonary hemorrhage have symptoms undistinguishable from those of hyaline membrane disease. The cause is unknown and treatment remains supportive.

Pulmonary Edema. As its name implies, this is the result of a buildup of fluids in the lungs when the lymphatic channels are overloaded, impairing the gas exchange. Two types of pulmonary edema are recognized: (1) *hemodynamic,* resulting from elevation of the pressure in the blood vessels in the lungs (sometimes as the result of heart disease) and (2) *permeability edema,* resulting from certain infections (usually severe) in which the integrity of the delicate membrane containing the walls of the air sacs and their capillaries are physically injured.

Pulmonary Air Leaks. These are relatively common and can cause serious problems. The most common is *pneumothorax,* which arises when air leaks into the pleural space between the lungs and the chest cavity, breaking the seal and collapsing a lung. (See figure 22.2.) This occurs most often in infants already affected by disorders such as meconium aspiration and hyaline membrane disease. There can be leaks in other areas, but only pneumothorax requires treatment (withdrawal of the air by needle), because the air can build up under tension, pushing the heart to the opposite side and compromising the flow of blood through the lungs.

Neonatal Pneumonia. This is very serious and frequently leads to death. It is most often caused by streptococcal bacteria inhaled at birth and is the principal cause of severe neonatal infection, affecting two to three births per thousand. Of those, one-half develop fulminating pneumonia, and of those,

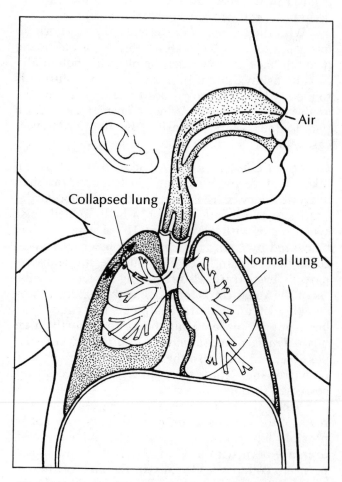

Figure 22.2. **A Pneumothorax (Collapsed Lung).**

only 25 percent are expected to survive. It is often hard to distinguish from hyaline membrane disease. The infant is usually very sick within six hours of birth. Treatment consists of large doses of antibiotics, some oxygen (to ward off cyanosis), and other drugs.

Other Abnormalities. These include obstructions caused by abnormalities of the heart and major arteries, which can be so big they impinge on normal respiratory function, and congenital *diaphragmatic hernias* (one in every 2,000 births); because the latter allows the intestines to move into the chest, compressing the lung during development in utero, the lungs may be severely underdeveloped. Surgery early in life is often required.

Tracheoesophageal Fistula. In the commonest form of this congenital abnormality the esophagus ends in a blind pouch so that there is no direct entry possible into the stomach. In addition there is a false passage between the airways and the stomach, so that naturally occurring acid from the stomach can regurgitate into the lung, causing serious injury. For these reasons early recognition and surgical correction is essential to avoid irreversible pulmonary damage.

INFECTIONS OF THE RESPIRATORY SYSTEM

INFECTIONS MAY STRIKE any part of the respiratory system. Based on symptoms and findings on physical examinations, physicians use a bewildering number of terms to indicate the site of infection. The initial separation is between upper and lower respiratory infections. Starting at the nose and mouth, there are infections of the sinuses (sinusitis), throat (pharyngitis), the entry to the trachea or epiglottis (epiglottitis), the vocal cords (laryngitis), the wind pipe or trachea (tracheitis), larger airways or bronchi (bronchitis), smaller airways or bronchioli (bronchiolitis), and the remainder of the lung consisting primarily of the tiny sacs involved in oxygen and carbon dioxide transfer (pneumonia). Sometimes more than one area is involved (in croup, for example, which is sometimes called laryngotracheobronchitis). Although the common cold is referred to as an upper respiratory infection, there is evidence that the lower respiratory tract may be involved even though clinically silent.

When the airways are irritated by infection or other causes, nerves in the walls are stimulated, leading to a cough. Further irritation or inflammation may stimulate the airways to produce increased mucus (phlegm) or may stimulate the muscles surrounding the airways to constrict, producing bronchospasm or wheezing. The former is often referred to as bronchitis, the latter as asthma, but there is considerable variability in how physicians apply these terms. Because these symptoms may represent a wide spectrum of the same condition, there is an increasing tendency to refer to this spectrum as reactive airways disease.

UPPER RESPIRATORY DISORDERS

ONE CHARACTERISTIC of the upper airways is that they tend to constrict and narrow slightly during inspiration (and dilate and expand during expiration). For this reason, any further narrowing of the airways potentially threatens the child's ability to get air into the lungs.

The most common upper respiratory infections are a manifestation of the most common disease—the cold.

Common Cold

The generic "upper respiratory infection" (URI) is caused by one of over 100 viruses that settle into one stretch of the upper respiratory tract or another, causing irritation and inflammation of the delicate membranes lining the upper air passages and an accelerated production of mucus. The infection is named by where it appears: *rhinitis* (the nasal passages and the back of the nose), *pharyngitis* (the back of the mouth leading to what we commonly call a "sore throat"), and *laryngitis* (which, when most acute, can bring on a temporary loss of speech).

The common cold is indeed common. People often get one or more per year throughout their lives. Young children often experience six to nine colds per year, which accounts for the fact that many parents complain that their children are always sick. Colds are spread by infected persons when they talk, cough, or sneeze, or through contact. Most colds are caught during the winter months, not only because chilling appears to be a predisposing factor, but also because people are more likely to be indoors in close proximity to one another. Being tired and having a poor diet are also thought to make one more susceptible to colds, but the evidence for this widely held view is slim at best.

Children, of course, get many more colds than adults. The symptoms will start to appear one to three days after the virus has taken hold, and will begin with a scratchy or sore throat, runny or congested nose, and with or without low-grade fever. When it takes hold in the respiratory tract and virus-fighting mucus accumulates, the child will often begin coughing to clear the mucus.

The only known "cure" for the common cold is common sense: acetaminophen to bring down the fever and adequate liquids. Although a variety of medicines including many nonprescription ones have been traditionally used for colds, they have rarely been subjected to well-controlled double-blind studies, so that their efficacy remains in doubt. They may, however, provide some symptomatic relief. Some of the most common types and their potential benefits and limitations are listed in the accompanying box on medicines for colds. One caution: a persistent cough may be the result of hyperactive airways disease or asthma triggered by colds, and may respond better to other medicines discussed later in this chapter.

Colds will usually pass in a few days and pose no threat to the respiratory system themselves.

MEDICINES FOR COLDS

While there are no cures for the common cold, non-prescription medicines can help lessen the effects of the symptoms such as cough, sore throat, fever, and congestion. There are several basic ingredients that are found, in various combinations, in most cold preparations.

Analgesics/Antipyretics

Acetaminophen is used to lower fever and to reduce aches and pains. Aspirin should not be used if a child is already taking anticoagulant medicine or has a bleeding disorder. It also should not be used to treat symptoms of flu, chicken pox, or other viral infection because of a possible link to Reye's syndrome.

Anticholinergics

These are used to help dry up nasal and sinus secretions by reducing the amount of mucus produced. Whether they are sometimes counterproductive by causing plugging or clogging remains unknown.

Antihistamines

Primarily used to treat allergic reaction, antihistamines may reduce the amount of mucus secreted, drying up the nose and sinuses, and reducing sneezing and runny nose. However, they are of limited usefulness with children, and may even make the situation worse by inducing drowsiness or irritability.

Antitussives

While they may quiet coughing, antitussives can also cause considerable drowsiness. Since cough is basically a protective mechanism, there may be hazards from using excessive amounts of cough medicines. If cough persists, causes other than the common cold should be sought.

Decongestants

As their name suggests, decongestants relieve nasal and sinus congestion. Often administered in spray form, they work by shrinking swollen mucus tissues. However, if used for more than a few days, they may actually produce a chemical irritation causing the passages to become congested again. Some of the newer sprays contain cromalyn or steroids and may be useful for allergic rhinitis.

Expectorants

In cases where the bronchi and bronchioles are congested, expectorants are widely believed to help loosen the mucus clogging them, so that coughing will work to clear the passages. Their efficacy also remains in doubt.

In general, the effects of these cold medicines are not dramatic, and yet they may reduce discomfort. The best bet for treating a cold still seems to be rest, acetaminophen for fever, and adequate liquids. If any medicines are taken, the cardinal rules are: *Check with your doctor to see what your child can and cannot take (certain conditions, allergies, and other medicines rule out the use of certain cold preparations)* and *follow the instructions on the package exactly, unless otherwise specifically instructed by the child's doctor. For infants, normal saline nosedrops are all that need be used. These are available without prescription and are both useful and safe.*

Their only danger is in taxing the immune system and lowering the body's resistance to other, more serious viral and bacterial infections such as pneumonia (discussed later), strep throat (an acute form of pharyngitis caused by streptococcal bacteria, which must be treated with antibiotics), whooping cough (a dangerous bacterial infection, now mostly eradicated by early immunization), and croup.

Croup

There are several types of croup, all of which result in inflammation or swelling of the membranes lining the larynx, trachea, or bronchi. They are all characterized by a stridorous or loud, noisy respiratory sound during inspiration, as well as a barking or brassy cough and hoarseness. The severity of croup can range from a mild viral case that lasts three to four days, to fulminating acute epiglottitis, which can completely obstruct the airway. Because croup is often quite insidious in its onset and appears deceptively mild it must be followed closely by both parents and pediatrician for signs of excessive airway obstruction. Obstruction is manifested by chest retractions (sucking in of the skin above and below the sternum or between the ribs) and irritability and fatigue as a herald of respiratory failure.

Viral Croup. This disease most often afflicts children between six months and three years in age and is most prevalent during the winter months. The child may have the infection two or three days before developing croupy or stridorous breathing.

There may be a low-grade fever and the infection may spread to the lower respiratory tract, but the child will often not appear all that ill. Indeed, in most cases, he or she won't be.

If the child is having little or no trouble breathing, and the pediatrician agrees, intake of adequate liquids and humidified air at home is usually sufficient treatment and the illness should pass within a few days. If, however, breathing is labored and the child shows any sign of oxygen deficiency (blue lips or fingertips), then he or she will have to be hospitalized. In the hospital, usually the child will receive humid air, and perhaps oxygen as well, delivered in a croup tent. Special drugs given by aerosol that shrink edematious or swollen membranes and relax the airways may help open up the narrowed passages.

Acute Epiglottitis. This bacterial rather than viral infection, caused by *H. influenzae* type B, usually afflicts children over the age of three. It requires prompt and aggressive treatment as it can progress from stridor to complete obstruction of the airway in from four to twelve hours. Once the diagnosis is made (usually after a quick examination to determine that epiglottitis is indeed the cause of the obstruction) a tube is placed in the trachea without delay and the child is put in intensive care and given appropriate antibiotics as well as oxygen. Sometimes an emergency tracheotomy is required. As serious as this sounds, and as serious as it is, if treated quickly it is rarely fatal. Children with epiglottitis act sick and usually drool because it hurts them to swallow.

Spasmodic Croup. This occurs repeatedly, usually at night, with severe obstruction usually lasting only a few hours. It is like viral croup in that its targets are young children and it can often be treated at home. One common household cure is to put the child in the bathroom with a hot running shower to breathe the steam. Use of prescribed aerosol inhalators that shrink swollen membranes and thus open the airways more widely may also speed the passing of the attack. If breathing is quite labored and continues to be so, an emergency visit to the hospital may be necessary. Often, in such a case, parents and doctors have noted that by the time the child reaches the hospital he or she may be over the worst of the obstruction, having been helped by the cool night air. Why such apparently diverse therapies as steam or cool air should be effective is not clear.

Diphtheritic Croup. This is fairly rare because of widespread immunization and is only considered in cases where the child has been hospitalized for several days with acute infectious croup, looks very ill, and hasn't been immunized against diphtheria, making it a possibility. As with epiglottitis, treatment must be immediate and aggressive, in this case using both a diphtheria antitoxin and antibiotics.

Other Disorders

Infants can be born with some form of airway obstruction—such as laryngeal webs, fused false vocal cords, or tumors or cysts. Most of these will be self-limiting and will not require medical attention, while others may necessitate surgery.

Children may acquire infections that are not specifically respiratory infections, but that may create difficulty breathing. For example, with tonsillitis and adenoiditis, the enlarged and inflamed tonsils or adenoids may obstruct the airway, especially during sleep; thus their effects on respiration must be considered.

LOWER RESPIRATORY DISORDERS

THE LOWER AIRWAYS consist of the lower end of the trachea, the bronchi, and the bronchioles. In direct contrast to the upper airways, lower airways are within the chest and hence tend to constrict and narrow during expiration and widen and expand during inspiration. If the narrowing is exaggerated in any way, a condition can arise where air can easily enter but not so easily leave: this air trapping produces an overinflated lung or part of a lung (lobe), a condition known as *lobar emphysema*. If the air trapping and hyperinflation is severe, the over-expanded lung may press on other contents of the chest, causing a medical emergency. When obstruction is complete, the lung in that area will be deprived of the normal cleansing movements of mucus, making it prone to infection and collapse or airlessness (atelectasis).

Other than congenital structural defects, there are four main types of problems that can develop in the lower airways: the aspiration of foreign bodies, inflammation, bronchoconstriction, and edema (a buildup of fluids).

Foreign Bodies

Infants and young children will put anything to their lips that they can get their hands on. If it is small enough to fit in their mouths, it may be small enough to be aspirated. Out of 1,000 cases of foreign-body aspiration covered in one study, bones accounted for 20 percent of the items swallowed; hardware, 15 percent; nuts, 14 percent; coins, 14 percent; and safety pins, 11 percent. Peanuts are especially dangerous because they are smooth and can slip into the airways; they produce an especially destructive chemical irritation of the airways and surrounding lung.

Large objects can partially or completely block the large airways and often quickly cause acute respiratory distress. Often they can be removed by placing the child head down and applying a firm blow to the back. They may require the use of *bronchoscopy* (the insertion of a tube into the airways) or even surgery for removal.

Smaller objects can go farther into the respiratory system and may not be so immediately noticeable. Unbeknownst to a parent, a small aspirated object can block off a portion of a lung. The first symptoms might be a cough and a mild fever. Infection and abscess may develop, along with hyperinflation or emphysema.

That this is being caused by an aspirated foreign object will only become apparent from a chest X ray, and only then if the object is radio-opaque (shows up on X ray). Non-radio-opaque objects such as pumpkin seeds, nuts, and popcorn are very hard to see and may only be suspected by their effects on the lung, for instance, overinflation, partial lung collapse (atelectasis), or recurrent infection or pneumonia. Complications due to infection and inflammation may remain for long periods even after the small foreign body is removed.

Parents should keep all small objects that may be potentially aspirated out of the hands of their children, and they should be particularly vigilant about insisting that children be still and not jump around while eating.

Influenza

Influenza, commonly called the flu, is an acute respiratory illness that is caused by two viruses: Types A and B, with many different subtypes. Influenza A is the most frequent cause of the illness and the one responsible for most of the epidemics, outbreaks that are confined to a region—whether that be a city, county, or country. Epidemics of influenza A usually occur every two to four years. Pandemics (outbreaks that start in one area, but extend to all parts of the world) are caused by new strains of the virus to which few people have an immunity.

While the symptoms of influenza can mimic those of other viruses, for example, the common cold, there are two features of flu that distinguish it from other diseases: it occurs in epidemics and it can result in death from pulmonary complications.

(The greatest pandemic of influenza occurred in 1918–19. Worldwide it was responsible for 21 million deaths; with 549,000 dying from the disease in the United States.)

Often the first indication of a flu epidemic is the increased number of children with febrile respiratory illnesses. A pattern of increased school absenteeism of young children is a later indication of a flu epidemic.

Flu is spread via respiratory secretions when an infected person sneezes, coughs, or talks. The influenza A virus appears to favor low relative humidity and low temperatures, which may explain why outbreaks occur almost exclusively in the winter months. (In the Northern Hemisphere the flu season is between October and April; in the Southern Hemisphere, it occurs from May through September.) The virus attaches itself to the lining of the respiratory tract and begins replicating itself. After an incubation period that varies from 18 to 72 hours, symptoms appear.

The onset of influenza A or B is abrupt, with symptoms of fever, chills, headaches, muscle aches, lethargy, and a dry cough. Fevers in children can reach as high as 104 degrees F. Small infants may only exhibit a fever, cough, and fussiness. While these systemic symptoms usually last for three days, the usual duration of the fever, they may last anywhere from one to five days. Less common symptoms involve the eye and include tearing, burning, and pain. Although the incidence of flu is higher in children (presumably because they have less immunity against strains of the virus) than it is in adults, the incidence of pulmonary complications among children is lower than it is for the general population.

A diagnosis of flu in a child is most often made by a parent, who is aided by the knowledge that the illness is "going around." There is no specific treatment for a child with flu, except bed rest, and restricted activity for 24 to 48 hours after the fever has subsided. To control the fever, acetaminophen (but not aspirin) can be given. The child should be given plenty of fluids to prevent dehydration. Steam may be helpful in relieving nasal congestion.

Most cases of flu in children resolve themselves within five days with no complications. Occasional secondary complications include bronchial pneumonia and otitis media (an infection of the middle ear), most often caused by the bacteria *Staphylococcus aureus*. These should be treated with appropriate antibiotics. Bacterial infections should be suspected if the cough persists or the fever remains elevated for more than four days. Primary complications are rare but can include encephalitis (a serious disease caused by a virus infecting and inflaming the brain cells) and myocarditis (an inflammation of the heart muscle). Viral pneumonia, which was responsible for many of the deaths during the pandemic of 1918–19 is also an occasional complication and usually occurs during a pandemic of influenza A, and mostly afflicts children suffering from cardiovascular disease. There have been outbreaks of Reye's syndrome among children during influenza B epidemics. Because the possibilities for serious complications do exist, any child with flu should be carefully watched. Symptoms that warrant medical attention include febrile convulsions, chest pain, and a continued fever.

Improvements in the flu vaccine have increased its effectiveness while reducing the frequency and severity of its side effects. Still, vaccination is not appropriate for all children; it is only recommended for those with chronic respiratory or cardiovascular disease. The vaccine should be given in the fall. Immunity develops in about two weeks, lasts only one or two years, and extends only to specific strains of the virus. Children are more likely than others to experience a local or systemic reaction to the vaccine; however, this is not common and most reactions are minor.

The prescription drug amantadine can prevent infection (especially in individuals who have been immunized) from influenza A. It is not effective against influenza B. During an epidemic of influenza A, it may be given to children who are at high risk, especially those who have come into contact with infected persons. Such prophylactic use can extend to members of a family with a high-risk child, whose members have been exposed to the virus. During an epidemic, children who are at high risk (those with chronic cardiovascular or respiratory diseases) who have not been vaccinated, should be vaccinated while they are receiving amantadine. The dosage for young children must be administered by a doctor according to body weight. If the vaccine is given, the drug should be discontinued after three weeks. Children who have not received the vaccination may have to receive amantadine for the duration of the epidemic, which usually lasts around two months.

Asthma

Asthma is a condition that is characterized by chronic, recurring obstruction of the airways. It differs from most other chronic lung conditions in that the airway obstruction is reversible, either spontaneously or as the result of treatment. The primary symptoms during an attack are shortness of breath, wheezing, and coughing; the severity of symptoms ranges from mild and almost undetectable to severe and unremitting, as in status asthmaticus, the most severe, but fortunately less common, form of the disease.

Asthma is the most common chronic lung disorder seen in children in this country. Depending on how the disease is defined, there are approximately 9.7 million asthmatic patients in the United States, and 3 million of these are under 18 years of age.

Although the death rate from asthma in those over 65 has increased from 1979 to 1987, it has remained relatively constant in those 5 to 35 years old. In 1987, the death rate for blacks was nearly twice that of whites; among 10- to 19-year-olds, the death rate for blacks was three to nine times that of whites. In children, hospitalization for asthma has increased more than four-fold.

In 1983, there were 459,000 hospitalizations for asthma, and the large majority of these were children. The disease is somewhat more common among males; it is also more common among people living below the poverty level and among persons in the South and West.

Generally, but not always, there will be a family history of asthma. Often there is also a history of atopy (allergies) in several family members. What has made the relationship between allergy and asthma difficult to determine is the observation that one can have allergies without asthma, asthma without apparent allergies and, of course, often both together. Thus, the demonstration that a child is sensitive to a particular substance (for example, a particular food) as judged by skin tests, does not prove that the child's asthma is caused by that food allergy.

About half of the youngsters with childhood asthma will develop the disease before the age of three. Asthma tends to be more serious in children who develop it at this early age, especially if they have frequent episodes of wheezing in the first year of the disease. Many asthmatic children tend to lose the manifestations of the disease with age; for example, youngsters who develop the asthma after the age of three are often free of symptoms by the age of ten. The disease may, however, recur during adulthood.

A Modern View of an Old Disease. When the airways are injured and the membrane lining of the airways becomes inflamed, nerves in the walls of the airways are stimulated, producing coughing. Airway injury and inflammation also stimulate the mucous glands in the walls of the airways to produce more mucus or "phlegm," which in turn leads to a loose cough that brings up mucus-containing sputum. Finally the inflammation may stimulate the muscles in the walls of the airways to contract, narrowing the lumen of the airways, making it difficult for air to move in and out of the airways and producing wheezing. Traditionally when there is only coughing or coughing with sputum, physicians have referred to the condition as bronchitis (literally inflammation of the airways), and when there is also wheezing, they have called it asthma. In adults, this distinction is still made since bronchitis and emphysema result in lung destruction while asthma is a reversible condition. In children, physicians now believe that these are all part of a spectrum of the same conditions and refer to the spectrum as reactive airways disease. For reasons not fully understood those who get reactive airways disease have airways that hyperreact when injured or inflamed.

What Happens During an Attack.

In recent years, a great deal has been learned about the changes that take place in the airways of people with asthma. At one time, it was thought that a tightening or spasm of the bronchial smooth muscles was the major factor in producing symptoms. Although bronchospasm, due to increased bronchial responsiveness to such stimuli as viral infections, exercise, allergens, cold air, noxious fumes, among many others, is generally present, it is now recognized that other factors can contribute to the airway obstruction. For example, there is an increased manufacture of thick tenacious mucus, which contributes to the airway obstruction. Injury to the epithelial cells that line the inner surface of the airways may destroy cilia, the tiny hair-like cells whose rhythmic beating helps cleanse the airway of mucus and other debris. Injured epithelial cells also may be shed into the airways, thus thickening the bronchial secretions and further clogging the airways. Inflammation of the cells lining the airway stimulates the release of potent chemical substances or medication which magnify the amount of inflammation, leading to swelling or edema of the airway mucous membranes. Inflammation within the airway walls is now known to be a major factor in the asthmatic process because it sets in motion a vicious cycle. The inflammation induces increased bronchoconstriction and the release of powerful chemical mediators, which in turn causes further injury to cells within the airways, resulting in increased inflammation and so on. (See table 22.1 for a listing of early warning signs.)

The events described earlier lead to the coughing and wheezing that is characteristic of asthma. In addition to the increased difficulty in getting air into the lungs, it is also harder to exhale, leading to a buildup of stale air within the chest. Early on, there is incomplete oxygenation of the blood. The body responds by "overbreathing," but as the ob-

Table 22.1 **EARLY WARNING SIGNS OF ASTHMA**

Cough
Tight chest
Wheezing
Labored breathing
Increased amount of mucus coughed up

struction becomes more severe, this may no longer be possible, leading to respiratory failure.

Acute Versus Chronic Asthma.

The fact that the airways of those who have asthma hyperreact to a variety of stimuli even during periods of no symptoms indicates that asthma is a chronic condition. In the past the focus has been to care for the asthma attacks, and consequently the treatment has been episodic. More recently physicians have begun treating individuals between acute attacks as well in an attempt to decrease the frequency and severity of acute episodes as well as the degree of hyperreactivity. Thus, as discussed below, regular programs of treatment are found to be more effective in the long run.

Establishing a Diagnosis.

Asthma is not the only condition that produces coughing, wheezing, and noisy or labored breathing. Before establishing a diagnosis of asthma, it is important to eliminate other possible disorders that produce similar symptoms. These include congenital lung defects, bronchiolitis, cystic fibrosis, pneumonia, an inhaled foreign object, and swollen tonsils and adenoids. If there is any doubt as to the diagnosis, the child may undergo a challenge test in which he or she is exposed either to a suspected asthma trigger (for example, exercise or cold air) or methacholine, a substance that produces bronchial constriction.

Asthma-Triggering Factors.

An attack of asthma can be triggered by a wide variety of inciting agents, which may be a specific allergen, a nonspecific irritant, exercise, environmental factors (including cold air), certain medications (including aspirin), and an infection (usually a respiratory virus). Because asthma threatens the ability to breathe it may induce fear and panic. Many specialists believe this may increase the severity of the attack. However, it is extremely difficult to find conclusive evidence that psychological and emotional factors initiate the asthma episode. There is considerable debate among experts regarding the relative role of each type of agent in producing asthma, and the extent to which each factor provokes an attack depends upon the individual person and the offending agent.

Respiratory infections and allergies are common triggering factors in all age groups; occupational factors are common triggering factors in adults. The role of indoor and outdoor pollution is ill-defined but could be very important.

At times, it may seem that virtually everything can provoke an attack of asthma. Very often, however, specific triggering factors can be identified and steps taken to avoid or minimize exposure to them. Some triggering factors are more universal and irritating than others. For example, cigarette smoke will worsen most asthma, and it is important that parents of an asthmatic child maintain a smoke-free home environment. Animal dander is another common triggering factor, and one that asthma specialists find particularly hard to eliminate. Understandably, most people find it difficult to part with a beloved pet, such a dog, cat or even bird. Since one can never be certain whether a child will develop sensitivity or allergy to animal dander, it is prudent that an asthmatic child not live in a household with a furry or feathered pet.

Identifying triggering factors can be difficult and time-consuming. Skin tests and other tests for specific allergens may be useful, but not all people with asthma have demonstrative allergies, and not all individuals with positive skin tests or allergies have asthma. Keeping a careful diary of asthma attacks and relating the attacks to possible triggering factors can be useful. For example, does the child invariably start wheezing when entering a certain room? Can attacks be associated with particular foods? Exercise? Activities? Specific environments?

In individuals who have hyperreactive airways characteristic of asthma, cooling and drying of the airways is a common trigger for coughing and wheezing. Because exercise is accompanied by deep and rapid breathing through the mouth (short-circuiting the nose where air is warmed and humidified) it is common in individuals with asthma for exercise to induce coughing or wheezing. In the past this has led to severe restrictions of a child's activity. With good medical management and the use of appropriate inhalers, it is possible for most individuals with asthma to engage in active sports. (This includes some well-known Olympic champions.)

Although vaporizers have been found to be very useful for the treatment of croup, there is no evidence that they help asthma. Furthermore, since humidity tends to encourage the growth of molds, a common trigger for asthma in some children, vaporizers and humidifiers may be counterproductive or harmful.

Many misconceptions abound regarding asthma, and one of the most persistent is that the disease is of psychological rather than physical origin. Although asthma is often associated with emotional problems—not just for the child, but for other family members as well—the primary cause is in the lungs, not the head. Furthermore, an attack of asthma can be very frightening to both the victim and parents. Understandably, parents will go to great lengths to prevent a child's attack. The tendency is to restrict the youngster's normal activities and to become over-protective. The child in turn may become manipulative. While it is very important to recognize the early warning signs of an asthma attack and to take appropriate preventive action, it is also important to work out treatment programs that make it possible for a child to lead as normal a life as possible. In addition to drug therapy, psychological counseling for child and family may be useful.

Treatment. Effective management of asthma entails a combination of treatment to both prevent and stop an attack. Chest physical therapy, in which the back is pounded while the child is placed in different positions to promote the drainage of mucus and secretions from the lungs, may be helpful, especially if coughing is impaired.

Since inflammation of the airways is among the earliest events in asthma, medications that prevent or minimize inflammation are especially useful. Cromolyn (Intal) has been especially effective in some asthmatic children in preventing inflammation and even in preventing attacks. Once inflammation is present, corticosteroids ("steroids") are among the most powerful antiinflammatory agents. Although they can have serious side effects when used on a daily basis for prolonged periods, physicians have learned how to use them in ways that maximize their benefits while minimizing their side effects. In addition, there are now steroids that can be given by inhalation with relatively little absorption into the body.

When asthma proceeds to the stage of bronchoconstriction, adrenalin and a host of adrenalinlike substances (called catecholamines) are especially effective. These too can now be given by inhalation. The correct dose is important because the catecholamines not only relax the muscles in the airways, relieving bronchospasm, they also may produce stimulation producing jitteriness, irritability, and a rapid heart beat.

Another agent that has been used for decades to reverse airway obstruction in an asthmatic is called theophylline. Here, too, the dose is very important since too much can upset the stomach as well as produce excessive stimulation and headaches. Fortunately, it is possible to measure the blood level and adjust the dose accordingly. In addition, there are sustained-release or long-acting preparations that are especially useful for individuals whose asthma is worse at night or in the early morning.

Several other agents have been developed that show promise of being effective in the control and treatment of asthma. Some of these like ipratropium (Atrovent) are designed to block the parasympathetic nerves much like atropine but with a greater margin of safety.

Since asthma is a chronic condition, focusing simply on the treatment of the child when symptoms are severe is not nearly as good as working out long-term programs that minimize the extent of the underlying inflammation. In the modern era, physicians are tending to use some medicines prophylactically, for example, cromolyn-adding catecholamines and theophylline at the earliest signs of worsening or in anticipation of exposure to known triggers, including exercise. When chronic inflammation is resistant to other forms of therapy, steroids (preferably given by inhalation) have been found to be helpful. With such approaches, the need for emergency-room care can be reduced. Use of a regular regimen in place of purely episodic treatment also makes it possible for a child to lead a normal life, including participation in sports. Older children can learn to use a peak flow meter to detect early bronchospasm.

For those individuals with asthma in whom the primary triggers are allergic and in which avoidance is not practical or possible, careful allergic management is essential and may involve the use of immunotherapy, that is, repeated injections of small amounts of the offending agent to stimulate the body to develop an immune response. Although antihistamines have been considered potentially harmful in asthma because of the concern that they may lead to even more secretions, this area of pharmacology is undergoing some reevaluation even as this chapter goes to press. There is early evidence that some newer types of antihistamines may be helpful for some individuals in whom allergies play a major role in the triggering of asthma attacks.

Long-Term Outlook. Many parents fear that asthma invariably leads to long-term lung damage. In fact, about 50 percent of those who have asthma in childhood are symptom-free in adult life, about 25 percent have mild symptoms in adult life, and 25 percent go on to have severe symptoms as adults. In general, the changes that take place during an acute asthma attack are reversible, and once an attack is controlled, the lungs generally return to their normal state. An attack may last for a few minutes or, in severe instances, for several days. In some cases, the attack may be prolonged and progressively

worsen, leading to a serious condition called status asthmaticus. In this life-threatening circumstance the obstruction to breathing is so severe that the child may not be able to exchange enough fresh air with each breath. This is a medical emergency that requires prompt hospital treatment.

In a typical case, asthma develops at some point during childhood, and it may be severe during the early growing years. With the approach of adolescence, it usually lessens and often seems to disappear completely. Even though there may be no symptoms, lung studies will show that the airways are still hypersensitive or hyperreactive—a person does not actually outgrow the disease, as is commonly thought. Sometimes the symptoms will reappear during adulthood, often on the heels of a respiratory infection.

Even though asthma does not produce permanent damage to the lung, as indicated above, it can produce a life-threatening emergency. For those who have frequent and severe symptoms, it can interfere seriously with a normal life, with frequent absences from school or work. Modern *programs* of treatment and education are designed to minimize these disruptions, and when adhered to regularly make it possible for most individuals to lead a normal life.

Role of Health Education. Because of the complexity of the causes and treatment of asthma, health education programs for patients with asthma or, in the case of children with asthma, for both parents and children, have been shown to be an important adjunct to the treatment and prevention of asthma. Such programs (sometimes referred to as "self-management") provide a great deal of factual material about causes and consequences of asthma as well as its treatment. They emphasize the importance of avoiding known triggers of asthma and adhering to the medical regimens prescribed by physicians and, of course, maintaining a healthy life-style.

These programs also stress the importance of trying to keep the asthmatic child's environment calm and helping the child to relax and avoid panic. Information about self-management programs can be obtained from the local chapter of the American Lung Association.

Bronchitis

With bronchitis, the mucous membrane lining the bronchi becomes irritated and inflamed. This is a defense reaction to the irritation or infection, and the inflammation and production of mucus presumably serves a function. The mucus, however, can partially obstruct the bronchi. Together with swelling of the membranes lining the airways and constriction of the muscles surrounding the airways, this can lead to narrowing of the airway lumens and create air turbulence as the child breathes, producing wheezing. The child will cough to clear the mucus away. Some children, especially during the early years of life, will get bronchitis only as the complication of a cold or other respiratory illness. In this case, the bronchitis usually is not serious and will run its course within a few days. In many cases bronchitis is believed to be part of asthma or reactive airway disease and may therefore be indistinguishable from asthma. In any case a bronchodilator and antiinflammatory agents may be helpful in hastening recovery. (See section on asthma above.)

Bronchiolitis

Bronchiolitis is a viral infection with greater potential for danger than bronchitis. It affects the tiny bronchioles of the lungs, partially or completely obstructing them. It usually comes in epidemics during winter and spring and at first may appear to be a simple respiratory infection. After a few days, however, as the bronchioles become partially blocked, there is a quick onset of ever more rapid breathing. Portions of the lungs trap air and hyperinflate.

The infection is usually self-limited and clears up in a few days. If it becomes severe, there will be chest retractions, signaling airway obstruction, and irritability, suggesting inadequate supply of oxygen to the tissues, in which case hospitalization may be necessary. If the child's lips appear blue, indicating cyanosis, medical attention should be sought immediately. The child can appear dangerously ill and should be carefully monitored, but will usually improve in 12 to 24 hours when treated in the hospital with oxygen and provided with adequate but not excessive hydration. Full recovery may take several days.

Bronchiestasis

Bronchiestasis is almost the reverse of other inflammatory diseases: instead of a constriction of the airways it is actually a persistent dilation of the bronchi. The major causes are chronic infection and inflammation in the walls of the airways as the result of cystic fibrosis, congenital immune deficiency conditions, or presence of an aspirated foreign body. In the case of an aspirated object, the bronchi usually return to normal after the object is removed. If the cause is chronic infection with excess mucus

production, however, the problem can be self-perpetuating unless treated with antibiotics. Once the walls of the airways are destroyed by chronic infection, the normal cleansing activities of the airways, including the effectiveness of cough, are impaired. This can lead to chronic infection of the lung or pneumonia.

Cystic Fibrosis

Cystic fibrosis (CF), the most common cause of suppurative (pus-forming) lung disease in children, is eventually fatal. It is characterized by dysfunction of the exocrine secretory glands, leading to obstruction of the ducts of mucus-secreting glands throughout the body. This affects the lungs most severely, resulting in chronic infection and mucus buildup and reducing the effectiveness of the lungs as a gas-exchanging organ.

Cystic fibrosis is an inherited disorder, carried in a recessive gene. If both parents have the gene, there is a 25 percent chance that each child born to them will have cystic fibrosis. In the United States, the disease strikes one in 2,500 Caucasian children, but only one in 12,000 black children.

In many instances, the disease is first apparent with an early cough. In infants the clinical signs may be indistinguishable from bronchiolitis. A child with cystic fibrosis is also more likely to come down with bronchitis and bronchiolitis. With some children, these manifestations may only appear after the first decade of life. The condition, however, is present from birth. The abnormal mucus secretion also blocks the pancreas from secreting its digestive enzymes, so that malabsorption and failure to grow despite taking in large amounts of food is an early sign of cystic fibrosis. It is also characterized by very high concentrations of sodium and chloride in the sweat. These abnormally high levels are present from day one and form the basis for the most reliable test of whether or not someone has cystic fibrosis. Unfortunately, it may not be possible to collect adequate specimens of sweat in the first few months of life. Recent developments in genetics and molecular biology, including the discovery of the gene and its abnormal protein product, offer promise of new and better ways to make the diagnosis in early life and perhaps a cure for the disease.

Treatment for the pulmonary aspects of cystic fibrosis includes the use of antibiotics, physiotherapy and, more recently, the use of antiinflammatory drugs. The antibiotics are needed to battle the risk of infection posed by the accumulation of mucus in the lungs and the susceptibility to bacteria that do not generally infect subjects without cystic fibrosis. Because of the use of antibiotics, the threat of cystic fibrosis is not a sudden catastrophic infection, but rather a long-term infection that slowly destroys the lungs. The physiotherapy consists of pounding and vibrating the child's chest to loosen up the mucus so it can be expelled. Children with cystic fibrosis also need extra salt to make up for the large amounts they lose in their sweat (especially in hot weather), as well as pancreatin, a substance that helps them digest their food. Engaging in regular and vigorous exercise seems to be helpful in a general way and may also be effective by promoting deep breathing and drainage of chest secretions.

Cystic fibrosis drastically alters the life of the entire family, demanding almost as much of parents and siblings as it does of the child who has the disorder. For many children with the disease, however, the quality of life can be very good for long periods of time. Every year treatment improves and life expectancy is extended. The median age of survival is almost 20 years; many survive well into their twenties and some into their thirties and forties. There have been some dramatic scientific breakthroughs in our understanding of this genetic abnormality and in our understanding of the salt-and-water defect. Scientists have identified the abnormal gene on chromosome 7, offering promise of finding better solutions to cystic fibrosis.

Congenital Structural Defects

There are a number of congenital structural defects that can affect the lower respiratory tract. These include:

Tracheomalacia. In this disorder, the support systems for the airways are not mature or strong enough and the airways tend to narrow more than they should, obstructing the entrance of air, especially if there is any obstruction on the level of the nose or mouth. This condition may generally clear up as the child grows, and the airways become larger and stiffer.

Tracheal Stenosis. This is a rare disorder in which the tracheal lumen itself may be congenitally too narrow, often because it is impinged upon by a complete cartilaginous ring. It is also possible, although rare, that *vascular anomalies*—such as deformed or malpositioned arteries—may compress the trachea or bronchi, requiring early surgery. Tumors in the lower airways are quite rare in childhood, but congenital obstructing cysts are recognized from time to time and may simulate asthma (hence, the aphorism well known among doctors, "all that wheezes is not asthma").

Parenchyma Disorders. The parenchyma is that part of an organ responsible for the primary function of the organ. In the case of the respiratory system, the parenchyma comprises primarily the gas-exchanging sacs, the alveoli, and the capillaries within their walls—all of which are used in the crucial exchange of oxygen and carbon dioxide. In addition we now recognize that the cells of the lungs also produce or control the level of a variety of naturally occurring chemicals that have effects on the circulation, the immune response, and other functions. The severity of disorders of the parenchyma depends on how many of the alveoli are affected and how much of the gas exchange is impaired.

Bacterial Pneumonias

Once an often fatal illness, pneumonia is now treated relatively easily with antibiotics. The need for hospitalization, even for the smallest child, is declining. It is, however, still potentially a very severe illness. While the respiratory system's defense mechanisms are extremely efficient, they can be weakened by a viral infection, opening the door for bacteria. Bacterial pneumonia develops in one or more of the lobes, and the alveoli quickly fill with inflammatory fluid and cells, reducing gas exchange and making breathing difficult. There are several types of bacterial pneumonia.

Pneumococcal Pneumonia. The organism causing this disease (streptococcus pneumonia) is the most common cause of community-acquired pneumonia (and incidentally the second most common cause of bacterial meningitis and responsible for more than 50 percent of middle-ear infections in children). Usually preceded by an upper respiratory infection, its onset is abrupt, with fever, chills, chest pain, and shortness of breath. Within 24 to 48 hours, the alveoli of the affected area will be filled with infection. Expectorated mucus may be tinged with blood early on, but this may pass as the lobe fills and consolidates.

Penicillin is the preferred antibiotic for treatment. The initial doses are generally injected, while the remaining doses may be taken orally over the following few days. Supportive care includes rest and adequate fluids to prevent dehydration. Aspirin or acetaminophen are usually sufficient to reduce fever and take care of the aches and pain. Hospitalization and administration of oxygen may be needed if lung capacity is considerably diminished by the extent of the infection (which may be indicated by labored breathing and cyanosis). Bloodstream infection (or bacteremia) is always a serious complication and can occur in as many as 25 percent of cases. Early treatment with antibiotics usually is effective in clearing up this pneumonia within a few days and only very rarely is there any long-term damage.

Staphylococcal Pneumonia. This is less common, but quite serious and progresses rapidly, either from aspiration or by spreading through the bloodstream. It is preceded by an upper respiratory infection or influenzalike illness. It then progresses into fever, short and rapid breathing, rapid heartbeat, and cyanosis. The chest X ray may show multiple thin-walled abscesses of the lung. The child will be lethargic, irritable, and acutely ill. Special semisynthetic penicillin may be required. Air in the chest cavity surrounding the lung (a condition known as pneumothorax) may occur in the first two days and the lung may have to be decompressed. Other complications include pus surrounding the lung (pleural empyema) as well as infections of the bones or joints. As serious as it sounds, most children recover fully with appropriate antibiotic treatment.

H. Influenzae and Friedlander's Bacillus. These are two rare bacterial pneumonias that look like pneumococcal pneumonia but don't respond to penicillin. Ampicillin, chloramphenicol, and the newer cephalosporins work on *H. influenzae*, while kanamycin or gentamicin are effective treatment for Friedlander's bacillus.

Chlamydial Pneumonia. Chlamydial infections cause pneumonia in infants. Chlamydia is now considered a special type of bacteria. About 2 to 6 percent of pregnant women have the organism in the genital tract at the time of delivery, thus exposing the newborn infant. Peak incidence of the disease is between three to six weeks of age, and the clinical illness can last for weeks. The infection is characterized by staccato coughs followed by a deep inspiration, resembling whooping cough. The infection is usually treated with erythromycin.

Mycoplasma Pneumonia (Primary Atypical Pneumonia). Serious diseases of the respiratory tract usually occur in older children or young adults, with milder infection in young children. The organism is acquired from infected persons by means of infected respiratory secretions. The pneumonia is usually mild, with fever, cough, and malaise, and only a small percentage of children require hospitalization. Other causes of atypical pneumonias include psittacosis (from infected birds), Legionnaires' disease, and respiratory viruses. Erythromycin or tetracycline are usually effective drugs.

Viral Pneumonias

Many viruses—such as rhinovirus, adenovirus, influenza, respiratory syncytial virus, and parainfluenza—can cause pneumonia. Usually viral pneumonias attack the spaces between the alveoli (called interstitial spaces) and only occasionally the alveoli themselves. Like other pneumonias, a viral pneumonia is usually preceded by a few days of an upper respiratory infection. It is characterized by a sudden onset of rapid, shallow breathing, a nonproductive cough, low-grade fever, and malaise. Upon examination, the physician may find a reddened pharynx and will hear diminished breath sounds with crackles (called rales) when listening over the infected lungs.

There is no specific treatment for viral pneumonias, and no cure as miraculous as penicillin is for bacterial pneumonias. The best bet is the basic rest, fluids, and aspirin or acetaminophen. If airways become obstructed, bronchodilating drugs, like those used for asthma, help to open the passages. If cyanosis appears, oxygen may be needed.

The mortality rate for viral pneumonias is low, but the convalescence may take a very long time, because they can cause extensive damage in the lungs.

Chemical Pneumonias

When damaging chemicals are inhaled they can cause another form of pneumonia. The most common case is *hydrocarbon pneumonia*, which is caused when a hydrocarbon chemical (such as kerosene or charcoal lighter fluid) is swallowed and some of it is aspirated. This fills the alveoli with a blood-tinged fluid and can produce all the symptoms of the other pneumonias.

If it is known that a child has swallowed such a chemical, but it is not known whether he aspirated any, vomiting should *not* be induced, as it can increase the possibility that more of the liquid will be aspirated. The child should be closely observed for the following 48 hours to be certain that lung disease does not develop.

If indeed the child has breathed in some of the chemical and it has caused pneumonia, the symptoms of fever and shortness of breath will develop. There is no penicillinlike cure for this. Treatment will largely be supportive: oxygen (if a large part of the lung is affected and gas exchange is impaired), physiotherapy, maintenance of nutrition and normal fluid intake. Whether antibiotics will be effective to ward off a secondary bacterial infection remains controversial. In general the child should recover completely.

The prognosis for children who inhale other chemicals can be worse. *Silo-fillers' disease* (rare, but not unheard of in children), is caused by the high levels of nitrogen dioxide found in recently filled silos. The onset of this pneumonia is swift and the mortality is high. Inhalation of *paraquat*, a deadly herbicide, almost always causes serious damage to the lungs, leading to acute respiratory failure. The swallowing or inhalation of many chemicals can cause serious and potentially fatal health problems. All such hazardous material must be kept locked away, out of the reach of children.

Other Pneumonias

Mycotic Infections. These are fungal infections that can cause pneumonia. There are two types. One infects children with normal resistance, causes little more than flulike symptoms, and usually requires no treatment. Another type infects children whose immune system is suppressed, for example, by cancer, prolonged use of steroids, or by AIDS. Some fungi, such as aspergillus, can cause hypersensitivity lung disease. Fungal infections may also occur in those who take antibiotics. Such an infection can be far more serious and may require treatment with amphotericin B, a drug that must be monitored carefully because it can have adverse side effects.

Tuberculosis

In spite of dramatic development of effective drugs against tuberculosis, including INH and rifampin, tuberculosis continues to be a serious and widespread disease in many Third World countries. Many new cases, especially in urban settings in this country, can be traced to disease in recent immigrants from Southeast Asia. Tuberculosis also is on the increase in individuals (mostly adults) with immune defects from AIDS. An effective vaccine has never been developed, although BCG is used in many Third World countries.

Loss of Lung Tissue

Agenesis. Absence of parenchymal tissue can reduce the functioning of the lungs. Agenesis is a quite severe defect in which the tissue fails to develop in the fetus. In most cases, though, survival is possible because only one lung is missing.

Hypoplasia of the Lung. This occurs when the lungs are too small and fail to develop to full size, sometimes because of a genetic defect and sometimes because something is impinging on the lungs (the chest cavity may be too small or the bowel may herniate through a congenital defect in the diaphragm, compressing the lungs). Survival is questionable with hypoplasia and depends on how small the lungs are and how impaired the gas exchange is.

Lobectomy and Pneumonectomy. These are surgical procedures used to remove parts of the lungs for a variety of reasons. Because they result in a decrease of overall lung volume, they may lead to overdistension of the remaining lung and increased resistance to blood flow through the lung.

Accessory Lobes and Sequestered Lung. These are conditions in which part of the lung may be cut off from the bronchial system or supplied solely by the systemic circulation and not the pulmonary circulation as in the normal individual. This may pose no problems, as long as the sequestered lung remains uninfected. If there is chronic recurring infection, it may be necessary to remove the abnormal lung.

The function of the parenchyma can also be reduced by lesions that take up space in the lungs. *Cysts* are not uncommon in the lungs of children, but only cause problems if they are large and reduce gas exchange, impinge on the airflow in the airways, or become infected. In such cases they should be removed.

Primary Tumors

These are rare in the lungs of children, but do occasionally occur. Metastases to the chest from elsewhere in the body are not rare and are just as serious as in the adult.

Neuromotor Diseases

Although rare now in the immunized population, *poliomyelitis* (commonly, polio) can so disable the respiratory system that mechanical respiration is required. *Guillain-Barré syndrome*, also rare (but now more common than polio), is a disease characterized by progressive, gradual paralysis, which can be fatal if it reaches the respiratory system. Complete recovery is expected in most cases, however. *Muscular spinal atrophy* (Werdnig-Hoffman disease) is a rare but lethal disease in which certain cells in the spinal cord wither away, proving fatal in most children before the age of five. As the respiratory muscles weaken, deep breaths become difficult, cough is impaired, and these children become vulnerable to pneumonia, lung collapse, and respiratory failure. In *muscular dystrophy*, much the same sequence follows, and respiratory failure occurs as progressive weakness develops.

Structural Abnormalities of the Thorax

Structural abnormalities of the thorax may only present cosmetic problems and have no effect on the respiratory system. Spinal malformations, however, such as *scoliosis* (curvature of the spine), while not causing any problems initially, may lead to serious respiratory trouble later on if not corrected early in the child's life. Sternal depressions or *funnel chest* (pectus excavatrum) may cause no symptoms. If it is severe, however, there is now evidence to suggest that function may be impaired (especially while exercising) by the second or third decades of life. Although surgical correction of the depressed sternum was once thought to be merely cosmetic, some experts now believe that pulmonary function can also be improved by surgery.

Pleural Diseases

The *pleura* are duplicate and delicate membranes that surround the lungs and separate them from the chest wall. Air or fluid may break the seal between the two pleural membranes, leading to a collapse of the lung. This leak is known as *empyema* if the invading substance is a purulent or infected fluid and *hemothorax* if it is blood. If it is an air leak, it is called pneumothorax, which can be a spontaneous condition in children, usually just causes chest pain, and is self-healing. If it is more serious, the air may have to be withdrawn by needle or chest tube, the leak sealed, and the lung if collapsed allowed to reexpand. It is also possible for the disease to scar the pleura, which in turn could envelop the lung in a fibrous tissue, limiting lung expansion.

SUMMING UP

THE RESPIRATORY SYSTEM is a frequent site for health problems in infants and children. During the neonatal period, much of the trouble stems from the fact that the infant's lungs are not fully mature; the airways are small and more easily blocked than those of an adult. The growing child is a target of the myriad viral and bacterial infections that batter the defense of the respiratory system every day. Normal host defense systems, including the cilia, cough, and the immune system, protect the lungs.

Most respiratory infections are mild and require only the basic treatment given to colds and the flu. However, simple infections often weaken the defense, paving the way for more serious trouble, such as croup, pneumonia, or asthma; so care should be given to see that the child has fully recovered from an infection before being exposed to other infectious agents.

Parents should always be on the lookout for the basic symptoms of respiratory trouble; a harsh or persistent cough, a change in breathing (speeding up or becoming more labored), a change in breathing sound (stridor or wheezing), visible retractions or sucking in of the chest on inspiration, or cyanosis. While in some cases there will be nothing serious, these signs and symptoms nevertheless should be taken seriously and reported promptly to the child's doctor.

23 Gastrointestinal Disorders

*Richard J. Deckelbaum, M.D., and
Joseph Levy, M.D.*

INTRODUCTION

THE GASTROINTESTINAL SYSTEM is commonly called the digestive tract. Its purpose is to process food, so that it can be absorbed and utilized by the body, and to eliminate waste products. In essence, the gastrointestinal system is a hollow tube beginning at the mouth and ending at the anus. Branching from this tube are the digestive organs and glands—the liver, gallbladder, and pancreas. (See figure 23.1.)

Twelve to fifteen feet in length at the baby's birth, the digestive tract is divided into several sections, each with distinct functions, both mechanical and chemical. The digestive process begins in the mouth, where liquids and solids are mixed with saliva. Produced by the salivary glands, saliva contains amylase and lipase, the first two of many digestive enzymes released along the digestive tract. As the saliva is mixed with liquids and solids in the mouth, it begins the breakdown of starches and fats into simpler elements used for body fuel and other important metabolic processes.

As milk is sucked or food is chewed, it is pushed to the back of the mouth by the tongue. The epiglottis closes to prevent food from getting into the windpipe, and the milk or food bolus passes through the funnel-shaped pharynx into the esophagus, a muscular tube that empties into the stomach. The esophagus passes through an opening, the hiatus, in the diaphragm and joins the stomach just below this flat muscle that divides the chest and abdominal cavities. At the junction of the esophagus and the stomach is a valvelike mechanism called the lower esophageal sphincter, an area of increased muscle tone that opens to allow food to pass into the stomach and then closes to prevent the backflow of food into the esophagus. Rings of muscles in the esophageal wall push the food along by contracting and expanding in wavelike motions called peristalsis. This same peristaltic process occurs along the entire digestive tract.

The stomach, a soft muscular bag shaped like a pear, is usually situated on the left-hand side just below the ribs. The wide upper portion is called the

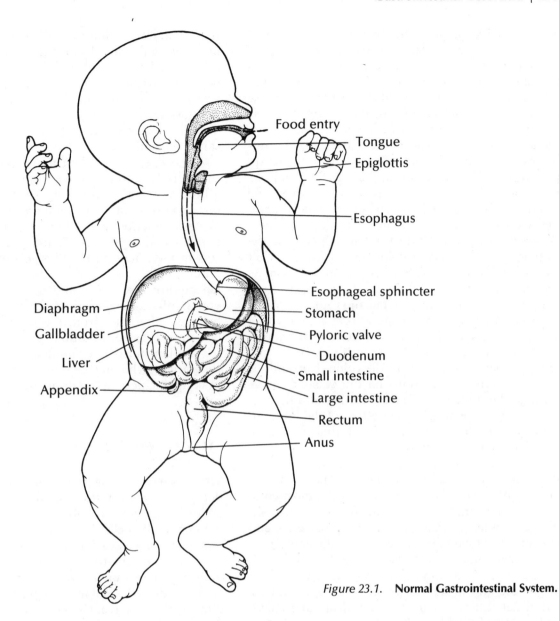

Figure 23.1. **Normal Gastrointestinal System.**

fundus, and the tapering portion is the antrum and pyloric canal, which pumps partially digested food from the stomach into the duodenum, the first section of the small intestine. The stomach, which can stretch to hold up to six ounces at birth and almost a quart of food at maturity, gently churns its contents with the hydrochloric acid and digestive enzymes it secretes to continue breaking down nutrients (carbohydrates, proteins, and fats) into their component parts. Hydrochloric acid is a strong chemical that could eat through the stomach wall were it not protected by a mucus coating. In addition to its other functions, hydrochloric acid kills most of the bacteria in foods.

The stomach empties gradually as the pyloric valve opens periodically to release about 1 percent of the stomach contents at a time. Signals produced by food chemicals, motion, and pressure are sent to the brain via the vagus nerve and then back to the pyloric valve causing it to relax and open. This process can continue for as much as three or four hours if the stomach is quite full.

In the small intestine the digestive process is completed and the nutrients now broken down into molecules are absorbed from it. In the adult, the small intestine is about twenty-two feet long. It lies coiled beneath the stomach and is surrounded by the large intestine (colon). It is divided into three sections (duodenum, jejunum, ileum), divisions more anatomical than functional. The presence of food in the small intestine stimulates the production of hormones which, in turn, cause digestive juices from the pancreas and bile from the liver and the gallbladder to flow into the duodenum. The surface area of the intestinal walls through which food passes into the bloodstream or the lymph channels is expanded greatly by the presence of millions of tiny fingerlike projections called villi.

What remains after the absorption of nutrients through the villi are water, leftover enzymes, mineral salts, and indigestible plant fibers. This refuse is moved from the ileum into the cecum, the first section of the large intestine, or colon, located on the lower right-hand side of the abdomen. (The vermiform appendix, a small closed tube with no apparent function, extends from the cecum.) The large intestine is divided into four sections. The ascending colon travels from the lower right side of the abdominal cavity where it turns and becomes the transverse colon, running from right to left behind the stomach. The descending colon moves down the left side and curves into the S-shaped sigmoid colon. As the waste products pass through the colon, salts are absorbed and water is extracted and returned to circulation. This changes the stool from a liquid to a solid form that acquires its color from bilirubin pigments and its odor from decomposition of fecal material by bacteria present in the colon. Normally it can take from 12 to 18 hours for this waste to move through the three or more feet of colon into the rectum, the storage area at the bottom of the large intestine. Here it is collected for a time and then expelled through the anus.

Branching off the digestive tract are the liver, the gallbladder, and the pancreas. The liver, the largest internal organ, is also one of the most complex, having some 5,000 separate functions. It manufactures bile, cholesterol, vitamin A, proteins, and clotting factors; it stores glycogen, amino acids, fats, blood, iron, and other minerals, and fat-soluble vitamins A, D, E, K and B_{12}. It regulates the amount of glucose and protein distributed to body tissues, and it detoxifies alcohol and other drugs and chemicals. The gallbladder, whose function is to concentrate and store bile, is attached to the liver and to the duodenum by small ducts.

The pancreas, about eight inches long, lies behind the stomach adjacent to the duodenum. Most of this gland is devoted to producing digestive juice containing enzymes necessary for digesting carbohydrates, proteins, and fats. Its other products include insulin and glucagon, two hormones essential to the regulation of blood sugar and the metabolism of carbohydrates, which are produced in tiny clusters of islet cells scattered throughout the gland and secreted directly into the bloodstream. (See chapter 30, Endocrine Disorders.)

It is possible to remove all or portions of each section of the digestive tract, the gallbladder, and the pancreas and still maintain almost normal digestion. For example, there is sufficient duplication of function along the digestive tract to allow portions of the small intestine and all of the stomach, the colon, and the gallbladder to be removed if necessary without seriously compromising the ability to lead a normal life. If the pancreas is removed, the hormones and enzymes it produces can be supplied by medication. The liver, however, is necessary to sustain life.

The digestive system as just described is one that is fully mature. In the normal, full-term infant, all the components of the digestive tract are present, but several months are required before all of them begin to function in a fully mature fashion. The gastrointestinal problems of very young children are somewhat different from those of older children and adults. First, the problems that result from birth defects are discovered and dealt with in the very young infant. Second, the immature digestive tract behaves differently from the mature tract in some circumstances. In addition, gastrointestinal symptoms often must be evaluated without the help of the patient, who may be too young to communicate, making diagnosis more difficult.

DEVELOPMENTAL FACTORS

THERE APPEAR TO BE four interacting factors that determine gastrointestinal development: genetic endowment (what is inherited), biological and developmental clocks (the natural sequence of developmental processes for human beings in general), regulatory mechanisms (hormones, for example), and environmental influences (for example, infections, maternal smoking during pregnancy, or dietary variations in early life).

Genetic endowment is determined by the DNA molecule. This can be changed by genetic mutation. For example, if both parents are carriers of a genetic disorder, meaning they both have a recessive gene for some disorder, they may produce a child that is normal, a child that also has the recessive gene as they do, or a child that has the disorder, which neither of them has but which they can transmit. Examples of genetic disorders include inborn errors of metabolism such as the absence of an enzyme. For example, persons with a genetic lack of the enzyme glucose G phosphate dehydrogenase (G.G.P.D.) will be unable to digest fava beans and will become ill from them. However, these same persons will be less susceptible to malaria. Over time, through selection, such disorders can predominate in certain geographic areas or populations, as seen in genetic disorders common to one racial or ethnic group.

The "biological clock" governs the sequence of events in the formation of the digestive tract. Under normal circumstances, the human gastrointestinal tract will be anatomically complete after 20 weeks of gestation. The developmental clock, which regulates the appearance of various enzymes and digestive processes, is not synchronized. Certain enzymes do not appear until after three months of life; some digestive processes are incomplete until after six months; and some muscle functions will not be capable of voluntary control until later still. This accounts for the different dietary needs and bowel functions in infants and young children.

An example of a regulatory mechanism that can affect the development of the digestive tract is the role of certain hormones. The biologic clock can be slowed down in the absence of adrenal or pituitary gland activity. And sometimes, even when certain hormones are present, they have no effect because the cells they ordinarily regulate are not receptive.

Superimposed upon these interactive processes is the environment. Infection of the fetus in the first trimester by a virus can cause both retarded growth and physical anomalies. After delivery breastfed babies are in general better protected from intestinal and other infections than bottle-fed babies.

CONGENITAL DEFECTS

WHEN SOMETHING GOES WRONG in any of the developmental processes, congenital defects may occur. Such defects are rare, but they are mentioned here because they demonstrate what happens when there is a disruption of normal developmental sequences, whether because of a problem in the mother (poor nutrition), in the placenta (perhaps caused by maternal diabetes or kidney disease), or in the fetus (genetic, infectious, or toxic substance damage). When such defects occur, they are usually discovered in the newborn period or early infancy. Frequently they constitute an emergency.

Defects of the Mouth and Esophagus

Cleft Lip and Cleft Palate. These defects can occur together or separately. (See figure 23.2.) Although they are thought to be hereditary, they can occur without a family history of the defect. Cleft lip with or without cleft palate is more common in males while cleft palate alone is more common in females. There are many variations of this defect, and in all cases surgery is required to correct the problem.

These defects create problems with feeding, upper respiratory and ear infections, as well as speech and dental development. As the child grows, there may also be problems related to self-image. Parents often experience feelings of guilt, fear, and even revulsion because of the unsightly defect and may find it difficult to want to establish the close relationship that is necessary to the baby's well-being.

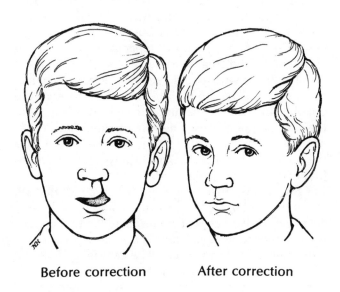

Before correction   After correction

Figure 23.2. **Cleft Lip.**

Feeding a newborn is usually a pleasurable and fulfilling occasion for parents, a primary bonding event. However, with these babies, feeding may be difficult, frightening, and perhaps unpleasant for the parent. Whether the baby is fed with a soft, disposable bottle or a specially designed feeder will depend upon how well he can suck. The feeding method is determined in the hospital and taught to parents before the baby goes home. Since these infants may swallow a great deal of air while feeding, there is an increased chance of choking and coughing and a need for frequent burping. Feeding requires vigilance, skill, and patience.

Surgery to close the lip is usually done at three or four months of age, while palate surgery is usually delayed until about 12 to 18 months. Additional surgery may be required later to correct nose deformities, to revise or repair as the child grows, or to reconstruct the nasopharynx to improve speech. Although correction of the defect may be long and arduous, results are usually quite good cosmetically, and since no other part of the gastrointestinal tract is involved, once repairs are complete the child is able to live a normal and full life.

Esophageal Atresia and Tracheoesophageal Fistula. These difficult-to-pronounce deformities, although rare, are frequently seen together. The former is an interruption in the continuity of the esophagus (foodpipe) between the mouth and the stomach. The latter is an abnormal opening between the esophagus and the trachea (windpipe). This can happen in diverse ways, but in the most common type the esophagus is in two parts with a closed pouch at the top and a second section opening into the trachea at the top and into the stomach at the bottom. This creates a serious emergency in the newborn, and the prognosis depends upon the speed of diagnosis and treatment.

The baby with this defect is in great danger of inhaling digestive juices into the lungs through the opening in the trachea and through overflow from the upper pouch, causing pneumonia and other complications. When the baby cries, air rushes into the stomach through the trachea, causing abdominal distention and vomiting.

Surgery is always required. The type of surgery, the number of operations required, and how the surgery is staged are dependent on many factors including whether or not the infant is premature, the exact nature of the deformity, etc. The goal is to close the fistula and to reconstruct the esophagus. Although the outcome can be poor, especially for those babies who have pneumonia, most children will recover fully. In many cases, the recovery process can be lengthy.

Congenital Esophageal Stenosis and Webs. Occasionally an infant will be born with a constricted or narrowed esophagus or with a kind of webbing that obstructs the passage of food. These disorders are not always detected immediately, since the symptoms of difficulty in swallowing and vomiting of undigested formula or food usually begin only after the esophagus becomes inflamed and swollen due to continuous retention of portions of feedings above the obstruction. Webs may not be discovered until solid food is introduced.

Sometimes the condition can be corrected by dilating or expanding the narrowed area with a bougie (a long flexible instrument). If this procedure is not successful, then the constricted area is removed surgically and the esophagus is rejoined. If children with such problems are otherwise healthy, the prognosis is quite good.

Intestinal Obstructions

The most common birth defects in the intestines are obstructions that appear at various sites along the tract and arise from different causes. Some of these are discussed in detail in other sections of the chapter and will be only briefly mentioned here.

Pyloric Stenosis. This is an obstruction to the outlet of the stomach that prevents the passage of food into the small intestine. (See figure 23.3.) It occurs frequently in newborns (one in every 200 births), in males about three times more often than in females, and most often in firstborn children. The most common symptom is forceful, projectile vomiting. This is quite unlike the spitting up seen in most babies. The baby may appear to be eating normally but then will suddenly vomit up everything. The vomiting usually appears by the second or third week of life, but occasionally not until after two months. The cause is a thickening of the pyloric muscle accompanied by spasm, which contributes to the forceful vomiting. A few children have been treated successfully with antispasmodic drugs, but almost all undergo surgery. The operation is a simple one and generally corrects the condition completely and immediately.

Atresia. This is the failure of a hollow organ to open properly. Intestinal atresia is the most common cause of intestinal obstruction in the newborn. Atresias occur most frequently in the duodenum and ileum, then in the jejunum, and least often in the colon. There is no apparent genetic cause, but they arise from the maldevelopment of the bowel during pregnancy. The symptoms, which include the vomiting of bile, abdominal distention, and the absence of bowel movements, will vary depending on the location of the atresia. The condition is corrected by removing the affected section of the intestine and

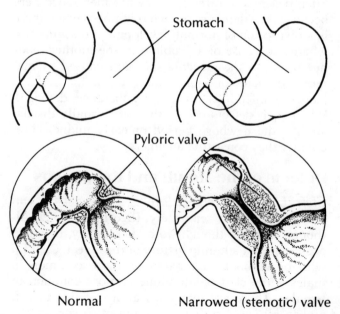

Stomach

Pyloric valve

Normal

Narrowed (stenotic) valve

Figure 23.3. **Pyloric Stenosis.**

rejoining the healthy portions of the bowel. If there are no other anomalies and the area to be removed is not extensive, the prognosis is good.

Hirschsprung's Disease.   This is a condition in which certain nerve cells that regulate propulsion in the colon are missing. This causes a portion of the rectum or lower colon to remain contracted, resulting in dilatation of the bowel above the functional obstruction. Hirschsprung's disease accounts for about one in 10,000 hospital admissions and it appears four times more frequently in males than in females. A temporary colostomy—an artificial opening in the abdominal wall to permit exit of fecal wastes—is constructed to allow the bowel to decompress and the child to grow before definitive surgery. When the baby has reached the age of 12 months the constricted segment of the colon is removed and the normal bowel is brought down to the anus ("pull through" operation). Although this is a major procedure, a complete cure can be expected in about 95 percent of cases.

Anorectal Malformations

Imperforate anus is the general name applied to three different types of anorectal anomalies. Some children are born with stenosis, or narrowing of the anus. This condition can often be corrected by widening with a narrow dilator or physician's finger or by a small incision to widen the opening. In others, the anus is closed by a membrane growing across the orifice. This can be removed easily. However, in some infants the rectal pouch has failed to descend to the skin. In this event, the rectal pouch must be pulled down and brought to the skin through the sphincter muscle at the end of the anal canal. Sometimes it is necessary to do a temporary colostomy, postponing definitive surgery for 6 to 12 months. In most cases, normal anorectal function and continence can be achieved. In other cases, there may be a fistula, or connection, from the rectum to the urinary bladder, which also can be corrected surgically.

Liver and Gallbladder Defects

The liver has hundreds of physiologic functions. If any one of these functions is deficient—for example, if only one enzyme is missing or is incorrectly formed—the child will have what is known as an inborn error of metabolism. These are chemical defects, some of which can be life-threatening if undiagnosed and untreated. Some can be treated by dietary management; some require both diet and drug therapy; still others may be cured only by liver transplant.

There are also physical defects associated with the liver and gallbladder. The ducts leading to or from the liver or gallbladder may be missing, closed off (biliary atresia), or unnecessarily duplicated. The gallbladder may be missing altogether or improperly located. The liver may be invaded with cystic disease. Some of these physical anomalies are treated with appropriate surgical procedures. The outlook for the various surgical procedures is often very good, though some anomalies are beyond repair.

Jaundice, a condition in which the skin becomes yellow, is common in newborns. In most cases this represents the transient inability of the young liver to excrete adequate amounts of bilirubin, and it clears up spontaneously within a few days as the liver matures. In other cases jaundice results from incompatibility of blood type between mother and baby. However, since jaundice may also be a symptom of liver disease, any baby with this problem should be closely watched and promptly examined if the jaundice persists. With many liver disorders early diagnosis is essential in order to prevent irreparable damage such as cirrhosis or mental retardation. As more and more tests for these disorders are being perfected and administered as a routine part of newborn screening, the outlook for early diagnosis and successful management continues to improve. (See section on jaundice later in this chapter.)

COMMON SYMPTOMS AND THEIR MEDICAL SIGNIFICANCE

THERE ARE A NUMBER OF digestive symptoms that commonly occur in infants and children. Some of them have little medical significance and will disappear in time without special treatment. Others may not be serious but nevertheless need specific attention in order that they not become a big problem. And some may point to conditions that require immediate treatment, medical or surgical, to ensure the health or survival of the child.

For parents, knowing when to call the doctor immediately, when to wait a while, and what to report can be confusing and frightening. Some parents tend to be frightened at the smallest thing; others may fail to pay attention to potentially important symptoms. Following are the most commonly reported problems in infants and small children with indications of what can be taken in stride and what requires immediate action.

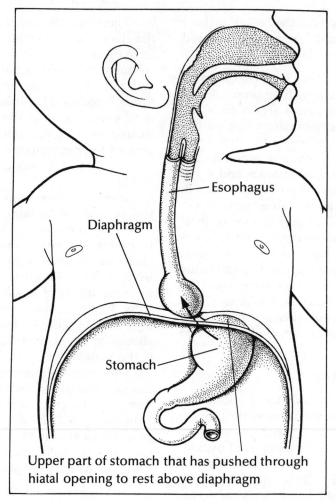

Upper part of stomach that has pushed through hiatal opening to rest above diaphragm

Figure 23.4. **Hiatal Hernia.**

Feeding Problems

Parents find feeding problems particularly frustrating. While many of the problems have a simple cause, others may result from significant gastrointestinal or nonintestinal problems. Among the most benign causes are colic, inadequate frequency of breastfeeding, overfeeding of formula, formula intolerance, and an inadequate nipple. In general, breastfeeding avoids many of the feeding problems described here. Bottle feeding, partly because it is so easy for the baby, has its own problems. For example, the most common cause of infant vomiting is overfeeding of formula. Overfeeding and inadequate nipple require only adjustments in the amount of food given or the size of the opening in the nipple. Formula intolerance may be associated with a specific protein allergy, or with sugar malabsorption. Colic, discussed later in detail, disappears with time. In a baby who appears to be well, the doctor will look first for some of these causes.

Some physical conditions are characterized by feeding problems. These include cleft lip and palate and large adenoids; neurological problems such as cerebral palsy; and other conditions resulting in abnormal swallowing mechanisms. Parents are given special training, usually by hospital nursing staff or a feeding therapist, to help them learn necessary techniques.

Infants with malabsorption caused by metabolic disorders may experience pain, cramps, and abdominal distention when they are given certain foods, and the end result may be a child who resists being fed. These babies do not grow properly and require prompt evaluation to avoid serious developmental damage. The feeding problems usually disappear when the condition is diagnosed and proper diet and treatment are begun.

A child with marked vomiting and failure to thrive from insufficient intake is likely to have gastroesophageal reflux, a condition in which the contents of the stomach flow back into the esophagus. This is sometimes aggravated by a hiatal hernia, a condition in which the hiatus—the opening in the diaphragm through which the esophagus passes to connect to the stomach—becomes weakened, so that a portion of the stomach squeezes through the opening and rests above the diaphragm. (See figure 23.4.)

Crying, vomiting, refusal to take the bottle, irritability, taking a few gulps and then stopping, along with poor weight gain, may be symptoms of reflux. However, these same symptoms may be present with several other conditions, and investigation is sometimes necessary to clarify the relation between symptoms and reflux.

Vomiting and Regurgitation

Spitting up (regurgitation) in a thriving infant is usually no cause for concern. In some babies, the valve mechanism between the esophagus and stomach does not work perfectly at first, allowing small amounts of milk to return from the stomach and spill from the mouth. If this happens immediately after feeding, the food will be exactly as it was when taken. If it occurs an hour or so later, the acid in the stomach will have acted upon the milk and it will be sour.

Babies with a tendency to spit up should not be overfed or vigorously moved about immediately after feeding. Sometimes it helps to carry or keep the baby sitting up for twenty minutes or so after feeding. These simple precautions may reduce the amount of spitting up, but there is no need to worry if the baby is growing normally and is not ill. The spitting up usually stops when the child begins to walk.

Spitting up that is accompanied by choking or any sign of illness such as fever, poor appetite, or slow weight gain should be reported to the physician right away, as this can be the first sign of a number of different problems.

Vomiting is the forceful expulsion of the contents of the stomach through the mouth. It is not dangerous in and of itself unless the child is unconscious, in which case the vomitus may seep back into the lungs. However, small infants and even very young children can quickly become dehydrated from vomiting, a dangerous condition in which too great a loss of body fluids causes a salt and water imbalance.

Babies and small children frequently vomit when they have upper respiratory infections, flu-like infections, or gastroenteritis. If it is apparent that a well infant or child has such an infection and the vomiting subsides without commencing again with the gradual introduction of fluids, there is no need for concern. However, if vomiting persists, even if it seems to be related to some ordinary illness, the doctor should be contacted. It may be necessary to

take precautions against dehydration or to examine the child to rule out some other underlying cause.

Since vomiting may be the first symptom of a host of diseases or disorders, the process of diagnosis is often one of ruling out problems in the absence of certain other positive symptoms either through observation or through testing. One of the first clues is the nature of the vomitus itself. It is important to report whether the vomitus contains blood or bile, is curdled or contains bits of undigested food, for example. Other important information includes when the vomiting occurs, what and how much has been eaten.

About 50 percent of infants exhibit spitting or vomiting as an isolated complaint, but less than 5 percent have significant underlying disease. In most cases it reflects physiologic immaturity, improper feeding, or a disturbed relationship between baby and mother. In older children vomiting is commonly attributable to respiratory infections (ear, throat), gastritis, gastroenteritis, and least often, hepatitis; generally it disappears on its own. Rarely it may be a symptom of a major gastrointestinal disorder such as Crohn's disease or a psychological disorder as in the case of bulimia. In newborns and young infants gastrointestinal disorders that may be heralded by vomiting include pyloric stenosis (see Congenital Defects), milk protein allergy and lactose intolerance, intestinal obstruction (see Congenital Defects), and a long list of inborn metabolic diseases.

Persistent vomiting accompanied by increasing lethargy and other symptoms also may be a symptom of Reye's syndrome, a relatively rare but potentially life-threatening disease that causes brain swelling and fatty liver. Reye's syndrome occurs most often in children who are recovering from a viral infection, especially chicken pox or flu. If Reye's syndrome is suspected, the child should be taken immediately to an emergency room, preferably at a teaching hospital or medical center where there are likely to be physicians experienced in the care of this serious condition.

Acute Diarrhea

Depending upon the season, as many as 50 percent of a pediatrician's patients may be troubled by diarrhea. There are many causes of this symptom, but in older infants and children, it is most commonly associated with viral or bacterial gastroenteritis (stomach flu), is self-limited, and has little significance. However, in newborns and young infants there are two causes for concern. Certain diseases that are present with diarrhea require immediate attention because they are unique to the small infant and because dehydration and acidosis, conditions that can be very dangerous in early life, may occur within hours in the very young.

The normal stool of a breastfed baby will be quite soft and yellow or mustard in color. In the bottle-fed infant, the stool will be darker and firmer as a rule. Some babies move their bowels after every feeding, others once a day or even less frequently, especially after the first few months. Toddlers and young children have fewer bowel movements, perhaps one a day or every other day. In fact, a wide range of elimination patterns may be considered normal in a well child as long as the pattern is consistent.

In simple terms, diarrhea represents an increase in frequency of bowel movements or an increase of stool fluidity. It is important to note the size and consistency of the stool, the presence or absence of blood or mucus, the color (green, black, or pale), and the odor (acid, foul, or rank). Another significant fact is whether this represents a sudden change (acute) or whether it has been going on for some time (chronic). This information offers important clues to the illness causing the diarrhea.

Except for newborns, the most common cause of acute diarrhea is viral or bacterial gastroenteritis. It is accompanied by such symptoms as fever, abdominal pain, and perhaps upper respiratory infection. Often other members of the family have a similar illness. It is important for the doctor to be informed if the child spends much time in a daycare center, because in such cases the possibility of a parasitic infection exists. These illnesses usually respond to treatment quickly and the child is back to normal in a few days. In these instances, as with all forms of diarrhea, it is important that the child get sufficient fluids to counterbalance what is being lost through frequent bowel movements, in order to guard against dehydration (see box, above right).

Oral rehydration therapy, the replacement of fluids and electrolytes (sodium, potassium, bicarbonate) lost during acute diarrhea, has become commonplace both in this country and in developing nations, where it has had a major impact on the prognosis of children with infectious diarrhea, a major cause of infant death in these countries. As long as the child is not having severe vomiting along with the diarrhea, it is possible in most cases to replace the deficits. (A severely dehydrated child may need intravenous hydration.)

Unless the physician advises otherwise, a nonprescription solution such as Pedialyte can be used to maintain electrolyte balance. Unfortunately, the commonly recommended "clear fluids" (such as ginger ale and flavored gelatin) are not adequate because they lack electrolytes. Oral rehydration so-

---

SIGNS OF DEHYDRATION

Estimated Percent of Dehydration

5 percent
Dry mucous membranes
Decreased urine production
Concentrated urine
Decreased tears
Slightly increased heart rate (10 percent above base)

10 percent

Worse than above
Sunken eyeballs
Depressed anterior fontanel ("soft spot")
"Loose" skin (decreased turgor)

15 percent

Much worse than above
Decreased blood pressure (shock)

---

lutions should only be continued for a day or two because they do not provide sufficient calories to prevent malnutrition. The use of lactose-free formulas or a BRAT (bananas, rice, applesauce, tea) diet is popular among many practitioners in the recovery phase. It may be advisable to avoid high carbohydrate juices, such as grape or apple. In any case, the important thing is to provide sufficient calories.

Other causes of acute diarrhea in a previously well child include contaminated food, poisons (iron, arsenic, insecticides), laxatives, specific food intolerances, emotional stress, and constipation with fecal soiling. In a sick child possible causes include antibiotics, acquired sugar intolerance, Hirschsprung's disease, milk protein allergy, or quite commonly either an upper respiratory tract or a urinary tract infection. (See table 23.1.)

Table 23.1 **CAUSES OF ACUTE DIARRHEA IN CHILDREN**

In an otherwise well child:
  Dietary indiscretions
  Infections
  Contaminated foodstuffs
  Antibiotics
  Poisons
  Laxatives

In a sick child:
  Viral or bacterial gastroenteritis
  Carbohydrate intolerance
  Milk protein allergy
  Inflammatory bowel disease

Chronic Diarrhea

Chronic diarrhea sometimes presents a more difficult diagnostic puzzle. Some babies and young children develop chronic diarrhea that has no apparent cause and does not seem to be medically serious. The child continues to grow and develop normally despite having several loose, runny stools a day. Although it may be troubling to the parents, this type of chronic diarrhea is not a problem as long as the child is eating and growing normally.

The most common cause of chronic diarrhea in well children between the ages of six months and three years is the irritable bowel syndrome, also called nonspecific diarrhea of infancy and childhood or toddler's diarrhea. Another cause is acquired lactase deficiency or rarely, milk protein intolerance. Both problems may begin or become worse after another intestinal infection. Food allergies also may cause diarrhea and other symptoms. Considerable detective work may be involved; keeping a careful diary of foods and other factors that may be related to the symptoms often helps pinpoint causes. Dietary changes usually suffice and the condition is ultimately outgrown.

In the infant or child who is not thriving, chronic diarrhea is apt to result from a serious condition. Some of the more common disorders are cystic fibrosis, celiac disease, and immune deficiency disease. Maternal deprivation syndrome can result in malnutrition and failure to thrive. Celiac disease and cystic fibrosis will be discussed in more detail later in this chapter. (See table 23.2 for a list of causes of chronic diarrhea in children.)

Specific Causes of Failure to Thrive

Failure to thrive is a condition that describes an infant or child who does not grow or gain weight at the expected rate. Since it is a gradual deceleration and not a sudden drop in weight or the total absence of growth, parents do not always notice right away, or they may assume that the child is just small. The critical importance of the weighing and measuring that is part of each physical examination in infancy and childhood is not appreciated by many parents as one of the key indicators to the child's health and well-being.

There are three patterns of failure to thrive. The first two are related to serious conditions such as severe birth defects or endocrine problems. In these cases, retardation in terms of stature is usually more severe or equal to failure to gain weight. However, the majority of infants who fail to thrive belong to the third type, in which malnutrition is the underlying cause. In these cases poor weight gain is more

Table 23.2 **CHRONIC DIARRHEA IN CHILDREN (PARTIAL LISTING)**

1. Infection
    Bacteria
    Viruses
    Parasites

2. Sugar Intolerance
    Congenital
    Acquired
        Lactose
        Sucrose-Isomaltose
        Glucose

3. Allergies
    Cow's protein
    Soy protein
    Gluten (Celiac disease)

4. Pancreatic Insufficiency
    Cystic fibrosis
    Schwachman's syndrome

5. Immune Deficiencies

6. Metabolic
    Abetalipoproteinemia
    Hormonal tumors

7. Anatomic Abnormalities
    Partial obstruction
    Enteric fistula
    Short Bowel syndrome
    Pseudo-obstruction syndrome

Adapted from "A Practical Approach to Pediatric Gastroenterology" by Joseph Levy, M.D. Year Book Medical Publishers, 1988.

prominent than failure to grow in height.

Malnutrition may result from inadequate caloric intake, caloric losses from gastrointestinal disease, or impaired peripheral utilization, a condition arising from infection, disease, or an inborn error that prevents the proper utilization of nutrients by the cells. Often there will be an interplay among the three causes. In addition, environmental, social, and cultural forces may play a role in failure to thrive caused by malnutrition.

At least half of those babies who fall into the malnutrition category suffer only from inadequate caloric intake and will grow normally when the amount of food given meets their needs. Babies may not get enough calories in families where poverty is so severe that there is not money enough to purchase adequate food for the nursing mother or formula and food for a bottle-fed baby. This problem has been largely relieved by the U.S. Department of Agriculture's Women, Infants, and Children (WIC) Program, which provides both food coupons and nutritional counseling for pregnant women and those with children up to age five. Malnutrition can also be a problem where the mother is very young, without the necessary knowledge or ability to properly nurture her baby, or where she has a psychiatric disorder or drug or alcohol dependency. Sometimes the baby is not wanted or is neglected by an overwhelmed, isolated, or sick parent. However, even stable, mature mothers (both nursing and nonnursing) who adhere to dietary cults or strict vegetarian diets may also compromise their babies' nutrition. While such dietary regimens may be adequate for adult family members, they may deprive infants and small children of necessary nutrients.

There are several ways in which an infant or child can lose calories even though adequate amounts are being taken. The most obvious are vomiting and diarrhea, which have been discussed earlier.

In addition, there is a whole group of disorders called malabsorptive states that prevent adequate nutrition because digested food cannot be absorbed from the small intestine into the lymph channels or veins, from which it is distributed through the body. (See figure 23.5.) Defects in transport occur in a variety of ways. Certain enzymes may be missing or functioning improperly within the absorptive cells of the intestine either through inborn error or acquired disease. Or these cells may be hindered in their work by disease processes that affect the tissues, disturb motility, permit excessive bacterial growth, or block the normal passageways. If a sig-

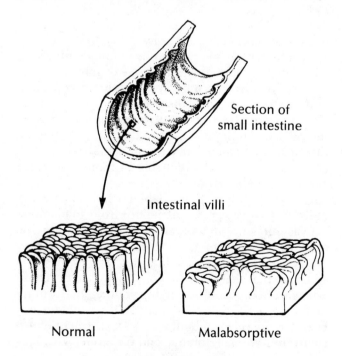

Section of small intestine

Intestinal villi

Normal   Malabsorptive

Figure 23.5. **Anatomy of Malabsorption.**

nificant portion of the small intestine has been surgically removed, malabsorption may occur because of inadequate bowel surface.

Celiac Disease. Celiac disease (gluten enteropathy) and cystic fibrosis (see next page) together comprise the most common causes of malabsorption in infants and children in the United States. In those with celiac disease, foods containing gluten—most notably wheat products—damage the lining of the small intestine. Just how and why this occurs is not clear. It was once thought to be the result of a metabolic defect in which an intestinal enzyme that detoxifies gluten is missing. Now it is believed that celiac disease may be an immunologic disorder in which gliadin (an extract of gluten) produces an injurious immune response in the intestinal mucosa. There are still many questions about the relative importance of genetics and environment (for example, the age at which gluten is introduced into the diet).

Celiac disease often occurs in several members of one family, and it is more common in Europe and in Canada than in the United States, the highest incidence being in Ireland. It is uncommon in blacks and Asians.

Celiac disease usually appears in children between the ages of 8 and 24 months, most commonly between 9 and 12 months of age. Often it is not diagnosed immediately, and by about 18 months the child will have a history of several months of diarrhea, both height and weight will be well below normal, the limbs will be wasted in contrast with a round face and a distended abdomen. The child will have a poor appetite and exhibit constant irritability. This is a typical picture, but some children will be asymptomatic, some will be suddenly desperately ill, and others will not have the pale, fatty, foul-smelling, and bulky stools that are characteristic of the disease. In older children, short stature may be the only visible sign. Because celiac disease affects children in a variety of ways, a definitive diagnosis can only be established through a process of intestinal biopsies, positive response to diet changes, and worsening after rechallenge with wheat.

The critical factor in treatment is a gluten-free diet. Because no series of patients has been followed through life, there is still no definitive proof that rigorous adherence to the diet throughout life is essential. Indeed, it is very hard to convince parents to maintain the diet because it is difficult to do so as the child becomes more socially independent and because the obvious symptoms of celiac disease sometimes disappear. When gluten is introduced later in life, there may be subtle changes that are not observable either to the child or to the parent. However, there is strong evidence that abandoning the diet results in either relapse of the disease or growth retardation, anemia, or softening of the bone. Those who maintain the diet can lead a normal life.

Cystic Fibrosis. Cystic fibrosis is an inborn error of metabolism in which an enzyme essential to the normal functioning of the body is missing. It is caused by a single recessive gene, meaning that both parents must carry the defective gene, although neither will have any symptoms of the disease. In the United States it is estimated that one person in every 20 has the gene for cystic fibrosis, but this is primarily within the white population. Black children are occasionally affected, Asian children rarely.

Only 30 years ago, cystic fibrosis was considered a rare disease universally fatal in childhood, often before age two. Now it is known to affect about one in every 1,500 to 2,000 white children (although only one in 17,000 black children). There is no cure, but improved treatment has dramatically extended life expectancy so that 80 percent of those with cystic fibrosis now live beyond the age of 20.

Cystic fibrosis affects the body's exocrine glands, which control the production of mucus, saliva, and sweat. Children with cystic fibrosis produce an abnormally gluey mucus that blocks the pancreas, preventing the transport of essential digestive juices to the intestines and interfering with the digestion of food. This same type of mucus clogs the lungs, causing breathing difficulties. And because the excessive sweat contains a high concentration of salt, there is a danger of dehydration and salt depletion in hot weather.

It is the unusually high salt content in the sweat that provides the first clue to diagnosis. Most babies born with cystic fibrosis appear normal and healthy at birth. Only about 5 percent show any signs of the disease in the newborn period, and in these babies the intestine becomes clogged with meconium, causing an emergency that must be corrected immediately by surgery.

In some children, digestive problems appear first and predominate, while in others lung problems cause more distress. Those with greater lung problems have a poorer outlook. Treatment is largely symptomatic. The pancreatic enzymes are replaced by a commercial supplement, and a nutritious diet must be maintained. These children often require twice the amount of food normal children eat to maintain near-normal weight and growth. Their stools tend to be large and full of undigested food particles, and passing these bulky stools often irritates the rectal area. Sometimes the mucous membrane of the rectum may push out through the anus (rectal prolapse).

A variety of complications may appear. Peptic ulcers can occur at any age. Those who survive to adulthood may develop diabetes. And all males with cystic fibrosis are sterile. Even so, the outlook for those with cystic fibrosis is rapidly improving, and the hope is that the defect will be identified and that it can be treated as many other genetic diseases are.

Other Causes of Malabsorption. Malabsorption in children may also be caused by milk protein intolerance; disaccharidase deficiency, which blocks the chemical reaction needed to digest some sugars; immunologic deficiencies; parasitic infestation; liver disease; congenital anatomic defect of the bowel; and inflammatory bowel disease, though the latter is seldom seen in children under age five.

One of the most common of these is lactose intolerance, caused by the lack of the enzyme lactase, which is necessary to digest lactose, the sugar found in milk. Between the ages of six and twelve, many peoples of the world lose this enzyme. For example, lactose intolerance affects 75 percent of Africans and nearly 100 percent of Asians. In fact, only Northern Europeans and other ethnic groups with pastoral heritages are relatively unaffected. For those affected, the degree of intolerance varies. Some, for example, are able to drink one glass of milk, but experience cramps with the second glass. Others can tolerate no more than a half glass or none at all.

Constipation and Fecal Soiling

Constipation may be defined as a decrease in the frequency of defecation, hard stools, and/or painful defecation. Although it occurs frequently in infancy and childhood, and is a great source of concern to parents, constipation is seldom medically significant in this age group. In the newborn period, however, constipation is always considered significant, because it may indicate that there is some intestinal obstruction or malformation.

Early introduction of solid foods or a change from breastmilk to cow's milk may cause the stools to be fewer in number and harder. A change in environment or an illness may also cause temporary constipation in the infant or small child. If hard stools have caused an anal fissure, the subsequent pain in passing stools may cause the baby or child to hold back and further complicate matters. Very often the condition can be managed by the addition of high fiber foods such as bran to the diet or the use of stool softeners or both.

If constipation does not respond to dietary changes, the physician will look for other symptoms, since constipation alone rarely signals a serious disorder. It may well be the first symptom noticeable to the parent, however. One disorder (although rare) for which obstinate constipation may be the only, obvious symptom is Hirschsprung's disease, described above in this chapter, under Congenital Defects.

Severe constipation with fecal soiling (encopresis) may occur when a physiologic problem causes excessive dehydration of the stool within the intestine. This hard stool, which is difficult and painful to pass, becomes impacted, and then liquid stool seeps around the impaction and is expelled involuntarily. This condition may also occur because of coercive toilet training, or in an older child as a result of psychosocial factors. A child with this problem is usually well and has already been fully toilet trained. Often the child will try to hide the problem, and parents sometimes assume it is a "training" problem and fail to report it promptly.

Other symptoms usually accompany fecal soiling. They include painful defecation, fissures, occasional passage of a very large stool, urinary frequency, loss of appetite, and abdominal pain. The condition can be helped with guidance, and it is important to do so not only from a physiologic point of view but for psychological reasons as well.

When fecal soiling occurs in the child who has never achieved continence or fails to respond to usual therapeutic measures, other factors such as neurological or psychological disorders may be involved.

Abdominal Pain

The precise diagnosis of abdominal pain is often difficult and elusive. First of all, the pain may be nonspecific, and it may be referred pain originating from another site. In addition, the characteristics of pain may be perceived differently by different people. This problem is compounded when the patient is too young to discuss the nature of the pain or when the pain is described by a parent. The physician must try to determine whether the pain is acute or chronic, whether there is any ongoing or underlying condition that might produce the pain, and, if possible, the location, character, duration, and radiation of the pain. These clues, combined with information including the age and sex of the child, the nature of the onset, the accompanying symptoms, and the physical exam form the base from which the diagnosis will be made. Fortunately, most abdominal pain in infants and children is self-limiting and has no lasting significance.

Colic, a group of symptoms that often appear in the newborn period and usually disappear by the time the baby is three or four months old, is a common cause of apparent abdominal pain in early infancy. The cause is unknown. Though intestinal allergy, overfeeding, and swallowing air have been proposed as possible factors, a temporary immaturity of the peristalsis mechanism in the intestines is currently believed to be the most likely candidate. Babies with colic typically cry frantically, apparently from acute abdominal pain. They may draw their legs up and clench their fists, and nothing the parent does seems to have much effect.

Colicky babies generally continue to gain weight and otherwise thrive. However, their irritability and frequent bouts of crying, typically at the same time each day, can cause great physical and psychological stress for the parents. Babies will sometimes be relieved by being placed stomach-down across the parent's knees, on a lukewarm hot-water bottle while their backs are gently massaged, or carried after feeding in a soft baby carrier (such as a Snugli) for 15 to 20 minutes. Some babies seem better after a bowel movement or passing gas. Parents can and should seek relief by leaving the baby in competent hands for a few hours of entertainment or relaxation as often as possible.

Colicky behavior that is fairly constant may signal a milk allergy. In such cases the doctor may recommend changing to a different formula for a bottle-fed baby or he may suggest that the nursing mother avoid milk products.

Unless the colic attacks are suddenly accompanied by vomiting or abdominal bloating, which might indicate some more serious problem, parents need not worry. However, any sudden change in the pattern should always be reported immediately.

In an older infant (typically 6 to 24 months of age), the sudden onset of severe colicky pain may be the first symptom of intussusception, a telescoping of one section of the intestine into the next. Additional symptoms may include bile-stained vomitus or stools that resemble currant jelly. Intussusception can occur in a well child, but it is frequently associated with a recent intestinal infection, surgery, or an injury. If the intussusception has not been present for more than 24 hours, the condition can sometimes be corrected by administration of a barium enema. If this is unsuccessful, or if some predisposing condition such as a Meckel's diverticulum (see below, under Bleeding), a polyp, or a tumor must be corrected, then surgery is indicated. The repair is generally simple, hospitalization is usually brief, and most children have no recurrence or complications.

In preschool children, gastroenteritis is the most frequent cause of abdominal pain. It is generally suspected by both parent and physician in the presence of accompanying symptoms of fever, vomiting, and diarrhea, particularly when a similar illness is widespread in the community. Other conditions that may look like stomach flu at the outset are appendicitis and, rarely, pneumonia. Sometimes the correct diagnosis can be made only when the flu-like infection does not follow a normal course.

Vague abdominal pain may be an indication of a genitourinary problem, especially in girls. Pain that is more localized may indicate some organic problem such as liver or gallbladder disease or ulcers. Other causes for abdominal pain in both infants and children are sugar intolerances and a whole array of drugs, including aspirin, nonsteroidal antiinflammatories, antibiotics, and theophylline.

Bleeding

Parents and children old enough to be aware of such an incident are truly alarmed by the vomiting of blood or the passing of blood rectally. Consequently, such an event is promptly reported to the physician. Since the number of conditions associated with blood in the vomitus or the stool is impressive, the initial information provided to the doctor can be most helpful in arriving at a diagnosis.

The effects of some substances can simulate rectal bleeding, and a quick mental check of what the child has ingested should be undertaken before assuming that the color in the stool is actually blood. Food coloring, beets, fruit drinks, gelatin desserts, and drugs such as ampicillin syrup can look very much like blood. If these can be ruled out, it is important to note the color of the blood (bright red, dark red, or tar colored) and whether the blood is only on the outside or is mixed into the stool. Also significant is the amount of blood (streaks, drops, a teaspoonful or a cupful). Last, are there any other symptoms such as pain, pallor, diarrhea, constipation, fever, or vomiting? These facts, along with the child's age and medical history, will help the physician in the diagnostic process.

In the newborn period, rectal bleeding is often associated with the birth process. Maternal blood swallowed by the baby during the course of labor may be passed. Certain drugs taken by the mother before delivery may predispose an infant to hemorrhagic disease or stress gastric ulcers, or hemorrhagic gastritis may result from a difficult labor and delivery. In addition, infectious diarrhea (bacterial) is usually accompanied by bloody stools. All of these conditions occur within the first few days of life, and except for the presence of swallowed maternal blood, which has no medical significance, prompt diagnosis and treatment may be life-saving.

From age one month onward, the leading cause of rectal bleeding in infants and children is anal fissure. Fissures are caused by the passing of very large or hard stools. When later stools are passed a small amount of red blood may streak the outside of the stool, and a drop or two of blood may also appear after the stool is passed. The presence of a fissure may cause considerable discomfort or pain and should be treated promptly to prevent intentional holding of stool to avoid pain.

Small amounts of red blood both on and within the stool may indicate an inflammation of the anus or rectum. And small amounts of blood in the stool are frequently caused by infectious diarrhea. In an infant with a family history of milk intolerance, bloody stools may be the first clue to this condition, though other symptoms such as eczema, colicky pain, and vomiting may be present.

For toddlers and preschool children, the most frequent cause of rectal bleeding after anal fissures is juvenile polyps. This condition will be suspected if a well child begins to pass small amounts of bright red blood both within and on the outside of the stool. Juvenile polyps are not precancerous, but depending on the number and location of the polyps, the physician may recommend that they be removed during childhood, since adult polyps are frequently dangerous. The procedure is a simple one and is often done on an outpatient basis.

The passage of a large amount of blood, especially in a child under age two, suggests the presence of a Meckel's diverticulum. This is a small outpouching of the intestinal wall near the end of the small intestine where a duct between the intestine and the navel that is present before birth fails to disappear completely. If it becomes irritated and bleeds profusely or perforates, it must be surgically removed.

The passage of blood clots or a dark red (currant jelly) stool probably points to intussusception, described above under the topic Abdominal Pain.

Children who are taking or have just completed a course of oral antibiotics sometimes develop antibiotic-associated colitis. In such cases, bright red blood in the stools, accompanied by abdominal cramps, diarrhea, and abdominal distention is the typical pattern. Effective medical therapy is available.

When blood is vomited (hematemesis), just as in rectal bleeding, it is useful to review what the child has eaten or drunk in the past few hours to rule out red food dyes and other substances that might be mistaken for blood. Also, the color and quantity of blood vomited, as well as other symptoms, if any, should be noted and reported.

Small amounts of bright red blood in the vomitus of a child who is suffering from prolonged vomiting or retching can arise from blood vessels in the esophagus. This bleeding will stop when the vomiting has subsided.

When suffering a nosebleed, children sometimes swallow considerable amounts of blood. If this blood stays in the stomach for even a short time, it may look like coffee grounds when vomited. If the amount of coffee-ground vomitus is very small and follows a nosebleed or dental work, there is no cause for concern. Occasionally small amounts of coffee-ground materials will appear with viral gastritis or after taking aspirin. However, this type of hematemesis is usually related to an ongoing illness or abnormality and is reason to seek immediate medical attention if the cause is not clear.

In the newborn period, the causes of vomiting blood are for the most part the same as for rectal bleeding and are often related to factors in labor and delivery. Except for the swallowing of maternal blood as a cause of hematemesis, all other causes are serious and require rapid diagnosis and immediate treatment.

After the newborn period and during the first year, the most common cause of vomiting large amounts of bright red blood is a bleeding duodenal or gastric ulcer. In children aged three to five, this symptom is more apt to result from esophageal varices (varicose veins in the esophagus). However, either condition may occur from infancy forward. Both disorders usually occur in children with some underlying cause that predisposes them to the problem. Children with esophageal varices are often otherwise asymptomatic, while children with ulcers usually have other symptoms as well.

More often the amount of blood vomited is small and is of the coffee-ground type. The most likely causes for this type of bleeding are peptic esophagitis and gastritis (inflammation and irritation of the foodpipe and stomach, respectively). In addition to disease states that cause esophagitis and gastritis, in small children the swallowing of foreign objects and caustic substances can produce these inflammations. If a child swallows a caustic substance, it is important to determine the exact chemicals involved if at all possible. When the substance can be identified, an immediate call to the nearest Poison Control Center should be made for emergency instructions even before going for medical assistance. If the substance cannot be identified, medical aid should be sought promptly. Foreign objects are somewhat easier to deal with since most can be detected by X-ray examination.

Jaundice

Bile pigment (bilirubin) is the product of the breakdown of hemoglobin in the red blood cells when they are destroyed. If the liver is unable to excrete the bile pigment for some reason, or if the pigment is produced at a faster rate than the liver can handle, the bilirubin will accumulate in the serum of the blood, causing a yellow discoloration of the skin and eyes, a condition called jaundice.

There is a long list of possible causes for jaundice in the newborn. Fortunately, many are relatively rare and three of the most common causes are not considered dangerous. However, because a large number of conditions causing jaundice can be life-threatening, it should never be taken lightly.

Jaundice appears in a significant number of newborns when they are three or four days old. It occurs because the immature liver cannot excrete adequate amounts of bile pigment. This is called physiologic jaundice, and it clears spontaneously in a few days as the liver begins to function normally. Occasionally a factor in breastmilk can interfere with one step in the process of handling the bile pigment, causing hyperbilirubinemia. And certain drugs may be responsible for an elevated bilirubin. Jaundice from these causes appears in well babies and usually has no medical significance.

Among the more serious causes of jaundice in the newborn are isoimmunization disorders such as ABO and Rh-factor disease, blood poisoning (septicemia) caused by a major infection, hemolytic anemia, birth deformities of the bile ducts, and a host of conditions affecting the liver (see preceding section, Liver and Gallbladder Defects).

Sometimes jaundice will not be noticed until the six-week examination. Most frequently this is breastmilk hyperbilirubinemia, but if the baby is producing pale, clay-colored stools and dark urine, some form of obstructive jaundice or viral hepatitis are likely causes. Obstructive jaundice occurs when the flow of bile into the intestines is completely obstructed, either by the absence of ducts, by a cyst or tumor pressing on the ducts, or by swelling inside the liver due to infection closing the intrahepatic channels. The appearance of pale stools and dark urine are always cause to seek immediate medical attention.

SURGERY OF THE GASTROINTESTINAL TRACT

Hernias

A hernia is the protrusion of a part of the intestinal tract through a weak spot in the structure that normally confines it. The most common hernias in infants are umbilical hernias and inguinal (groin) hernias. Umbilical hernias occur more frequently in girls than in boys, and in black children more often than in white. Inguinal hernias are somewhat more common in boys.

The vast majority of umbilical hernias cause no pain and eventually close naturally by the time the child is one or two. It was once thought that these hernias should be strapped or taped to assist in closing, but this is now thought to be useless or perhaps harmful. On rare occasions a loop of intestine may become incarcerated in the hernial sac, causing pain and vomiting. If this should happen, surgery is required to correct the problem.

Inguinal hernias can occur at any time in life. In male babies they are usually discovered as a bulge alongside the penis or in the scrotum, and in females the mass will appear in the groin area beside the external genitals. Often there is a tendency for inguinal hernias to appear on both sides.

Ordinarily there is no pain associated with these hernias, but if a loop of bowel gets into the hernial sack there may be considerable discomfort. If the bowel is caught in the sack (incarcerated), the pain will increase and the child may vomit. If the circulation to the incarcerated loop is cut off (strangulation), the child will become very ill and probably vomit. A strangulated loop can become gangrenous in a matter of hours, so prompt treatment is in order.

In the case of incarceration or strangulation, surgery will be performed immediately, no matter what the age of the infant. However, if these conditions are not present the physician may prefer to wait until the baby is three or four months of age. The procedure is simple and safe, recovery is complete, and there is rarely a recurrence after repair.

On rare occasions a baby is born with a defect in the diaphragm that allows the abdominal contents to protrude into the chest cavity. This is a true emergency requiring immediate surgery if the child is to live. An incision is made in the upper abdomen, the protruding organs are properly placed, and the rent in the diaphragm is closed. If the abdominal cavity is too small for the contents being placed there, the outer layers of skin and tissue will be closed leaving the muscular layers of the abdominal wall open, to be repaired a few months later after sufficient growth has occurred. When diagnosis and treatment are prompt, the outlook for these children is excellent.

Appendicitis

Appendicitis is more difficult to diagnose in infants and young children than in older children and adults because the symptoms are much less specific. Pain is rarely localized, and several of the symptoms might result from something else. Typical symptoms in a child with appendicitis include lack of appetite, immobility, irritability, moaning, fever, vomiting, keeping the legs flexed, and crampy pains that become constant.

Acute appendicitis is rare in very young children, and sometimes even the most expert doctor cannot be absolutely sure that the child has appendicitis. However, any stomach ache that persists for more than an hour should be reported. If there is serious suspicion of appendicitis, immediate surgery will be advised. The reason for this is that in young children an inflamed appendix tends to develop quickly and may burst within a matter of a few hours. When this happens the infection can spread throughout the abdomen. This is called peritonitis, and it is a serious condition, indeed, far more dangerous than the surgery.

Surgical procedures related to pyloric stenosis, esophageal strictures, and tracheoesophageal fistulas were discussed above under Congenital Defects.

DIAGNOSTIC TOOLS

IN ADDITION TO THE chemical and cellular analysis of blood, stool, and tissue samples used to diagnose medical conditions, pediatric gastroenterologists use a particular group of tests to determine what may be wrong within the intestinal tract. The most commonly used tests are these.

Upper GI Series. Barium, a contrast material similar to chalk, is given either by bottle, spoon, or tube in order to observe its progression down the esophagus and through the stomach. The test does not expose the child to excessive radiation and is very important in diagnosing anatomical problems with the esophagus, stomach, and upper intestine.

Small Intestine X Rays. The procedure is the same as above, except that the barium is followed every 30 minutes until it reaches the end of the small intestine, the site of inflammations such as ileitis.

Barium Enema. A "bowel prep" is required in order to clean the large intestine of fecal material. This is done by giving a laxative solution such as magnesium citrate or other salt solutions especially used for this purpose. With the new solutions, preparatory enemas are not necessary and the results are excellent. The procedure itself consists of placing a small tube in the rectum and dripping in barium to fill the large intestine. Air is sometimes blown into the intestine to provide better detail of the bowel walls. This test is useful in detecting inflammation (colitis) and polyps, or other congenital problems, including lack of ganglion cells (Hirschsprung's disease).

pH Monitoring of the Esophagus.

This is a relatively new test that determines the frequency and duration of acid reflux from the stomach into the esophagus when reflux is suspected in serious conditions such as apnea (intermittent halts in breathing), aspiration pneumonia, esophagitis, feeding difficulties, etc.

A small wire is placed through the nose into the esophagus allowing constant measurement of the acidity. This can be simultaneously correlated with the symptoms as they occur. Once the probe is in place, the child is rarely disturbed by its presence.

Breath Hydrogen Test.

This test is done to document carbohydrate intolerance. The child is given a dose of the sugar suspected of being malabsorbed. If this is the case, the sugar will progress to the large intestine where bacteria will digest it, producing hydrogen. This hydrogen is expelled in the breath and can be measured simply by collecting expired air in a special bag, or in an infant, by collecting air from the nostril. This test has taken the place of tolerance tests, which required frequent blood drawing to document the expected rise in the sugar level, proof that the sugar was digested and absorbed.

String Test.

A small gelatin capsule containing a cotton thread is swallowed, leaving the end of the string taped to the cheek. The gelatin is dissolved in the stomach and the string is carried into the upper intestine. After three or four hours, the string is removed and the mucus adhering to it is squeezed onto a glass slide for examination. This is the best test to detect certain parasites living in the duodenum that may be the cause of persistent diarrhea or other intestinal symptoms. The test is painless and gives better results than several stool examinations for parasites.

Endoscopy.

The literal meaning of endoscopy is "to look inside." It is possible to see the inside of the intestinal tract with the help of flexible tubes having a fiberoptic system. If the endoscopy is of the upper GI tract it is called esophagoscopy (esophagus), gastroscopy (stomach), or duodenoscopy (duodenum). In the lower GI tract, the terms would be proctoscopy (rectum), sigmoidoscopy (the beginning of the large intestine), and colonoscopy (the entire large intestine).

General anesthesia usually is not required, especially in the older child. Instead, an injection of medications such as diazepam or meperdine is given just before the test, which is done in the endoscopy suite or the operating room. The heart and respirations are constantly monitored by the doctors and the assisting nurse.

The upper endoscopy involves passing the tube through the mouth and advancing it under direct vision, observing the lining and noting sites of inflammation or bleeding. The flexible endoscope can be passed into the duodenum. If necessary, an ERCP can also be done. This stands for endoscopic retrograde choledoco pancreatoscopy and involves passing a small tube into the pancreatic or the bile duct and injecting contrast material while X rays are taken. Although these tests are not pleasant, they carry very little risk and the radiation exposure is extremely low.

Ultrasonogram.

In this test, a probe is passed over the skin after a soft jelly has been applied. Sonography permits accurate diagnosis of many intestinal conditions by detecting masses, stones, tumors, enlargement of ducts such as the bile ducts, ureters, etc. Abscesses, ovarian disease, and organ enlargement can be detected without exposing the child to radiation. This test is painless.

CT Scan.

Computerized tomography is a special type of X-ray study permitting precise visualization of the inner organs and their relations to other structures, as if a "cut" through the body had been done. It is useful in investigating tumors, masses, and organ enlargement.

Nuclear Scan.

A large variety of compounds can be injected into the body and are picked up by the bones and various organs such as the liver, spleen, and kidneys. Recently these compounds have been added to milk and solids to determine the rate of stomach emptying. The injected or ingested isotopes emit radiation that can be detected with a gamma camera. The patient lies quietly under a round detector until the image has been collected. It takes longer than an X ray, but the amount of radiation is very small.

Magnetic Resonance Imaging (MRI).

This technique uses magnetic fields to "scan" internal structures. It does not use radiation, and thus is safer than X rays, CT scans, or other such procedures. It is very costly and, at present, available mostly at large medical centers only.

24 Childhood Blood Disorders

Sergio Piomelli, M.D.

INTRODUCTION

AN ABNORMAL BLOOD TEST in a young child is not necessarily cause for alarm. Many abnormalities are slight or represent temporary reactions to infections. If, on the other hand, the condition requires expert attention, the child may be referred to a pediatric hematologist, a pediatrician who specializes in blood disorders of children. Even when they require further testing to rule out more severe disorders, most blood abnormalities turn out to be minor. And although some blood disorders are severe and life-threatening, many of these can be cured with proper treatment.

CHILDREN'S BLOOD

BLOOD CIRCULATES IN A one-way system, carrying life-sustaining nutrients and oxygen to cells throughout the body, and removing their waste products. Chem-ical messengers, particularly hormones, also travel through the circulation; thus, blood serves as a means for parts of the body, however distant, to communicate with one another. Blood also provides a vehicle for the immune system, which helps fight infection.

Blood is not the only fluid in the body's circulatory system: the other one is *lymph*. Fluid, formed after blood filters through the tissues of the body, drains into the lymph, which circulates through a network of lymph nodes and is then returned to the bloodstream. Lymph also contains antibodies (proteins that help protect the body against foreign substances), as well as white blood cells that have traveled through the walls of the blood vessels; both antibodies and white blood cells help fight infection. Swollen lymph nodes are often associated with infections.

When something goes awry with the circulatory system, effects are often seen throughout the body. Conversely, when disorders, including infections, affect tissues elsewhere in the body, they can often be discerned as abnormalities in the components of the blood.

Components of Blood

Blood consists of a variety of cells suspended in a liquid known as plasma. (Table 24.1 lists the different blood types.) The three kinds of blood cells are red cells, white cells, and platelets. Each type of cell plays a specific role in the overall functions of the blood.

Red Cells. Responsible for carrying oxygen, red cells (also known as red blood cells or *erythrocytes*) are the most numerous of the cells in the blood. They contain *hemoglobin*, an iron-rich substance that gives the color to these cells—and to blood itself. Each hemoglobin molecule has two components: *heme*, the iron-containing part, and *globin*, the protein portion. As blood passes through the lungs, hemoglobin picks up oxygen and retains it as the blood travels through the arteries. Not until reaching the capillaries, a network of tiny blood vessels that surround cells in tissues throughout the body, does hemoglobin release this oxygen, which is then used in cells' energy-producing activities. The blood then carries carbon dioxide, a waste product of these activities, back through the veins to the lungs, where it is exhaled, completing the cycle. Red cells, which have a lifespan of about 120 days, are continuously replaced. The iron salvaged from old red cells is recycled and used to make hemoglobin for new ones.

White Blood Cells. Helping to protect the body against disease-causing bacteria, viruses, and fungi, white blood cells (also called *leukocytes*) come in three main types: *granulocytes, monocytes,* and *lymphocytes.* Granulocytes (grainy cells, including *neutrophils, eosinophils,* and *basophils*) and monocytes all serve as a nonspecific kind of reserve army, rapidly increasing in number to respond to a variety of infections; they engulf foreign substances such as bacteria and also destroy worn-out red cells. Lymphocytes mount specific immune reactions to particular infectious agents. They include *B-cells,* which produce antibodies, and *T-cells.* T-cells and B-cells interact in complex ways to control the immune response to diseases. (For more information on immunology, see chapter 31, Allergies.)

Platelets. Responsible for coagulating (or clotting) blood, and thus protecting the body against prolonged bleeding when a blood vessel is damaged, platelets are not actually cells, but small, colorless fragments of large cells called *megakaryocytes.* Platelets aggregate (clump together) at sites of blood vessel injury where they begin to form a clot; formation of the clot is completed by other components of the clotting system (see Plasma below). The fully formed clot is a mass of clumped platelets held in place by a network of protein that forms around them, plugging up injured blood vessels.

Plasma. The yellowish liquid in which the blood cells are suspended is called plasma. In contrast, the term *serum* refers to the liquid that remains after blood that has been removed from the body coagulates and the clot is removed; so serum is plasma minus the coagulation factors, which are proteins in the plasma that collaborate with platelets and blood vessel walls to clot blood.

Development of Blood

All types of blood cells are produced, matured, and released into the blood through a process called hematopoiesis. In this process, most of the immature

Table 24.1 **BLOOD GROUPS**

Percentage of U.S. Population with Each Blood Type:

	O	A	B	AB	All ABOs
Rh positive	39	35	8	4	86
Rh negative	6	5	2	1	14
Both Rhs	45	40	10	5	

There are four major blood groups—A, B, AB, and O—with each one divided further into two Rh types, positive and negative. When patients receive blood transfusions, they get donor blood that has been matched with their own ABO group and Rh type.

Each blood group represents a different type of inherited antigen (protein) on the surface of every red cell. And people develop naturally occurring antibodies (immune proteins providing protection from antigens from outside the body) in their plasma against the type of antigens that are not present on their own red cells. If they received any blood containing antigens they lacked, their antibodies would immediately attack the "foreign" blood cells, make them agglutinate (clump together), and destroy them.

People with group A blood have A antigens on their red cells and antibodies against B in their plasma; and those with B blood have B antigens and anti-A antibodies. Those with AB blood, who have both A and B antigens but no anti-A or anti-B antibodies, are known as universal recipients, because they can receive blood from donors with any of the four ABO blood groups; and those with O blood, who have neither A nor B antigens but both anti-A and anti-B antibodies, are known as universal donors, because they can donate blood to any of the four groups.

Even though people with Rh negative blood do not spontaneously produce naturally occurring antibodies against the Rhesus antigen or factor that they lack, Rh matching is also important to them. Their first exposure to Rh positive blood will cause them to develop antibodies against the Rhesus antigen; and a second exposure to Rh positive blood could then cause serious complications and even death.

blood cells (called stem cells) are produced in the blood-forming tissue of *bone marrow* (the fatty material in cavities inside many of the body's bones). These undergo a process of maturation in the bone marrow; when fully developed, they are released into the bloodstream. For example, *reticulocytes* (a specific type of young red cells) are present in large amounts in the bloodstream of the fetus and they persist during the first few days of life. Reticulocytes are even more abundant in newborns whose birth was premature.

It is considered normal (that is, "physiologic") for the composition of the blood to change as an individual develops from a fetus into an infant, child, and adult. Red cell production and hemoglobin concentration fall dramatically during the first weeks of life; this normal process is called *physiologic anemia* of infancy. In premature infants this decrease, called physiologic anemia of prematurity, is even sharper, but it usually causes no problems.

The percentage of the blood's volume occupied by the red cells (called the *hematocrit*, or *HCT*) is about 60 percent in the newborn. As the infant matures, the HCT normally drops to about 32 percent at nine weeks, and then rises gradually through childhood to about 43 percent in adult women and 45 percent in men.

Hemoglobin normally changes in quality as well as quantity. Within the first six months of infancy, the composition of hemoglobin shifts from the fetal form (which is adapted to life in the womb) to the so-called adult form, in which one of the two types of globin chains is different. Each hemoglobin molecule contains two types of globin chains: the alpha- and gamma-globins in the fetal form; and the alpha- and beta-globins in adult hemoglobin.

White blood cells, like red cells, are present in high concentrations immediately after birth; their numbers decrease during the first week, then level off until one year of age when they start declining steadily until reaching adult amounts at about 21 years of age. The levels of white blood cells are quite labile because it is normal for them to increase during periods of infection.

Unlike red and white blood cells, platelets are present in the newborn in concentrations within the normal adult range. Although many of the plasma's coagulation factors are decreased in activity in the newborn, most reach normal adult levels within the first few weeks of life.

BLOOD DISORDER DIAGNOSIS

THE MOST COMMON BLOOD TEST is a *complete blood count (CBC)* which involves counting the number of each type of cell in a given volume of blood and examining the cells under a microscope to check for any abnormalities in their size or shape.

Interpretation of a child's CBC takes into account the age of the child because the normal numbers of the various blood cells change throughout infancy and childhood. Information from a CBC can help detect a variety of blood disorders. Frequently, however, more sophisticated tests will be required to confirm a suspected diagnosis.

The CBC includes a red cell count, calculation of the packed volume of red cells, the percentage of blood volume occupied by these cells (the hematocrit, or HCT), and the hemoglobin concentration (amount of hemoglobin present in a given amount of blood). If the hemoglobin concentration is below normal for a given child's age, anemia is present.

A white blood cell count is another part of the CBC. A high white blood cell count for the child's age does not necessarily signify any trouble. A temporary increase in production of white blood cells can be a normal—and even desirable—response to an infection. To check for disorders of specific white blood cells, a differential count measures the relative amounts of various types of white blood cells.

Other blood tests measure the number of platelets and the bleeding time (how long blood takes to clot). In addition, two other tests, the *prothrombin time (PT)* and *partial thromboplastin time (PTT)*, measure the function of different but overlapping groups of coagulation factors. If either of these is found to be abnormal, tests of individual coagulation factors will be conducted.

Samples for these tests are usually collected by drawing blood from a vein in the arm. However, blood for a complete blood count is sometimes taken from a fingertip or heel. Blood can also be obtained from the umbilical cords of newborns and even fetuses for certain types of tests. In addition, it is sometimes useful to obtain a sample of the bone marrow to diagnose disorders of blood cell production.

Examining Cord Blood

Diagnosis of blood disorders can start early. At birth, the newborn's blood is usually taken from the umbilical cord and sent for a series of routine tests. For fetuses at high risk of anemia, hemophilia, Rh factor disease, or a low platelet count, diagnosis can start even earlier with an experimental approach called *percutaneous umbilical fetal blood sampling* that involves advancing a needle through the uterus into a blood vessel in the umbilical cord. This is done under continuous ultrasonic monitoring to make sure blood is taken from the proper place.

Even earlier in the pregnancy, amniocentesis and other tests can determine whether the fetus has thalassemia, sickle-cell anemia, or hemophilia.

Examining Bone Marrow

Abnormalities in bone marrow function, including overproduction or underproduction of various types of blood cells, can be detected by examining bone marrow under a microscope. The marrow is usually obtained by inserting a needle into the back portion of the child's pelvic bone and aspirating (sucking out) a small amount of marrow fluid. This procedure is done under a local anesthetic. Often, at the same time as the aspiration, a bone marrow biopsy consisting of a small core of bone and marrow is also obtained. The bone marrow is examined for the presence of normal precursors of blood cells, which are counted, and a careful search is conducted under the microscope to detect any abnormal cells. Bone marrow examination is a crucial part of the diagnosis of leukemia and other disorders of blood cell production.

RED BLOOD CELL DISORDERS

THE MOST COMMON DISORDER of red cells is *anemia*, a condition in which the blood does not contain enough hemoglobin to carry adequate amounts of oxygen to the cells of the body. If the hemoglobin concentration is low for a child's age, anemia is present. A number of different disorders can result in insufficient amounts of hemoglobin.

Regardless of the cause of the anemia, the symptoms tend to be similar. They may be quite subtle, increasing in severity as the anemia gets worse. Signs and symptoms include pallor, fatigue, weakness, dizziness, shortness of breath, heart palpitations, and irritability. Pallor appears as paleness not only of the skin, but also of the gums, nailbeds, palm creases, and the undersides of the eyelids. Anemia in small children may even cause behavioral problems.

When anemia is suspected, a thorough history, a physical examination, and additional blood tests are obtained to reveal the underlying cause of the anemia. There are several different causes of anemia in children. Iron deficiency is the most common, but anemia can also be caused by lead poisoning, chronic disease, and inherited disorders of hemoglobin and the hemolytic anemias.

In iron-deficiency anemia, insufficient iron is available for the production of hemoglobin. Lead poisoning also interferes with hemoglobin production, but usually does not result in anemia unless a child is also iron deficient. Various infections and chronic diseases, including certain cancers, can lead to anemia by causing an underproduction of red cells. Anemia can result from defective hemoglobin production as in certain inherited disorders such as sickle-cell anemia and thalassemia. The red cell disorders known as *hemolytic anemias* involve a high rate of hemolysis (breakdown) of the red cells thereby shortening their lifespan. Anemia results when the bone marrow's production of new red cells cannot keep up with the rate of breakdown. Hemolytic anemias can be caused by inherited disorders such as glucose-6-phosphate dehydrogenase (G6PD) deficiency and other enzyme disorders.

In addition, many children have red cell abnormalities that do not necessarily cause illness but still may have important implications for the child's future. Such abnormalities, which can be detected by routine screening tests, provide clues used to pick up the carrier states of inherited red cell disorders.

Iron-Deficiency Anemia

Iron-deficiency anemia, by far the most common form of childhood anemia in the United States, is due to an inadequate supply of iron, restricting the production of hemoglobin. Although iron from old red cells is recycled into new ones, dietary iron is still necessary to make up for the small amounts of lost iron. Children require extra iron, as compared with adults, to allow for proper growth. Indeed, the factor that contributes most often to the development of iron-deficiency anemia in children is rapid growth. Blood loss usually plays a role in iron deficiency in children.

The prevalence of iron-deficiency anemia in the United States is highest during late infancy and adolescence with a peak between six months and three years of age. In addition, it is particularly prevalent in children from low-income families. Iron-deficiency anemia of infancy should not be confused with the normal process of physiologic anemia of infancy in which red cell production and hemoglobin concentration decline. (This occurs earlier and, as discussed above, is a normal condition.)

Symptoms of iron deficiency tend to appear gradually, and are similar to those of other anemias. Fatigue, decreased exercise tolerance, irritability, and loss of appetite are the most common. When the anemia is extreme, the heart may become enlarged and its rhythms disturbed. In chronic forms of anemia, including iron deficiency, the body undergoes some physiologic adjustment to the anemia. When a child has chronic anemia, the symptoms may not be as severe as those of another child with the same degree of anemia, but in an acute form (from hemolytic anemia or blood loss). Thus, a child with chronic anemia may be more anemic, yet not appear as sick as a child with acute anemia.

To make sure the child receives all necessary treatment, it is necessary to determine whether blood loss contributed to the iron-deficiency anemia, even in children with iron-deficient diets. Treatment usually consists of giving oral supplements using a form of iron called ferrous sulfate. It is important that iron be given in moderate doses (1–3 mg/kg/day). Excessive iron can induce gastrointestinal irritation, and in extreme doses, bleeding. An iron-deficient diet can be corrected by increasing the intake of foods such as meats, dark green leafy vegetables, and iron-fortified flour products including bread and cereals. The body's absorption of the iron tends to be enhanced when the iron-containing food or supplement is taken with citrus juice; absorption declines when it is taken with milk or tea.

Although breastmilk contains iron in a form that is particularly easy for the body to use, both breastmilk and cow's milk contain less iron than does a mixed diet. Therefore, some experts recommend that iron supplementation should start by six months after birth in term infants and two months in premature infants to prevent iron deficiency. For breastfed infants, iron-fortified cereal can be given; for formula-fed infants, iron-fortified formula and iron-fortified cereal are available. Iron drops are not recommended for normal children. Treatment with iron drops should be reserved for those children with proven iron-deficiency anemia. (See chapter 4, Nutrition in the First Year.)

Lead Poisoning

Lead is a toxic metal without any function in the body, but centuries of lead mining have released so much lead into the environment that most people have measurable amounts of lead in their blood. The major sources of lead for children in the United States are leaded paint (found mostly in old houses), air and dust lead (which are greater in urban areas), and food lead (which is greater in canned food). Drinking water that flows through old lead-containing pipes is another source.

Lead paint, of the type used before World War II, is the most concentrated source of lead. Children ingest lead from paint sometimes in the form of paint chips, but mostly as dust. Sources of air lead are emissions from cars using lead-containing gasoline and from lead-smelting factories. The lead in canned foods comes mostly from the lead solder used to manufacture the cans. Dietary intake of lead is additive to the ingestion of lead in dust.

Especially before they reach school age, children have higher blood lead levels than do adults sharing the same environment. Children breathe in more airborne lead than do adults. With their frequent hand-to-mouth activities, they also end up consuming more lead dust than do adults. A child will absorb several times as much lead for a given amount of body weight as will an adult fed on a diet with the same composition. This occurs because children require more calories per unit of body weight, and their intestines absorb more lead.

Low-level exposure to lead can exert adverse effects on hemoglobin synthesis and on the nervous system well before any symptoms become obvious. Lead interferes with the activity of a variety of enzymes all over the body, but particularly in the blood, including some of those that help produce the heme portion of hemoglobin. The heme-producing biochemical pathway can be affected even at blood lead levels as low as 14 micrograms per deciliter—well below the levels presently considered "acceptable." This interference is produced by lead competing with iron in the heme-production process, and when iron levels are low, lead is even more likely to do so.

Children's intestinal absorption of lead is increased by dietary deficiencies of iron. Thus there are two reasons why inner-city children in low-income families are particularly susceptible to lead's effects: they tend to be at highest risk for both iron-deficient diets and lead exposure (from peeling lead-based paint and car exhaust). Their susceptibility can be reduced by supplementing their diets with iron.

There are indications that hemoglobin-synthesis changes and other effects may start at lead levels too small to cause obvious symptoms. Amounts of lead in the body above 50 micrograms per deciliter of blood have long been linked to childhood learning problems; recent studies indicate that the presence of even small amounts of lead in the body can diminish children's cognitive ability and learning skills.

A standard screening test for lead in which a fingertip is pricked can detect lead's effects on red cells long before anemia becomes obvious. Severe lead poisoning of children first results in malfunctioning of the nervous system; the neurotoxicity of lead can cause encephalopathy (a disease of the brain), with seizures, coma, and even death before anemia develops. In children, as opposed to adults, anemia is a late effect of lead poisoning.

Treatment involves controlling the seizures and giving chelation therapy to remove the lead from the body. It is essential to identify the source of the lead in the child's environment and to remove it (or to remove the child).

Glucose-6-Phosphate Dehydrogenase Deficiency

There are numerous inherited abnormalities of red cell enzymes that cause hemolytic anemia, although most of them are rare. (In hemolytic anemia, older red cells undergo hemolysis, or breakdown, faster than the bone marrow can produce new red cells.) The most common example of this sort of disorder is deficiency of an enzyme called glucose-6-phosphate dehydrogenase (G6PD), which can be caused by a variety of defects in the gene for this enzyme.

The gene for G6PD, like those affected by hemophilia (discussed later in this chapter), is sex-linked (carried on the X chromosome). Therefore, the disease almost always affects boys, who have only one X chromosome, rather than girls, who have two. Men cannot pass G6PD deficiency on to their sons, to whom they give a Y, not an X, chromosome. Instead, it is passed from mother to son. Women who carry a defective G6PD gene usually do not have the disease, because they are protected by the normal gene on their other X chromosome; however, they may have somewhat less than the usual amount of the G6PD enzyme. On average, they will pass the trait to half of their daughters, who will be carriers, and to half their sons, who will have G6PD deficiency (the other half will be normal).

The disorder can occur in any ethnic group. It affects about 5 percent of Chinese and 10 percent of black American boys and men. It is also frequent in other races, particularly in populations from subtropical areas, such as the Mediterranean, Southern China, etc. Like the sickle-cell trait and thalassemia, the G6PD deficiency trait exerts a protective effect against malaria in areas of the world where the disease is or was common.

G6PD deficiency is always associated with a reduction in the lifespan of the red cells. Yet the symptoms depend on which type of defective gene is present, and they range from mild to severe. The types that appear in blacks tend to cause milder symptoms, whereas those in people of Mediterranean descent tend to cause more severe symptoms.

With the most common of the mutant forms, chronic hemolysis is usually mild, but with some other very rare types it can cause severe physical impairment with jaundice (yellowing) of the skin and the whites of the eyes and enlargement of the spleen (splenomegaly). Most types of G6PD deficiency are associated with acute flareups of hemolysis, usually provoked by infections or exposure to certain chemicals, including some drugs (which are harmless to most other people). Infants can be exposed to such medications from breastmilk (or, while still in the womb, through the placenta). These acute episodes involve increasing pallor, jaundice, dark urine, back pain—and in the most severe cases, shock, heart failure, and even death.

Except for avoidance of the substances that cause hemolysis in these children, no form of treatment for G6PD deficiency is available—or even required in the chronic state, except for the extremely rare severe mutant forms. The acute hemolytic episodes require supportive treatment, including removal of the causative agent (such as a medication) and blood transfusions if necessary.

Sickle-Cell Anemia

There are two major types of inherited disorders of hemoglobin; both involve the globin portion of the oxygen-carrying molecule. In one group, which includes sickle-cell anemia, an abnormal type of globin is made; in the other, which includes the thalassemias, a smaller than normal amount of the normal alpha (or beta) globin is made. Both groups cause a lack of functional hemoglobin and thus result in anemia.

Sickle-cell anemia is particularly prevalent among blacks, but it also occurs in people from Central and South America, India, Asia, and the Mediterranean region (including Greece, Italy, and Arab countries). In the United States, about 1,500 black babies are born with sickle-cell anemia each year; 1 in 600 blacks has the disease and 1 in 12 carries the trait.

Sickle-cell anemia causes the formation of abnormal red cells that look like sickles. When the abnormal hemoglobin molecules (known as hemoglobin-S) bond together they form rods that twist red cells into the sickle shape. Unlike normal red cells, which are round and flexible, the rigid sickle cells are easily damaged as they pass through small blood vessels. This damage causes chronic hemolytic anemia in which red cells are broken down at a high rate. Although in response the body expends more energy than normal on making new red cells, the blood still lacks sufficient functional hemoglobin. In addition, because of the malfunctioning of the spleen, children with sickle-cell anemia are much more susceptible to various infections, including certain types of pneumonia.

During acute episodes called sickle-cell crises, the rigid sickle-shaped cells can clog small blood vessels, causing severe bone pain or even death of tissue due to loss of blood supply. By the time the child reaches adulthood, these repeated crises can cause permanent damage to the kidneys, lungs, liver, and central nervous system. Crises can also involve acute anemia as a result of any of three causes: temporary decreases in the rate of red cell production in bone marrow (often caused by infection), increases in the amount of red cells sequestered by the spleen, or acute hemolytic anemia in children with both sickle-cell disease and glucose-6-phosphate dehydrogenase deficiency.

If the appropriate blood test is done at birth, sickle-cell anemia can be diagnosed in infants who have not yet shown any symptoms of the disease. Indeed it is highly recommended that screening for sickle-cell anemia be made available for all newborn babies. When screening is not limited to the particular ethnic groups at most risk, it is less likely to miss any cases of the disease. Newborn screening makes it possible to identify sickle-cell anemia at birth and allows for treatment to begin as early as possible. This treatment involves starting preventive therapy with the antibiotic penicillin when the child with sickle-cell anemia is four months old, and continuing it until at least five years of age. Any fever of 101 degrees F. or higher should be considered a life-threatening emergency for these children, even if there are no other symptoms of disease. They should also receive vaccinations to protect them from infectious diseases such as hepatitis, flu, and pneumococcal pneumonia.

The gene that causes sickle-cell anemia is recessive; that means two copies of it have to be present to cause the disease. People with only one copy of the gene, who are called carriers of the trait, do not have the disease. Instead, they are actually at an advantage in areas where malaria is common, because they tend to survive that disease better than do people without the trait. For this reason the sickle-cell trait is present in certain ethnic groups, such as that of the American black, who originated from areas of Africa where malaria was endemic for centuries.

People who know that sickle-cell anemia runs in their family are urged to get tested and to seek genetic counseling before pregnancy. It is also important for the spouses of carriers of the trait to be tested. When both members of a couple carry the trait, for each pregnancy the chances are one in four that the child will have sickle-cell anemia; two in four (or one in two) that the child will carry the trait; and one in four that the child will have neither sickle-cell anemia nor the trait. The disease can be diagnosed prenatally. (See chapter 3 in *The Columbia University College of Physicans and Surgeons Complete Guide to Pregnancy* for a more detailed discussion of genetic disorders.)

Thalassemia

There are two main types of thalassemia: alpha-thalassemia, in which an insufficient amount of the hemoglobin component called alpha-globin is produced, and beta-thalassemia, also known as Cooley's anemia or Mediterranean anemia, in which beta-globin is lacking. Since the beta-thalassemia genes are recessive, people with only one copy, who are said to have thalassemia minor or thalassemia trait, do not have the disease; two copies need to be present, as in people with thalassemia major, to cause the disease.

Beta-thalassemia. In beta-thalassemia, normal beta-globin is produced either in small amounts or not at all. Most Americans with the disorder are descended from families from the region around the Mediterranean Sea, including Italy, Greece, and Arab countries, as well as India and Southeast Asia. However, it also occurs in people of Middle Eastern, Southeast Asian, and African descent.

Infants with beta-thalassemia appear normal at birth. A few months later the first symptoms of the disease develop and then become increasingly more severe. The first signs and symptoms resemble those of other types of anemia, including pallor, weakness, irritability, and failure to thrive. Fever, feeding problems, diarrhea, and other gastrointestinal problems may occur. Without transfusions, these symptoms may lead to death.

Beta-thalassemia causes a severe form of hemolytic anemia; the hemoglobin-poor red cells are short-lived and broken down at a high rate, and the spleen and liver become enlarged. In some cases, the spleen may become less effective at helping to protect the body against infection. In response to the anemia, new red cells are produced at a high rate, causing expansion of the bone marrow cavity and weakening the bones; facial as well as other bone structures may become deformed. This overproduction of red cells, which are abnormal and most of which do not even reach the bloodstream, makes massive demands on the body's metabolic energy.

There is no cure, but with prompt diagnosis and proper treatment, people with beta-thalassemia may reach adulthood; without treatment, they would die in early childhood. Treatment involves repeated transfusions of packed red cells approximately every three weeks. These transfusions provide oxygen-carrying capacity to the blood. They also eliminate the bone marrow's production of red cells, thus preventing the associated drain of energy and possible bone deformities.

Unfortunately, however, the transfused cells carry iron, and with repeated transfusions iron tends to overload the body's vital organs. This complication can be lessened by nightly infusions of a chelating medication, which helps the body rid itself of the extra iron by converting it into a water-soluble state that can be eliminated. This treatment allows the vital organs to function longer without succumbing to iron overload. The prognosis may improve as therapy for iron overload gets better. Research into new treatment continues; bone marrow transplantation may be possible for some of these patients.

Carriers of the beta-thalassemia trait, which can be detected by a set of blood tests, are often detected through routine blood testing. Although some carriers may have some minor red cell abnormalities, they are never affected by any symptoms of the disease themselves. However, because beta-thalassemia is such a severe disease (even more so than sickle-cell anemia), this trait (like sickle-cell trait) has important implications when carriers consider having children. Their spouses should be tested for the presence of the trait. If one spouse has the trait but the other does not, with each pregnancy there is a 50 percent chance of passing the trait on to the child. If both parents carry the trait, with each pregnancy they have a one in four chance of passing on the severe form of this disease, beta-thalassemia major. Each of their children has a one in four chance of not inheriting even the trait. The disease can be diagnosed prenatally in the first trimester of pregnancy.

People with beta-thalassemia trait need to know that they have it and to remember that if they are going to have children, their partners should be tested for both beta-thalassemia and sickle-cell traits. A disorder called sickle thalassemia results in a fourth of the offspring of couples who include one person with sickle-cell trait and another with beta-thalassemia trait. Sickle thalassemia resembles sickle-cell anemia, but it is usually not as severe.

Alpha-thalassemia. This disorder, in which the normal form of alpha-globin is produced in smaller-than-usual amounts, is frequently found in Southeast Asia. In the United States it is less common than is beta-thalassemia. Because it appears that each person has four copies of the gene for alpha-globin, not just two, there are four different forms of alpha-thalassemia. They range in severity depending on how many copies are affected. These are (1) a silent carrier state; (2) alpha-thalassemia minor, or trait; (3) alpha-thalassemia major, also known as hemoglobin H disease, which involves relatively mild anemia (compared with beta-thalassemia); and (4) the most severe form, which usually results in fetal death.

WHITE BLOOD CELL DISORDERS

DISORDERS OF WHITE BLOOD CELLS can raise susceptibility to infection and lower resistance to a variety of other diseases. These white blood cell disorders fall into two categories: disorders of the function of various types of white blood cells and cancers of these cells.

The functional disorders include *neutropenia* (low amounts of the type of granulocytes called neutrophils) and several inherited immunodeficiencies that involve deficiencies in function of various types of white blood cells. Neutropenia, which is often a side effect of chemotherapy, creates a general susceptibility to overwhelming infections. Immunodeficiencies due to white cell disorders are quite rare and are recognized by a history of severe infections such as pneumonia. Neither an abnormal white blood cell count nor numerous minor infections are necessarily signs of an immunodeficiency.

In children, the most common type of severe disorder of white blood cells is leukemia, a cancer of blood-forming tissues (bone marrow, lymph nodes, and spleen) that causes overproduction of nonfunctional white blood cells and suppression of production of the other types of blood cells. Cancers other than leukemia that also involve the white blood cells include the *lymphomas* (cancer of the lymphoid tissue). The lymphomas include *non-Hodgkin's lymphoma* (which predominates in children) and *Hodgkin's disease* (more common in adults). Their first symptom is often swollen lymph nodes without an associated infection.

Leukemia

In leukemia, unusually large amounts of white blood cells are produced. These cells accumulate in the bone marrow, the lymph system, and the bloodstream, where they crowd out existing healthy cells. As a result of this crowding, the bone marrow cannot maintain production of sufficient numbers of red cells or platelets. The crowding also prevents the white blood cells from becoming mature enough to perform their infection-fighting functions.

The shortage of mature, functional white blood cells mars the body's ability to fight infections, and because of the loss of red cells, insufficient oxygen is delivered to vital organs. The lack of platelets leaves the body prone to easy bleeding and bruising. In addition, the abnormal blood cells are carried through the body by the bloodstream and lymph system to the vital organs, where they can impair normal functioning. By any or all of these mechanisms, leukemia leads to death when left untreated.

Leukemia is about as common in boys as in girls. Its causes are obscure; it has been difficult to prove that various suspected agents, including certain chemicals and viruses, are responsible for any specific cases. While certain chemicals are known to be able to cause cancer, only rarely is exposure to a certain chemical established as the cause in a specific case. Certain viruses are known to cause leukemia in animals, including cats; however, no viral cause of human leukemia has been found. There is some evidence of a genetically inherited susceptibility to leukemia; children with some inherited disorders, including Down's syndrome and congenital immunodeficiency syndromes, are at higher-than-normal risk of developing the disease.

Leukemia can occur in acute (rapidly progressing) and chronic (slowly growing) forms. In acute leukemia, the overproduced cells are all immature blood cells known as *blasts*, which are seen in bone marrow aspiration when the disease is diagnosed. The symptoms of acute leukemia usually appear suddenly. They include fatigue, weight loss, pallor, fever, repeated infections, chronic or severe bone and joint pain, and abnormal bruising (such as *petechiae*, which are small hemorrhages into the skin that appear as tiny red pinpoints) or bleeding. Symptoms of chronic leukemia are much like those of acute leukemia, but the prognosis is different. In the absence of any treatment, acute leukemia can be fatal within two months. In contrast, untreated chronic leukemia can last for years, because this form of the disease involves overproduction of mature, functional white blood cells as well as blasts. Unfortunately, in children acute leukemias are the rule. Chronic leukemias are exceedingly rare.

There are two main types of childhood leukemia: lymphocytic leukemia, which involves lymphocyte precursors formed in lymphatic tissue, and nonlymphocytic leukemia, which involves precursors of granulocytes or monocytes formed in the bone marrow. These two types can be distinguished by staining leukemic cells with dyes and measuring their levels of particular enzymes. About 98 percent of cases of childhood leukemia involve the acute form of the disease. Of these, a large majority are the acute form of lymphocytic leukemia; most of the remainder are the acute form of nonlymphocytic leukemia.

The goal of all treatment for leukemia is to produce a remission in which the body appears rid of leukemia cells with no more evidence of the disease. For long periods after remission begins, small numbers of leukemia cells persist, and without continued treatment (known as maintenance therapy), the full-blown form of the disease may recur. For most forms of leukemia, a remission that lasts five years after treatment is considered to indicate a cure.

Because of recent improvements in survival, acute leukemia is now considered a potentially curable disease. There are now many long-term survivors in remission who have never relapsed. However, despite these improvements, leukemia remains a killer of children between the ages of 3 and 14 years.

Acute Lymphocytic Leukemia (ALL). Also known as acute lymphoblastic leukemia, acute lymphocytic leukemia is sometimes termed "childhood leukemia" because it is the most common type of leukemia in children. Although it can occur at any age, it usually starts between the ages of 2 and 10 years and accounts for about 85 percent of leukemia in people under 21 years of age.

Childhood lymphocytic leukemia is the type of leukemia for which advances in treatment have been most dramatic. Indeed, it is one of the great success stories of cancer treatment. With the best treatment, as many as 75 percent of children with the disease survive—up from much less than 5 percent only two decades ago. This vastly improved outlook is attributed to the development of highly effective anticancer drugs, which usually are given in combinations. By combining chemotherapeutic drugs that have different toxic side effects and mechanisms of action, it has become possible to minimize the specific side effects from each individual drug and to prevent leukemia cells from escaping the drugs' actions by changing their genetic makeup. In addition, leukemia cells that seek sanctuary in the central nervous system can be destroyed by injecting chemotherapeutic drugs into the spinal column.

Also important is supportive therapy to treat the child until the chemotherapy takes effect. Supportive therapy includes transfusions of blood products as well as administering antibiotics and nutritional support. Sometimes radiation therapy is used to supplement chemotherapy; it may also be used (as may chemotherapy) to destroy a child's own bone marrow in preparation for bone marrow transplantation—a new approach to cases of leukemia that are particularly difficult to treat.

In bone marrow transplantation, the bone marrow is replaced with that of a healthy donor. To prevent the child's body from rejecting the donated marrow, this treatment demands finding a donor, usually the child's brother or sister, whose genetically determined *human lymphocyte antigens (HLA)* match those of the child. (These antigens, also known as human histiocompatibility antigens, are proteins found on the surface of white blood cells and most other cells in the body, and they dictate the probability that a transplant will "take.") However, in about two-thirds of cases no such HLA-matched donor is available.

When no HLA-matched donor can be found, there are two still experimental alternative approaches. Both are called autologous (same person) bone marrow transplantation because the donor and the recipient are the same person. One involves removing bone marrow from the pelvic bones while the disease is in remission, freezing it, and implanting it later if needed. The other involves removing some of the child's bone marrow, even during a relapse, but ridding it of leukemia cells in the laboratory (with the help of specific monoclonal antibodies that target the cells), and then implanting it back into the child.

Acute Myelogenous Leukemia (AML). Like acute lymphocytic leukemia, nonlymphocytic leukemia is treated using combinations of chemotherapeutic drugs. However, although remission and survival rates for acute nonlymphocytic leukemia are improving, therapy for this disease remains far less successful than that for lymphocytic leukemia, with remission achieved in approximately 70 percent of patients, lasting six to nine months, and average survival about one year. Approximately one in three children with this form of leukemia are cured. Because chemotherapy tends to be less effective for nonlymphocytic leukemia, bone marrow transplantation plays a larger role in its treatment. And because complications occur more often with nonlymphocytic leukemia than with lymphocytic leukemia, supportive therapy (including antibiotics and transfusions) is even more important for this form of the disease.

CLOTTING DISORDERS

BLOOD CLOTTING DEPENDS on a precisely orchestrated chain of events involving not only the platelets but also a variety of the plasma proteins called coagulation factors. The process starts with platelets adhering to the site of a new wound and then being held in place by a protein network that forms around them. The network is formed from a complex cascade of enzyme reactions involving the coagulation factors. In the cascade, each coagulation factor is, in turn, transformed from an inactive to an active form.

There are two main types of clotting disorders: those that involve platelets (including thrombocytopenia) and those involving coagulation factors (such as hemophilia and von Willebrand's disease). Clotting disorders in which platelets fail to function tend to cause the formation of petechiae (red pinpoints on the skin), whereas those involving disorders of the coagulation factors tend to cause bleeding deep into the tissues and joints.

Thrombocytopenia

Disorders of platelets usually involve thrombocytopenia, a deficiency of these cell fragments in the blood. The most common form is *idiopathic thrombocytopenic purpura (ITP)*. Although idiopathic

means "of unknown cause," most cases of childhood ITP are actually triggered by a viral infection, usually of the upper respiratory tract. Other cases can be triggered by medications or some other unknown factors. This triggering is thought to occur by way of the spleen's formation of antibodies against the body's own platelets, destroying them prematurely.

The bone marrow often compensates for the decline in the lifespan of the platelets by boosting its production of new ones. Because young, highly functional platelets may predominate in ITP, the blood's ability to clot is often better than would be predicted from the platelet count alone. However, children with ITP may suddenly develop "easy bruisability." They start bleeding into their skin, either spontaneously or after minor trauma, forming petechiae and purpura (larger hemorrhages into the skin, causing patches that start out red, turn purple, and then fade to brownish yellow). Nosebleeds are also common.

In about 80 to 90 percent of children with acute ITP, the platelet count returns to normal within one to three weeks, even without any treatment; other cases, which persist for over six months, are called chronic ITP. Occasionally ITP recurs years after the initial episode. Idiopathic thrombocytopenia affects about equal numbers of boys and girls (although it is seen more in women than in men). The peak age range for childhood idiopathic thrombocytopenia is two to five years of age, with progression to chronic ITP most common among older children (over nine years old), especially girls. In addition, the onset of idiopathic thrombocytopenia is usually related to the presence of another disease such as systematic lupus erythematosus, which is more common among older girls.

The most serious complications of thrombocytopenia, bleeding into the central nervous system and gastrointestinal tract, are rare. They are the main causes of death from the disease, but they occur in less than 1 percent of cases. The first month after the onset of acute thrombocytopenia is the period of greatest risk. Therefore, it is particularly desirable during this period to restrict the child's physical activity. More severe cases are treated with corticosteroid medications, and major blood loss is replaced with packed red cells or whole blood. Recently, therapy with intravenous gamma globulin at high dose has been very successful, both in acute and chronic cases. Chronic thrombocytopenia is sometimes treated with splenectomy (surgical removal of the spleen).

Hemophilia

Hemophilia includes a variety of inherited disorders of specific coagulation factors (proteins in the plasma that help blood to clot). The most common inherited coagulation factor deficiency, accounting for about 85 percent of hemophilia cases, is hemophilia A (also called classic hemophilia) in which there are insufficient amounts of the coagulation factor known as Factor VIII. Most of the remaining 15 percent of hemophilia cases involve hemophilia B (or Christmas disease) in which Factor IX is lacking.

Like G6PD deficiency (discussed earlier in this chapter), hemophilias A and B affect genes that are recessive and sex-linked (carried on the X chromosome), so the disease almost always affects boys, rather than girls. Girls who inherit a hemophilia trait are symptomless carriers, protected by the normal gene on their other X chromosome, although they may have somewhat less than usual of the clotting factor involved. Usually hemophilia occurs in families with a known history of the disease, passing from grandfather to grandson through a mother who is a carrier. Yet up to a third of new cases happen in families in which the disease has been "hidden" (with carriers only) for generations.

Children with hemophilia do not bleed any faster than others do, but their bleeding tends to last longer before a clot can form to stanch it. In addition their clots tend to be softer and less effective than usual at plugging up the injured blood vessel. Superficial external cuts often can be easily treated with pressure and a bandage; the major problem for hemophiliacs is uncontrolled internal bleeding.

In hemophilia, the severity of bleeding varies from child to child. The more severe forms become apparent early in life. Although newborns seldom show signs of hemophilia unless they are circumcised, marked bruising may develop beneath the skin as the infant starts to crawl, pull himself up, and walk. In its more severe forms, excessive bleeding happens often and sometimes spontaneously (without any apparent cause). However, in its mild forms, hemophilia may not manifest itself until later in life, and these bleeding episodes may happen only after surgery, tooth extraction, or major injury.

Blood from these episodes drains most often into the large joints, such as the knees and elbows, and the muscles of the arms and legs. It is important to stop these episodes promptly and prevent blood from collecting in the joint, where it can cause chronic pain, weakness, and even destruction of the joint (through a form of arthritis). Bleeding into muscles may put pressure on nerves, causing pain, stiffness, numbness, and eventually, if left untreated, permanent nerve damage and muscle wasting. When blood collects in the head, neck, or gastrointestinal system, it is usually even more serious.

All of these bleeding episodes are cut short only after the missing coagulation factor is replaced. The factor, derived from donated human blood, is usually supplied as purified coagulation factor concentrate (which is freeze-dried and needs to be reconstituted). It can also be supplied in the form of cryoprecipitate (which is prepared from fresh blood donations and stored in the freezer) or, for mild forms of hemophilia, as fresh frozen plasma. Any of these blood products can be infused (injected slowly into a vein) as soon as the child shows signs of bleeding. Additional clotting factor should be infused each time internal bleeding occurs. This can be done at home, and older children can even do it themselves. Although these blood products are expensive, they are necessary to prevent the devastating complications of uncontrolled bleeding.

With current medical treatment, people with hemophilia can approach a normal life expectancy. Although the disease is lifelong, it can be controlled, thereby allowing for a relatively normal life. However, depending on the severity of the hemophilia, it may be necessary to take extra care to minimize bleeding from sports injuries, surgery, and dentistry. In addition, sometimes hemophilia becomes more difficult to treat, because antibodies develop to the coagulation factor that has been infused.

Blood concentrates are prepared from the pooled blood of a large number of donors, so they may spread viral diseases such as hepatitis. In addition, people who received blood transfusions or blood product infusions between 1977 and 1985 are at some risk of having been infected with human immunodeficiency virus (HIV) which causes acquired immune deficiency syndrome (AIDS). However, since 1985, antibody testing of blood donations and heat treating of blood products have reduced this risk to near, although not quite, zero. (And, of course, it is safe to give blood donations, which are always needed, because a new, sterile, disposable syringe is used for each donor.)

Von Willebrand's Disease

Von Willebrand's disease is an inherited clotting disorder that occurs in both sexes. In most cases it takes a rather mild form, inherited as an autosomal (not sex-linked) recessive trait. The disease is caused by a defect in von Willebrand Factor, a coagulation factor that normally combines with Factor VIII to form an active complex. Without von Willebrand Factor, platelet clumping is impaired.

Unlike hemophilia, von Willebrand's disease is characterized by bleeding from the skin and mucous membranes, with nosebleeds and easy bleeding common. The symptoms of von Willebrand's disease resemble those of thrombocytopenia, because platelet clumping is impaired in both of these disorders. Treatment includes infusion of cryoprecipitate or fresh-frozen plasma, with the frequency of treatment depending on the severity of the bleeding.

SUMMING UP

THE EFFECTS OF the various blood disorders of childhood depend on which component of blood they affect. Those that affect red cells cause anemia; those that affect white blood cells impair resistance to infection, and those that affect platelets or coagulation factors in plasma cause bleeding.

Tremendous progress has been made in recent decades in treating these diseases. Advances in molecular genetics offer hope for new treatments for children's blood disorders. For instance, genetic engineering may allow production of coagulation factors for people with deficiencies of these factors, including hemophilia: within a few years, abundant and safe supplies of pure, virus-free Factors VIII and IX may become available. Researchers are also attempting to develop a new approach called gene therapy in which a normal gene would be inserted into the blood-forming cells of a child with any of several inherited blood disorders such as thalassemia and sickle-cell anemia.

In the future it may be possible to manipulate a newly available group of hormones, known as hematologic growth factors, to stimulate the bone marrow to make specific types of blood cells in desired amounts. These factors include erythropoietin, which stimulates production of red cells, and granulocyte-colony stimulating factor, granulocyte-macrophage-colony stimulating factor, and interleukin-3, which induce production of certain types of white blood cells.

FURTHER RESOURCES

For more information about children's blood disorders, contact the local chapter of the following organizations:

American Cancer Society (on leukemia)
4 West 35th Street
New York, NY 10001
(212) 736-3030

Cooley's Anemia Foundation
105 East 22nd Street, Suite 911
New York, NY 10010
(212) 598-0911

Leukemia Society of America
733 Third Avenue
New York, NY 10017
(212) 573-8484

March of Dimes
Birth Defects Foundation
(on Cooley's anemia, hemophilia, sickle-cell disease, and thalassemia)
1275 Mamaroneck Avenue
White Plains, NY 10605
(914) 428-7100

National Association for Sickle Cell Disease
4221 Wilshire Boulevard, Suite 360
Los Angeles, CA 90010
(213) 936-7205

National Hemophilia Foundation
110 Greene Street, Room 406
New York, NY 10012
(212) 219-8180

Sickle Cell Disease Foundation
209 West 125th Street
New York, NY 10027
(212) 865-1201

25 Urogenital Disorders

Martin A. Nash, M.D., and
Terry W. Hensle, M.D.

INTRODUCTION

IN BOTH SEXES—BUT especially in males—the organs of reproduction lie in close physical and functional relationship to the organs involved in excreting urine. For this reason, the two systems are generally referred to as one: the urogenital system.

The organs of the urinary system are the two kidneys, the two ureters, the bladder, and the urethra. (See figure 25.1, next page, for a drawing of the normal urinary tract.)

THE KIDNEY

LOCATED AGAINST THE back abdominal wall on either side of the spine at the level of the lowest ribs, each kidney is shaped like a lima bean. At almost every age, kidney size correlates with the size of the fist. At birth, each kidney weighs only 0.5 ounce; a 12-year-old's kidneys are 3.3 ounces each.

The kidney is a complex filtering system, one of whose most important functions is cleansing the body's blood supply of waste material and excess fluid and separating what needs to be retained in the body from what should be excreted in the urine. Moreover, the kidney functions as a gland, producing hormones important in the production of red blood cells, in regulating blood pressure, and in the formation of bone.

The filtering process works like this: Blood enters the kidney through the renal artery, a major branch of the aorta, the heart's main artery. Once inside the kidney, the blood passes through the *nephrons,* the kidney's functioning units. (Each kidney contains about one million nephrons.) A neph-

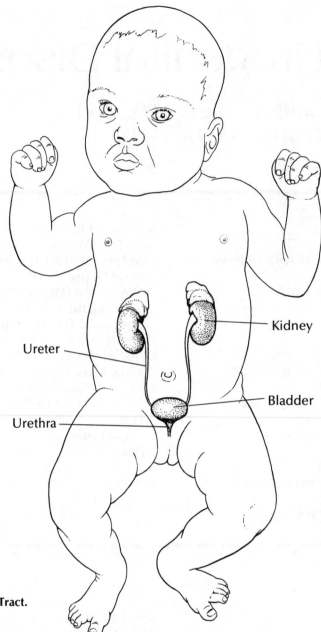

Figure 25.1. **Normal Urinary Tract.**

ron is made up of a cuplike receptacle containing a cluster of small blood vessels, the glomerulus, and a long tubule lined with specialized cells. First the blood passes through the *glomerulus* where everything but blood cells, protein, and large particles are filtered out. These unfiltered substances are returned to the bloodstream, while the fluid and the smaller particles—useful or not—pass through to the tubule. Here almost all (99 percent) of the water, salts, and nutrients is reabsorbed. Waste substances such as urea, creatinine, uric acid, and excess salt, water, and calcium empty into the center of the kidney (the pelvis) and from there into the *ureter*, the muscular tube connecting the kidney to the bladder. They are stored in the bladder until it becomes full

and are then eliminated through the *urethra*. The cleansed blood—containing salt, protein, sugar, calcium, and other substances vital to maintaining normal body chemistry—leaves the kidney through the *renal vein* and circulates throughout the system.

At any given time, one-quarter of the blood pumped from the heart is being filtered through the kidneys. Blood arriving at the glomeruli must be regulated to a precise pressure and flow. The nephrons accomplish this in part by sensing pressure and releasing an enzyme called *renin* into the total blood circulation. This results in the production of angiotensin, which causes constriction of blood vessels (arteries). If the pressure is too high, less renin will be released and the walls of all the blood vessels throughout the body will tend to relax. If the pressure is too low, increased renin causes the production of *angiotensin* and constriction of the vessels that will bring pressure up to normal.

Angiotensin also stimulates the production of the hormone *aldosterone* (itself a chemical messenger) in the adrenal gland at the top of the kidney. This hormone regulates the uptake of salt in the tubules of the nephrons. Retained salt and water raise the volume of plasma in the blood, and so increase the blood pressure. A new balance is then set as the higher blood pressure causes the nephrons to reduce their release of renin. It is easy to see that there is a close connection between diseases of the kidney and blood pressure.

DEVELOPMENT OF THE KIDNEYS AND URINARY TRACT

AT ABOUT FIVE WEEKS' gestation the kidney begins to form in the embryo. The development of the primitive ureter, the ureteral bud, begins simultaneously. The normal development of one is necessary for the normal development of the other. For example, if there is no ureteral bud, the kidney on that side also will be absent.

Even before birth, the kidneys manufacture urine. Excreted urine is partially responsible for the formation of amniotic fluid. If the fetal kidneys are abnormal, there may be a decreased amount of amniotic fluid. In utero, the *placenta* performs the major filtering function of the kidney. Waste products pass directly from the fetus's blood into the mother's through the placenta. At birth, the infant's kidneys must take over the whole responsibility for dealing with waste products in the blood.

Birth defects of the urinary tract usually involve an obstruction, most commonly where the different structures of the tract meet—the junctions between the kidney pelvis and the ureter, the ureter and the bladder, and the bladder and the urethra. Obstruction may also occur in the urethra itself. Any obstruction in the system puts a strain on the parts above the blockage. For example, if there is a blockage between the bladder and the urethra, accumulated urine will stretch the bladder, back up into the kidney pelvis, and distort the nephrons. If this is untreated, kidney failure may eventually result.

In a newborn, an enlarged kidney may be detected by touch, but a partial obstruction in the tract may not be felt and may not produce symptoms until the child is older. Sometimes a problem will not be apparent until an infection has occurred. Difficulty in urinating, a dribbling flow of urine, infection, and a complete failure in toilet training are signs of trouble and should be brought to a doctor's attention.

URINATION AND THE APPEARANCE OF URINE

FOR 90 PERCENT OF INFANTS, the first voiding occurs within the first 24 hours of life. After that, infants can generally be expected to urinate 8 to 20 times per day, with the total day's volume ranging from 1/3 to 1 cup. For young children, the frequency drops to 6 to 8 voidings in a 24-hour period, with the amount increasing from the one-year-old's 2-cup output to 1½ quarts for older children. The usual adult output is 1½ to 2 quarts a day.

Parents are often unduly concerned about the urine's color. As a rule, the color ranges from clear to pale yellow in early childhood. Parents may notice a faint pink stain in the diaper, which is the result of urate, a salt of uric acid, and not a cause for alarm. Similarly, some foods change the urine's color. The urine of a baby who has eaten beets, for example, may have a reddish cast, whereas infant vitamins may turn it orange. Occasionally, anxious parents rush to the pediatrician only to find that what they thought was brown urine in their child's diaper was actually spilled chocolate milk.

The urine of infants and very young children usually has little odor, but as the child grows, parents often notice an unpleasant smell. This in itself is not a sign of infection, although the urine of a child with a urinary tract infection may have a bad odor, and parents whose child has had numerous infections often become adept at detection simply by smelling the urine. The odor is that of ammonia, which is secreted by the kidneys into the urine and helps buffer acid. The longer the urine remains in the diaper and is decomposed by bacteria, the more the odor intensifies. The urine of children over two years old contains more ammonia than that of infants and therefore may have a more pronounced odor.

BLADDER CONTROL

MOST CHILDREN ACHIEVE daytime control of their bladders between the ages of two and three. Crucial to this control is a sufficiently developed relationship between the nerves at the base of the bladder and the sphincter that controls the flow of urine. Prior to age two, most children are not physically capable of holding their urine until an appropriate time. Control at night takes longer. Although bed-wetting is a frequent complaint among parents, it is a common condition, especially in children who sleep deeply, and most doctors would not be worried if it continued to occur in a child of four or five.

There are some physiological causes for the inability to control urination. Some children have a small or spastic bladder that cannot hold a normal amount of urine; others leak urine constantly as a result of underdeveloped nerves in the bladder, a condition known as *neurogenic bladder*. These children, however, are usually wet during the day as well as at night.

Before undertaking a major medical investigation for isolated bed-wetting without daytime wetting or infection, parents should examine whether the problem responds to simple measures, or could be an emotional response to something such as the birth of a sibling or the move to a new home. If the situation continues, however, consultation may be warranted.

Treatments for isolated bed-wetting include restricting fluids in the evening, waking the child up to go to the bathroom before the parent goes to bed, using an alarm that is triggered by the first drops of urine, and reward programs. While every method has its advocates and critics, it is clear that neither punishment nor humiliation is helpful. The best treatment usually is "tincture of time."

URINALYSIS

URINALYSIS IS THE examination of collected urine and is the first step in determining the presence of kidney or urological disease and in separating major from minor problems. A urinalysis is often part of the routine physical exam.

In the laboratory, a dipstick is used to determine the urine's acid level and to detect the presence of protein, blood, glucose, and ketones. The urine is then centrifuged so that its solid components are collected in the bottom of a tube. They are examined under the microscope for red blood cells, white blood cells, and casts.

If an infection is suspected, a culture of the urine is done. This involves growing the bacteria to determine the species, so that the appropriate antibiotic can be prescribed. An abnormal number of red or white blood cells may indicate an infection.

The collection of urine for culture is a simple procedure that may be performed by the parent. The genitals are first thoroughly cleansed with soap. For infants, a special bag obtained from the physician is placed over the genitals and promptly removed after the child voids. Children who are toilet trained are instructed to start urinating in the toilet. Halfway through the process the parent places a cup under the stream. This midstream approach is used to avoid collecting in the sample the bacteria that normally surround the opening of the urethra.

The presence of protein in the urine *(proteinuria)* may or may not indicate a kidney problem. Sometimes infants excrete protein during illnesses with high fever, but once the temperature returns to normal, the urine clears. Some children have *orthostatic proteinuria,* which means that there is protein in the urine if sampled while they are standing but none while they are lying down. While the cause of this anomaly is uncertain, these children are not at high risk for developing kidney disease. Children with persistent proteinuria regardless of body position should receive additional evaluation, even though the risk of a major kidney problem is small. They may require blood and radiological studies such as an intravenous pyelogram (a contrast X-ray procedure commonly referred to as an IVP) or a sonogram.

Blood in the urine also requires additional tests, although as an isolated finding it usually is not associated with major kidney disease unless there is a family history of kidney disease. The blood may cause the urine to appear redish or smoky, or it may be detected only with a microscope. When a urinalysis detects both blood and protein in the urine, a prompt and thorough investigation should be undertaken, as this finding frequently indicates kidney disease.

URINARY TRACT INFECTIONS

THE MAJORITY OF THOSE who suffer from urinary tract infections are female. Bacteria commonly enter the urinary tract by spreading up through the urethra (they may also be transported in the bloodstream). Generally the bacteria are *Escherichia coli,* normal inhabitants of the intestines.

Because the female's urethra is shorter than the male's, which runs the length of the penis, it is easier for bacteria to invade the bladder.

Typically, a urinary tract infection affects the bladder and does not infiltrate the kidney. With children, the usual symptoms are pain in the lower abdomen and burning during urination. Those who are toilet trained may suddenly start wetting the bed or having accidents on the way to the bathroom. Frequency of urination may increase, yet the amount at each voiding may be small. Sometimes blood is visible in the urine, or it will have an unpleasant odor. Some children, especially infants, may have a fever. In an infant with a urinary tract infection, however, fussiness may be the only symptom.

The only way to determine whether there is infection is to do a urinalysis and urine culture. Unfortunately, the tests are not helpful in determining whether the infection involves the kidney, a potentially serious situation, or is limited to the bladder. This is where a physical examination is important. The physician will check for fever, chills, and back pain, and if symptoms indicate kidney infection, the child may be admitted to the hospital, where antibiotics will be injected directly into the bloodstream.

Treatment for urinary tract infection consists of a 7-to-10-day course of oral antibiotics. Symptoms should disappear within 24 to 48 hours. A second culture is usually done after the medication is completed to ascertain that the infection has completely cleared. Thereafter, the urine should be checked several times a year. After several closely spaced infections, some children may be treated with a bedtime dose of an antibiotic over six months or more to prevent recurrence of infection. Some children may have bacteria in the urine without any other sign of disease. If appropriate tests are negative, these children should be checked annually for several years to make sure they remain healthy.

Following the first urinary tract infection, a child should be evaluated for an underlying physical abnormality. One-third of children with urinary tract infection have a backward flow of urine *(uretero vesical reflux)*. Thought to be a congenital abnormality of the point where the ureters enter the bladder, reflux allows urine to flow back up to the kidney. In itself, this is not necessarily a problem. The danger comes if the urine becomes infected, thus introducing infection into the kidney. Untreated this can lead to scarring and decreased function.

Reflux and other disorders of the urinary tract are detected by an X ray of the bladder and urethra, called a *voiding cystourethrogram (VCU)*. This is an outpatient procedure in which the patient is catheterized and fluid infused into the bladder. Whether the reflux has caused damage to the kidneys can be assessed by an intravenous pyelogram (IVP) or renal scan. The severity of reflux is graded from I to V, with the latter being the most severe. Eighty percent of children with grades I or II do well on low-dose antibiotic therapy, eventually outgrowing the problem. Those who have a more severe grade or who continue to have infection even while taking antibiotics may require surgery to reimplant the ureter, a procedure that is 97 percent effective in preventing reflux.

KIDNEY INFLAMMATION (ACUTE BACTERIAL PYELONEPHRITIS)

Most URINARY TRACT infections remain confined to the bladder and urethra. Occasionally, however, infection spreads to the kidneys, a potentially dangerous situation. This may occur when there is an obstruction in the tract or reflux (see above). Whatever the cause, the first indication of a bacterial infection of the kidneys is often a shaking chill with a high fever. Confusingly, there is seldom any urinary frequency or discomfort on urination, as with bladder infection. However, the kidneys will feel tender when the doctor does a physical examination. As the kidneys become more inflamed, there will be other symptoms typical of infection: pain, headache, nausea, and loss of appetite.

The urinalysis will show pus (white cells) and large numbers of bacteria. The child must be hospitalized for several days while antibiotics are given intravenously or intramuscularly. Once home, oral antibiotics must be taken for a further two weeks.

CIRCUMCISION AND ANOMALIES OF THE PENIS

Circumcision. In many cultures, the surgical removal of the foreskin covering the end of the penis, is routine shortly after birth. There is some increase in urinary tract infections in uncircumcised boys; however, the procedure is usually done because of the parents' personal or religious beliefs rather than medical indications.

Later in a boy's life, several relatively rare conditions may make circumcision necessary. One of these is *balanitis*, an infection underneath the foreskin that causes redness and swelling. While it usually responds to antibiotics, the condition often warrants circumcision. In *phimosis*, the foreskin of an uncircumcised boy is constricted and cannot be completely pulled back (this is normal in infants). Later, especially if the boy has had infection underneath the foreskin, scar tissue may develop, narrowing or even blocking the urinary opening. This problem may require circumcision to allow the urine to pass. *Paraphimosis* is a condition in which the foreskin becomes retracted and cannot be brought back again over the end of the penis. This requires immediate attention. A circumcision or partial circumcision (a dorsal slit) may be needed to reduce swelling and allow the foreskin to be brought back into place.

Hypospadias. Eight boys out of 1,000 are born with the urethral opening displaced, on the underside of the penis or even in the scrotum. The condition is usually associated with a down-curved penis, called *chordee,* and at times, with kidney abnormalities. Surgery is necessary if the boy is to be able to urinate normally and function sexually later in his life. One or more operations may be necessary to bring the urethral opening closer to the tip of the penis. These are best done early, usually at about one year of age.

Epispadias. In this rare disorder, the urethral opening is at the top of the penis, rather than underneath the tip. Like hypospadias, it may be associated with curvature of the penis. It can also be found in boys with an abnormal bladder and is often associated with exstrophy (See *Exstrophy of the Bladder* later in chapter under section, Malformations of the Lower Urinary Tract.) Surgery, although often more difficult, has the same goals as that for hypospadias.

Micropenis and Concealed Penis. A micropenis is at birth less than 3 centimeters (¾ of an inch) long in a full-term male infant. Sometimes a portion of the tissue that causes the penis to be erect may be missing. If the penis is extremely small or there is a defect in formation, the decision may be made to change the sex of the child to female and surgically alter the genitalia.

A concealed penis is a normal-size organ that is either "hidden" by fat on the pubis or tethered by overly tight skin after circumcision. Surgery can be done to remove some of the fat or release a tethered penis, but this is not usually necessary.

THE TESTES, SCROTUM, AND SPERMATIC CORD

Testicular Torsion. Torsion occurs when a testicle twists on the spermatic cord that suspends it in the scrotum and so cuts off its blood supply. This constitutes a true emergency because if not un-

twisted within a few hours the testicle will die. Torsion can happen at any age, although it is most common in adolescence. Sometimes it follows strenuous physical activity—but it can also occur during sleep. The main symptoms are pain in the lower abdomen and sudden pain and swelling of the scrotum.

Although the physician can sometimes untwist the cord by hand, as a temporary measure, surgery is usually done within hours to examine the testis and attach it to the scrotal wall so it will not twist again. This abnormality is a congenital condition and often shows up on both sides, so that both testicles must be examined and, if necessary, surgically anchored to the scrotum.

Torsion of the Appendix Testis. The appendix testis is a small appendage that protrudes from the upper portion of the testis. Occasionally this twists on itself and is destroyed. The major symptom is the same severe pain associated with testicular torsion. The child should be seen by a physician immediately. Often surgery is necessary to rule out torsion of the entire testis, and to relieve the pain.

Orchitis and Epididymitis. These are bacterial infections of the testes (orchitis) and the tube connecting the testes to the vas deferens (epididymitis). The symptoms of these conditions, rare in children, sometimes mimic those of testicular torsion, at times necessitating surgery to differentiate the two.

Typically, infections are treated with antibiotics for several weeks. A few days of bed rest with ice packs and elevation of the scrotum will help alleviate the pain.

Because the infections can be associated with abnormalities of the urinary tract, it is important that the child undergo an X-ray evaluation of the kidneys and bladder, once the infection has been cleared.

Undescended Testes (Cryptorchid Testes). Two months prior to birth, the testicles descend through a small opening in the abdominal muscles (the *inguinal canal*) into their normal position in the scrotum. The scrotum is cooler than the peritoneal cavity and allows more normal sperm formation. In about 3 percent of all newborn boys, one or both testicles have yet to descend. (See figure 25.2 on the next page.) In the first year, the problem corrects itself spontaneously in all but 0.5 percent.

Treatment of cryptorchidism is important for several reasons. Boys with undescended testis may also have hernias, because the opening in the abdominal muscles has not closed correctly, and may allow a portion of the intestine or bladder to slide through and become trapped. Moreover, fertility

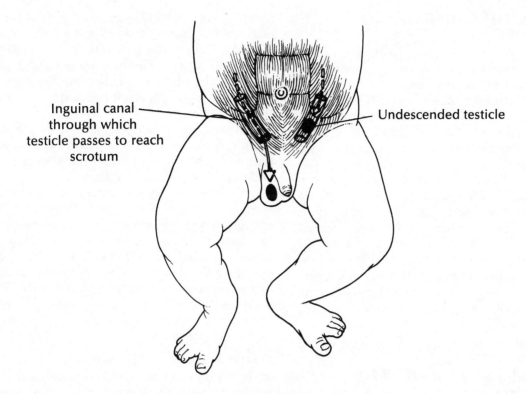

Figure 25.2. **Undescended Testicle.**

may be compromised, especially when neither testis has descended. Finally, the risk of cancer is much greater in a testicle that has not descended properly. While bringing the testis into its normal position does not reduce the risk of cancer, it does allow the testis to be examined more closely, thus enhancing the chance of early detection should cancer occur.

Sometimes the testes will be observed in the scrotum (especially when the infant is in a warm bath) and then disappear. These are called *retractile testicles* and almost invariably they descend into the scrotum on their own. No other treatment is necessary.

Some boys with both testes undescended are given a trial course of hormones (gonadotropins) to see if this will cause the testes to drop. If, however, at the end of a year, the testes still have not descended, statistics indicate that they probably will not and surgery is indicated. Generally, surgery for this condition is done between the ages of one and two.

Hydrocele. Boys are not infrequently born with a small amount of fluid surrounding the testes in the scrotum. This condition, hydrocele (see figure 25.3), is often associated with inguinal hernia. (See chapter 23, Gastrointestinal Disorders.)

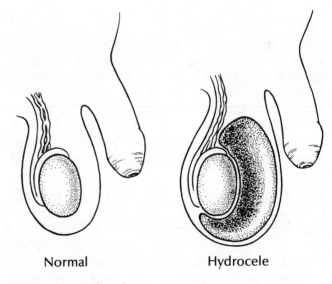

Normal   Hydrocele

Figure 25.3 **Hydrocele.**

A hydrocele is not painful or harmful and usually requires no treatment. However, if it does not disappear within a year, and especially if it is large, it indicates that the saclike projection of the peritoneum, the *processus vaginalis*, has not sealed off completely and that hernia is likely to occur (or may have occurred already). Because of the likelihood of a hernia, doctors usually recommend surgery for a large or persistent hydrocele.

VAGINAL DISCHARGE

IN THE FIRST WEEK OF LIFE, many infant girls have slight vaginal discharge, often tinged with blood. This is the result of the stimulation of the baby's uterus by maternal hormones (primarily estrogens) and is no cause for concern. Before menstruation starts, many girls have a normal clear discharge for which no treatment is needed, and which also is no cause for concern.

In the years between infancy and puberty, a vaginal discharge (often accompanied by itching and burning) may be associated with a urinary tract infection or may suggest that the girl has inserted something into her vagina that has been retained there. This foreign body must be promptly removed by a doctor. A vaginal discharge with irritation may also be associated with sexual molestation. Parents should take a close look at the girl's living situation.

MALFORMATIONS OF THE LOWER URINARY TRACT

IN BOTH BOYS AND GIRLS, congenital abnormalities are more common in the urinary tract than in any of the body's other organ systems.

Patent Urachus. The urachus is a tube that connects the bladder with the umbilicus in the early months of fetal life. In most, the tube disappears before birth. When it remains open (patent), problems occur. The infant may pass urine through the umbilicus, as in utero. If there is only a small amount of drainage, the urachus sometimes disappears spontaneously within a few days; otherwise it needs surgery.

Urachal Cysts. If the urachus is blocked near the umbilicus and near the bladder but the center portion of the tube is still open, fluid may collect in this cystic area, sometimes becoming infected and requiring surgical drainage and removal.

Sometimes infections in the area surrounding the umbilicus are confused with patent urachus. If an infection does not clear or drainage continues, X rays of the bladder and draining area should be obtained. If the child is found to have a patent urachus or a urachal cyst or infection, the urachus needs to be surgically removed.

Exstrophy of the Bladder. When the front part of the bladder and the muscles of the lower abdominal wall do not develop properly in utero, the child may be born with a bladder that opens directly onto the skin, a serious major anomaly called exstrophy.

Other abnormalities, such as abnormal separation of the pelvic bones, a short and curved penis, misplaced ureters, and a urethral opening on top of the penis (*epispadius*), may be associated with this condition of the bladder. In the male with exstrophy, sometimes the penis is not adequate for sexual function in later life.

Treatment consists of several surgeries to rebuild the bladder, penis or vagina, and urethra; to reimplant the ureters in other parts of the bladder; and to achieve urinary continence.

The first surgery usually is done within 48 hours after birth because the pelvic bones are still soft enough to be bent into the correct position. Most of the operations are completed before age six, although vaginal reconstruction is sometimes postponed until later. If a boy remains incontinent, further surgery is usually delayed until after puberty because changes in the urethra during this time can reverse the condition. Lifelong follow-up care is necessary.

Meatal Stenosis. This is a narrowing at the end of the urethra in boys which may cause the urinary stream to have the diameter of a pin. Frequently meatal stenosis is the result of irritation of the penis following circumcision. It can be treated with a simple procedure to make the opening larger.

Posterior Urethral Valves. This is a congenital obstruction in the urethra of boys. It is sometimes recognized by a characteristic dribble rather than a forceful stream during urination. The obstruction may lead to abnormal development of the kidneys in the fetus and can lead to kidney failure. The defect usually can be detected by prenatal ultrasound.

Disorders of the Ureter

Structural disorders of the ureter are usually caused by the failure of normal ureteral muscle to form, or by failure of the ureter to open into the correct part of the bladder.

Children with abnormalities of the ureters may be incontinent or have recurrent urinary tract infections. Diagnosis is made by X rays of the bladder and kidney, with all treatment aimed at preserving kidney function. There are a number of specific abnormalities:

Ectopic Ureter. The ureter does not open into the bladder in its proper location but may open elsewhere in the bladder or even in the vagina or urethra. Children with such conditions may have infection and incontinence.

Ureterocele. The muscular backing at the junction of the ureter with the bladder is missing and causes the end of the ureter to balloon (in girls, the balloon can protrude from the urethra). In either sex, there is urinary retention, infection, flank pain, and, if the condition is not corrected in time, loss of some renal function.

Megaureter. The muscle fibers of the distal ureter are abnormal, causing dilation of the ureter. This may obstruct the flow of urine from the kidney to the bladder. Children with this problem have infection and abdominal pain.

Ureteral Duplication. Two ureters supply one kidney. Often there are no symptoms nor is treatment required. Sometimes, however, the ureters enter the bladder in abnormal positions, causing obstruction in one part of the kidney and reflux in the other. A major indication of this problem is urinary tract infection.

SOLITARY KIDNEY

MOST CHILDREN born with a single kidney, or with only one healthy kidney, will go through life without kidney problems. In fact, the anomaly may not even be suspected, as the solitary kidney will work twice as hard as nature intended.

However, people with one kidney are at special risk if the organ becomes infected, if it is injured, or if cancer or stones occur. Any such strain on the kidney will greatly decrease its overall function.

MALFORMATIONS OF THE KIDNEY

SOME KIDNEY MALFORMATIONS have no symptoms and are often discovered in a routine urinalysis or during an investigation into some different problem. Others may gravely affect function.

Kidney Hypoplasia or Dysplasia. One or both kidneys may be small (hypoplastic) or abnormally formed (dysplastic). If only one kidney is affected, the child often maintains good kidney function. However, when both kidneys are hypoplastic, the eventual outcome is renal failure, necessitating kidney dialysis or transplantation. The main symptom is the frequent passage of a large amount of urine. The standard diagnostic tool is the IVP.

Multicystic Kidney. With this abnormality, one kidney is filled with cysts, giving it the appearance of a cluster of grapes. This nonfunctional organ usually atrophies, but because it carries a small risk of cancer, the kidney should be removed surgically if it does not disappear on its own. Multicystic kidney is diagnosed by renal sonogram. Most children with this malformation have normal kidney function throughout life.

Ureteropelvic Junction Obstruction (UPJ). A UPJ obstruction is a congenital narrowing of the site where the ureter joins the renal pelvis. This obstruction blocks the outflow of urine from the kidney to the bladder. In the newborn, the obstruction usually has been noted before birth in a prenatal ultrasonic examination. In an infant a UPJ obstruction is first found by the parent or pediatrician as a mass in the abdomen. In older children the first symptom is usually abdominal pain. Surgery is usually necessary to relieve the obstruction if the kidney function is affected by it. The surgery is best done as soon as the obstruction is discovered.

Polycystic Kidneys. Both kidneys have numerous cysts that cause the kidneys to enlarge while at the same time losing much of their function.

There are two forms of this disease—the infantile and the adult forms. Polycystic kidneys in the infant usually are discovered at birth by the presence of abdominal masses. Some of these children die as infants as a result of lung failure, which is associated with the malformation. Others have long-term disease with normal or near normal kidney function, but often have high blood pressure and liver problems. The disease is hereditary.

In an adult, polycystic kidney disease is inherited in a dominant fashion and often leads to kidney failure associated with hypertension, stones, and occasionally with liver problems, including cysts in the liver.

Medullary Cystic Disease (Nephronophthisis). In this rare hereditary disease, the cysts are in the inner portion of the kidney. Often a child with this condition will have anemia, and blood tests will show an elevated BUN (blood urea nitrogen) and creatinine, signs of decreased kidney function. The child may not grow at a normal rate, and there may be bone disease. This disease leads, usually very slowly, to kidney failure.

Horseshoe Kidney. In this genetic defect, the bottom ends of the two kidneys are connected, forming a horseshoe. This problem is one that is likely never to be detected unless the child has a kidney X ray. Children with horseshoe kidneys may occasionally have blood in the urine, kidney stones, or an increased risk of infection because of poor urine drainage, but the abnormality is generally benign.

Medullary Sponge Kidney.   This usually asymptomatic abnormality is a microscopic dilatation of the ends of the tubules. It can be seen on an IVP. While a medullary sponge kidney may be associated with blood in the urine or kidney stones, it is otherwise benign.

Duplication of Kidney.   The pelvis (or urine-collection part) of the kidney may be divided into two separate compartments with two separate ureters on one or both sides. The child may have no symptoms or may have obstruction of urine, reflux, and an increased risk of infection. Surgical treatment is then required.

DISEASES OF THE GLOMERULI

THE GLOMERULI are the kidneys' filtering units. They are tiny clusters of blood vessels, measuring no more than a millimeter in diameter, and numbering about a million in each kidney. When the filtering system goes awry, both kidneys usually are affected. The results may be temporary or permanent, depending on the cause of the problem.

A chronic inflammation of the glomeruli comes on gradually and may not be noticed until a routine urinalysis shows protein and blood in the urine. In an acute inflammation, on the other hand, the urine may be noticeably dark as a result of bleeding from the glomeruli and there is headache and swelling (edema) of the body tissues.

Acute Postinfectious Glomerulonephritis.   This is the general term for inflammation of the glomeruli occurring between one and three weeks after an infection. The reaction is not to the infection itself but to the antibodies produced in response to the bacteria. Poststreptococcal glomerulonephritis is an example.

Children with postinfectious glomerulonephritis have blood in the urine, giving it the appearance of tea or cola. Urine volume is decreased, swelling (edema) occurs because of excess body fluids, and blood pressure rises. The child also may complain of headache, blurred vision, and generalized aches and pains. The goal in treating the disease is to avoid problems associated with high blood pressure (hypertension) and edema. This requires stringent control over salt and fluid intake. The kidneys sometimes temporarily fail and dialysis must be undertaken until they resume normal function.

The prognosis for most children is good. The problem usually resolves itself and does not recur.

Berger's Disease or IgA Nephritis.   This inflammation of the glomeruli is often associated with a cold or other respiratory illness and involves recurrent episodes of dark or red urine. The only definitive diagnosis is made by kidney biopsy. Most children with Berger's (pronounced Berjay) have normal kidney function through life; a few have a gradual decline in function. There is no specific treatment.

Nephrotic Syndrome (Nephrosis).   Sometimes, for reasons that are not clearly understood, something causes a change in the ability of the glomeruli to retain protein in the blood. Protein molecules that were once too large to pass through are now leaked in large quantities into the urine. As a result, there is a marked drop in blood protein. In addition, the kidney's ability to excrete salt is affected, leading to fluid retention and the swelling of tissues all over the body.

Children with the nephrotic syndrome often have swelling around the eyes, later spreading to the feet and abdomen. Weight increases due to retained fluid. The problem occurs more often in boys than girls, with the average age of detection around three or four years. The syndrome is diagnosed with blood tests and urinalysis.

An estimated 75 to 90 percent of children under six who have the disease have what is called minimal change nephrotic syndrome, the most common form of the disease and one that seldom leads to structural damage or loss of function in the kidneys. Treatment consists of one to two months of oral doses of prednisone, a powerful drug whose side effects include increased appetite, weight gain, and facial puffiness. Even those who respond are likely to have relapses from time to time, which also can be effectively treated with prednisone. Some children, however, require so much of the drug that their growth rate is affected. An alternative for this group may be the drug cyclophosphamide. However, because the drug also has side effects, it is not the drug of first choice and should only be given to those who experience side effects from prednisone. In most patients who respond to prednisone, the disease eventually disappears in the late teens or earlier and kidney function remains normal.

In about 15 percent of children, nephrosis occurs in association with other types of nephritis. If a child with nephrotic syndrome does not respond to prednisone with a resolution of the proteinuria, a kidney biopsy should be done to determine the specific type of disease. These other types of glomerular disease include focal segmental sclerosis and mesangiocapillary glomerulonephritis (membranoproliferative glomerulonephritis). Both of these are likely to be progressive and to end in kidney failure. Several drugs have been tried but none proven definitely to be effective.

Henoch-Schoenlein Purpura or Anaphylactoid Purpura.
The symptoms of this disease are small red spots on the legs and buttocks, pain in the ankles and knees, abdominal discomfort, and blood in the urine and stool. The cause is unknown but the problem usually resolves itself without damaging the kidney.

Hemolytic Uremic Syndrome.
This syndrome (a group of symptoms) usually occurs in infants and very young children following a gastrointestinal or upper respiratory tract infection. A few days later the kidneys will fail, the urine turns brown, the child develops anemia and bleeds and bruises easily. This serious condition requires hospitalization. Sometimes a kidney biopsy is performed, particularly in severe cases, to determine the amount of damage. Because of the acute renal failure, dialysis through the abdominal cavity (peritoneal dialysis) may be required temporarily.

The mortality rate in hemolytic uremic syndrome is 5 percent, while another 10 percent may be left with chronic kidney failure or high blood pressure. Most, however, recover completely.

Hereditary Nephritis (Alport's Syndrome).
This inherited defect of the glomeruli, often associated with nerve deafness and, less commonly, with eye abnormalities, is much more severe in males. It is often diagnosed during a routine physical when urinalysis reveals blood or protein in the urine. This, combined with a family history of chronic renal failure, necessitates a thorough evaluation, which should include blood tests, radiological studies, and a kidney biopsy.

This is a progressive disease that often results in chronic kidney failure.

Renal Biopsy

Many of the diseases of the glomeruli require a kidney biopsy for diagnosis. During this procedure a small piece of kidney tissue is extracted with a needle through a tiny incision in the skin of the child's back. It is usually done with local anesthesia around the area, much like that used in the dentist's office. The exact location for the biopsy is often determined with an IVP or renal sonogram. The child usually remains in the hospital one or two nights to be certain there is no bleeding following the biopsy.

DISEASES AND DISORDERS OF OTHER TISSUES OF THE KIDNEYS

Congenital Tubular Disorders

In the tubules, water, nutrients and salts are selectively reabsorbed into the bloodstream while waste chemicals pass through in the urine to leave the body. A defect in this system can result in the loss of valuable minerals and other substances. In many cases, the tubular disorder is secondary to enzyme defects in many organs of the body or defects in the metabolism of proteins, sugars, and other substances.

A urinalysis performed on a child with a congenital tubular disorder often shows glucose, amino acids, or excess phosphate and bicarbonate—all substances that are normally reabsorbed. If left untreated, the child will develop rickets, a poor appetite, and a retarded growth rate.

Some children with these disorders can be treated with oral doses of the substance or substances the kidneys are mistakenly excreting. While the disorders usually do not result in serious kidney problems, they are often associated with other problems such as mental retardation and liver disease.

Renal Tubular Acidosis.
An early sign of this problem is failure to thrive (poor growth). It results from the tubules' inability to reabsorb bicarbonate, leading to an excess retention of acid. The problem is treated by giving the child sodium bicarbonate (baking soda) or a similar substance.

Vitamin D-Resistant Rickets.
Due primarily to huge losses of phosphate in the urine, vitamin D-resistant rickets results in poor growth and various bone deformities (such as bowing of the legs). This disease is usually hereditary and is treated by giving oral doses of vitamin D and phosphate.

Renal Glycosuria.
This describes the presence of glucose in the urine with no other abnormalities. These children's blood sugar is completely normal and they are not diabetic. Renal glycosuria causes no symptoms or impairment of kidney function.

Nephrogenic Diabetes Insipidus.
Here the defect is a lack of response in the tubules to the antidiuretic hormone that circulates in the blood. Bed-wetting is often an early symptom, as the child is constantly thirsty and drinks large quantities of liquids—and so produces large quantities of urine. In an infant, who cannot signal thirst, severe water depletion may occur, with vomiting and febrile convulsions.

Most children suffer no lasting effects from this

disease if they can drink enough water, but this is hard to manage (because of the volume needed) and inconvenient (because of the amount of urine produced). Salt restriction and thiazide diuretics may be useful as therapy.

Acute Interstitial Nephritis. In this condition, the spaces in between the glomeruli and tubules become inflamed. The most common cause is an allergic reaction to antibiotics or other drugs. To the body, a drug is a foreign substance; its reaction to a foreign substance is to try to expel it. Since the drug dissolves in body fluids, the route of expulsion is in the urine. And since urine formation involves the concentration of waste materials, the level of a drug in the kidney can be very high.

The child with this condition may develop fever, rash, and joint pains, and even have a transient decrease in kidney function.

Acute interstitial nephritis usually is completely reversible; when the drug is eliminated, the kidney heals.

HYPERTENSION

EVEN NEWBORNS CAN HAVE severe blood pressure elevations. The cause of hypertension in a child usually can be identified—which is not the case with the "essential" hypertension common to adults.

Any of the kidney diseases or malformations previously described can cause hypertension in a child. The combination of protein in the urine and hypertension may indicate kidney scarring as the result of reflux of infected urine from the bladder to the kidney. Other causes of hypertension include constriction of the aorta, the narrowing of the main artery to the kidneys, and various neurological and hormonal disorders.

Childhood hypertension should be investigated and its cause determined. Tests may include a sonogram of the kidneys, an IVP, hormone studies, a kidney scan, and catheterization of the renal arteries to check for blockage or constriction. The last procedure requires a one-day hospitalization.

KIDNEY FAILURE

BECAUSE THE KIDNEYS have much more functioning power than is necessary, symptoms of failure do not usually occur until 70 or 80 percent of function is lost. The loss may be gradual (chronic renal failure),

with the body able to adjust and to some extent compensate for the lack of function. Sudden loss (acute renal failure), on the other hand, happening in a few days or even hours, is an emergency situation.

Waste products accumulating in the blood result in a syndrome (a group of symptoms) called *uremia*. In both chronic and acute renal failure, the major symptoms of uremia are:

- upset stomach (ranging from loss of appetite to severe pain and vomiting)
- fatigue and weakness
- dry and sometimes itchy skin
- pallor due to anemia
- shortness of breath, due to hypertension, heart muscle weakness, and retained fluid
- edema
- a urinelike smell on the breath

Acute Renal Failure

There are many causes of acute renal failure, ranging from dehydration or blood loss to adverse drug reactions. The first sign is usually a decrease in urine output, although some children may have a normal or even increased output. Potassium builds up in the blood and without treatment may cause serious heart problems.

The treatment consists of close monitoring of intake and urinary output and the concentration of potassium in blood. More specific therapy depends on the underlying cause. This may include rehydration or removal of an obstruction or discontinuation of an offending drug.

Occasionally an artificial kidney must be used to take over kidney function until the damaged organ can repair itself.

Chronic Renal Failure

Chronic renal failure, the gradual and permanent loss of kidney function, is the eventual outcome of some of the serious diseases previously discussed, particularly those affecting the glomeruli.

Unlike many diseases, kidney disease is often silent and there is little that can be done in the way of prevention. Many children reach a low level of kidney function before their problem is diagnosed.

When kidney function, as measured by the level of creatinine in the blood, reaches 20 to 30 percent of normal, uremic changes begin to take place that require medication. As harmful waste products accumulate, growth is retarded or even ceases altogether. Attention span may diminish and school performance worsen. The child may tire easily, have poor appetite, and be pale and listless.

At this stage, treatment usually involves diet changes such as restricting phosphate (contained in dairy products and other foods) and possibly protein; the use of oral calcium, vitamin D, and sodium bicarbonate supplements; and medications that reduce the absorption of phosphate from the intestine into the blood. Controlling the blood pressure is important. Drug dosages must be adjusted for the amount of kidney function that remains.

Although some children remain stable with only 30 percent kidney function, for most the disease is progressive. When kidney function has deteriorated to between 5 and 10 percent of its normal capacity, the condition is called "end stage renal disease" and it is time for dialysis or transplantation.

TREATMENT OF CHRONIC RENAL FAILURE

Dialysis

Most of the children on dialysis are in their early teens or older, although occasionally even infants require it. Children on dialysis must adhere to a special diet, reduce fluid intake, and take regular medication.

There are four different types of dialysis.

Hemodialysis. This is done at a hospital or dialysis center two or three times a week; sessions last about four hours. During that time the dialysis machine—the artificial kidney—assumes the function of a working kidney. Initially a surgical procedure is necessary to create a shunt or fistula in the arm or leg, allowing access to the bloodstream. This involves connecting an artery to a vein. After the wound heals, the arm looks normal, although the vein may stand out somewhat.

During dialysis the patient's blood is pumped out of the body into a cellophane-like membrane that works like the kidneys' glomeruli, prohibiting large particles from passing. A solution in the machine, dialysate, helps to regulate chemicals in the blood and remove excess fluid and wastes.

Intermittent Peritoneal Dialysis. This form of dialysis also is done at the hospital. It is most often used for acute renal failure where quick recovery is expected. The peritoneal cavity, with its huge capillary-filled surface, can take on the same task as the hemodialysis machine. First, a catheter is surgically inserted into the abdomen. Then the cavity is in-

fused with dialysis solution. The small blood vessels in the membrane surrounding the inner abdomen filter waste products and water into the dialysis solution, which is then drained. The process is repeated every hour for 24 to 48 hours.

Continuous Ambulatory Peritoneal Dialysis (CAPD). This is similar to intermittent peritoneal dialysis except that the abdominal cavity is infused only four or five times a day, with the solution remaining within the cavity for four to six hours. This form of dialysis is done at home, and the child is free to go about his or her normal activities while undergoing treatment.

Continuous Cycling Peritoneal Dialysis. This technique is a variation of CAPD. While the child sleeps, a machine infuses the peritoneal cavity and drains the solution several times over the course of the night.

The type of dialysis used is geared toward the individual. The choice depends also on how much responsibility the parents want to take for treatment. Most of the cost of dialysis is paid by Medicare.

Transplantation

Like dialysis, kidney transplantation is not done until failure has reached the end stage. For children in particular, transplantation is preferable to dialysis because it enables them to lead a healthier and more normal life. It must be emphasized, however, that kidney transplantation is not a cure. No matter how successful the transplant, these children need frequent medical follow-up. They will require medication for the rest of their lives, and they are prone to infection. As with dialysis, one disease is, in essence, replaced with another.

The first step, once a transplant is deemed appropriate, is finding a kidney whose donor's tissue matches as closely as possible that of the potential recipient. This is critical because the body's defense system, its immune response, naturally attacks all foreign substances. It is less likely, however, to attack a kidney that closely matches the native kidneys. Compatibility is determined by blood tests that provide genetic information, including blood type, and assess the body's antibodies.

The best match—one in which the chance of rejection is lowest—is with a close relative, preferably a sibling. A kidney transplanted from a parent has an 80 to 90 percent chance of survival two years after surgery, whereas one from a sibling carries with it a success rate of 90 to 95 percent. The greatest risk of rejection is during the initial two years.

While a brother or sister is the best donor, sometimes this isn't feasible. Donors must be 18 to give consent and that eliminates many potential donors for young transplant candidates. When an older relative is not available, tissue-typing centers throughout the country are called upon to help find acceptable matches from accident victims and other recently deceased persons who have donated their kidneys. The two-year success rate of a cadaver transplant is between 65 and 80 percent.

The actual transplantation is not a complicated procedure. If the kidney comes from a living donor, the organ is removed from the donor and implanted in the child immediately. Kidneys from cadavers must be transplanted within about 48 hours after death. Either way, the operation lasts about four hours and the child is in the hospital anywhere from 10 days to 6 weeks, depending upon how well the body accepts the new organ.

The major problems following surgery are rejection and infection. In recent years, rejection has become less of a problem because of cyclosporine, a drug that suppresses the body's immune system and so lowers the chance of rejection. Suppression of the normal immune response, however, makes even a minor infection potentially life-threatening. Fortunately this risk decreases sharply after the first year as the dosage of immunosuppressant drugs is gradually lowered.

The expenses of both the donor and the recipient of a transplanted kidney are paid by Medicare.

KIDNEY STONES

WHILE KIDNEY STONES are found more often in adults, children also can suffer from this painful ailment. In the great majority of cases, stone disease is what doctors call idiopathic—of unknown origin. Other cases are due to metabolic problems affecting the whole body or structural problems in the kidneys themselves. Whatever the underlying reason, a kidney stone forms when the concentration of one or more substances in the urine becomes too high and the substance precipitates. Phosphates, calcium, urates, and other substances in the urine crystallize, forming a hard mineral deposit that is often the size of a small pebble.

Usually the only symptom is severe pain, beginning over the kidney area on one side. The pain (renal colic) comes in waves as the stone is pushed along gradually. As the stone moves, the pain travels from the flank, around to the front, and down to the groin. When the stone reaches the bladder, the pain stops. Usually the stone passes with the next urination.

Most often a stone passes in this way, without intervention. It may take weeks, or even months, and there will be intermittent pain, but as long as there is no infection, waiting is not dangerous. Sometimes surgery is necessary to remove the stone, however, or it may be pulled out by means of a basket-tipped caliper inserted through the urethra.

A stone that passes on its own may break up into pieces the size of grains of sand. As it is passed, the urine should be strained to collect the crystals. Chemical analysis of these will show what substances are present and suggest what should be done to prevent another attack. If, for example, the stone is calcium, a low-calcium diet may be recommended. Sometimes medication is prescribed. Because water decreases the urine's concentration, thus impeding the formation of crystals, most kidney stone patients are advised to increase their intake.

TRAUMA

THE TESTES AND SCROTUM frequently are injured during sports and other activities. The testes may rupture but often can be surgically repaired. In severe trauma, surgical exploration is necessary if radiological studies and physical examination cannot determine the nature of the damage.

There can also be injury to the kidneys caused by direct trauma, the most common symptom of which is blood in the urine *(hematuria)*.

TUMORS

Testicular Tumors. Often discovered as painless lumps, several types of cancerous tumors can invade the testicles. For this reason, frequent testicular examination is crucial in all boys and men.

Any hard lump in the testicle should be brought to the attention of a physician. If a lump is suspicious, it will be removed surgically and biopsied. If cancer is found, the child may undergo chemotherapy, radiation therapy, or further surgery to treat the malignancy. Fortunately, with early detection, a boy with testicular cancer has almost a 100 percent chance of leading a nearly normal life.

Wilms' Tumor. This is the most common tumor of the urinary tract, accounting for 95 percent of malignancies in that area in children under 14. Located in the kidney, Wilms' tumor occurs in approximately eight of every one million children under age 14. Ninety percent of the children afflicted are seven or younger.

Most children with Wilms' appear healthy initially. However, physical examination reveals an abdominal mass. A few have blood in the urine, poor appetite, fever, or anemia. The tumor may also be associated with deformities of the ears, skull, or tongue, hernias, undescended testes, hypospadias, and abnormal kidneys.

When a mass is felt, the child must have an abdominal sonogram and other tests, including an IVP, computerized tomographic (CT) scans, and various laboratory studies. The object of the tests is to confirm the diagnosis and define the extent of the tumor.

Treatment includes removal of the mass, chemotherapy, and possibly radiation. Sometimes the tumor is too large to be removed in one operation; a second procedure will be done after chemotherapy.

Prognosis is very good when the tumor has not spread. If it has metastasized, the outcome varies. Overall, however, 85 to 90 percent of children with Wilms' are cured when treated with a combination of therapies.

Mesoblastic Nephroma.   This tumor usually occurs in very young infants. Like Wilms' tumor, it is detected by the presence of an abdominal mass; diagnosis is with the same tests. Usually removal of the kidney is the only treatment necessary for long-term survival.

26 Eyes, Ears, Nose, and Throat

Kenneth Pituch, M.D.

INTRODUCTION

ENCLOSED WITHIN a relatively small area of the head and neck, the eyes, ears, nose, and throat provide us with most of our information about the outside world. Four major senses—sight, hearing, smell, and balance—depend on the elaborate, interrelated structures of these organs. The nose and throat also provide gateways for vital air, food, and water, and the throat contains the larynx, which enables us to cry, speak, and sing. All of these begin to function at —or perhaps even before—birth. Sight, at first poor, improves rapidly in the first few months of life.

The pediatrician or family doctor is the appropriate physician to consult for most diseases of the eyes, ears, nose, and throat. He or she should check the baby's hearing and vision frequently during the first years of life. Eye problems will be referred to an ophthalmologist.

If there is a problem with ears, nose, or throat, the child's doctor will suggest a visit to a specialist. An audiologist or speech therapist checks hearing; an otolaryngologist or ENT specialist (a subspecialty of surgery) diagnoses and prescribes therapy for more complex ailments.

THE EYES

A Living Camera

In many ways the eye is like a supersensitive camera, transforming incoming rays of light into information for the brain. One way to understand the eye and its diseases is by following a ray of light into the eye to see the structures inside.

A circle of bone called the orbit forms a protective casing around the eye. In front, it consists of the eyebrow, cheekbone, and bridge of the nose; a bony hollow in the skull completes the circle behind the eye.

The eyelids form a softer, more flexible shield, protecting the eye from dust, too-bright light, and dryness. We are all born with a reflex that slams the eyelids shut at the sight of an approaching object.

Tears, produced by tear glands inside the upper eyelid, and propelled by the blinking eyelids, moisten and clean the eyes many times every waking minute. Under the protective eyelids, tears keep the eyes moist during sleep, when drying out could harm them. After passing across the eye, tears accumulate in a structure called the lacrimal sac, which drains into the nose, making it necessary to blow the nose after crying.

The eyeball is connected to the outer skin by a single layer of tissue, the *conjunctiva*, which begins at the eyelashes, runs underneath the eyelids, then folds and returns over the white surface of the globe. This white layer of tissue is called the *sclera*. Many tiny blood vessels nourish both conjunctiva and sclera. Red eyes usually result from swelling or rupture of these blood vessels due to injury, infection, or irritation.

Thousands of times a day, six muscles attached beneath the conjunctiva rotate each eyeball toward whatever catches the attention. These muscles synchronize the movement of both eyes without any conscious effort. In sleep, rapid tiny movements of these muscles signal the occurrence of a dream.

At the front of the globe is the *cornea*, a transparent membrane that provides most of the eye's focusing power. Although it is extremely sensitive to pain, it is tough. In many cases, even after an injury painful enough to be treated in the emergency room, the outer layer of the cornea is often regenerated in only a few days, usually without scarring.

The *anterior chamber*, behind the cornea, helps protect the eye from injury by absorbing impact with a clear, watery liquid called the *aqueous humor*. The back wall of the anterior chamber is formed by the iris and the lens. (The *pupil* of the eye is not actually a structure. It is merely the opening in the iris that allows light to pass through to the back of the eye.)

The *iris* corresponds to the aperture-setting device of the camera, controlling the amount of light that enters the eye. Involuntary muscles can widen the pupil to 25 times its minimum size in a minute or so as we go from sunlight into a dark room. Excitement, attractive sights, and many drugs can also dilate the pupil, while other drugs can make it smaller.

The color of the eyes depends on the amount of pigment in the iris: brown eyes have more pigment than blue. Most Caucasian babies have bluish eyes at birth, but in six months most will have mud-colored eyes that eventually turn brown. Black and Asian babies are generally born with brown eyes.

Behind the iris is the *lens*, shaped like the lentil bean for which it is named. It is a mass of long, elastic fibers that expand and contract to provide a third of the eye's focusing power and the variable portion of it. It was once thought that newborns could not see immediately, but it is now known that, even before leaving the delivery room, a baby can focus on the mother's face.

The *vitreous chamber*—the round space behind the lens—is the largest part of the eyeball. Vitreous humor, a clear, colorless, gelatinous liquid, permits light to reach the retina at the back of the eyeball. Leftover bits of material from prenatal development of the eye may become opaque. Called floaters, these are one cause of spots before the eyes. They are usually harmless and do not seriously interfere with vision.

At the back of the vitreous chamber is the *retina*, a transparent network of cells thinner than paper. Like the film of a camera, the retina perceives light and color with its *rod* and *cone cells*, respectively. The light that stimulates rod and cone cells is converted into electrical impulses sent through the *optic nerve* to the *visual cortex* at the back of the brain. There the signals are converted into a picture of the outside world. Damage to the visual cortex can cause an optical illusion—the famous "stars" seen after a blow to the head.

The Eye Examination

Children should have an eye examination before the age of three, and then again before starting school. (See box on Eye Care Professionals, next page.) A visit to the doctor is also warranted if these signs of eye trouble develop:

- wandering of one eye in or out, up or down
- frequent eye-rubbing
- closing or covering one eye
- inability to do close work or see distances
- blinking or squinting or unusual complaints about bright lights
- red, watery, or burning eyes

Parents should remember that children don't know what "normal" vision is, but abnormal vision

EYE CARE PROFESSIONALS

Ophthalmologists have the longest training of any eye care professionals. They are physicians (M.D.s) specializing in diagnosing and treating diseases and conditions of the eye. The techniques involved may include medications and surgery. They may also prescribe corrective lenses. *Oculist* is an old term for ophthalmologist.

Optometrists also have special training, in a school of optometry. They are doctors of optometry (O.D.s) specializing in corrective lenses. They examine the eyes, test eyesight (visual acuity), and determine the proper prescription for glasses or contact lenses. They may also find other signs of disease in the eye—especially in the retina—but many states do not permit optometrists to use a full range of eyedrops for diagnosis.

Opticians do not examine eyes at all. They specialize in grinding lenses and fitting them into frames to fill the prescriptions of ophthalmologists and optometrists.

EYE SIGNS AND SYMPTOMS

Red spots. "Subconjunctival hemorrhages" are small, bright red spots that appear in the white of the eye, usually after a small injury, coughing, or sneezing. They usually resolve in two weeks and need no special medical attention.

"Spots before the eyes." Doctors call them "floaters." White or gray ones are bits of debris floating in the vitreous humor, and are not cause for concern. A heavy shower of brown or red spots are danger signs: they may signal leakage of blood from the retina into the vitreous chamber. Retinal detachment, heralded by sparkling spots and the feeling that a curtain is being pulled across the vision, may follow. The patient should see an ophthalmologist or go to an emergency room immediately.

Pain. Many people, especially fair-skinned ones, find bright sunlight painful. Sunglasses are one solution.

Minor injuries and foreign bodies. These are other common causes of eye pain. If the cause of pain is not obvious, however, it should be investigated by an ophthalmologist.

Protruding eyes. Gradual protrusion of one or both eyes over a month or more may be due to hyperthyroidism or tumor. Sudden protrusion of one eye is generally due to infection or hemorrage in the orbit behind the eye.

Rolling or jerking eyes. The medical term is *nystagmus*. The condition may result from one of a variety of unusual abnormalities of the eye itself or the nervous system controlling eye movements. Certain drugs (alcohol, anticonvulsants) are occasional culprits. The underlying condition should be evaluated and treated immediately.

Double vision. When the brain cannot reconcile the two pictures it receives from the two eyes, the result is double vision, or diplopia. Injury or weakness of the eye muscles are common causes. Double vision always requires immediate investigation.

can cause problems in education and even in social situations. (See box for common Eye Signs and Symptoms.)

Eye doctors use a variety of examinations, depending on what the first few basic tests reveal. Starting with a general medical history (including medications taken regularly, eye problems, and activities), the examination should include testing of eye muscles. How straight are the eyes when looking at objects in the distance and up close? How well do the eyes fix on objects moving toward them? Can they track up and down, as well as right to left? How well do they work together to perceive depth and blend two images into one? Are pupils normal in size and in their reaction to changes in light? The doctor uses moving fingers to test peripheral vision.

The outer layers of the eye should be examined with a slit-lamp microscope for signs of injury or disease. An ophthalmoscope—a hand-held device with a bright light—is used to examine the retina for a variety of abnormalities, such as detachment, infection, and signs of a number of diseases that affect the whole body. Diabetes and high blood pressure cause changes in the blood vessels at the back of the eye. The eye also serves as a window through which increased pressure inside the skull can be detected.

With small children, the doctor uses pictures of animals or tumbling Es instead of the alphabet to test visual acuity. Further testing to detect refractive error may involve a *phoropter*—a black metal mask into which different lenses are inserted. The child tells the doctor which lens makes vision clearest. There are no "wrong" answers on this test; the doctor determines the proper lens almost entirely from the physical examination. The patient's answers merely provide confirmation. The examiner will use additional lenses or repeat the question if there is any doubt.

Testing a Baby's Vision at Home

We all begin life nearsighted. At four to six weeks, babies can focus on faces about 8 to 12 inches away, and begin to smile when they recognize their mothers at this distance. At three months, babies should be able to follow with their eyes the movement of a favorite toy dangled in front of them.

Small babies lack the coordination to move both eyes together and may occasionally look wall-eyed or cross-eyed. When this is intermittent in the early months there is no cause for alarm. If it is continuous, or persists beyond the sixth month, however, parents should check the baby to be sure both eyes are looking straight. Broad folds of flesh at the side of the nose may confuse the issue in children with normal vision.

A parent who suspects an abnormality can confirm it by watching the child's eyes as he or she looks at a penlight or candle. If the child has normal vision, the two spots of light will be symmetrical, over the pupils. If the spot of light in one eye lies off-center, over the iris, the child has *strabismus*, the medical term for cross-eye or walleye. Another sign of strabismus is fussing and crying when the good eye is covered. An older child may also rub or cover the less effective eye. Catching this abnormality early is important in preventing loss of vision in the affected eye. (See section on Strabismus and Amblyopia, later in chapter.)

An eye test that parents can use to check out the vision of preschoolers is available without charge in English or Spanish from the National Society for the Prevention of Blindness (P.O. Box 426, New York, NY 10019).

Color Vision and Color Blindness

All the information the brain receives about color comes from the cone cells in the retina. Cone cells are specialized by color: different kinds perceive red, blue, and green. Less than 5 percent of the cells in the retina are cone cells, and they need more light to function than do the rod cells. This is why colors fade so rapidly as the light dims.

Most color blindness is caused by a defect in red-perceiving cone cells. Reds—and especially pinks and other pastel shades—appear greenish or brownish. Another form of color blindness involves a similar confusion between blues and yellows. Cards marked with multicolored dots are used to diagnose the condition. They reveal different words or numbers, depending on whether they are seen by normal-sighted or color-blind people.

About 3 percent of the population is color blind. Luckily, it almost never presents any difficulty in life. Most defects are hereditary and carried on the X chromosome: almost ten times as many men are affected as women. Women may be carriers, however, and pass the defect on to their sons.

Eye Safety

American emergency rooms see approximately 35,000 eye injuries each year. According to the National Society for the Prevention of Blindness, nine out of ten of these injuries are avoidable, mostly through the use of such safety measures as proper instruction in the use of tools and equipment and the use of protective goggles.

Sports involving racquets, sticks, and balls; bicycling; swimming; gardening; sunbathing; and do-it-yourself projects are responsible for most of these injuries. BB guns and sling shots are potentially dangerous, as are "Superballs," which bounce back faster than expected. The majority of accidents occur in warm weather when these leisure activities are more common and when children are more likely to be engaged in unsupervised play. A few precautions may prevent an injury that results in hospitalization, or even loss of vision.

When parents play tennis or softball, hang around the pool, or use power tools—especially the lawnmower—they should be mindful of their children's whereabouts. What passes harmlessly around an adult's knees may go straight into a toddler's eyes.

Sunburn. Lying in the sun or under an ultraviolet lamp, or exposure to welding equipment without eye protection can cause painful sunburn of the corneas. Twelve to 24 hours after exposure, the eyes feel very painfully gritty. Painkilling drugs are often required, and an eyepatch. An ophthalmologist should be consulted to determine the extent of the damage. With proper care, the cornea can heal itself in a matter of days.

Children generally prefer not to wear sunglasses. Those whose eyes are sensitive to bright light may want to wear them for comfort. For normal sunny days, sunglasses that let only 30 percent of the light through are good. (The light-transmission factor is usually listed on the label.) For glare from sand, water, or snow, 10 to 15 percent is better. Gray, brown, or green lenses generally give adequate protection. A strap around the head or wires over the ears will help prevent the glasses from being broken or lost.

Sunglasses that allow for tanning of the eyelids shield the eyes from visible light but let through ultraviolet rays, which are the most harmful to the retina. These lenses are dangerous and should not be used by adults or children.

Eclipse Burns. Staring directly at the sun causes the rays to focus on the retina. The result is the same as using a magnifying glass to focus the sun on a piece of paper: heat. The paper will catch fire; the rod and cone cells of the retina will be permanently damaged, causing loss of vision. To avoid solar burns, children (or anyone else) should not stare at the sun, during an eclipse or at any other time. Smoked glass and exposed film give inadequate protection; optical instruments such as telescopes may even hasten the burn by further focusing the sun's rays.

Water-Related Problems. Goggles are an inexpensive way to prevent a number of injuries. Infections (most common in fresh-water swimmers) and chlorine irritation can both be avoided by watertight goggles that may cost as little as five dollars. Goggles should not be used for skindiving below the surface; proper instruction in use of mask and snorkle is preferable.

Eye Injuries and First Aid

Despite precautions, eye injuries caused by blows, foreign particles, cuts, burns, and chemicals are common in children. First aid, especially within the first few minutes after an accident, may prevent a trivial accident from becoming serious, or a serious injury from destroying sight.

Bruises and Cuts. When the flesh over the circle of bone protecting the eyeball is bruised, it is called a black eye. An icebag or other cold compress placed over the eye may lessen the extent and darkness of the bruise, but only if applied immediately after the injury. There is no medical reason to use a piece of expensive, messy steak. Later, heat in the form of warm soaks may decrease discomfort and help the eye heal.

Bleeding from a cut near the eye may be controlled by applying pressure. A severe injury that results in a bad cut or black eye warrants a complete ophthalmologic examination to check for neurological damage or bleeding behind the cornea. This is especially important if the child complains of pain in the eye, or double or blurred vision.

In severe injuries, the eyelid may swell up, closing firmly over the eyeball. No attempt should be made to open the eye or to press on it in any way. If the eyeball is perforated, the eyelid may be the only thing holding it together. Opening the eyelid prematurely may cause loss of its contents, before an ophthalmologist can try to suture the fragments together in a sterile operating room.

Careful testing is necessary to evaluate the nature and extent of damage after a serious eye injury. Painkilling drugs may be necessary. Fortunately the cornea and conjunctiva are very resilient, and often heal in a few days. Blobs of blood under the conjunctiva (hemorrhages) will vanish without medical treatment within a few weeks. An eyepatch, antibiotics, and oral painkillers may be needed to prevent the eye from moving or becoming infected.

If vision in one eye is irreparably destroyed, the ophthalmologist may suggest removing it. This painful decision is necessary to prevent a mysterious condition called "sympathetic ophthalmia." Although no one is certain why, leaving an injury-blinded eye in position for more than 12 days occasionally results in loss of vision in the remaining eye, sometimes years later. The increasing rarity of this tragedy is another unanswered question: its incidence, as high as 2 to 4 percent during World War I, is now down to 0.1 percent of cases.

Foreign Bodies. From the painful but harmless eyelash to the dangerous sliver of steel or wood, foreign objects in the eye are important causes of eye injury.

Removing an eyelash or bit of grit can be easy, but improper attempts at removal can exacerbate the injury. Being careful not to rub the eye, the parent should try to shift the object toward the inside corner of the eye, where it can easily be removed. Sometimes a few hard blinks can move a lash off the cornea into the corner. If the object is visible in the child's eye, it should be wiped toward the corner with a clean handkerchief moistened with water (not saliva). Do not persist if the object does not move easily.

Another technique is to grasp the eyelashes of the upper lid and pull the lid slightly away from the eyeball and down over the lower lashes. This not only promotes tears to wash the object out, but allows the lower lashes to sweep the inside of the upper lid, which may dislodge the object. Next, the procedure is reversed, using the upper lid to free anything stuck to the underside of the lower lid.

If the problem persists, the child should be taken to a physician or hospital emergency room without delay. An ice cube or cold compress over the eye can lessen the pain during the trip.

Small fragments of wood or metal can cause serious damage or infection. Only mild pain and little external injury may result from the quick penetration of the eyeball by a machine-propelled splinter. Sometimes infection or a delayed reaction even years later destroys sight in the affected eye. In this type of injury, no first aid is possible. The eye should be covered with an eyepatch and the child taken to an ophthalmologist. An expert with a magnet may be able to remove iron-rich bits of metal.

Corneal injuries due to foreign bodies usually heal rapidly with help from an eyepatch to immobilize the eye, as described above. Wood splinters usually take a little longer to heal.

Chemical Burns. First aid for chemical burns consists of water, which may be poured directly over the eye. Attempts to "counteract" the irritant with another chemical will only worsen the injury. The child's head should be positioned with the injured or more-injured eye lower. The eye should be rinsed gently for at least 5 to 10 minutes. With an older child, the face can be immersed in a large bowl of clean water and the eyes kept open.

If the inner layers of the cornea are still transparent, the damaged outer layers may regenerate, and even very painfully injured eyes may be restored to full vision—sometimes with just a few days of rest. Painkillers and antibiotics may be prescribed, and the eye may be covered by a patch for a while.

Unfortunately, in many cases the damage is more severe, resulting in a white, opaque cornea and consequent loss of vision. Corneal transplants are the only current method for restoration of sight, and sometimes the eye is too severely burned for even this technique to succeed.

Strabismus and Amblyopia

In the first six months of life occasional strabismus—the medical term for all forms of cross-eyes, wall-eyes, or other eye deviation—is no cause for concern. The baby just hasn't yet learned how to focus both of his or her eyes together. But if the condition persists into childhood, it can result in amblyopia—the loss of sight in the "wandering" or "lazy" eye. Luckily, treatment, sometimes including surgery, is available if the condition is diagnosed early enough.

Strabismus (see figure 26.1) is usually caused by a delay in development of fusion (the use of both eyes as a team) or by farsightedness. The signs of wandering eye may show only occasionally, for example when the child is tired or ill. Rubbing the eye, tilting the head to see, or covering one eye are also warning signs. (See preceding section on Testing a Baby's Vision at Home.)

If the problem is not treated before the age of four, the brain will ignore the blurred, distorted, or poorly aligned signal from the weaker eye. By relying solely on information from the stronger eye, the brain avoids double vision, but eventually loses the ability to receive signals from the weaker eye. Without information from both eyes, binocular vision—and stereoscopic vision—are lost. If the problem is

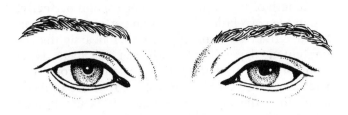

Figure 26.1. **Warning Sign of Strabismus.**

Light reflected from a penlight is asymmetrical, with the pinpoint centered in the pupil of one eye, but off-center in the other.

not diagnosed until grade school at the age of six or seven, the loss will probably be permanent.

Treatment. The earlier amblyopia is diagnosed, the simpler the treatment. Sometimes an eyepatch over the stronger eye is enough. As the vision improves, a blurring eyedrop may be used in the better eye. Special eyeglasses with one corrective lens and one filmed one may be used to force the child to rely on the "lazy" eye. Surgery may be necessary to tighten or loosen the muscles holding the eyeball before the child can align the "lazy" eye.

The longer the young brain lives with amblyopia, the harder it is to overcome. Treatment for the amblyopic child should begin before the age of three. Even at the age of seven or eight, exercises may help restore vision. In older children, surgery may enable the eyes to move symmetrically, but this cosmetic improvement will not restore binocular vision.

Visual Acuity and Refractive Errors

Visual acuity, or sharpness of vision, is the ability to distinguish small differences between similar images. In children, acuity is commonly tested by having the youngster identify pictures or letters of varying sizes at a distance of 20 feet. Normal acuity is the ability to make out an image of standard size at this distance. Thus, 20/20 vision means that at a distance of 20 feet, the child correctly identifies the standard-size image. A child with 20/80 vision can at 20 feet just make out those images that a child with "normal" eyes can identify at 80 feet. Causes of poor acuity include cloudy corneas, or any opacity in the anterior chamber, lens, or vitreous, as well as abnormalities of the retina, nerves, or brain.

The most common cause of poor acuity is refractive error. The lens and cornea of each eye bend (refract) the light passing through them to make the parallel rays focus sharply on the retina. To operate perfectly, the curvature of the lens and cornea and the length of the eyeball must correspond perfectly. When the correlation is less than perfect, the person has a refractive error and is either nearsighted or farsighted, depending on whether the focus is in front of or behind the retina. When the cornea is irregular, so that only some of the rays are in focus at a time, the eye is astigmatic. It is not known whether these conditions are due to heredity or environment, but in most cases, they can be corrected with lenses. Diet and exercises are completely ineffective in correcting refractive errors.

Myopia. In a nearsighted, or myopic eye the cornea and lens bend light too sharply, usually because the eyeball is too long. Light from a distant image focuses in front of the retina and the images appear blurry. The myopic child sees objects clearly when they are close to the face. Symptoms of this "nearsightedness" include inability to recognize faces at a distance, sitting too close to the television screen, and squinting.

Eyeglasses usually correct the problem. Since myopia often increases rapidly until maturity, requiring changes in prescription as often as every six months, frequent examinations, at least annually, are recommended. Corrective lenses for myopia are concave—thicker around the edge—to push the focusing point back toward the retina by spreading the rays of light before they reach the cornea.

Hyperopia. Farsightedness in children—hyperopia—is usually congenital. Rays of light converge behind the retina because the eyeball is too short. In most cases, no correction is needed until middle age. (Hyperopia is not the same as presbyopia, the farsightedness that makes almost everyone invest in reading glasses or bifocals in middle age. Presbyopia is caused by changes in the lens, not the shape of the eyeball.)

Some farsighted children have an occasional crossing of one eye when they attempt to focus. It is important that this be treated before the crossing becomes constant.

Corrective lenses for farsightedness are thicker in the center—convex—to bring the focus forward by forcing the light rays to converge before they enter the farsighted eye.

Astigmatism. In astigmatism, an irregularity in the curve of the cornea makes vision blurry. The condition may be complicated by near- or farsightedness. Lenses with a thickness distributed along one axis, called cylindrical lenses, may be combined with concave or convex shapes in order to correct the problem.

Red Eyes

Conjunctivitis. When allergy or infection (bacterial or viral) irritates the covering of the eye and lining of the eyelid, the result is "pink eye," or conjunctivitis. The whites turn red as tiny blood vessels enlarge, and the eyes feel hot or gritty. Pus may appear and even "glue" the eyelids together. Conjunctivitis often develops along with a cold or sore throat. Like them, it may be contagious and could quickly infect an entire daycare center.

The treatment for infectious conjunctivitis involves placing antibiotic drops or ointments in the eye. If virus or allergy is the cause, drops to constrict the blood vessels may help minimize discomfort.

Occasionally an eye infection will be present at the same time the child has an ear infection. The same bacteria is generally the cause of both problems. The antibiotic given by mouth for the ear infection will enter the tears via the bloodstream. Additional eyedrops are unnecessary.

A word of warning about eyedrops: Many prescription eye medications contain hydrocortisone or other steroid drugs. While steroids are a helpful component in treating many inflammatory eye conditions, for certain problems steroids can cause dangerous reactions. For this reason eyedrops prescribed for one family member should never be used for another without your physician's approval.

Neonatal Conjunctivitis. Conjunctivitis with drainage of pus is common in newborn infants. The infection may be caused by microbes picked up from the mother's vagina during birth. Another common cause is the silver nitrate placed in the newborn's eyes soon after birth. This practice, a legal requirement in some states, is a standard way of preventing damage to the baby's eyes should the mother have a gonorrheal infection. The drops may cause irritation that develops within six to eight hours and disappears without treatment within a day or two.

Treatment of conjunctivitis due to infection depends on which microbe is the culprit. Accurate diagnosis is essential. In many cases the infant must remain in the hospital. Gonorrheal infection is treated with up to a week of intravenous antibiotics, while chlamydial infection, often associated with nose and throat infections or even pneumonia, requires two or more weeks of an antibiotic.

Corneal Ulcer

Ulcers of the cornea are most often caused by infection after an injury due to accident or a foreign body, but they can also follow other eye diseases. The eye becomes painful, especially in bright light. Tearing, the feeling that something is in the eye, and eyelid spasm are also common. Sometimes the grayish ulcer is visible.

Corneal ulcers should be treated without delay by an ophthalmologist. Depending on the cause of the ulcer, antiviral or antibiotic therapy may be necessary.

Eyelid Problems

Blepharitis. Infection or allergy can cause this irritating disease of the edges of the eyelids. Sties (see below) and seborrhea also may precede it. Itching, burning, and scaling near the eyelashes are characteristic. The eye also may become red and teary. Sticky secretions may glue the lids together at night.

The treatment is warm compresses, followed by antibiotic ointment. Associated conditions—dandruff, boils, or other *Staphylococcus aureus* infections—must be treated as well. Many cases are resistant, and require steroids or oral antibiotics or both.

Sty. A sty, or hordeolum, is an infection in a tiny skin gland, usually at the base of an eyelash. Pain, redness, and tenderness develop into a small, round, hard point. The eye may be teary or light-sensitive, or feel as if something is in it.

Hot compresses can often help the sty come to a head and drain spontaneously. Unfortunately, sties tend to recur and occasionally need to be drained and the infected gland removed by an ophthalmologist.

Chalazion. Some chalazions start out like sties, with lid swelling and irritation. In other cases, the chalazion itself—a painless round lump in the eyelid—is the first sign. They are caused by blockage of a small gland in the eyelid. Although generally harmless, they may grow.

Hot compresses may help the chalazion resolve. If it doesn't, an ophthalmologist can remove it in a simple office procedure.

Droopy Lids. An upper lid that hangs over one eye needs prompt evaluation. Called *ptosis*, the condition can occasionally be caused by a serious disorder of muscle or nerve. More commonly, it represents an isolated muscle weakness.

Surgery for ptosis present at birth is usually delayed until after age three when accurate measurements of muscle action can be made.

Retinal Problems

Detachment. If the retina becomes separated from the blood vessels at the back of the eyeball, rod and cone cells will die, resulting in permanent loss of vision. In children, retinal detachment is generally caused by injury. The condition is painless, but it does include such symptoms as a shower of dark spots, light flashes, or loss of peripheral vision.

This is an emergency, requiring immediate ophthalmologic treatment. The ophthalmologist will use a laser, a cryoprobe (a very cold instrument), or other techniques to reattach the retina. In the majority of cases, the patient's vision is restored at least in part after a week or so in the hospital.

Retinitis Pigmentosa. About a million people in the United States have retinitis pigmentosa, a hereditary condition involving slow, gradual, patchy degeneration of the retina. About 23,000 of these people are legally blind. Rod cells are the first and most severely affected, so that reduced night vision may be seen in early childhood. Peripheral vision is lost next. Central vision may be retained until adulthood.

There is no treatment in most cases. Experimental precision-optics devices enable some older patients to gain a wider field of vision. Parents and siblings of a child with retinitis pigmentosa should receive genetic counseling.

Choroiditis. The retina is nourished by an underlayer of blood vessels, the *choroid*. An infected choroid can infect the retina, leading to scars that permanently impair vision. *Toxoplasma gondii*, a microbe carried in the feces of cats, is a common cause. Children may pick up the infection by playing where cats defecate. More severe disease is caused when the infection is transmitted to a fetus in the mother's womb.

The main symptom is blurred vision. There is no pain. Vision impairment can result from choroiditis in one eye. Medical therapy—usually steroid drugs—should begin as soon as possible, to reduce the likelihood of scarring. Drugs to suppress the immune system may be necessary in babies born with the disease.

Retinopathy of Prematurity. The blood vessels of the retina are undergoing their final remodeling in the last stages of fetal development. When a baby is born prematurely, the normal formation of blood vessels easily can be upset. Infection, anemia, changes in blood pressure, and either too high or too low a concentration of oxygen in the vessels can contribute to abnormal formation and reactive changes in the retina. The level of oxygen is a key determinant of these changes, although the reason is not completely understood. When oxygen is needed to treat a premature infant's lung disease, the level of oxygen in the blood is monitored and adjusted to decrease the risk to the eyes. Premature infants should be examined for retinal changes regularly

EYE MYTHS

Overusing the eyes will injure them permanently. An open eye is an eye in use. Reading without glasses, in poor light, or for too long will not cause nearsightedness or other eye injury. Eyestrain, a tired feeling from holding the same focus for too long, can be avoided or alleviated by gazing off into the distance or unfocusing the eyes for a few minutes every half hour or so.

Over-the-counter eyedrops will help eyestrain. Eyedrops may soothe eyes irritated by dust, smoke, or air pollution. They should be administered by having the child lie down, squeezing a few drops into each eye, and letting them wash across the eyeball. These medications are often overused. Bacteria may contaminate them after opening, and some people become allergic to them. Eyedrops should not be shared and should be thrown out when they are old. Most important, they should not be used when professional eye care might be more appropriate.

Children with crossed eyes will outgrow them. Babies in the first few months sometimes cross their eyes in the course of learning to use them. But after six months, crossed eyes can be a sign that the baby is relying on one eye and not using the other. Neglect of this problem can lead to loss of sight in the weaker eye.

during the first year of life. At its worst, the retinal damage may include severe scarring and retinal detachment. Milder disease may cause blurred vision but is amenable to treatment.

Retinoblastoma. A malignant tumor of the retina, retinoblastoma accounts for 2 percent of childhood cancers. Both eyes are often affected. Crossed eyes or a light reflection inside the pupil (like that in a cat's eye) is usually noticed before the child is two. The ophthalmologist may find many small tumors on close examination. The danger is more than loss of vision—the tumor could spread up the optic nerve to the brain.

More than four out of five cases are curable, but at a cost. If only one eye is affected, it will be removed, along with much of the optic nerve. If the disease attacks both eyes, the eye with more tumor will be removed, and the other treated with lasers, cryotherapy, radiation, or chemotherapy—often in combination. Frequent reexamination by an ophthalmologist is necessary, as well as the full range of tests for possible metastasis (spread). Because nearly half of all cases are hereditary, genetic counseling and frequent examinations are advised for the patient's parents and siblings.

Problems of the Orbit

Orbital Cellulitis. Infections of the sinuses or teeth can spread to the eye area. The result is a very painful, bulging, swollen eye. This is an extremely serious condition, with blindness from pressure on the optic nerve and meningitis as possible complications. Hospitalization is required for the administration of antibiotics and for the surgery that is occasionally necessary. Other treatment includes hot compresses, bed rest, and painkillers.

Protruding Eyeballs. Possible causes of this condition, called *exophthalmos*, include hyperthyroidism, tumors, hemorrhage, and infection. Treatment depends on the underlying condition.

THE EARS

Inside the Ear

The complex structures of our ears do more than just hear (see figure 26.2); they also help us keep our balance and literally tell us which way is up. The inner ear connects with the throat via the *eustachian tubes*, making the ear the uppermost part of the respiratory tract.

Anatomists divide the ear into the outer ear, the middle ear, and the inner ear. The outer ear comprises the earlobe, or *auricle*, and the external canal, to the eardrum, or tympanic membrane, a thin layer of tough tissue stretched across the ear canal. Sound waves in the air are funneled through the earlobe and down the external canal until they hit the eardrum, making it vibrate.

Behind the eardrum is the middle ear. Inside the middle ear are the *ossicles*, three small, connected bones with names that describe their shapes. These magnify the vibrations and pass them inward. The hammer, or malleus, is attached to the eardrum and transmits its vibration to the *incus*, or anvil. The inner end of the incus attaches to the *stapes*, or stirrup, which in turn transmits the vibration to the inner ear via the oval window.

Another feature of the middle ear is the eustachian tube, a pipe connecting the back of the nose with the ear. Swallowing or yawning in elevators and airplanes widens the tube to equalize pressure between the ear and the surrounding environment. Long and narrow in adults, the eustachian tube is relatively shorter and less rigid in infants and children, a factor partly responsible for the frequency of ear infections in young patients.

The inner ear is filled with fluid. The many tiny hairs of the *cochlea*, a snail-shaped structure, perceive sound vibrations. The auditory nerves at-

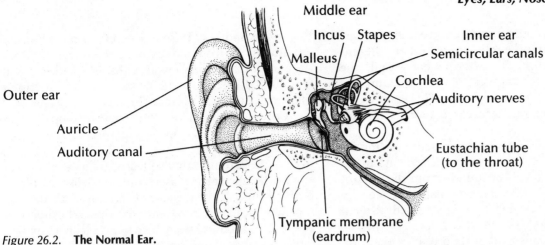

Figure 26.2. **The Normal Ear.**

tached to the cochlea send the resulting signals to the brain, which interprets the sound.

Our sense of balance is also housed in the inner ear, in a fluid-filled structure called the *labyrinth*. This consists of two connected chambers and three semicircular canals perpendicular to each other. Moving the head or body causes the fluid to move around, or come to rest. The changes in position of these fluids are interpreted by the brain—in conjunction with information from the eyes and muscles—to give a sense of balance. Dizziness and vertigo (the sensation that the world is spinning) generally result from a disorder or infection of the labyrinth.

Testing a Baby's Hearing at Home

Most babies are born with good hearing, and they will be startled by loud noises and soothed by the sound of conversation. Hearing can be tested at home by clapping or crinkling up a piece of paper or aluminum foil out of sight about 12 to 18 inches behind the baby's head. The baby who hears normally will act startled. At three months, the baby will blink or throw out his or her arms. By six months, he or she should turn to look for the source of the sound.

A baby's hearing should be evaluated professionally soon after delivery, at four to eight weeks, and at regular checkups thereafter. Because hearing is essential to development of speech and other communications skills, more frequent testing is recommended for babies who are at high risk for hearing loss (see section later in chapter on Sensorineural Hearing Loss). Parents should also observe the baby's reaction to voices and household sounds, and discuss any questions with the pediatrician. (See box on Ear Signs and Symptoms.)

The Hearing Examination

Simple hearing tests can be performed by the pediatrician or family physician. If a hearing problem is

EAR SIGNS AND SYMPTOMS

Ringing in the ears (tinnitus). Besides ringing, this very annoying symptom may sound like buzzing, hissing, or roaring, or a combination of sounds that fluctuates over time. Only the patient hears it, and it is often associated with hearing loss. The cause ranges across the list of ear diseases, from earwax accumulation to medication overdose and serious illnesses. Usually, but not always, it clears up when the underlying cause is treated.

Besides diagnosis and therapy of the underlying disease, there is no specific therapy for tinnitus. Background music—played even when the child goes to sleep—may mask the ringing. A special devise called a tinnitus masker, worn like a hearing aid, replaces the tinnitus with more pleasant sounds.

Earache. Pain in the ear requires prompt attention from a physician. The most common cause in children is otitis media (see Eardrum and Middle Ear Problems, later in this chapter), for which antibiotics should be started immediately.

Vertigo. Vertigo is the sensation that the world is spinning around one. In severe cases, it can cause loss of balance or nausea and vomiting. A disorder of the labyrinth in the inner ear, such as a viral infection, is usually responsible. Prompt medical evaluation is advisable. Therapy involves diagnosis and treatment of the underlying disease.

detected, more complete evaluation should be performed by a specialist. Different tests may be used to diagnose different conditions.

Audiometry is a hearing test that involves listening through earphones in a soundproof room. Each ear is tested for perception of different frequencies, from deep to high, and from soft to loud, to determine the hearing range.

Tympanometry involves a special probe placed

inside the ear to bounce sound waves off the eardrum. By measuring the reflected sound at different air pressures within the external ear canal, the probe determines the tautness of the eardrum, and thus the pressure in the middle ear. This enables the specialist to deduce the nature and severity of middle ear disease.

In infants under six months, hearing testing involves watching the baby's body movements in response to varying levels of sound. From the ages of six months to two years, hearing can be tested by illuminating a toy after a tone is sounded. After a brief training period, the child will look for the toy if he or she hears the sound. After a year, perception of speech can be monitored by having the child point to parts of the body.

Older children can be told to put a toy into a box in response to a tone. A four- or five-year-old can simply raise a hand to indicate perception and direction of sounds.

Brainstorm auditory-evoked response (BAER) is similar to an electroencephologram (EEG). It measures the brain waves produced in response to sound and is an excellent test for the very young.

External Ear Problems

Protecting the Ears. Children have very delicate eardrums that can be perforated by a slap on the ear or a cotton swab. Loud noises can cause damage to the inner ear and result in hearing loss. Children should be protected from overexposure to jackhammers, aircraft, loud music, and other sources of extreme noise.

Obstructions. It is a rare youngster who survives childhood without getting something stuck in the ear: water at the very least; insects that fly or crawl in; and, not uncommonly, seeds, pebbles, or beads the child places there.

The first rule for parents is to stay calm. The eardrum will prevent the foreign object from penetrating to the middle or inner ear. Many objects can be dislodged by tilting the head, with the affected ear down, and shaking gently. This is effective for water as well. A clearly visible object may be removed with tweezers. A live insect in the ear canal can be drowned in mineral oil to stop its buzzing.

For removing all other ear obstructions, a special forceps is necessary. Jabbing with a cotton swab or bobby pin will only force the object further in, possibly damaging the eardrum. The child should be taken to a physician or hospital emergency room.

Earwax. Secreted by special glands, earwax protects the external ear canal. There is a wide variation in the nature of earwax—from brown and oily to grayish and dry. Different people produce different amounts—from almost none to enough to block the ears entirely every few months. Blocked ears will feel stuffed, hearing will be poor, and sometimes there will be ringing or buzzing.

Cotton swabs merely push the wax up against the eardrum and may even puncture it. The proper tool for cleaning the ears is a pinky finger wrapped in a cloth. Parents can also learn to flush the child's ear with lukewarm water squirted from a rubber bulb syringe. If these methods do not clear the ear, a physician can remove earwax. Special drops will soften the accumulation before an electric suction device, warm-water flushing, or probe eliminates the problem.

Otitis Externa. When the protective wax is scraped or washed from the canal, or when contaminated material sits in the ear, an infection of the skin may result. Symptoms include severe pain, tenderness to any touching or pulling on the ear and occasionally, an ear discharge. This otitis externa or "swimmer's ear," will require antibiotic or anti-inflammatory eardrops, or both; occasionally they can only be applied via a wick of cotton inserted by a physician into the tightly swollen ear canal.

Eardrum and Middle Ear Problems

Perforated Eardrum. A child's eardrum can be easily perforated as a result of trauma. The symptoms can include sudden, severe pain, hearing loss, ringing in the ears, and bleeding from the ear. A discharge of pus may begin immediately or within a day or two of the accident.

In many cases, the eardrum will heal in less than two months without medicine or surgery. But other cases may require antibiotics. It is important to keep the ear dry to avoid infection.

Acute Otitis Media. Infection in the middle ear space is the most common illness diagnosed in young children. Most patients are between six months and two years, but older and younger children are also frequently affected. In the healthy child the middle ear space contains air that enters via the eustachian tube. This tube opens and closes during swallowing and fluid does not collect in the middle ear. A common cold or an attack of respiratory allergy, however, may cause a swelling around the eustachian tube, causing it to function improperly.

When the small eustachian tube of the young child malfunctions, fluid and germs become trapped in this middle ear space. The bacteria or viruses in this fluid produce more inflammation and further swelling. The result is earache and a mild, temporary hearing loss, often accompanied by fever, nausea, or vomiting.

When the doctor looks at the eardrum through an otoscope, he may see a red and bulging tympanic membrane with cloudy-colored pus on the other side. This *purulent* (pus-producing) *otitis media* will require antibiotics to eliminate the bacteria. If untreated, the pus may rupture the eardrum, relieving the pain but producing a draining ear that will contain a mixture of pus, fluid, and blood.

Often, however, the fluid behind the drum does not appear cloudy. But even clear middle ear fluid will very often contain bacteria. As in purulent otitis media, antibiotics are a necessary first step. The bacteria in the middle ear contribute to the ongoing inflammation and keep the eustachian tube from recovering its normal function. When the infection is brought under control, the fluid will gradually disappear as the eustachian tube begins to open and close normally again.

In most children, pain and fever decrease significantly within 48 hours of starting an antibiotic such as amoxicillin, which is effective against the bacteria most frequently found in infected ear fluid. Persistence of symptoms for more than three days usually indicates failure of the initially chosen drug to kill the bacteria in one or both ears. A change to an antibiotic that is active against other, less frequently found bacteria will be appropriate.

Occasionally it may be necessary to perform a myringotomy—an incision of the eardrum, permitting the outflow of fluid—to avoid a spontaneous rupture. This procedure will relieve pain and pressure and the small cut will heal better than a rupture. The fluid can be sent to a laboratory for specific identification of the germs.

Persistent and Recurrent Otitis Media. In nearly all children, the middle ear space will become normal within two weeks to three months following successful treatment of acute otitis media. The "ear recheck" following therapy may reveal either complete resolution or persistent signs of inflammation, requiring another course of antibiotics. Often, however, appearance of the eardrum falls somewhere in between. The middle ear fluid may contain no more bacteria, but may remain for many weeks. As long as the fluid is there, hearing may be decreased, and true infection may return at any time. Decongestants and antihistamines are not helpful in eliminating the fluid.

Frequent bouts of acute otitis media, or persistence of fluid for more than three months, requires special consideration, especially in the small child in whom full or partial hearing loss may interfere with the development of normal speech. Prolonged courses of low-dose antibiotics may be prescribed to prevent recurrent attacks, or myringotomy may be performed to drain the fluid. Small "ventilation tubes" will usually be inserted during *myringotomy* surgery to allow air to reenter the middle ear and prevent recurrence of fluid and inflammation. (See figure 26.3.)

Whether antibiotics, ear surgery, or time alone have any long-term advantage over the other approaches in preventing hearing loss remains

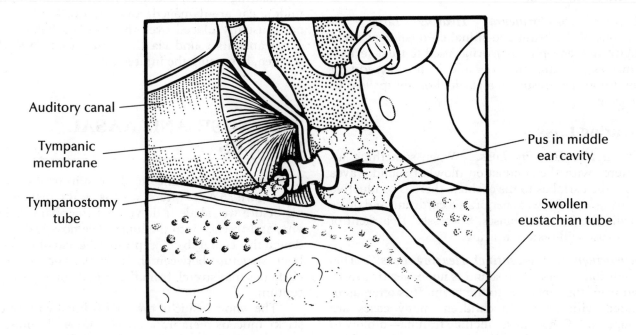

Figure 26.3. **Insertion of Tube to Relieve Otitis Media.**

Auditory canal

Tympanic membrane

Tympanostomy tube

Pus in middle ear cavity

Swollen eustachian tube

unsettled. Pediatric ear specialists are presently conducting large comparative trials to determine which approach may be best for specific children.

A generation ago chronically draining ears, and infection of the nearby bones or even of the inner ear structures were common sequellae of untreated otitis media. Fortunately these complications are now rare.

Another common complication of middle ear disease is *cholesteatoma*. This is a noncancerous growth on the eardrum that can enlarge and invade the surrounding bones. It can only be treated through meticulous surgery and often requires repeat procedures.

Inner Ear Problems

Congenital Sensorineural Hearing Loss. Hearing loss can occur in newborns whose mothers had rubella (German measles) or took certain drugs during pregnancy. It can also be the result of birth injuries, Rh-negative disease, or any number of hereditary conditions—or it can occur without a known risk factor. Babies with known risk factors should have their hearing tested frequently.

Without hearing, a child cannot learn to speak. If a child does not begin to speak normally, expert analysis may be necessary to distinguish whether deafness, mental retardation, aphasia, or autism is responsible. If the cause is deafness, the child should begin wearing a hearing aid as early as eight or nine months. (See Hearing Aids.) Special education is necessary as well, and should begin before the age of two or three years.

Acquired Sensorineural Hearing Loss. Infections of the brain and spinal cord (such as meningitis and encephalitis), drugs used to treat serious illnesses, certain tumors, and a few hereditary conditions can result in a gradual or abrupt loss in hearing.

Hearing Loss

Conductive Hearing Loss. When something interferes with the conduction (flow) of sound waves from the earlobes to the cochlea, there is conductive hearing loss. Earwax, perforated eardrum, and otitis media are frequent causes. Successful treatment of the cause will restore hearing.

Sensorineural (Perceptive) Hearing Loss. This condition occurs when sound is no longer transmitted from the inner ear to the brain. It is often associated with aging. In children, many cases are congenital. Other causes include trauma—a blow to the ear or too much loud noise. Sensorineural deafness can also result from certain drugs or can follow infections of the brain or nerves. Prolonged exposure to noisy machinery, airplane noise, or so-called "rock and roll deafness" from overamplified music at concerts or through headphones may all be responsible.

Hearing loss can often be helped by the proper hearing aid, but an improperly fitted one can be worse than none at all. Although in most states hearing aids can be sold over the counter, it is best to have one fitted by an audiologist, a specially trained professional.

Hearing Aids. There are six types of hearing aids. The most powerful is the body aid, in which a plastic case houses the battery and amplifier, with a thin wire connection to the ear. The case can be carried in a body harness or shirt pocket.

The *postauricular* (or *behind-the-ear*) *hearing aid* contains a tiny amplifier and battery, connected over the ear to an earphone that fills up the entire earhole so that no sound is lost.

Eyeglass aids are like postauricular aids built into the temple bar of eyeglasses. These are only useful to the child who must wear eyeglasses continually.

In-the-ear aids are the least noticeable, with the whole apparatus contained in the earlobe and external ear canal.

The *contralateral routing of signals (CROS) aid* helps those with hearing loss in only one ear by rerouting sounds that hit the deaf ear into the functioning ear.

The *bone-conduction aid* helps remedy conductive hearing loss, for example when the bones of the middle ear are damaged. An oscillator (a vibrating pad), usually placed over the mastoid behind the ear, transmits sound via the bone structure to the cochlea, bypassing the injured area.

THE NOSE AND NASAL SINUSES

THE NOSE is the entrance to the respiratory system. (See figure 26.4.) It filters, warms, and moistens the air before we inhale it down past the pharynx, larynx, and trachea into the lungs. The nose is divided down the center by a septum (the cartilage-and-bone structure between the nostrils) and six bony curlicues that stretch from the outside in toward the septum.

The whole inside of the nose is lined with thick, sticky mucous membranes over a layer of temperature-sensitive erectile tissue. When cold, dry, or polluted air enters the nose, the tissues swell, slowing

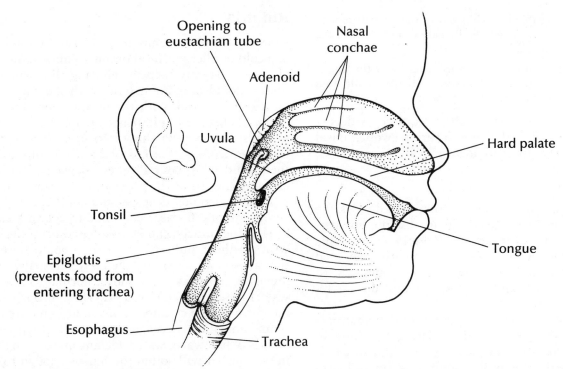

Figure 26.4. **Normal Nose and Throat Structures.**

the passage of air so that it can be more thoroughly warmed, humidified, and filtered. The swollen tissues produce large amounts of mucus, and the nose runs.

Bacteria and bits of dirt and pollution are trapped in the mucous membrane, or washed out by the flow of mucus. Tiny hairlike cilia wave the foreign particles to the back of the nose and throat, where they can be swallowed, or forward to the front of the nose, where they can be blown out.

The *olfactory bulb*, in the roof of the nose, contains the tiny, sensitive hairlike ends of the olfactory nerve. This transmits information about odors up to the brain, which compares it for identification to memories of previous smells. Our sense of taste is almost entirely dependent on the sense of smell, so that any interference with the sense of smell will greatly interfere with the enjoyment of food.

The *paranasal sinuses* are parallel pairs of air-filled spaces in the bones of the face. The *maxillary sinuses* are located in the cheekbones, the *frontal sinuses* are under the eyebrows, and the *ethmoid* and *sphenoid sinuses* are behind the nose and under the eye socket. Like the nose, the sinuses are also lined with sticky mucuous membrane that may become infected.

Fractures

The bones and cartilage of the nose are more fragile than the other facial structures, and a broken nose should be suspected in any injury or fall causing a nosebleed, or an injury that is followed by a stuffy nose. The rapid swelling of soft tissue may make it difficult for a lay person to detect the break. The child should be taken to a physician or hospital emergency room for evaluation at once. An untended nasal fracture, or even a blood clot beneath the lining of the nasal passages may lead to infections, abscesses, and destruction of the cartilage.

General anesthesia is required to set a child's broken nose. The nose may require packing and splinting to hold the fracture in place while the bones "knit." Fractures of the septum are difficult to hold in place and may require a second operation later.

Foreign Bodies

Young children commonly stuff things up their noses. Sometimes the object is unnoticed until it begins to rot; in other cases, mineral salts in the mucus gradually accumulate on the object, producing a stonelike covering.

Poking at the object with a swab or toothpick will only push it back into the nose. The following methods may work with a recently inserted object and a calm, cooperative child:

- Ask the child to breathe through the mouth, not the nose.
- Have the child blow his or her nose a few times. This may push the object forward. Do not ask for forceful or repeated nose-blowing.

- An object visible right in front of the nostril may be removable with tweezers. Be careful not to push the object further in.
- If these techniques are unsuccessful, or if the object was inserted hours or days ago, take the child to a doctor or hospital emergency room.

General anesthesia is often required. A decongestant, applied to the nose to shrink swollen nasal passages, may also facilitate removal.

Deviated Septum

The nasal septum is the partition that divides the nostrils. It is never exactly in the middle nor perfectly straight, but it deviates more in some people than in others. A child may be born with a deviated septum or it may be the result of an injury. Most cases cause no trouble whatsoever and do not require treatment.

In some cases, however, the deviation obstructs the flow of air in one nostril, hindering breathing. In others, it blocks a sinus, leaving the child susceptible to sinusitis. It may also predispose him or her to frequent nosebleeds.

A deviation that is causing problems or that noticeably affects appearance can be surgically repaired, a procedure that involves paring away extra or asymmetrical cartilage. In older children, the operation may be performed in conjunction with rhinoplasty, surgery to reshape the appearance of the nose.

Nosebleed

Sometimes the cause is obvious—a blow to the nose, a bad cold, dry air, nose-picking. But often there is no obvious reason when *epistaxis*—the medical term for nosebleed—begins, usually in only one nostril. Some children have them more frequently than others. Although the blood may seem alarming, in most cases no significant amount of blood is lost during a nosebleed, and it is rarely a symptom of serious disease.

To stop a nosebleed, the child should be seated with the head forward. The bleeding nostril should be pinched closed with firm pressure and held for 5 to 10 minutes while the child breathes through the mouth. This should enable a clot to form. The child should avoid blowing the nose for 12 hours to permit the clot to heal. This method is more direct than use of ice or a cold pack to constrict blood vessels.

If this technique does not stop the bleeding, a visit to a physician or hospital emergency room is the next step. Packing the nostril with medicated gauze applies pressure to the injured blood vessels. Cautery—coagulation with an electrical device or with silver nitrate—may be used in some instances.

Rhinitis

Rhinitis, simply a runny nose, is usually the result of a cold or allergy. Nasal decongestants in the form of nosedrops may help in relieving the symptoms. These should be administered with the child lying on his or her back with the neck extended so that gravity helps the liquid penetrate the swollen nasal passages. Nosedrops should be used sparingly. In less than a week, the nose becomes habituated to them, and a "rebound" effect develops, with increasing rhinitis as the previous dose wears off.

Medicated nosedrops should not be used in very young infants. If nasal congestion prohibits eating or sleeping, mucus can be evacuated from the nose with a rubber bulb syringe (care should be taken that air is not blown into the baby's nostrils). If the mucus is too sticky to remove, normal saline (salt water) nosedrops can be used. These drops can be bought over the counter or made at home by combining one-quarter teaspoon of table salt with eight ounces of lukewarm water. Placing one or two drops in one nostril will soften the mucus enough to permit removal with the bulb syringe. Or the baby may sneeze in response to the nosedrops and so clear the breathing passages.

Over-the-counter and prescribed decongestants may help convert a drippy nose to a stuffy nose, but these drugs do not hasten the end of a common cold. Avoidance of nonspecific irritants is advisable. Cigarette smoke, dust, and very dry air will aggravate rhinitis. The home vaporizer is helpful in seasons and homes with low humidity. Cool mist vaporizers are effective even without added medications and present no danger of hot water scalds to children. Floor humidifiers do an adequate job with less work since they only require refilling every three to six days. These devices must, however, be kept clean or molds can develop. The goal with any of these is to maintain relative humidity at 40 percent or more.

Sinusitis

The sinuses (see figure 26.5)—air-filled spaces in the front of the skull—are sometimes blocked during viral infections such as cold or flu. Sinusitis, usually a bacterial infection, can be the painful result.

The main symptom is a headache, behind the cheekbones or forehead or eyes, depending on whether the maxillary, frontal, or ethmoid sinuses are involved. The pain also may be perceived as originating in the teeth or the back of the head. The mucosal tissue lining the nose becomes red and swollen; the nasal discharge may contain large quantities of yellow or green pus.

Inhaling steam may constrict the nasal blood vessels enough to allow the sinus to drain, but the

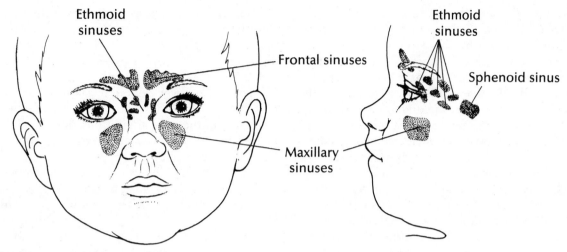

Figure 26.5. **Normal Sinuses.**

condition should be treated by a physician, who can provide antibiotics. Nosedrops (see Rhinitis, above) are also helpful. In severe cases, drainage through irrigation is necessary. In this procedure, the sinus is "washed out" when the physician injects fluid through an "accessible" area of the sinus and lets it flow out through the nose. If recurrent attacks of sinusitis are due to a deviated septum, surgical correction will help prevent them.

THE THROAT

THE THROAT, or pharynx, is a long tube ringed by muscle and cartilage. It begins at the back of the nose and branches below the mouth to convey air to the windpipe (or trachea) and food and drink to the esophagus.

At the lower end of the pharynx is the voicebox or larynx, which contains the vocal cords, two lengths of tissue that are stretched thin, so that air passing over them vibrates, creating the sounds of crying, singing, and speech.

On top of the larynx is the epiglottis, which serves as a lid for the trachea. It closes automatically upon swallowing, so that food and water cannot fall into the trachea. The tonsils and adenoids are other important parts of the pharynx.

The throat, the larynx, the epiglottis, the tonsils and adenoids—all are subject to infection. In fact, infection is the most common cause of throat diseases in children.

Pharyngitis (Sore Throat)

Tonsillitis, pharyngitis, and laryngitis are common causes of a sore throat in children and adults.

Tonsillitis and pharyngitis are slightly different entities but are similar enough to be considered together. The tonsils are the irregular protrusions of pink tissue at the sides of the throat. They are a first line of defense against infection of the throat by viruses and bacteria and therefore are often the most visibly affected part of the infected pharynx. The term *pharyngitis* indicates a less specifically located inflammation of the back wall of the throat, the soft palate (the rear portion of the roof of the mouth), the uvula (the punching-bag-like structure hanging from the palate), and the tonsils.

Often the terms *tonsillitis* and *pharyngitis* are used interchangeably. The causes and symptoms are indeed the same, whether or not the tonsils are the only targets. Pharyngitis is used here to include both conditions.

Pharyngitis is usually caused by one of a small group of ubiquitous viruses. As with the common cold, this viral illness is self-limited, running its course in several days. Unlike common-cold associated viruses, which produce runny nose, cough, an irritated throat, and usually no fever, the viruses producing pharyngitis will give the child a more severe sore throat. Also common is a fever of 101.5 degrees F. or more, with or without a runny nose. Swallowing may be difficult and the appetite diminished, especially for milk and acidic juices. Symptomatic relief can be obtained from acetaminophen, which decreases both pain and fever, and from gargling warm salt water. Trouble breathing or swallowing should always lead to evaluation by a physician.

Streptococcal Pharyngitis

Fewer than half of the pharyngitis cases seen in children are caused by a bacteria known as the Group A beta hemolytic streptococcus (G.A.B.H.S.). *"Strep throat"* can produce symptoms identical to those caused by viruses: sore throat, fever, trouble swallowing. There are two reasons to try to find out if the infection is caused by this streptococcal bacteria, however. First, the strep throat can be treated with antibiotics—penicillin, amoxicillin, and erythromycin are all effective—and the symptoms will abate more quickly. But second *and more important*, a small percentage of patients with untreated strep throat will go on to have complications. Early complications of untreated strep pharyngitis include abscesses behind the tonsils, sinusitis, and middle ear infections. (See figure 26.6.) Complications that occur in the weeks following recovery from the sore throat include kidney damage and rheumatic fever. Rheumatic fever causes inflammation of the heart, skin, joints, and nervous system and can result in permanent damage to heart valves. This condition can be completely avoided if a strep throat infection is treated within a week after onset of symptoms.

It is prevention of rheumatic fever that has led to current recommendations for the diagnosis and management of sore throats. Because viral and strep pharyngitis may cause the same symptoms, sore throat with fever should be evaluated medically. Physical findings such as white pus on the tonsils, very tender lymph nodes in the front of the neck, and red spots on the soft palate suggest a greater likelihood of finding the Group A streptococcus. A throat swab will usually yield a positive result in 12 to 48 hours, the time it takes for strep bacteria to multiply on a special "culture plate" and be identified.

If the suspicion of strep is not high, the throat culture can be taken and no antibiotics need be started. If the culture in one or two days confirms that there was no strep, no further test or treatment is needed and symptoms by that time have usually disappeared. If strep is present, however, an antibiotic is necessary to prevent the later complication of rheumatic fever. Even if symptoms are completely gone, a 10-day course of an orally administered antibiotic or a single injection of long-acting penicillin will be necessary to prevent this unusual but serious complication.

Recently, rapid tests have been developed to detect the presence of streptococcus in the throat in less than an hour. A positive "rapid test" would lead to presumptive use of an antibiotic. Rapid tests are still being evaluated. For now, the throat culture remains the standard for diagnosing strep throat and determining treatment.

During the two to four days that a child is ill with pharyngitis, rest and fluids are the only supportive care needed. After the first 24 hours of antibiotic therapy, strep throat is no longer contagious. Children may return to school when the fever has been gone for one day.

Scarlet fever is "strep throat with a rash." Some strains of the G.A.B.H.S. bacteria produce a toxin that circulates through the body and causes a red, sandpapery total body rash in addition to the sore throat. Several days later the skin will peel. A person who has had scarlet fever develops an immunity to the toxin. He or she may get strep throat again, but the rash will never return.

In children under three years old, strep throat is uncommon and rheumatic fever is extremely rare. Therefore, if a child of this age has pharyngitis, the

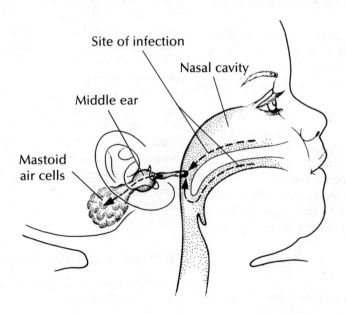

Figure 26.6. **Spread of Infection.**

doctor may refrain from testing and treating with antibiotics.

Tonsils and Adenoids

A half a generation ago tonsils and adenoids were removed frequently in children who had "breathing troubles," "eating problems," and "too many infections." More careful study of the benefits of these operations as well as acknowledgment of the risks and costs is leading to more specific indications for surgery.

The adenoids and tonsils are parts of a ring of tissue encircling the back of the throat. The adenoids, in the back of the nose, constitute the upper part of this ring. The tonsils are on the sides, and a "lingual tonsil" exists on the rear of the tongue. This ring acts as a sieve, or filter, protecting the lower respiratory tract from microorganisms that enter the mouth and nose.

The tonsils and adenoids are relatively large in young children and usually decrease dramatically in size after age eight. Why some children's tonsils are enlarged, often touching each other, is unknown. Most swollen tonsils are the result of infection with a virus or bacteria (see above) and will shrink back down as the infection subsides.

Medical indications for removal of tonsils are enlargement that interferes with normal breathing, swallowing, or speaking, or frequent attacks of proven strep throat. Tonsillectomy may not decrease the number of sore throats because the other tissues of the pharynx can still be invaded by viruses and bacteria. Another indication for tonsil removal is an abscess within or adjacent to a tonsil.

Prolonged enlargement of the adenoids can cause chronic mouth breathing, excessive snoring, and muffled, "nasal" speech. Temporary enlargement is usually related to infection and may cause blockage of the eustachian tubes and lead to otitis media. Breathing dry air through the mouth can cause an irritative cough, compounded by draining secretions from the back of the nose. Evaluation for adenoid enlargement may include palpation of the roof of the mouth, examination with a mirror, or an X ray.

Rarely, the obstruction of breathing is profound enough during sleep to cause inappropriately long pauses in respiration. These pauses can lead to overstressing the lungs and then the heart. Therefore, if the cause of the enlarged adenoids is not found, they may need to be removed. The tonsils need not be removed if they are not causing problems of their own.

While tonsils rarely return once removed, adenoids do occasionally grow back, as they cannot be as completely excised during surgery.

Laryngitis and Croup

A sore throat may not involve the tonsils or pharynx at all. Some viruses prefer to infect the voice box and upper trachea. In addition to an irritated throat, hoarseness is the major symptom. The infant and toddler will often have a barky cough as well. If the child can drink and is not having trouble breathing, treatment consists of rest, plenty of liquids, and humidified air via a vaporizer or "shower steam." High fever, trouble drinking, drooling, or difficulty breathing are reasons to seek medical attention promptly.

Retropharyngeal Abscess

The retropharyngeal lymph nodes behind the pharynx can become infected as a result of infections in the pharynx, sinuses, adenoids, nose, or ear. An infection with pus can lead to an abscess. The symptoms are painful swallowing, fever, swelling of the lymph nodes in the neck and, in more severe cases involving blockage of the airway, difficult, noisy breathing.

The treatment includes surgery to drain the abscesses and antibiotics.

Velopharyngeal Insufficiency

If the back of the throat and palate are not properly formed, the two sections of the pharynx below the mouth and the nose cannot move in the well-coordinated manner necessary for swallowing and for speech. This usually is a result of a cleft palate or other birth defect.

In very severe cases, swallowed food and liquid are regurgitated through the nose. This defect is recognized immediately in newborn infants. Many babies can eat well despite this defect. A larger hole in the nipple of their bottles may temporarily solve the problem for bottle-fed babies. In more severe forms, the baby requires a special plate for the roof of the mouth during feeding, or a brace for malformed gums.

In less severe forms, swallowing is normal but speech is impaired. Treatment involves surgical correction. Plastic surgery is usually performed when the baby is about a year old—before the development of speech. The surgery requires a general anesthetic and a five-day hospital stay. Some patients need speech therapy as well.

Epiglottitis

Although its symptoms are initially somewhat like those of a severe bacterial sore throat, epiglottitis is a medical emergency. Luckily it is rare. This disease occurs when the "lid" of the windpipe (or trachea) becomes infected. The healthy epiglottis closes over the trachea during swallowing to prevent saliva, food, or drink from entering the lungs. The infected epiglottis can become so swollen that it prevents air from entering the lungs, with potentially fatal results.

Symptoms begin rapidly, with a severe sore throat, high fever, and difficulty breathing. The pain of swallowing is so great that the child will not eat and drools rather than swallowing saliva. Rapid, audible breathing is common, but there is no crouplike cough.

A child with these symptoms should be rushed to the hospital emergency room. Treatment begins with maintaining an airway, either by passing a tube from the nose to the trachea or, rarely, by making an opening in the trachea through the front of the neck. Intravenous antibiotics will help eradicate the infection. Usually the tube to hold the airway open can be removed within two days, and the patient usually improves dramatically within this period.

SUMMING UP

EYES, EARS, NOSE, AND THROAT are the source of vision, hearing, smell, and speech, by which the child learns about the world and how to communicate with it. Parents should therefore be alert to trouble signs, such as eye-rubbing or earaches, that might signal serious disease. The child's doctor should check hearing regularly. To avoid loss of sight due to amblyopia, vision should be tested when the child is three and again before school.

Most problems of the ear, nose, and throat are caused by viral or bacterial infections, and are either self-limiting (like a cold) or easily treated with antibiotics from the pediatrician or family physician. The ear, nose, and throat specialist provides medical and surgical expertise in more difficult cases.

27 Disorders of the Bones and Joints

David Roye, M.D.

INTRODUCTION

MOST PEOPLE think of bones as being static and, once growth is achieved, relatively unchanging. In reality, however, the tissue that forms the body's bony framework grows, develops, and replaces itself throughout life. The rigid nature of our skeletal system helps to protect internal organs and the brain as well as to support the body itself.

Normal Growth and Development

A child's skeleton constantly adapts to the process of growth and to the demands of movement. Normal growth of the skeleton depends on the smooth functioning of the muscles, tendons, ligaments, joints, and individual bones. A child's ability to move every part of his or her body also depends on the normal development of the nervous system, which carries messages from the brain to the muscles.

Bone growth from childhood to adulthood is a highly dynamic process. At birth an infant's body contains 270 bones—a far greater number than the 206 bones in the adult body. In fact, many of these bones, such as those in a newborn's spinal column, are composed mostly of *cartilage*, the flexible connective tissue that, in some parts of the body, turns into bone as the child develops. By adulthood, too, a number of childhood bones have become fused.

A newborn's spine curls inward, without the four curves that characterize an adult's spine. Within three months of birth, the neck (or cervical) curve develops, allowing the head to be held up. By six months of age, the baby's lower back has a lumbar curve that develops as the child starts to sit. The sacral curve at the base of the back starts to form as the child begins to walk.

From birth to about age 4, children undergo the period of most rapid growth. During these four years, the skeleton doubles its size from an average of 20 inches to about 40 inches. Growth progresses at a slower pace from age 4 to late childhood and then speeds up again during adolescence. Accelerated growth begins in girls around age 10 and in boys around age 12. During the adolescent growth spurt, which ends by about age 15 or 16 in girls and by about age 18 or 19 in boys, the skeleton reaches its full height.

In early childhood, the cartilage surrounding each vertebra of the spine is replaced with bone. These bone segments join together to form a single cylindrical bone (*vertebra*) by ages three to six. When the 33 vertebrae are aligned, they house the vertebral column, which protects the delicate spinal cord.

During the teenage years, the growth process continues in each vertebra. The spine continues to grow until the skeleton reaches maturity. By this time, the last remaining part of the cartilaginous backbone has developed into bone. The five bones that form the sacral vertebrae at the base of the spine fuse to make one bone—the *sacrum*. When the fusion of all bones is complete, the mature skeleton has a total of 206 bones.

The bones of the spine, limbs, and hips change in shape, size, and length as a child grows. *Growth plates* in each bone control length. These plates serve as *ossification*, or bone-forming, centers, where cartilage is produced and transformed into bone. Bone is also formed inside the membranes of the connective tissue that covers the surface of the bone. Here, new bone is set down around existing bone while old bone cells dissolve below.

Because bone is living tissue, it continually renews itself. New bone replaces existing bone at a rapid rate during childhood and adolescence. Although replacement slows down during the adult years, bone tissue continues to remodel itself throughout life.

Certain cells inside each bone are responsible for the regular turnover of bone tissue. *Osteoblasts*, or bone-creating cells, make bone tissue from the connective tissue protein (*collagen*), chains of carbohydrates, and calcium. At the same time, bone-destroying cells called *osteoclasts* dissolve old bone and replace it with new bone cells.

All of a child's bones contain marrow, a substance that manufactures red blood cells. In a mature skeleton, the marrow is found only in the trunk. Bone also serves as the body's main storage region for calcium and phosphorus.

Trauma, disease, malnutrition, and congenital abnormalities can affect the normal growth and development of a child's bones, muscles, and joints. For instance, injury to the growth plate at the end of a long bone may impair growth and development. Delays in the development of motor skills can point to a neurological disorder. Growth hormone and sex hormones accelerate growth, while malnutrition, deficiency of vitamin D, and long-term illness slow down growth. Certain drugs also can impair growth. Common childhood bone injuries and disorders are described in the following section.

TRAUMA

Sprains and Strains

Active children commonly suffer sprains and strains. The ankles, for example, are especially vulnerable to sprains. A *sprain* injury tears the ligaments that surround the affected joint, whereas a *strain* is an injury to muscles or tendons that results from excessive stretching in a particular region.

Pain, swelling, and bruising may occur in both sprains and strains. Because the symptoms are similar, it is important to watch the injured region for the first 24 hours. If a child cannot bear weight on the ankle, for example, or if the ankle appears swollen and misshapen, it is possible that there is a severe sprain or a fractured bone. A severely sprained ankle, a fracture, or a chipped bone may require a cast.

Strain injuries usually occur in the upper arm, upper leg, or back when the muscles have been overworked in sports or play, or by a fall. Unlike a sprain, which allows little or no weight-bearing on the injured region, a strain does not prevent a child from walking.

When a child appears to have strained a muscle, apply cold compresses to the region for the first 24 hours. Have the child rest the injured region for at least a day. Cold compresses help reduce pain and swelling only during the first 24 hours after an injury. On the second day, heat will provide relief from pain. The pain, swelling, and stiffness usually disappear in a few days.

Dislocations

An adult may inadvertently cause a partial dislocation (subluxation) of a child's shoulder or elbow during play or while yanking on a child's hand to keep the child from falling from a curb or a step. Swinging a toddler by the arms can result in a dislocated shoulder, just as pulling on the hand of a child about to fall can snap the youngster's elbow out of place. When a joint is partially dislocated, the ends of the bones are out of alignment but they still touch. (See figure 27.1.)

Some children experience recurring full dislocation (*luxation*) or partial dislocation of the kneecap. This condition often begins in early childhood but may not become apparent until adolescence. Pain occurs while a child is running, breaking into quick movement sideways, or ascending and descending stairs.

Dislocations of the finger or thumb often occur when a child falls or suffers a strong blow, such as from a ball, that may jam the finger backward and out of its socket.

Because a partial dislocation of the elbow is painful, the injured child may be unable to use his or her arm fully. A doctor can manipulate the limb and restore the joint to its proper position. A sling is then applied for 24 hours. Normal range of motion returns to the limb within a few days. When a serious dislocation or fracture occurs, X rays and a longer period of immobilization may be necessary. Parents should avoid attempting to reposition a dislocated shoulder or elbow. If the limb is injured, place the arm in a sling until medical help is available.

When a young patient's kneecap undergoes recurring partial dislocation, exercise is prescribed to strengthen the quadriceps muscles in the thigh. If a full dislocation occurs, the limb is immobilized for about four weeks. After this, a series of isometric exercises to strengthen the supporting muscles is prescribed in an attempt to prevent future dislocations. If the patient does not respond to this treatment, the problem usually can be corrected surgically.

Fractures

When a child fractures, or breaks, a bone, the bone responds differently from an adult's broken bone. Because children's bones are still growing, they are resilient and can crack without breaking. Even if the bone is broken, realignment of the broken pieces of bone to their proper position, a process called *reduction*, is rarely necessary in a child unless a joint or the bone's growth plate is affected. The bone heals and remodels itself back into a normal position—usually within 12 weeks.

If a fracture produces an injury to the growth plate at the end of a long bone, this injury can result in a growth deformity. When the growth plate is crushed, it can stop developing and there may be a shortening of the bone. When an injury partially de-

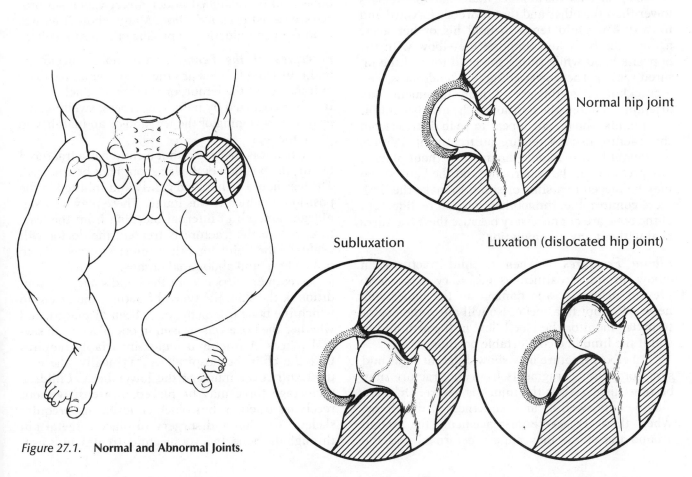

Normal hip joint

Subluxation

Luxation (dislocated hip joint)

Figure 27.1. **Normal and Abnormal Joints.**

stroys the growth plate, a deformity of the bone or joint can result.

Treatment of fractures depends upon the type of injury. Most fractures can be treated by orthopedic manipulation and immobilization in a cast. Children's fractures heal so quickly that manipulation of the broken bone often is impossible one week after the injury occurs because the bone has partially healed. The following are some of the more common fractures:

Collarbone Fractures. The bone most frequently broken by children is the *clavicle*, or collarbone. This fracture typically occurs when a child falls onto his or her outstretched hand, elbow, or the side of his or her shoulder.

A child may be born with a partially broken collarbone after an especially difficult delivery. There may, however, be no signs of a broken collarbone during the routine examination in the delivery room. If a newborn is unable to move an arm spontaneously, the clavicle is examined for swelling, tenderness, and any grating sounds. Often an incomplete fracture of the collarbone is first diagnosed when a lump is noticed at the end of the bone. The lump disappears as the fracture heals.

When a child has a complete fracture of the clavicle, parents may notice that one shoulder is lower than the other and that it droops forward and inward. The child tends to hold his or her arms against the body and supports the elbow with the opposite hand while tilting the head toward the injured region. There is swelling and tenderness, and a crackling or grating sound upon movement. Any attempt to change the position of the arm is painful.

Infants who do not appear to be in distress from the fracture usually require no treatment. Parents are taught how to handle the infant without placing any pressure on the collarbone, and the baby's arm may be placed in a sling or splint to make the limb more comfortable. Immobilization and realignment of the bone are not necessary because these fractures heal without any manipulation.

Elbow Fractures. When a child fractures an elbow, prompt treatment is necessary in order to prevent deformity and damage to the underlying nerves. Prompt treatment also will allow the doctor to better monitor the blood flow in the arm and to splint the limb in a comfortable position.

An elbow fracture may show different signs and symptoms. Bone fragments from the fracture may become displaced, if the injury is severe. Or there may be only swelling and tenderness of the elbow. When there is severe displacement, the region around the elbow may appear deformed and the arm may look shorter. The arm may be cool or pale or may have a decreased pulse, reduced sensation, or even paralysis. There also may be increasing pain.

When treating a fractured elbow, the doctor first monitors the nerves and the circulation and then splints the arm, to make it comfortable. Instead of placing the arm at a right angle, it is splinted into an extended position to ensure the continued flow of blood to the region.

Treatment varies, depending on how much the elbow has been knocked out of its normal position and the amount of both swelling and nerve damage. When the bone is broken but not out of position, the arm can be placed in a splint for four weeks. During this time, the parents should watch the arm for signs of increased pain or an inability to move the fingers.

When a fractured elbow is partially out of place, the bones may need to be realigned, which will require administering anesthesia. Afterward, a cast is placed on the arm so that proper healing can take place.

If there is marked swelling, a period of traction or elevation may be necessary before a cast can be applied. If the bones cannot be realigned successfully, the patient is placed under anesthesia and the doctor surgically opens the fracture site so that the bones can be realigned under direct vision—a procedure called *open reduction*. Many elbow fractures require open reduction to produce the best results.

Fractures of the Femur. Automobile accidents and falls from heights are the most common causes of fractures of the femur, or thighbone. Such a fracture is recognized by pain, tenderness, swelling, deformity, shortening of the leg, and/or an inability to move the leg.

When it is suspected that a child has a fractured femur, the position of the leg should not be changed. The leg should be handled gently and splinted in the position in which it was found. There may be a significant amount of internal bleeding from the fracture. Before the fracture is treated, the doctor will evaluate the child for other injuries, especially to head, chest, and abdominal organs.

Treatment depends on the child's age, the condition of the skin, the type of fracture, the extent to which the bone fragments have been displaced, and whether the bone was broken in one place or in several places. A fractured femur invariably requires that the child be hospitalized. Typically, the cast used will cover much of the lower body. Children under age three may be placed in a cast without receiving traction, but older children may require skeletal traction and surgery to place a metal pin through the bone. In a young child, treatment is usually less complicated and healing is quicker than in an older child.

Fractures of the Tibia and Fibula.
Fractures of the tibia, or shinbone, and the fibula, or the smaller bone in the shin, are somewhat common in children.

Toddlers occasionally undergo twisting injuries from what may appear to be a simple fall, with a resulting fracture or a spiral fracture of the shinbone. In these cases, the injury may be difficult to detect. Parents of a toddler with such a fracture often bring the tot to the pediatrician because the child is irritable, cries persistently, and refuses to walk.

Shinbone fractures in older children are usually produced by trauma from contact sports, skiing, or automobile accidents. Generally these patients require more treatment and experience more complications than do younger children with similar injuries.

A toddler with a spiral fracture is treated with a soft or hard cast that must be worn for two to three weeks. When the bone is displaced as the result of a more serious accident, reduction and immobilization may be necessary. If the doctor suspects there is any damage to the nerves and blood vessels, the child may be hospitalized for observation.

When the leg swells following a fracture of the tibia, the swelling can cause damage to the nerves and blood vessels. This problem can be treated successfully by surgically releasing the fascia, a band of connective tissue in the affected region.

Three kinds of fractures may require surgical treatment: those that do not realign easily under manipulation, those that are unstable, and those that affect the growth plate. Open fractures, or breaks in which the bone juts out through the skin, also require surgery.

The major complication of a fractured tibia or fibula is the swelling that can result in damaged nerves and blood vessels. Careful observation is necessary to ensure that any damage is prevented.

Skull Fractures.
Injuries of the head are particularly common among children and any severe head blow or skull fracture must be treated immediately. Surgery may be necessary to control bleeding or to ease pressure on the brain. Severe head injuries that are left untreated can cause mental retardation and seizures. (See chapter 28, Neurological and Neuromuscular Disorders, for a more detailed discussion.)

Prevention of Fractures

Physical exercise should be encouraged in children at an early age. A toddler who learns to enjoy exercise is more likely to be active than one who has little exposure to healthy activities. Because children are such active explorers, extra care should be taken to prevent accidents in the home. Safety gates should be placed at the top and bottom of stairways to prevent falls—and broken bones. Open, unguarded windows offer special hazards to exploring toddlers. Play regions should also be made safe to minimize the danger of injury.

Children are particularly vulnerable to injury in automobile accidents. Infants and children (as well as adults) should be properly restrained. Car seats of approved design should be used for children weighing up to 40 pounds and restraints used for larger children. Infants and children should never be held in a parent's lap. (For more information, see chapter 1, Before the Baby Is Born.)

Equipment of all kinds can present orthopedic hazards for children. Strollers and carriages should by sturdy and well designed. Folding models should have safety devices to prevent their collapse while a child is inside and to keep little fingers from getting caught in hinged parts. Tricycles and bicycles should be well made and equipped with reflectors; safety training for children riding bicycles is a must. Motorized vehicles such as motorbikes, all-terrain vehicles, and snowmobiles are not meant for small children.

Children who participate in sports have a higher risk of bone, muscle, and ligament injury. For this reason, proper training, conditioning, and supervision are necessary to prevent accidents and injuries. An active child who complains of persistent and sharp pain following participation in sports should be seen by a doctor. In some circumstances, extremely stressful movement may damage growing bones and joints. (For more, see chapter 14.)

First Aid for Broken Bones

When an injury, fall, or sudden movement causes a great deal of pain and the inability to move the affected limb, a broken bone should be suspected and the child taken to a hospital emergency room. If the child cannot be moved, an ambulance should be called. A few basic first-aid guidelines are outlined on the following page, in the box on First Aid for a Possible Broken Bone.

Child Abuse

Child abuse, or the battered child syndrome as it used to be called, is the result of deliberate physical injury to a child, frequently by a parent or other person responsible for the youngster's care. Broken bones, bruises, burns, and cuts may appear on many parts of the child's body. An abused child also may

FIRST AID FOR A POSSIBLE BROKEN BONE

While transporting the child or awaiting emergency assistance, here are a few basic first-aid guidelines to follow:

1. When there is pain upon moving the bone, deformity, tenderness to the touch, and swelling, the injury is most likely a fracture. If there is bleeding from the wound, control it by placing a clean cloth pad on the injury and applying direct pressure.
2. If an ice bag is available, place it on the injured region to reduce pain and swelling.
3. Do not give the child anything to eat or drink in case general anesthesia is needed to reset the bone.
4. If the child has fallen from a significant height and may have a back injury, do not try to move him or her without the aid of someone trained in moving accident victims. If there has been a spinal injury, improperly moving the child can cause permanent neurological damage.
5. If you must move the child, immobilize the limb by applying bandages or splints. A splint will provide enough support to prevent further damage to the region. In an emergency, a number of items can make an effective splint: A pillow, a rolled-up newspaper, a folded blanket, a coat, or a board will provide temporary immobilization until help is available.

be underweight, malnourished, and slow in development. The child's behavior is often extreme—either passive or extremely aggressive.

Children also suffer injuries through parental neglect—lack of supervision that results in children playing in the street or near unguarded open windows or riding in cars without infant seats or seatbelts.

Injuries can damage such internal organs as the pancreas, liver, and spleen, can cause abdominal bleeding, and can result in death. Very often, fatalities occur because the person responsible for the child's care delays seeking medical care. Most abused children are under the age of three and a large number of them are younger than six months old. Premature infants and stepchildren tend to be at increased risk for child abuse.

When a doctor, teacher, or other person suspects that a child is a victim of abuse, the youngster may undergo extensive X rays to identify new injuries as well as old ones. In some cases, the child is hospitalized for a complete evaluation, which includes tests for such disorders as leukemia, hemophilia, rickets, bone infections, and sexually transmitted diseases.

Fractures are common among abused children. The most frequent sites of fractures are the long bones of the arms and legs, the ribs, and the skull. When fractures repeatedly assault the growth plates, the injury can produce deformity of the affected limb.

Abusive parents who bring a child into a hospital for treatment tend to be vague or inconsistent when explaining the circumstances that caused the injury. It is common for an abusive parent to attribute the child's injury to a fall, such as falling out of bed, tumbling down the stairs, or being hurt on playground equipment. However, young children who fall from bed rarely fracture a bone. Similarly, it is unlikely that a child who has not begun to walk will suffer a fracture. It is true that some babies suffer broken bones at birth, but healing usually takes place within a few days or weeks.

Doctors and other health professionals are required by law to report all suspected cases of child abuse. All cases are investigated and counseling is provided to the families by the hospital's social services department.

Prompt action in suspected cases of child abuse often can prevent future abuse and injury. During an investigation, the parents are questioned, as are other children in the home, babysitters, and staff and students at daycare centers. Depending upon the circumstances, action is aimed at preventing further abuse. This may entail removing the child from the home and entering the parents in special child-abuse prevention programs. (See section on Child Abuse, chapter 15.)

ARTHRITIS

MOST PEOPLE think of arthritis as a disease of older people; in fact, there are forms of arthritis that can strike at an early age. Arthritis is an umbrella term to describe inflammation of one or more joints. There are more than 100 different types of arthritis, but not all affect children. Although the cause of noninfectious arthritis is unknown, researchers classify the condition as an autoimmune disease. For unexplained reasons, antibodies that usually fight off disease turn against the body's own tissues. In arthritis, this autoimmune response results in inflammation and damage to the surrounding tissue, including cartilage, bone, and ligaments. Inflammation is persistent in most forms of arthritis and causes further damage to the joint. The most common types of juvenile arthritis are described below.

Still's Disease or Juvenile Rheumatoid Arthritis

According to the Arthritis Foundation, as many as 200,000 children in the United States suffer from juvenile rheumatoid arthritis, a disease that is similar to but also quite different from the adult form. (Some doctors prefer to drop the "rheumatoid" from the disease name to avoid confusion.) The disease is somewhat more common in girls than boys, and it varies considerably in severity and characteristics.

There are three broad subtypes of juvenile rheumatoid arthritis. In about 20 percent of the cases, the disease comes on with a *systemic* attack that affects many parts of the body in addition to causing joint inflammation. High intermittent fevers are common, and there is a pale pinkish rash. There may be an enlarged liver and spleen as well as swollen lymph nodes. Sometimes the heart is involved, and severe anemia also may occur. The acute attack usually subsides in a few weeks, but about half of the children will suffer future systemic flare-ups. The joint inflammation and pain is usually worst during a systemic attack, especially when there is fever. But about 25 percent of children with systemic juvenile arthritis develop chronic joint pains that persist even when the acute phase passes.

A second major subtype is referred to as *polyarticular onset*, so named because it starts with severe inflammation of several joints. The polyarticular type is more common than the systemic form, accounting for about 40 percent of cases. Any of the joints, including the spine, may be affected. As in adult rheumatoid arthritis, the joint involvement is often symmetrical—if one knee is affected, for example, the opposite is also likely to be involved.

The affected joints are swollen and painful, with the symptoms being more severe in the morning or after periods of rest. This type may be accompanied by a low-grade fever, anemia, weight loss, and other symptoms. Blood tests often show the presence of *rheumatoid factor*—a substance present in adult rheumatoid arthritis. In these children, the joint symptoms and long-term destructive effects are more severe than in cases with a negative rheumatoid factor test.

The third general subtype is referred to as *pauciarticular onset*. It also accounts for about 40 percent of juvenile arthritis cases. It may come on at an early age, usually before six, or alternatively, may begin somewhat later. The early-onset form is more common among girls, whereas the later form is seen more in boys. The joints most affected are the knees, ankles, and elbows; the spine is spared in the early type, but boys with the later form may go on to develop a chronic type of back arthritis.

Systemic symptoms are absent or mild, but iridocyclitis (inflammation of the iris and other parts of the eye) is a common feature of juvenile rheumatoid arthritis and should be checked by the physician.

Overall, the outlook for children with juvenile rheumatoid arthritis is good. About 75 percent of cases go into long periods of remission with little or no permanent damage. Some children, however, develop chronic arthritis and suffer recurrent flare-ups. Growth may be hampered, and children with the more severe forms of the disease may miss a good deal of school and develop a variety of emotional problems associated with having a chronic disease.

Treatment is aimed at relieving the symptoms, preventing long-term complications (especially when the eyes, heart, and other organs are affected), and retaining as much joint and muscle function as possible. Many of the medications used are the same as those taken for adult arthritis. Aspirin remains the most commonly used agent—when taken in large enough doses, it eases the joint inflammation and thereby helps prevent joint destruction. If aspirin is insufficient or is not tolerated, one of the other nonsteroidal antiinflammatory medications may be given. Gold salt therapy may be tried in cases where aspirin or other antiinflammatory agents are not enough. The use of systemic steroids is discouraged unless necessary in order to control the disease because these powerful medications have many undesirable side effects, including growth retardation. Occasionally steroid injections may be used to ease the inflammation and pain in a severely affected joint, and topical steroids may be prescribed to prevent eye damage.

Physical therapy is an important part of the overall treatment. Exercise is vital to retain as much joint and muscle function as possible, but the exercises should be carefully designed since the wrong type of activity can also cause joint damage. Splints may be worn at night to help prevent deformities.

Although juvenile arthritis can be trying for both the child and family, every attempt should be made to lead as normal a life as possible. The large majority of children can attend regular school, and they should be encouraged to participate in as many childhood activities as possible. A child who is unable to run and engage in sports that cause extra wear and tear on the joints may be able to swim or find activities that use joints and body parts that are not affected by the disease. In some cases, assistive devices may be needed, especially during flare-ups, but most children with arthritis can get around on their own and should be encouraged to do so.

Juvenile Ankylosing Spondylitis

Ankylosing spondylitis affects mostly the spine, although it often begins in other joints and is easily mistaken for pauciarticular arthritis in its early stages. The disease is more common among boys, and usually does not begin before the age of eight or ten. It tends to run in families, and sometimes accompanies other disorders, such as inflammatory bowel disease.

Treatment is aimed at easing symptoms and preventing as much spinal deformity as possible. In the past, victims of ankylosing spondylitis often ended up with a severe permanent stoop, unable to stand straight. Bracing can help prevent this deformity, although the spine may still be rigid and movement restricted.

Infectious Arthritis

Infectious arthritis and osteomyelitis (see following section) require prompt diagnosis and treatment in order to prevent permanent damage and the destruction of a growing child's joints and bones. Certain strains of bacteria, viruses, and fungi all can cause infectious arthritis when they travel through the bloodstream and lodge in a joint, causing inflammation and other symptoms.

The symptoms of infectious arthritis are characterized by their sudden onset. Any sudden swelling and inflammation of a joint on the heels of an infection, for example, a strep throat, indicates possible infectious arthritis.

A wide range of bacteria cause infectious arthritis: Staphylococcal and streptococcal bacteria are the main sources of infection. Children who receive tick bites can also develop a form of infectious arthritis known as Lyme disease. The infected tick carries a bacterium that travels to various parts of the body and causes inflammation and pain. When Lyme disease is not treated properly, it can lead to recurring flare-ups of the arthritis.

The hip joint is often the target of infectious arthritis in both infants and older children. In very young babies, there may not be any obvious symptoms of arthritis. Older children are able to complain about their pain or difficulty in moving, but this is not the case with young babies. In any instance, however, prompt diagnosis and treatment are important, especially when a hip is involved, because the infection quickly results in the dislocation and destruction of the entire hip joint.

Infectious arthritis is diagnosed via physical examination, X rays, blood tests, and analysis of a small amount of fluid from the joint to identify the infectious agent that is causing the inflammation. Treatment is by antibiotics, which are administered intravenously (directly into the veins) in the hospital. Drainage of the joint helps ensure the removal of any remaining infection.

The arthritis produced by such viruses as rubella, influenza, mumps, and infectious hepatitis usually disappears without treatment. This form of infectious arthritis is treated with aspirin or other antiinflammatory agents because antibiotics are ineffective against viruses. Infections by fungi are rarely the cause of infectious arthritis in children in this country.

Arthritis Associated with Other Diseases

A number of conditions begin with arthritis-like symptoms but are actually caused by another disease. The presence of fever and enlargement of the lymph nodes and spleen may suggest juvenile arthritis. When a blood test fails to confirm this diagnosis, additional tests are necessary. Because leukemia begins with a high fever and joint pain, a test of bone marrow cells can help in making a diagnosis. Such diseases of the connective tissue as systemic lupus erythematosus and scleroderma also may masquerade as arthritis in their early stages.

OSTEOMYELITIS

OSTEOMYELITIS, an infection of the bone tissue, occurs when bacteria enter the bloodstream via a wound in the mouth or throat, or through a region of broken or infected skin. Usually these bacteria are killed by the body's immune system, but in children they occasionally pass through the bloodstream to the long bones, where they cause infection. Children are more susceptible to osteomyelitis than are adults because children's immune systems are not completely programmed to kill all invading bacteria. The anatomy of the growth plate also predisposes children to osteomyelitis.

A child with osteomyelitis will look ill and have a fever, loss of appetite, and severe pain near the affected region. If the infection affects the hip, knee, or ankle, the child will not want to uses the limb and either will refuse to walk or may limp while walking. Similarly, the child will refuse to use an arm if the infection has settled into that part of the body.

Diagnosis includes X rays and blood tests, including an ESR (erythrocyte sedimentation rate), which is a measurement of the rate at which red blood cells fall to the bottom of a tube. Frequently the ESR is abnormal when osteomyelitis is present and the child's white blood cell count is high. Making a diagnosis in a newborn may be difficult because the young infant may not have the usual symptoms of the infection.

Early recognition and treatment of osteomyelitis is essential in order to prevent bone destruction, arrested growth, and deformity of the affected bone, and spread of the infection to other regions. Antibiotics are administered directly into the veins (intravenously) to control the infection. However, if diagnosis is delayed or the infection does not respond to the antibiotics within the first two days of treatment, surgical drainage of the region may be necessary. Antibiotic treatment usually continues for two to six weeks, or even longer if the infection becomes chronic.

DISORDERS THAT BECOME APPARENT WITH GROWTH

Scoliosis

Scoliosis is a lateral abnormal curvature of the spine that can occur during childhood or adolescence and progress throughout adult life. Idiopathic scoliosis is the most common form, and curves may appear during infancy or early childhood, but they tend to be most apparent during the growth spurts that occur in the preadolescent years. The large, progressive curves that accompany scoliosis are more common in girls than in boys. However, small curves appear with the same frequency in both boys and girls. Most curves are small and never require more than observation; in fact, surveys have found that about 5 percent of ninth graders have small curves.

A pediatrician or school nurse can often identify the initial curves of scoliosis during a routine examination or a school health screening. The doctor or nurse evaluates a child for scoliosis by checking the general posture and the alignment of the spine. The signs of this disease include shoulders that are not level with each other, a prominent shoulder blade, asymmetrical creases at the waist, and a high hip. It is important that scoliosis be detected as early as possible because its course is usually insidious. When a child tests positive for curves, X rays

are taken to measure the curvature. The child is then followed until growth is complete to ensure that there is no dangerous progression of the curvature.

In mild cases, no special treatment may be required. Exercises aimed at strengthening the back muscles are often recommended. In more severe cases, a brace may be prescribed to halt the course of the curvature. Some of the newer lightweight braces are barely noticeable under clothing and are more acceptable to self-conscious adolescents who must wear them. In recent years there have been a number of reports in the media describing therapy that uses electrical stimulation in an attempt to straighten the curve. Further investigation by the Scoliosis Research Society has determined that electrical stimulation does not influence the natural course of scoliosis.

The abnormal curvature may appear in the thoracic region in the upper back or in the lumbar spine, in the lower back. As scoliosis progresses, it causes the vertebrae to rotate toward the concave part of the curve. As a result, the ribs are crowded together on one side of the chest while there are wide gaps between the ribs on the other side. Severe scoliosis can cause abnormal posture and gait as well as cardiac and lung problems when the child becomes an adult.

The most common form of scoliosis is idiopathic, meaning that the exact cause of the disease is unknown, but it is known to be inherited. Other cases result from poorly formed or missing bones in the spinal column (congenital scoliosis), muscle imbalance caused by paralytic or spastic disease, or disorders of the connective tissue, such as Marfan syndrome and osteogenesis imperfecta.

Before beginning treatment, the doctor determines the degree to which the spine decompensates as a result of the curvature. In most cases, regular follow-up exams during the adolescent period of growth are sufficient. When a curve progresses beyond the 25-degree marker in a growing child, wearing a brace may be recommended.

If the child's skeleton has not yet reached maturity, a spinal brace molded to fit the body is the first choice of treatment. In about 85 percent of the cases, braces have arrested a spinal curvature. Most children remain in the brace for 16 hours a day. The duration of treatment depends upon the nature of the curve and the individual child.

Surgery may be recommended if the curve goes beyond the 40- to 45-degree mark. There are several surgical procedures; selection depends upon the severity and type of scoliosis and the experience of the orthopedic surgeon. Some of the new procedures require only short hospitalization and do not entail wearing a body cast as was common in the past.

Bow Legs

Bowing of the legs is a normal stage of development in almost all babies. By 18 months to two years of age, most children's legs remodel themselves into a normal position. Because the condition usually corrects itself, no treatment is necessary. A child who is bow-legged at age two may well be knock-kneed by age 4. But as the child grows, his or her knees and ankles become more aligned and usually look normal by the teenage years.

Abnormal bowing of the legs may result from a neurological problem; a metabolic bone disorder, such as rickets; or a specific growth problem, such as *Blount's disease*, a rare disorder of growth that causes severe bowing and is found in West Indian populations.

A diagnosis of bow legs can be made after a physical examination and an X ray. The bowing of the legs is often accompanied by an internal torsion, or twisting, of the shinbone. When the bowing results from a neurological or a growth problem, a brace may be prescribed or surgery may be necessary. When rickets is present, the bowing resolves itself after the metabolic and nutritional problem has been corrected.

Uneven Limb Length

Discrepancies in the length of limbs are common in children. Before the poliomyelitis vaccine was availble in this country, childhood polio frequently caused discrepancy in the lower-limb length as well as paralysis. Today, uneven limb length has a number of causes—congenital disorders, infection that causes a growing bone to grow slower or faster, trauma, and tumors. Some children who have a slight shortening of one leg (say, three-quarters of an inch) may require only a special shoe lift as treatment. Others who have severe shortening—more than seven inches—often can be treated by surgical correction or amputation of part of the limb, followed by use of a prosthesis, or artificial limb.

The doctor first determines how much of a discrepancy is present and then ascertains the skeletal age of the child. Determining a young patient's skeletal age is important because it allows the doctor to decide whether the problem should be corrected by lengthening or by shortening the limb. In an adolescent whose skeleton is approaching maturity, it is possible to correct the discrepancy by surgically adjusting the growth plate in the lower limb to arrest growth. Young children require a different approach, which may consist of one of these courses of treatment: mechanically lengthening the leg by surgically implanting a rod inside the bone and gradually lengthening the bone over a period of weeks or months; amputating part of the limb and applying a prosthesis; or surgically removing a portion of bone to shorten the limb.

In some children, discrepancies of limb length may suddenly stabilize and correct themselves, thus requiring no treatment. More likely, the discrepancy will be progressive. Doctors follow the growth of the affected limb by using a growth-remaining chart. This chart serves as a guide for estimating how much growth can be expected in the femur, or thighbone, and tibia, or shinbone, in girls and boys at different skeletal ages.

Flat Feet

From birth until about age three, all normal babies have flat-looking feet. Little pads of fat occupy the arch region and hide the normal bony contour of the foot. As the child learns to stand and walk, the muscles that allow the foot to arch upward off the ground are developed. However, some children have foot muscles that collapse under their own weight as they walk and stand, resulting in flat feet.

A child whose arch is flat when he or she stands up but returns to an arched position when weight is off the foot has a supple flat foot. This condition usually is related to an inherited laxity of the ligaments. No treatment is needed for a supple flat foot.

Older children with very flat feet may have difficulty running and may experience discomfort. This can be treated by modifying the child's shoe or by placing an orthotic insert inside the shoe.

A severely flat foot may require surgical correction. Adjustments can be made to the soft tissues around the foot—this includes moving tendons and releasing tight tissues. Surgeons may also cut and fuse bone to align the foot better.

In some children, flat feet may be caused by a neurological or general orthopedic disorder. When this is the case, orthotic shoe inserts are prescribed to prevent a permanent deformity.

Toeing In

Infants frequently curve their feet inward, or toe in, as a part of their normal development. Toeing in usually disappears without requiring any treatment. When the problem persists or begins to develop in a baby whose feet had been parallel, the doctor examines the foot and leg and prescribes a course of treatment.

Often the foot can be corrected by stretching or by placing it in a cast. When the tibia, or shinbone, is affected, the leg may also bow and turn in between the knee and the ankle. In a normal child, the problem usually corrects itself during the growth-and-development process.

A child who stops toeing in at 20 months but adopts the position again at 26 months, for instance, is only following the instructions of genetic programming. While this particular type of toeing in is frustrating to parents, it does not call for any special treatment. As the child grows and develops, the foot placement gradually improves. Occasionally a child may not be able to run or walk properly because of severely limited outward rotation of the legs through the hip joint. In these extreme cases, surgery may be recommended to place the leg in a more normal alignment. Neither braces, casts, nor corrective shoes can prevent the need for surgery when the leg and foot are abnormally skewed.

Toeing Out

Babies frequently are born with their legs turning out. This is thought to be due primarily to intrauterine position. In general, external rotation gradually but spontaneously corrects itself. Occasionally this external or outward rotation persists through the age that babies pull themselves up to stand and start to walk. As with internal rotation (toeing in), toeing out is affected by hereditary factors. For the most part treatment is not indicated for the positional or hereditary forms of toeing out. If the condition is severe, persistent, or only affects one side, it should be evaluated by a physician.

CONGENITAL ABNORMALITIES

CONGENITAL DISORDERS and deformities of the bones, muscles, and joints call for early recognition and treatment in order to prevent a lifetime of disability. A condition is considered congenital if it is present when an infant is born. Not every congenital disorder is hereditary. A congenital disorder can indeed be inherited—for instance, when an abnormal gene is transmitted from a parent to the child in dwarfism. But abnormalities can also result from conditions that occurred within the uterus during pregnancy.

Several congenital conditions are caused by both genetic and environmental influences—among these are clubfoot and dislocation of the hip. Finally, when there are abnormalities within the chromosomes—the structures housing the genes inside the cells—disorders such as Down's syndrome can appear in a child. The congenital orthopedic disorders, many of them rare, are discussed below.

Achondroplasia

Achondroplasia, a form of dwarfism, is a disorder characterized by short and stubby arms and legs. The long bones are primarily affected, although the spine and other bones may also be affected.

A child with achondroplasia tends at birth to have a trunk noticeably disproportionate with limbs. The child's head is enlarged, the face broad, and the forehead prominent. There may be an exaggerated curve in the lower back, and a tendency toward kyphosis, or hunchback. When the child begins to walk, the lower legs look bowed and the walk resembles a waddling gait.

Most children with achondroplasia are healthy and can be expected to have a normal life span. When complications occur, changes in the spinal column can cause deformity and compression of the spinal cord. Symptoms include pain in the back, buttocks, or legs; weakness of the legs; falling; and complaints of decreasing endurance.

There is no specific treatment for the genetic defect in achondroplasia. If severe bowing of the legs occurs, surgery can be performed to improve the gait and to prevent damage to the knee. When spinal column deformities progress, the child may need surgery to fuse the vertebrae to prevent compression of the spinal cord.

About 90 percent of children with achondroplasia are born to normal parents. The abnormal gene that the child carries is due to a spontaneous mutation. Genetic counseling for parents and children with achondroplasia is important. The child should be taught the risks of genetic transmission when he or she reaches an appropriate age. Women with achondroplasia can bear normal children, but because of the abnormal configuration of their pelvis, they are prone to spontaneous abortions. If they carry their pregnancies to term, delivery must be by cesarean section.

Arthrogryposis Multiplex Congenita

Arthrogryposis multiplex congenita is a syndrome in which any number of joints are rigidly fixed into position. Because the muscles are incompletely developed, the joints look large and spindly. The cause of arthrogryposis is unknown, but the syndrome appears to result when the fetus is unable to move for a long period of time inside the uterus. Such a lack of movement apparently leads to poor or incompletely developed joints in a fetus that is otherwise normal. This condition is not progressive. With a program of manipulation, physical therapy, and corrective braces and splints, the outlook for an infant with arthrogryposis is promising.

This disorder usually can be diagnosed right after birth. An infant with arthrogryposis has shoulders that turn inward, elbows that are fixed in a slightly bent or straight position, bent wrists, and hands that point away from the body. The fingers tend to be slender and poorly developed with no creases where they normally would bend. The hips are often dislocated and usually have contractures, or irreversible shortenings of the muscle fibers, so that the mobility of the joints is reduced. The knees may be bent or straight, and the patella, or kneecap, may be dislocated. Clubfoot is also frequently present. Usually both arms and legs are affected, but the syndrome can affect any combination of the limbs, or it can affect only one limb. Port wine stains sometimes appear on the forehead. As the child grows, severe scoliosis, or abnormal curvature of the spine, may develop. In rare cases, children with arthrogryposis can develop congenital heart disease or kidney disease.

This disorder has been divided into three major types. The first is associated with a lack of nerve tissue, a condition that leads to a lack of muscle tissue and rigidity in the joints. The second type causes the muscles themselves to undergo fatty degeneration without any neurological involvement. The third type is a combination of the other two.

There is no preventive treatment for arthrogryposis as its cause is as yet unknown. Early diagnosis allows a total rehabilitation program to be started at an early age. Treatment of the infant with arthrogryposis begins in the nursery with passive exercising of the contracted, or shortened, joints. Parents are taught to continue the movement therapy at home so that the child can develop as much range of motion in his or her limbs as possible. In addition to developmental and eventual occupational therapy, the child will probably require braces and splints at an early age.

Delays in reaching such milestones of early childhood motor development as standing and walking can be prevented in children with arthrogryposis if there is surgical correction before age two. However, surgery should not be undertaken until it has been determined that the condition is actually interfering with development. Surgical correction can take various forms, depending upon the joints involved.

Correcting a deformity of the foot, such as a clubfoot, can enable the child to maintain a normal foot position while walking. Surgery also may be helpful when arthrogryposis affects the knees. Braces and splinting are usually necessary to maintain a bent knee that has been surgically corrected.

A dislocated hip in a child with arthrogryposis multiplex congenita is much more complicated than the usual case of congenital hip dislocation. Because the hip may be extremely stiff, the surgeon may correct portions of soft tissue in the region instead of operating on the bone.

Children with arthrogryposis often have great difficulty walking and severe hyperlordosis, an exaggerated curve of the lower back that is a form of swayback. As they grow older, they often develop degenerative arthritis.

Before any surgery is begun on the upper body, the extent to which the child can use his or her hands and arms must be fully evaluated. In some cases, surgery is not advisable. Surgery on the upper body is performed mostly to increase the use of hands and thus enable a child to achieve independence in eating and performing other routine tasks. Pediatric orthopedic surgeons usually correct one limb first and then evaluate the results before operating on the other limb.

Congenital Absence of Limbs

When a child is born with a missing limb or a missing portion of a limb, it is difficult for a doctor to determine the cause. In some cases, missing limbs have been attributed to the ingestion of drugs by pregnant women (for example, some pregnant women took thalidomide during the 1960s and bore infants without arms). The problem, however, existed long before most prescription drugs were available. Maternal illness, radiation, and intrauterine problems have also been blamed for the congenital absence of limbs.

Children born with missing limbs should be treated as early as possible. A team consisting of a surgeon, a physical therapist, a prosthetist (a specialist who makes artificial limbs and braces), and a psychologist or psychiatric social worker can help the child and family members respond well to prosthetic rehabilitation.

Treatment of absent or poorly developed limbs in the upper body can be managed with a myoelectric prosthesis that the child can use in performing the activities of daily living.

Congenital absence of all or part of the foot, lower leg, or thigh can produce significant problems that may require surgical treatment. Reconstruction usually calls for amputation of the foot to allow for rehabilitation with a prosthesis below the knee. The primary goal of the pediatric orthopedic surgeon is to make the limb as useful to the child as possible. This may be accomplished by use of a prosthesis or by surgically straightening and lengthening long bones.

Since the cause of congenital absence of limbs remains unknown, it is still unclear how this problem can be prevented. When a woman learns she is pregnant, she should obtain good prenatal care and avoid exposure to dangerous elements in the environment. No medications should be taken without the advice of the obstetrician.

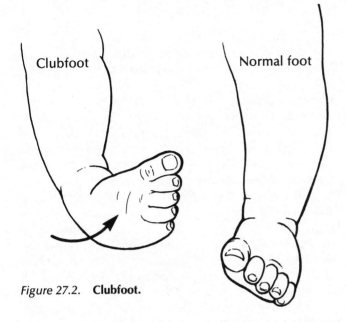

Clubfoot   Normal foot

Figure 27.2.   **Clubfoot.**

Congenital Clubfoot

One of the most common deformities of the bones is clubfoot, or talipes equinovarus. (See figure 27.2.) Clubfoot is characterized by an abnormal development of the soft tissue on the instep that causes one or both feet to twist in and to point downward or upward. As a result, the foot's range of motion is limited and walking is impaired. This bony deformity is more common in boys than in girls.

In the past, a diagnosis of clubfoot spelled a life with a permanent handicap for a child. But clubfoot can now be reversed when it is treated during infancy—thus enabling the child to walk normally.

In some cases, heredity or a neurological disease is responsible for clubfoot. Often the cause is unknown. Theories about the causes have pointed to such prenatal factors as compression within the uterus during fetal development. When clubfoot is detected at birth, the doctor must determine its cause before beginning treatment.

Early diagnosis and treatment immediately after birth are essential to the correction of clubfoot. When the doctor makes a diagnosis, he will determine whether the child has a true clubfoot or a postural clubfoot.

The *"true"* clubfoot is a rigid deformity that can be partially corrected with casting, regular manipulation, and braces. The *"postural"* clubfoot is flexible and easier to correct by regular manipulation of the foot. X rays will help to determine which of the two forms has affected an infant's foot. When a true clubfoot is present, X rays reveal an abnormal relationship between the bones in the back of the foot.

The first stage of treatment for both conditions includes corrective casting and splinting, which is also called strapping. The doctor gently manipulates the foot to correct the deformity and then applies a plaster cast to hold the correction in place. When treatment is first begun, weekly manipulation and casts are required. If the foot responds completely to casting over a period of months, the doctor will consider the condition a postural clubfoot and will prescribe a special shoe or a special shoe and bar for the child.

If the foot does not respond well to this treatment, and X rays show that a true clubfoot exists, surgery may be recommended. Pediatric orthopedic surgeons usually suggest that surgery be performed between four and twelve months of age. Surgery consists of lengthening the heel cords, tendons, and muscles, releasing the joint capsules, and transplanting tendons. Surgery on the bones of the foot is reserved for extremely severe cases in young children or for children over six years of age. After surgery, a cast is applied to hold the corrected foot in the proper position. The length of time the foot must remain in the cast depends on the type of surgery performed and the child's age.

There is no known way to prevent clubfoot. However, when a child is receiving treatment for clubfoot, it is important that parents work with the doctor to help achieve the best possible results and to prevent any complications. Parents usually are taught how to prevent damage to the cast and how to recognize when the cast is too tight in order to avoid any problems with circulation. Once the cast is removed, parents should learn how to manipulate the foot so that the child can have complete range of motion.

Congenital Dislocation of the Hip

Congenital dislocation of the hip is a somewhat common orthopedic problem of childhood in which the ball-shaped upper end of the femur, or thighbone, does not fit properly in its place within the socket of the hip joint.

While the cause of congenital dislocation of the hip is unknown, many factors indicate that it may be hereditary. The position of the unborn child in the uterus also has a definite influence on the incidence of congenital dislocation of the hip—children born in a breech position are more likely to have this disorder. The incidence of congenital dislocation of the hip is high in cultures where babies are swaddled or strapped with the legs extended. It is important that parents with a family history of this disorder have their infants carefully examined, especially the females, because girls are more likely to have a congenital dislocation of the hip. Children born from the breech position should also be examined carefully.

Although congenital displacement of the hip is usually present from birth, it is not always possible for a doctor to recognize the problem. Detection and treatment of this condition in early infancy produce the best results. Treatment consists of placing the baby in a Pavlik harness for about 12 weeks to allow the hip joint to return to its proper position. If the problem is not recognized early, treatment is more difficult because it involves traction to stretch the soft tissues around the hip, then surgery, and, finally, wearing a cast for up to 12 weeks.

Pediatricians routinely check infants for congenital displacement of the hip, but parents may notice certain signs that should be brought to the doctor's attention. These include: asymmetrical skin folds on the buttocks and thighs when the infant lies on the stomach; limited ability to move one leg at the hip joint (this is apparent during diaper changes when the infant has difficulty spreading one leg); and a decreased ability to move the affected leg spontaneously. If the problem is not diagnosed before the baby starts standing or walking, parents may then notice that the child will appear to sink down a bit when using the hip and to move the body toward the hip bearing the weight.

With early treatment, the hip returns to a normal position and the child is able to walk properly. Late detection that requires surgical correction may produce complications and problems with walking later in life.

Down's Syndrome

Children with Down's syndrome typically have a number of skeletal abnormalities, including a round head that is flat in the back, a broad and short neck, double joints, flat feet, short hands and feet, as well as other characteristics of the syndrome.

Among the orthopedic problems that afflict children with Down's syndrome are congenital dislocation of the hip and the kneecap as well as overly elastic joints. Foot deformities may also be present, but usually can be modified with a corrective shoe.

X rays from the side of the neck should be taken of all Down's children on a routine basis to screen for instability of the cervical spine. If instability is discovered, surgical fusion of the cervical spine may be recommended to prevent any neurological damage. Parents should be alert to even such vague symptoms as decreasing endurance in walking, clumsiness, or an increased tendency to fall. Such symptoms require a doctor's attention.

Osteogenesis Imperfecta

Osteogenesis imperfecta is an inherited disorder that is associated with brittle bones that fracture easily. This disease also affects the connective tissue, which provides the framework for the body.

When the disorder occurs in its severe form, it is apparent at birth because it leaves the infant with multiple fractures as a result of the delivery or of uterine contractions. The limbs appear shortened, and grating sounds can be heard in all of the regions where there are fractures. These infants have large soft skulls and often suffer from hemorrhage within the skull. Very few infants survive this form of the disease, called *osteogenesis imperfecta congenita*.

Osteogenesis imperfecta tarda, the other form of this disorder, is less severe. One type, called the *gravis form*, is characterized by fractures that occur during infancy. Because the child's long bones are deformed and bowed, braces, special devices to help with walking, and surgery often are needed to help the child gain some use of the affected region.

In the other type, known as the *levis form*, fractures occur in later years and with less frequency.

Fragile bones and multiple fractures are the major symptoms of osteogenesis imperfecta. A diagnosis of this disorder usually includes other symptoms. For instance, the sclera, or whites of the eyes, tend to be blue, the stature short, the joints very lax, and the teeth appear glassy. Hernia—inguinal, umbilical, or diaphragmatic—is also common. After a child passes puberty, the prognosis often improves because fewer fractures occur. This decrease may be due to hormonal changes or to the greater carefulness of older children, who are thus less likely to suffer fractures.

Careful orthopedic management has enabled many children with osteogenesis imperfecta to lead relatively normal lives. Among the concerns of the doctor are the treatment and prevention of acute fractures, the treatment of any deformity, and the child's quality of life. When acute fractures have occurred, the doctor pays close attention to preventing any deformity while aligning the bone. However, overtreating a broken bone is not wise either, because immobilization and disuse can cause atrophy and loss of bone. For this reason, when a bone is broken and its use is restored promptly, the loss of bone tissue is minimal.

The goal of treatment is to keep the young patient as mobile and active as possible. Often the child receives an outer skeleton of custom-molded polypropylene that allows the movement of joints while providing extra support for the long bones that are prone to fractures.

When there is a deformity of the leg, surgery may be necessary to correct it. Surgery entails cutting the shinbone (tibia) or the thighbone (femur) and inserting a metal rod, which may be expandable to allow the rod to expand as the child grows. Children with rods may, however, require braces in order to walk.

Scoliosis, or abnormal curvature of the back, is

difficult to treat in children with osteogenesis imperfecta. The curves tend to progress rapidly and fail to respond when spinal braces are applied to halt them. Surgical implantation of a spinal rod is difficult because the bone is so fragile. When it has been determined that the scoliosis is progressing, surgical fusion of the bone may be the best treatment.

Parents of infants with osteogenesis imperfecta must learn how to hold their children without causing injury. Attention must also be given to helping the child achieve such various developmental milestones as standing and walking and, at the same time, parents must minimize the chances of fractures. To avoid atrophy from disuse, parents must learn to gently exercise the child's limbs. The potential for fractures can be decreased by carefully applying and removing braces.

In most families, there is about a 50 percent chance that the offspring of a parent with osteogenesis imperfecta will also have the disease. In some cases, a family history may point to severe incidence of the disease. Genetic counseling is advised for those families who have a child with osteogenesis imperfecta.

BONE TUMORS

BONE TUMORS in children are often discovered by chance. Typically a child or adolescent who has been injured in sports or during play requires an X ray of the painful region and a bone tumor is detected. Less commonly, the child may suffer severe pain in one of his or her limbs or have difficulty moving that region. While examining the child, the doctor may discover what appears to be a mass. When such symptoms are present, X rays are taken as the first step toward diagnosis. A biopsy of the bone tissue is needed, however, to determine the nature of the tumor and whether it is malignant or benign.

When a tumor is detected in bone, it may be an indication that a malignancy is present elsewhere in the body. Bone tumors can originate in bone-forming cells and in marrow cells.

Osteogenic sarcoma is the most common malignant tumor in children, occurring most often between the ages of 10 and 20. Early diagnosis and treatment are essential. An osteogenic sarcoma usually develops on the inside part of the bone in the leg, usually at the bottom of the thighbone (femur) or the top of the shinbone (tibia). This type of tumor easily metastasizes, or spreads to other parts of the body. Amputation is the recommended treatment

for osteogenic sarcoma. Radiation therapy and/or chemotherapy may be administered in conjunction with the surgery.

Ewing's sarcoma, which originates in the bone marrow cells, is the second most common malignant bone tumor that affects children. Pain and swelling characterize this tumor, which can invade the entire shaft of a long bone. Cancerous cells from Ewing's sarcoma migrate to other parts of the body during the early course of the disease. Ewing's sarcoma is treated with radiation therapy and chemotherapy.

A *chondrosarcoma* is a malignant tumor of the cells that form cartilage. This type of tumor must be surgically removed.

A variety of benign bone tumors can appear during childhood. Among them are: *osteochondromas*, which occur in the cartilage-forming cells; *exostoses*, or outgrowths of cartilage, that grow from the end of a long bone; and *osteoid osteomas*, which arise in the bone-forming cells and commonly grow in the middle of long bones.

Bone cysts can also appear in the bones of children. The most common is the simple *solitary bone cyst*, which appears in children between ages five and fifteen. It usually affects the long bones. This cyst can be treated surgically or with corticosteroid therapy.

METABOLIC BONE DISEASE

Rickets

Rickets is a metabolic bone disease of the growing skeleton in which the bone does not absorb calcium properly. When the disease is caused by a vitamin D deficiency, it is called *nutritional rickets*. This form of the disease is rare in the United States, although it is sometimes seen in breastfed babies of vegetarian mothers, especially if they are dark-skinned. Such women should consult their pediatricians about vitamin D supplements.

A condition called *vitamin D-resistant rickets* is the primary cause of the disease in this country. This hereditary metabolic disorder interferes with the body's ability to absorb, utilize, and store vitamin D, which aids in the body's absorption of calcium.

Children with rickets are irritable, restless, and indifferent. They may show delays in development. Respiratory infections and diarrhea often occur. The children's teeth may appear late and have defective enamel or early decay. The head may look large and square, the chest may be narrow and protruding, and the ends of the ribs appear to be bent. Ankles, knees, and wrists are thick, and the long bones are soft, causing the legs to bow. Children with rickets also develop spinal deformities.

Treatment with vitamin D and a diet rich in milk, eggs, and liver may be sufficient to cure rickets in many young patients. The vitamin D-resistant form is treated with premetabolized vitamin D that can be given to the child to bypass the missing or malfunctioning enzyme. Treatment usually results in normal development; however, if a permanent deformity has occurred, the child may require surgery to straighten the bones.

HORMONAL DISORDERS

THE BODY'S ENDOCRINE system, which manufactures and regulates hormone production, plays an important role in the growth of the skeleton. When there is a deficiency of growth hormone, a substance produced by the pituitary gland, bone growth is stunted. Deficiency of growth hormone may be caused by a pituitary tumor, disease, or malnutrition, or its cause may be unknown. When growth hormone deficiency is present in a child, it becomes apparent between ages two and four. In some cases, a deficiency affects only growth, while in others it impairs the function of other glands, such as the thyroid and the gonads, or sex glands. A pediatrician can order tests to determine whether there is a hormonal deficiency. After a child has been diagnosed, he or she can be treated with human growth hormone at regular intervals until adolescence.

When the pituitary gland produces too much growth hormone, it results in rapid growth of the skeleton. A child or adolescent who experiences excessive growth should be taken to a doctor immediately. Usually such abnormal growth is caused by a pituitary tumor, which can be treated with radiation therapy or by surgical removal.

Premature sexual development also can result in growth abnormality and short stature. If there are signs of premature sexual development, the child should be evaluated promptly to learn the cause of the problem and to undergo treatment before the sex hormones cause the growth plates to close and halt future growth.

28 Neurological and Neuromuscular Disorders

Darryl De Vivo, M.D.

INTRODUCTION

THE HUMAN NERVOUS system is one of the body's most complex, and, because of its interaction with other systems, it plays a vital role in almost every bodily function. The nervous system controls our intellectual processes and conscious activities—such as movement or speech—as well as numerous involuntary functions, including respiration and heart rate. Thus, when something goes awry with this system, the effects can range from barely noticeable to catastrophic.

The system is divided into two parts: the brain and spinal cord make up the *central nervous system*, and the vast network of nerves that extends to every part of the body make up the *peripheral nervous system*. The nervous system is often likened to a sophisticated computer or electrical network. Although there are many similarities, in reality it is much more complex than either of these models.

The brain and spinal cord are formed, during the first eight weeks of pregnancy, from the neural tube, which arises from a group of cells that extend along the back of the embryo. It starts as a strip of cells that rapidly curls inward to form a tubelike structure. The upper end expands into what eventually becomes the brain, and the length of the tube becomes the spinal cord. During the time that the central nervous system is being formed, the embryonic brain and spinal cord are especially susceptible to damage that can result in a wide range of disorders. For example, large amounts of alcohol and certain other drugs consumed by the mother during this early developmental stage can result in mental retardation and neurological damage, as well as other defects. Failure of the tube to close properly can lead to spina bifida and other congenital defects.

The brain (see figure 28.1), which resembles a large walnut, is divided into several parts, each with distinct functions. The largest is the *cerebrum*, which occupies most of the skull and is the center of intellect and memory. The cerebrum is divided into two hemispheres, with the right hemisphere controlling the left side of the body and vice versa. The hemispheres also are divided into lobes, and have many infoldings and fissures that increase the surface area. Specific functions, such as vision, hearing, smell, speech and so forth, are controlled from certain geographic areas of the cerebrum. Thus, a speech problem may be traced to the specific area of the brain that controls that function.

Situated deep within the cerebrum are the thalamus, a structure that acts as a relay station for the body's major sensory pathways, and the hypothalamus, which controls many endocrine functions. The basal ganglia, masses of gray matter that control motor function, also are located within the cerebrum. Just below the cerebrum is the *cerebellum*, which is instrumental in muscle function and balance. The *brain stem* forms a continuous connection between the brain and spinal cord.

Overall, the nervous system is made up of billions of units called *neurons*. A neuron consists of a cell body, from which structures called axons and

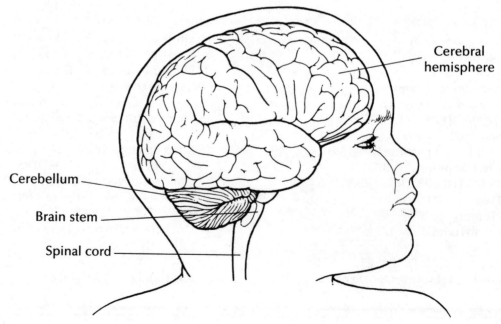

Figure 28.1. **Normal Brain.**

dendrites project. An axon, which may be several feet long, usually carries impulses or messages away from the cell body, and the dendrites, which are shorter than axons but still may be several feet long, accept messages from other neurons through special connecting points called synapses. Unlike an electrical circuit, which carries electricity in over an unbroken wire, neurons do not directly connect with each other. Instead, they form a pathway with many breaks over which messages or impulses travel via an electrochemical process, jumping from one to another to reach their destination. A number of body chemicals as well as sodium, potassium, and calcium are instrumental in conducting nerve impulses to either the brain or spinal cord, where they are processed and acted upon. Many of these impulses deal with the autonomic, or "automatic" nervous system, and require no conscious action. The autonomic system is divided into the sympathetic and parasympathetic systems, which produce opposite and counterbalancing effects to keep the body running smoothly.

Even today we do not understand exactly how the nervous system works. We do know that once the nervous system is fully developed, the body ceases to make new nerve cells. Thus, when a neuron is destroyed, it does not regenerate as is the case, for example, with the skin and certain other body structures that are constantly renewing themselves. Although a certain number of neurons "wear out" as we age, fortunately there are more than enough in reserve to last a lifetime, barring disease, injuries, or other unusual destruction.

Since the nervous system is so extensive and so instrumental in so many bodily functions, it follows that neurological disorders take many forms. Some are the result of birth defects or early neurological insults (for example, maternal infection or exposure to toxic substances); others may be caused by tumors, disorders of the brain's blood supply, injury, infections, metabolic disorders, or genetic diseases. Neurological disorders can produce a variety of symptoms, including seizure disorders, neuromuscular defects, paralysis, involuntary tics or movements, headaches or other pain syndromes, behavioral symptoms, and mental impairment. Any disorder that affects the nervous system is potentially serious, but it would be a mistake to equate all with disaster or doom. Indeed, there are effective treatments for most of the diseases discussed in this chapter, and some do not require any treatment at all. However, early and proper diagnosis is often crucial, especially when dealing with childhood neurological problems. All parents should be aware of warning signs of possible neurological problems and seek prompt and appropriate medical attention.

THE NEUROLOGICAL EXAMINATION

Patient History

In diagnosing neurological disorders, both the patient history and family history are important. The doctor will want to know if there is a history of neurological disorders among other family members, and about the events leading up to the present problem. When appropriate, the doctor will take as much of the history as possible from the child. Obviously this is impossible with babies or children too young to talk, or with children incapacitated by their illness.

Some neurological problems are readily apparent, but often the disorder involves subtle differences between normal and abnormal. Throughout a neurological examination, the patient is gauged according to the average: Is the child at an appropriate stage of intellectual development? How do reflexes, head size, and other parameters compare with the average? Are coordination and motor skills appropriate for the age?

Physical Examination

The precise order and areas of concentration of the physical examination will vary according to the symptoms, but these are some of the key areas that are included in most neurological examinations.

Mental Status. The child's memory, orientation, intellect, judgment, attention span, and behavior are among the factors that will be examined. Exact procedures vary depending upon the age of the child.

Craniospinal Examination. The size and shape of the head will be measured. The contour of the spine also will be examined. Functions related to the cranial nerves—eye movement, vision, hearing, taste, smell, swallowing, and facial muscle control, among others—will be checked. Sensation is tested with pin pricks, light touches, vibration, and exposure to objects of different temperatures. If age appropriate, the child will be asked to touch a finger to the nose with eyes closed.

Muscle Function and Coordination. Muscle tone and strength will be tested. For example, the doctor may ask the child to push away a hand or foot to test strength. Both fine and gross motor control will be measured; a child may be asked to hop on one foot, walk in a straight line, pick up certain objects and fit them into specific slots.

Tendon Reflexes. This includes the familiar tapping of the knee with a small rubber hammer. The child also will be tested for the *Babinski sign*—the sole of the foot is stroked firmly to see if the big toe arches up instead of clenching inward with the other toes, as it should. The upward arching is often an indication of a neurological disorder.

Special Tests and Examinations

Whether additional tests and examinations are needed depends upon symptoms and results of the physical examination. For example, if the child has a fever and other signs of possible meningitis, a *spinal tap* may be needed. A small amount of cerebrospinal fluid is withdrawn and examined. If a concussion, tumor, or other such abnormality is suspected, a *CT (computerized tomographic) scan* may be ordered. In fact, the development of computerized tomography has revolutionized the diagnosis of brain disorders. A CT scan involves taking a number of X-ray images and combining them to provide a cross-sectional view of the brain (or other body structure being examined). It can detect a variety of abnormalities and can be used to examine even very tiny babies. A dye may be injected into the circulation to make the brain's blood vessels more visible on a CT scan.

CT scans have largely replaced older examinations, particularly *pneumoencephalography* in which some of the cerebrospinal fluid was withdrawn and air was injected into the spaces of the brain to make them visible on an X ray. This examination can still provide much useful information about brain structures and also locate tumors, but is not used very much today because it can be very uncomfortable for the patient. Instead the doctor is more likely to rely on a CT scan, which involves a certain amount of radiation exposure and may be somewhat frightening to a patient who finds the machinery intimidating, but otherwise is not uncomfortable.

Magnetic resonance imaging (MRI) (formerly referred to as nuclear magnetic resonance) is another new examination. It uses two elements—computer-controlled radio waves and magnetic fields that are vastly stronger than the earth's magnetic field. By measuring the amount of energy released by atoms, the instrument can produce an image of the body's internal structures. During an examination, the patient is placed on an examining board atop a large, circular magnet. The examination is painless, but during it, the patient will hear sounds created by the magnetic fields. Since the test does not use radiation or dyes, it is even safer than a CT scan, and occasionally may find abnormalities that cannot be detected with the CT scan. It is particularly useful in examining the brain and spinal cord.

An *electroencephalogram*, an examination that records the brain's electrical activity, may be used to diagnose a seizure disorder. Neuromuscular function may be tested with *electromyography*, which measures the electrical activity of the muscles. Other electrical techniques, called *evoked potentials*, can measure the rate at which impulses are conducted along the peripheral nerves or along the pathways in the spinal cord and brain.

An *intrathecal scan* may be done to check the flow of cerebrospinal fluid. This test entails withdrawing some of the fluid and injecting radioactive isotopes, which are then followed in a series of scans.

A *myelogram*, performed by injecting a dye into the spinal canal, outlines the spinal cord and the nerves and is useful in revealing abnormalities in this region.

Even though there are many special tests for central and peripheral nervous system function, they frequently are not needed. In some instances, however, the symptoms could indicate a number of different problems, so special tests may be required to eliminate other possibilities and arrive at a definitive diagnosis.

PRENATAL AND DEVELOPMENTAL DEFECTS

THERE ARE SEVERAL critical periods in early embryogenesis and fetal development when prenatal defects may arise. During the first week after conception there is active cell division. Differentiation of the cells into two primary tissues, the ectoderm and the endoderm, occurs during the second week; and the third primary tissue, the mesoderm, develops during the third week of pregnancy with the early formation of the heart and blood vessels. Later in the third week and the fourth week the rudimentary elements of the nervous system appear with formation of the neural tube. By the end of the first month after conception the neural tube has formed and its two ends have closed, and the events of neural organogenesis then follow.

Proliferation of brain cells in the fetus occurs during the first three months of pregnancy, and brain cells migrate to distant regions between the third and fifth months. Organization of brain cell networks and formation of synaptic connections proceed during the third trimester and continue after birth, as does the myelination (formation of the protective *myelin* sheath) of the sensory and motor pathways. The major events underlying brain development are nearly complete by the child's second birthday.

Gross malformations of the nervous system such as anencephaly and myelomeningocele can be dated to early neurulation (neural tube) defects in the first month of pregnancy. Abnormalities of brain size or contour involve aberrations of cellular growth and migration between the second and fifth months of pregnancy.

Abnormal Head Size

Abnormal head size may be detected before birth by the use of ultrasound, but if the abnormality is only moderate, it may not be noted until birth. Small variations from the norm often are not a cause for worry—in some families, for example, babies may tend to have somewhat larger or smaller than average heads and be perfectly normal.

A very small *head*—microcephaly—indicates a small *brain* (micrencephaly) and consequently, a number of serious problems, including mental defects, cerebral palsy, seizures, and others. Causes for microcephaly include chromosomal errors, improper implantation of the embryo during early pregnancy, infection, malnutrition, or the use of certain drugs. Women who have a history of infertility or miscarriages have an increased risk of giving birth to a baby with microcephaly.

A large head does not necessarily indicate a large brain. Indeed, the brain could be normal size or even small, with the remaining space taken up by fluid, as in the case of hydroencephaly, or by some other growth or substance. True megalencephaly, an oversized brain, is a rare disorder that can result in mental deficiency, seizures, or movement disorders.

Hydrocephalus

Commonly called "water on the brain," hydrocephalus is an accumulation of the cerebrospinal fluid in the cranial cavity. It is a relatively uncommon condition that occurs when there is an imbalance in the production and absorption of the fluid. Usually the production is normal, but there is a problem in fluid absorption, causing it to accumulate and creating the oversized head that is characteristic of this disorder. The fluid buildup causes the skull bones, which are loosely connected in the developing fetus and newborn baby, to spread apart. If the condition is untreated, it can cause serious brain damage and also increase the risk of infection. Hydrocephalus can be caused by a maternal infection during pregnancy or a developmental malformation, such as aqueductal stenosis. Hydrocephalus after birth can result from tumors, cysts, infections, or bleeding. (Figure 28.2 shows a normal ventricular system of the brain; figure 28.3, on the following page, shows hydrocephalus.)

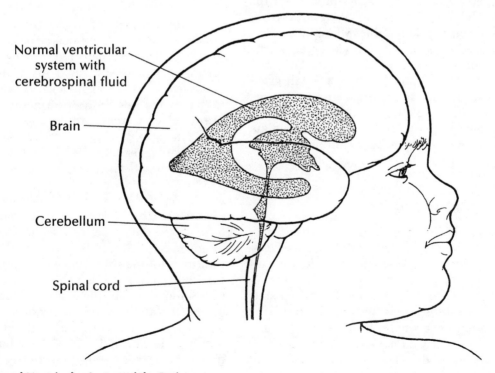

Figure 28.2. **Normal Ventricular System of the Brain.**

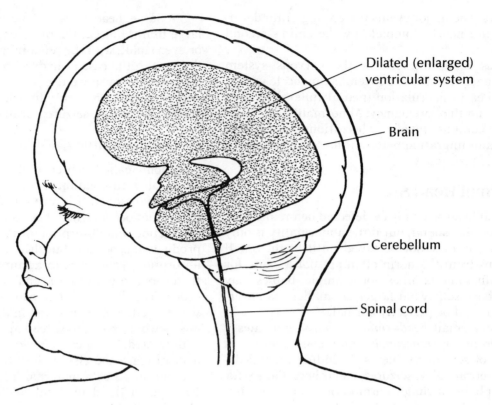

Figure 28.3. **Ventricular System in Hydrocephalus.**

Depending upon the cause, hydrocephalus often can be treated, preventing lasting brain damage. The most common treatment entails surgically inserting a shunt to drain the excess fluid from the brain to the abdominal cavity where it will be absorbed into the circulation. Babies who have undergone this procedure should be checked frequently, often every month or so. Typically, as the fluid balance is restored to normal, the head size will gradually return to normal as the child grows. Parents should be diligent in watching for any signs that the shunt is not working properly, and seek immediate medical treatment for the child. Symptoms include mood changes, lethargy, irritability, and persistent vomiting.

Other Congenital Defects

There are a number of congenital defects that may occur during the fetal stage when the head and central nervous system are being formed. In rare instances, parts of the brain may fail to form. This is often accompanied by severe facial defects, such as deformed eye cavities, forehead, mouth, and ears. The babies often have small brains, and when the defects are severe, they do not survive beyond early infancy. (These facial deformities should not be confused with the more common cleft palate, cleft lip, or split nose, which are not ordinarily related to

brain development except in those cases where they are associated with mild retardation.)

Spina Bifida

Sometimes the neural tube fails to close properly, which can cause a number of defects. Neural tube disorders can be detected during pregnancy by testing the mother's blood for a substance called *alpha-fetoprotein*. A high level of alpha-fetoprotein indicates the possibility of a neural tube defect or brain defect. Careful examination of the fetus with ultrasonography usually (but not always) can confirm whether the fetus has spina bifida or other congenital anomalies.

Spina bifida, or *myelodysplasia*, involves a malformation of the spinal cord and vertebral column. (See figure 28.4.) Typically it is characterized by a lesion over the spine, usually in the lower region. There may be paralysis and loss of sensation from that point of the spine on down. Children born with this condition may not be able to control bladder or bowel function, but the degree of handicap depends on the extent of the spinal damage. Some cases are barely noticeable, with only a slight indentation or bump at the affected area of the spine. Other babies may have a large membrane-covered bulge protruding through the gap in the vertebral column or an abnormally curved spine. In such cases, there is an

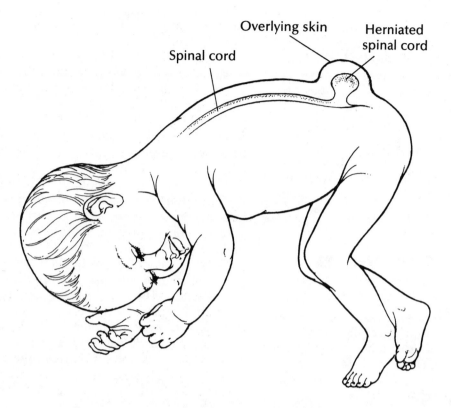

Figure 28.4. **Spina Bifida.**

increased risk of infection, as well as a danger of injury to the exposed membrane. Spina bifida also carries an increased risk of urinary tract infections.

Although the damaged spinal cord cannot be repaired, much can be done to help babies with spina bifida. For example, there are operations to increase protection for the exposed membrane and to reduce the risk of injury or infection. Some children, especially those with mild deformities, achieve normal bladder and bowel control without difficulty. Others may be helped by surgery, but many will remain incontinent. Depending upon the degree of the deformity, a child may be able to walk, either normally or with the aid of braces and physical therapy. Severe cases may be confined to a wheelchair. If the spina bifida is accompanied by hydrocephalus, there may be varying degrees of mental impairment. Many children, especially those whose defect is confined to the lower spine, have normal mental development and should be encouraged to attend regular school and participate in as many normal childhood activities as possible.

Anencephaly

Anencephaly is a catastrophic condition in which portions of the brain are missing. It is caused by gross failure of the neural tube to close. In most instances, the fetus is either aborted spontaneously or the baby is stillborn. Those that are born alive die shortly after birth.

Encephalocele

An encephalocele is a herniation of the membrane that covers the brain, resulting in a protrusion through the fontanel (soft spot) before the skull bones are formed and closed. The baby is born with a bulb of tissue on the head. The bulb contains fluid with or without brain tissue. If there is no brain tissue in the herniated matter, there usually are no mental deficits. If, however, brain tissue bulges through the herniation, there may be mental retardation, seizures, spasticity, blindness, or other neurological problems. Surgical closure of the herniation, if possible, is the treatment of choice.

Other Neural Tube Abnormalities

Other disorders, most of which are quite rare, include:

Hydromyelia.   This is a dilation, or widening, of the central canal containing the spinal cord, permitting a buildup of cerebrospinal fluid in the area.

Syringomyelia.   In this condition, a fluid-filled sac forms in the spinal cord, usually in the neck or shoulder area. It results in a loss of pain and temperature sensitivity in the affected area, but touch and other sensory functions usually are preserved. Depending upon the location and extent of the defect, there may be a wasting of muscles in the hands or arms. Syringomyelia may be present at birth, but more commonly it develops later, sometimes as a result of an injury. Surgical decompression of the fluid-filled cavity often is effective.

Occult Spina Bifida. This occurs when a part of the spinal column fails to fuse properly. It can result in skin-covered lesions over the spine, which may hinder the flow of blood to nerve tissue in the area.

ACQUIRED NEUROLOGICAL DEFECTS

MOST NEUROLOGICAL PROBLEMS are not congenital; instead they arise after birth as a result of infection, injuries, metabolic disorders or other diseases. The more common are described below.

Intracranial Hemorrhage

Intracranial hemorrhage is a term used to describe any bleeding inside the cranium. The bleeding can occur at any level of the brain's protective sheathing or in the brain itself. The most common sites seen today are in the subarachnoid and intraventricular areas. In the past, a number of babies suffered *subdural hemorrhage*—bleeding under the dura or hard tissue enclosing the brain—during the birth process, but today this is uncommon. The hemorrhage occurred when blood vessels in the head were torn during difficult deliveries, for example, breech or forceps-aided births, or simply when the head was too large or the birth canal too narrow to permit easy passage. If the bleeding is not too extensive, the body will absorb the blood without causing serious problems. Not uncommonly, however, a clot forms, pressing upon brain tissue. Symptoms may range from lethargy to seizures; permanent damage or even death can result if the clot compresses enough brain tissue. The clot usually can be surgically removed.

Hypoxia and Ischemia of the Brain

Hypoxia is a lack of oxygen, which can result in death of tissue—a situation that is particularly serious if the brain is the affected organ. Sometimes the umbilical cord can become knotted or twisted during the birth process, depriving the baby of adequate oxygen-rich blood. Or if the newborn's lungs are not functioning properly, there will not be enough oxygen in the baby's blood. Other causes include anemia and abnormalities of the brain's vascular system.

Hypoxia commonly is associated with an inadequate supply of blood (ischemia) to the brain. Hypoxia and ischemia are additive insults to the brain and may contribute to cerebral palsy.

Until the 1970s, when better means of early diagnosis and treatments for hypoxia affecting the brain were developed, this was the leading cause of death among newborn babies. (Now it is respiratory distress syndrome.) Symptoms of hypoxia are particularly difficult to spot in a premature baby. Full-term babies will show poor responses to stimuli and will be short of breath. Symptoms in older babies include stupor, respiratory problems, muscle weakness, and difficulty in swallowing. The outcome depends upon how quickly the problem is detected and reversed. The first 36 hours are crucial—if the baby appears normal or is progressing toward a normal oxygen level in that period, the prospects of survival are good. The degree of permanent brain damage depends upon the extent and length of hypoxia. Serious hypoxia must be treated within minutes if irreversible brain damage is to be avoided.

Low Blood Sugar

Glucose, or blood sugar, is the brain's major fuel; proportionately, a baby's brain needs more glucose than an adult's. If a baby develops *hypoglycemia*, the medical term for low blood sugar, it can affect many organs, but particularly the brain. A newborn baby may develop hypoglycemia if the mother suffered poorly controlled diabetes during pregnancy. The fetus responds to the mother's high blood sugar by increasing its own insulin production. Excessive insulin can result in hypoglycemia, among other problems. Hypoglycemia also can be caused by inadequate glycogen (which the body converts to glucose) stores in the baby. Symptoms of hypoglycemia include convulsions, lethargy, disorientation, jitteriness, breathing irregularities, muscle laxness, and possible coma. Blood sugar levels can be quickly corrected by glucose infusions if necessary; and they can then be adjusted by frequent feedings.

Drug Exposure

Most drugs readily cross the placental barrier and enter the baby's bloodstream. In the past, when many mothers were given a general anesthetic during childbirth, the babies would be born with varying degrees of neurological effects such as lethargy or excessive sleepiness. These were usually temporary and did not produce lasting damage. Today, however, most women use a minimum of anesthesia during childbirth, and their babies are born more alert and eager to feed and observe their surroundings than when a general anesthetic was used.

Babies born to drug-addicted mothers are usually addicted themselves, and they will suffer withdrawal symptoms and varying neurological effects. Drug overdoses among older children are usually accidental; for example, a toddler consumes a bottle of tranquilizers, sleeping pills, or other medication left within reach. If the drugs affect the central nervous system, they can cause a variety of neurological symptoms, such as lethargy, agitation, delirium, convulsions, vomiting, dilated pupils, and so forth.

Lead and Other Heavy Metal Poisoning

Neurological damage can result from chronic ingestion or exposure to certain household chemicals or poisons. One of the more common is chronic lead poisoning, which can be caused by eating chips of lead paint. Lead poisoning also can be caused by exposure to lead-laden fumes or dust. For example, high lead levels have been found in children living near expressways or industrial plants that burn leaded gas. House renovation that entails scraping, melting, or burning off leaded paint also carries a risk of excessive lead exposure. Recently, lead poisoning has been traced to drinking water from deteriorating lead-lined pipes.

Symptoms of lead poisoning are often subtle and easily confused with other disorders. Irritability, weight loss, abdominal discomfort, and constipation are the more common early signs. As the poisoning progresses, mental deterioration occurs. There are blood tests that can detect high lead levels; many urban health departments now offer free lead testing. Early detection and treatment with drugs to clear the lead from the system are important to prevent behavioral disorders, permanent brain damage or, in severe cases, death.

Mercury poisoning, which is relatively rare in this country, can cause severe irreversible brain damage. Pesticides, especially those that contain neurotoxins, also can produce lasting damage. Obviously, no one should be exposed to these substances, and this is particularly true of babies and young children. If exposure does occur, early treatment is vital.

Fluid Balance

There are two disorders involving the amount of fluid in the brain. With *hyponatremia*, there is too much water in the brain tissue and, concomitantly, too little sodium. The cause is usually a failure of the kidneys to excrete the excessive water. It also may be caused by hormonal disorders. If allowed to persist, the excessive fluid in the brain can cause water intoxication and brain swelling. Symptoms include changes in mental status, lethargy, and, as the condition progresses, increasing muscle twitching, convulsions, and possible coma. Treatment depends upon the underlying cause; if sodium levels are low, a sodium chloride solution will be given. A diuretic may be given to help rid the body of excess fluid. Sometimes reducing fluid intake for a few days to give the body a chance to adjust its fluid balance is all that is needed.

An opposite condition, *hypernatremia*, is characterized by too little water and, consequently, too much sodium in the brain tissue. Hypernatremia in babies can be caused either by excessive fluid loss, for example, during a high fever or persistent vomiting or diarrhea, or by excessive salt intake. Sometimes a newborn undergoing light therapy or a preterm baby in a radiant warming unit will become dehydrated if fluid replacement is inadequate. Accidental overdosing with sodium, for example, substituting salt for sugar in preparing a formula or putting too much salt in fluids given to treat dehydration, can be particularly dangerous for babies and young children. Parents should avoid altering formulas or the oral rehydration solutions given during bouts of diarrhea or vomiting.

Symptoms of hypernatremia include irritability, listlessness, twitching, convulsions, and coma. Treatment entails *gradual* increase in body fluids, usually by administering an intravenous glucose solution. Care must be taken, however, that the rehydration is not too rapid, which can cause problems of its own.

INFECTION

A NUMBER OF DIFFERENT infections—viral, bacterial, fungal, or parasitic—can affect the nervous system. Sometimes the baby is exposed to the infectious agent before birth, as in the case of rubella (German measles) and cytomegalovirus. Exposure to syphilis and AIDS also can have devastating effects on the fetus.

Fetal viral infections can cause serious damage, especially if they occur during the early embryonic period when the organ systems are being formed. Except for rubella and cytomegalovirus, most viral infections suffered by the mother during pregnancy are not particularly serious to the fetus, even though the fetal immune system is too immature to be protective. Because the fetal inflammation response is also immature, the cellular damage from the viral infection is not accompanied by an inflammatory reaction.

Exposure to viruses in the mother's body during the birth process also can pose serious problems for a newborn baby. Since newborns have an immature immune system, they are particularly susceptible to disorders such as herpes virus, cytomegalovirus, human immunodeficiency virus (the infectious agent that causes AIDS), or other infective agents that may be present in the mother's genital tract. Often the baby will appear healthy at birth, but then a few days or weeks later will show signs of lethargy, poor muscle tone, fever, and other symptoms, depending upon the type of infection.

Following are some of the more common infectious diseases that can produce neurological effects. The listing is alphabetical, and not necessarily in order of seriousness or incidence.

Viral Infections

Acute Cerebral Ataxia. This disorder often follows a viral infection, such as chicken pox, and is characterized by progressive loss of equilibrium and balance. Over a period of days, the child will lose his or her ability to walk in a coordinated manner. There are no other symptoms. It is most common in young children, and although it can be very disturbing, it is self-limited. Spontaneous recovery usually begins a week or two after the onset of symptoms and is complete within a few months.

Acute Polyneuritis. This disease, commonly referred to as *Guillain-Barré syndrome*, attacks the peripheral nerves. It usually follows a viral respiratory infection, but it also has been linked to Lyme disease, tetanus antitoxin, and rabies vaccine. It is believed to be an autoimmune disorder in which the immune system attacks the body itself. In this disease, the myelin sheathing, which covers the nerve fibers, degenerates, resulting in sensory loss, muscle weakness, and in severe cases, paralysis. It can be life-threatening if the muscles that control breathing are affected. In most cases, the nerves eventually recover, and there is only minor lasting damage. In some, however, there may be lingering impairment, especially of the lower limbs and hands.

Acute Viral Encephalitis. There are two types of viral encephalitis—one attacks the brain cells and the other is an autoimmune disorder in which the myelin covering of the brain's nerve fibers is attacked. In either instance, it is a frightening, potentially devastating infection. Symptoms include headache, vomiting, lethargy, an inability to eat, hallucinations, memory loss, combativeness, and other personality changes. Seizures are not uncommon; there may or may not be a fever.

Hospitalization and constant monitoring are required to provide needed supportive care. Survival depends upon the type of virus involved. Herpes encephalitis has a high mortality rate of 60 to 80 percent, and survivors often have permanent neurological damage. New drugs, however, can improve the outcome and lower mortality. In contrast, victims of certain other types often recover fully with no lasting effects. Some types are spread by mosquitoes that have picked up an equine virus from horses. This type is seen mostly during the summer months when mosquitoes are plentiful. In rare instances, viral encephalitis may follow measles, chicken pox, or other viral infections, or it may be triggered by a vaccine. Generally, children who survive an attack of viral encephalitis recover fully, but it may take months or even years to regain full neurological function.

Aseptic Meningitis. This is not a specific disease caused by a single infective organism; instead, it can be caused by a variety of agents. This type of meningitis is not contagious and it is not as serious as other forms of the disease. It usually strikes in the late summer or early fall, and although it can afflict people of any age, it is more common in babies and children. In the newborn and infants, the symptoms are nonspecific. Older children usually have a headache that comes on suddenly, fever, vomiting, lethargy, and a stiff neck—a characteristic sign of any type of meningitis.

Aseptic meningitis can last up to two weeks, and there are no lasting effects. There is no specific treatment, and hospitalization usually is not necessary unless the symptoms are very severe or the diagnosis is in doubt.

Acquired Immunodeficiency Syndrome (AIDS). About half of the babies born to women carrying the AIDS virus are expected eventually to develop the disease, which may affect the brain. As of this writing, there is no cure for AIDS. Women who are at risk of carrying the virus are advised to be tested before becoming pregnant.

Childhood Demyelinating Disease. This is the childhood form of multiple sclerosis and fortunately is quite rare. The cause is unknown, but it frequently follows a chronic viral infection and is thought to be somehow linked to the immune system. The symptoms are similar to those of the adult disease, often beginning with disturbances of vision, eye movement, and coordination, and loss of sensation. As in multiple sclerosis, the progression is variable, with periods of remission followed by flare-ups. Overall the course of the disease is one of gradual decline, often over a period of several decades.

Poliomyelitis. Fortunately, with the development of the polio vaccine, this is now a rare disease. It is still seen, however, among children and others who have not been immunized, especially in developing countries. It may begin as aseptic meningitis, or it may start as myelitis, an inflammation of the spinal cord. This proceeds to muscle pain, weakness, and paralysis. Any muscle group can be affected; it is particularly serious when the respiratory muscles that control breathing are attacked. Typically the disease peaks within a few days and is followed by a slow recovery. Severely hit muscles may recover only half or even less of their original function; those that are only moderately affected may recover 90 percent or more of function. There is no specific treatment for polio—the best approach is to make sure that all children are immunized at an early age. Rehabilitation therapy can help restore weakened muscles, but in severe cases there may be residual damage or paralysis.

Reye's Syndrome. This is another disease whose cause is unknown but which follows a viral infection, frequently flu or chicken pox. In the United States most cases occur in the fall, winter, or early spring; most victims are under the age of 18 although there have been a few reports of Reye's syndrome in adults. Typically the child will be recovering from a bout of flu, chicken pox, or other viral infection when suddenly he or she develops persistent, forceful vomiting that is unlike that which occurs with an upset stomach or other disorders. This is followed by a change in mental status that varies from lethargy to periods of disorientation, agitation, and combativeness. This stage can quickly progress to coma with a high risk of death or irreversible neurological damage.

Two organs are the major targets of Reye's syndrome—the brain, which swells due to a buildup of fluid, and the liver, which develops fatty streaks. If allowed to progress, Reye's syndrome has a high fatality rate—80 percent or higher among children who have seizures, arrested breathing, and coma. Thus, early emergency treatment is crucial. Any episode of unusual vomiting and mental changes coming on the heels of a viral infection warrants emergency treatment, which entails giving drugs to reduce the brain swelling, careful monitoring and adjustment of body chemistry and blood gases, and other treatments, such as renal dialysis or transfusion, depending upon individual circumstances. Since an increased risk of Reye's has been linked to aspirin use, parents are advised not to give children aspirin during a viral infection.

Systemic Herpes. This is caused by herpes virus Type 2, the major cause of genital herpes. If a mother has an active genital herpes lesion at the time of delivery, the virus can be passed to the baby as he or she passes through the birth canal. The disease can have a devastating effect on a newborn's nervous system. The development of effective drugs to treat systemic herpes has reduced the high mortality rate (up to 70 percent in the past), but death is still a possibility if the virus attacks the baby's central nervous system. Mental retardation and other irreversible neurological damage also may occur.

The best approach is preventive. Since about 40 percent of mothers with active genital herpes pass the virus on to their babies during vaginal deliveries, it is particularly important that the woman be examined carefully for any signs of a herpes flare-up near or at the time of delivery. If there is any possibility of exposure, a cesarean section is advised. Transmission of the virus during a cesarean section has occurred, but it is rare.

Transverse Myelitis. This is a spinal disease that comes on suddenly. The cause is unknown, but it frequently follows a viral infection. It attacks one area of the spine, causing inflammation of the myelin sheathing and resulting in loss of motor control and sensation below the level of attack. It begins with severe back pain, which is followed by muscle weakness, flaccid paralysis, disturbances of bladder and bowel function, and progressive spasticity. Many victims recover all or most function; only 10 to 15 percent are left with severe lasting damage.

Bacterial and Other Nonviral Infections

A variety of bacteria, fungi, and parasites can attack the nervous system. Most of these can be eradicated with proper diagnosis and treatment with an appropriate antibiotic or medication designed to work against the invading organism. Some of the more common of these infections are described below.

Bacterial Meningitis. This is the most common form of meningitis that affects children. Group B streptococci and *E. coli* are the bacteria most often implicated in the newborn, but almost any bacteria can invade the central nervous system and produce meningitis. The meningitis from *H. influenzae* is particularly dangerous—one reason why HIB vaccine is so important.

Symptoms depend upon the age of the child and length of the infection. Babies will most often show irritability, vomiting, lethargy, suppressed appetite, and seizures. After about the age of four months, the child will also have a fever and the characteristic stiff neck. Still older children may also have a headache and will suffer from confusion. Within 12 to 24 hours, their necks will become quite rigid. About 30 percent will suffer seizures. Two signs aid in diagnosis. One is the *Kernig sign*, in which the child lies down, with a leg bent at the knee. Attempting to straighten the leg to a vertical position will produce extreme pain. The other is the *Brudzinski sign*, in which the hip will flex spontaneously when the neck is passively flexed.

The progression of meningitis varies considerably from child to child. In some the worst will be over in a couple of days, and in a relatively short period the child will recover completely. Others will worsen rapidly, going into a coma followed by death. Mortality varies according to the type of bacteria, age of the child, duration of the infection, and condition of the child at the time of diagnosis. The mortality with group B streptococcus meningitis is about 50 to 60 percent, compared to 10 to 20 percent or less with *H. influenzae*. Long-term consequences are the most common if the meningitis occurs within the first two months of life. Hearing loss, mental retardation, behavior disorders, seizures, and hydrocephalus are among the long-term effects that may be encountered. Most older children who survive will recover completely, with few if any long-term effects.

Fungal Infections. For a healthy child, most fungal infections are relatively harmless. But a child who has a serious underlying disease, for example, cancer or certain metabolic disorders, or has undergone an organ transplant, is often more vulnerable to a fungal infection. The fungus may normally inhabit the body, or enter through inhalation or some other route. The most common fungal infections are aspergillosis, histoplasmosis and candida. If these fungi invade the central nervous system, they can produce symptoms simliar to those seen in meningitis: fever, headache, vomiting, lethargy, and stiff neck.

There are now a number of highly effective antifungal medications that can eradicate these organisms. The important thing is to arrive at a proper diagnosis and start treatment promptly.

Parasitic Infections. The brain and other parts of the nervous system are rarely the primary site of a parasitic infection, but there are some notable exceptions. Toxoplasmosis, a parasite that can be contracted from cat feces or undercooked meat, is an example. This parasite is most commonly passed to the fetus via an infected mother. The woman may not experience any symptoms, or symptoms may be misinterpreted as a mild flu. About 70 percent of the babies who contract toxoplasmosis in the uterus will be born without symptoms;10 percent will have

some sort of eye involvement, which may include blindness; and the remaining 20 percent will have a systemic illness that may include neurological damage. Many of these babies die, so it is important that a pregnant woman avoid contracting the parasite. She should let someone else empty a cat's litter box and also avoid eating undercooked meat. Even babies who do not have symptoms but are known to harbor the parasite should be treated in an attempt to prevent later complications.

Rickettsial Infections. Commonly known as Rocky Mountain spotted fever, rickettsial infections are spread by ticks and occur most often during the spring and summer. The disease-spreading ticks are by no means confined to the mountain states; they are found in most areas of the United States. About two-thirds of the victims are children, usually four to eight years of age. The infection takes two to twelve days to incubate, then appears abruptly with a high fever, vomiting, headache, and muscle pain. The symptoms worsen over the next two to four days, and at that point, the characteristic rash appears, covering the entire body. Neurological symptoms include confusion, delirium, and disorientation; there also may be a stiff neck and hearing loss.

Prompt diagnosis and treatment with antibiotics are crucial to prevent progression of the disease to paralysis and possible death. Early treatment can end the infection within three to four days; untreated, however, it can go on for weeks and often lead to death. Frequently, the child or parents will be unaware of any tick bite, or a tick may be found buried in the scalp and hidden by hair. When treated in time, the mortality rate is fairly low, usually 5 to 10 percent, but it is much higher if allowed to progress. (See chapter 20 for further discussion.)

Brain Abscesses or Focal Infections. Focal infections can be located in the brain or spinal cord and are very serious. They usually are an outgrowth of some other infection, such as a dental abscess or mastoid sinus infection. They can produce severe neurological deficits and death; early diagnosis and treatment are crucial.

Symptoms depend upon the size and location of the abscess. An *epidural abscess* is one that occurs between the dura—the protective sheathing of the brain—and the skull wall. This is usually the result of an infection of the mastoid sinuses or a dental abscess. Subdural abscesses, which lodge under the dural sheathing, also are frequently the result of a sinus infection, although they can result from an inadequately treated infection following surgery or an injury. They carry a high mortality rate of about

40 percent, so early treatment is paramount. Any sinus infection followed by headache, fever, and altered consciousness should raise the suspicion that it has spread to the subdural region. Treatment entails draining the abscess and administering intensive antibiotic therapy that can penetrate the brain and bone.

Brain abscesses are also usually the result of an inadequately treated primary infection, particularly in the sinuses or ear. Symptoms are generally due to the mass of the abscess in the brain and not from the infection itself. They include lethargy, anorexia, vomiting, headache, and seizures. Treatment involves antibiotics to fight the infection and surgery to remove as much of the abscess mass as possible. Brain abscesses carry a 30 to 45 percent mortality rate, with the likelihood of death or serious aftereffects increasing the longer the abscess is permitted to expand.

Spinal abscesses usually arise from an infection of the lungs or kidneys. They progress rapidly; in some cases it is only a matter of hours between the first symptoms and paralysis. The progression of symptoms is usually from backache and local tenderness over the spine to a loss of sensation, leg weakness, a loss of bowel and bladder control, and then paralysis. Treatment entails prompt surgery to drain the abscess and remove the mass, and aggressive antibiotic therapy.

STATIC NEUROLOGICAL DISORDERS

A STATIC NEUROLOGICAL disorder is one that is a result of an injury or insult to the central nervous system, usually during gestation, birth, or shortly thereafter. They are called "static" because they are relatively stable and not likely to progress or worsen with time. Cerebral palsy and attention deficit disorders are relatively common examples of static disorders; these and others in this category are discussed below.

Cerebral Palsy

Cerebral palsy is not a specific disorder, but instead is a term used to describe a group of diverse, nonspecific syndromes that are characterized by motor disorders and, in some cases, accompanied by seizures, learning disabilities, or mental retardation. Cerebral palsy is most often due to an insult or injury suffered before birth. It also can result from too little oxygen during birth, prematurity, or a brain hemorrhage. Other causes include radiation expo-

sure, maternal disease, and exposure to alcohol or certain drugs that affect the developing brain before birth.

Milder cases are characterized by varying degrees of *spasticity*, which may affect either the limbs on one side of the body or both arms or both legs. *Spastic diplegia* commonly is associated with prematurity. The spastic muscles in the affected area are weak and there is a problem with the way in which they contract. A common manifestation is toe-dragging with the affected foot, which may be so slight that it is barely noticeable or severe enough to cause problems walking or running. In contrast, *dyskinetic cerebral palsy* is characterized by involuntary movements of the face, neck, or extremities. In *ataxic cerebral palsy*, the person has a wide-spaced gait and experiences difficulty in turning. In some cases, these forms may be mixed; a child who is spastic may also experience dyskinetic movements or have difficulty turning.

Mental retardation or learning disabilities are common among children with cerebral palsy. A fourth to a third may have epilepsy, depending on the type and severity of palsy.

Cerebral palsy is usually evident shortly after birth. The baby may have difficulty breathing, sucking, or swallowing. In the toddler, walking is usually delayed, and the gait may be jerky or in a scissors-like motion. Not uncommonly, the arms may be normal or minimally affected, but the fingers may be spastic, making it difficult to write, self-feed, and perform other tasks that require eye-hand coordination.

Speech may be delayed and slurred; bowel and bladder control also may be delayed. Later the child may have difficulty learning to read, write, and perform other school tasks, even if intelligence is normal. Emotional problems arising from frustration over not being able to express oneself or other aspects of the disorder, or simply from being different from other children also are common.

The disorder does not progress, but may take different forms as the child grows. For example, the spasticity may not be evident until the child starts trying to crawl or walk. There is no specific treatment, but a number of measures can reduce the disability. Physical therapy to improve coordination and strengthen or relax muscles can improve motor control. The use of orthopedic devices can make it easier to walk. Drugs, such as anticonvulsants to prevent seizures, or muscle relaxants to prevent the involuntary movements, also may help. Speech therapy, special learning aids, and other approaches can help minimize the defect. With proper training and therapy, many victims of cerebral palsy can lead near-normal, independent lives.

Attention Deficit Disorders

These are basically behavior and learning problems that are associated with attention difficulties and impulsiveness. In the past a number of different names have been applied to this constellation of problems, including hyperactive child syndrome and minimal brain damage or dysfunction. More recently, it has been renamed attention deficit disorder, either with or without hyperactivity as a major component. The cause is unknown, although there has been speculation that it can result from factors arising during gestation. For example, children born to women who smoke, use alcohol or certain drugs have a higher incidence of attention deficit disorders. There also may be a hereditary aspect, since it seems to run in families. Tension in the home can also be a factor.

There are no laboratory tests or diagnostic standards; instead, each child must be evaluated individually. Frequently the problem is not considered "serious" until the child starts school, although parents usually recall that the youngster has a longstanding history of behavior difficulties. Children with the hyperactive component always seem to be "on the go"; they have difficulty sitting or playing quietly. Adjectives frequently used to describe these children include: fidgety, impulsive, easily distracted, combative, disorganized, inattentive, among others. In school they have difficulty sitting still, they will rush through an assigned task, often turning in incomplete or sloppy work, even though they have the intellectual ability to do better. They frequently disrupt a class or playgroup and have difficulty adhering to rules. In diagnosing the problem, however, it is important to distinguish between those children who truly have an attention deficit disorder and those who are normally more talkative, curious, or active than other children. In some families and classroom settings, for example, a "good" child is one who is respectful and quiet; a normally rambunctious youngster can easily be labeled a behavior problem in these situations.

Attention deficit disorders are ten times more common in boys than girls. Most children outgrow the problem by the time they reach adolescence, but others never seem to fully overcome some of the characteristics, such as impulsive actions or difficulty completing a task. Many of these children have normal or even above-average intelligence, but they still have difficulty learning; others have varying degrees of mental retardation.

Treatment includes counseling, special schools, and, in some instances, drug therapy, usually with methylphenidate (Ritalin). This drug is a central-nervous-system stimulant, but for unknown reasons it has a calming effect when given to a hyperactive child. In recent years, the increased use of Ritalin has become controversial, with some groups charging that it is being overused in lieu of trying to understand and redirect a child's behavior.

A number of anecdotal reports also have linked certain characteristics of attention deficit disorders to diet, especially such items as food dyes, additives, and sugar. The Feingold diet, a regimen that eliminates suspected foods or additives from the child's diet, has gained considerable attention as a possible treatment for hyperactivity. Scientific studies have failed to document its value, but some doctors suggest a three- or six-month trial of diet therapy to see if this helps. (For more information, see section on disruptive behavior in chapter 29, Psychiatric Disorders.)

Cognitive Disorders

There are a number of specific problems related to cognitive, or intellectual, development. These include:

Autism. This is a serious disorder characterized by an inability to relate socially with other people. Autistic children frequently engage in ritualized, repetitive movements and have late-developing or noncommunicative speech. Many never speak at all. Mental retardation is frequently associated with autism, but some afflicted children are of normal intelligence, although their ability to conceptualize is impaired.

The causes of autism are unknown, although it is thought to result from a structural abnormality in the brain. Treatment is generally unsatisfactory, although there have been some promising results from intensive one-to-one therapeutic relationships. Drugs are sometimes used to control behavior, which is often self-destructive.

Developmental Aphasia. This is the inability to acquire language skills. It is caused by an abnormality in the part of the brain that processes auditory information, and should not be confused with speech difficulties linked to retardation, autism, or hearing loss. Some children with developmental aphasia have trouble with listening, while others have problems with both listening and speaking.

Dyslexia. This is characterized by difficulty in recognizing certain letters or in sounding out unfamiliar words. Frequently the child will have difficulty learning to read, or reading skills may lag considerably behind age and intellectual ability. When asked to read aloud, the child will often omit, add, or distort words. A common characteristic is reversal of characters—24 becomes 42; "the" is written as "hte." The problem can be diagnosed by the history, and by comparing scores on verbal IQ tests with those of written tests. Often the child will have an average or above average score when tested verbally, but will have a low score on written tests.

Treatment includes using special teaching techniques to overcome the dyslexia. Most will eventually learn to read, although they still may find it easier to use a typewriter than to write by hand, and will learn better through the spoken word than by reading.

Clumsy Child Syndrome. Although this is a rather unscientific label for a disease, it is the term used to describe children who have significant coordination problems. Their fine motor control will be minimal; they often have difficulty orienting themselves spatially to their surroundings. The cause is unknown, although there are some indications that it may be genetically transmitted. Treatment involves physical therapy and special education programs.

TUMORS OF THE CENTRAL NERVOUS SYSTEM

Brain Tumors

Childhood brain tumors, especially during the first year of life, are rare, but they do occur. The tumors may be either benign or malignant; in both cases, they can produce similar symptoms because the mass grows within the confines of the skull and inevitably impinges on normal brain tissue. Symptoms of increased pressure within the skull include headaches, which are usually recurrent and increasing in severity as time passes; vomiting, which may be intermittent and variable; double or generally impaired vision; head enlargement; paralysis of facial muscles; personality changes; loss of muscle control; and seizures. The tumor usually can be diagnosed by computerized tomographic (CT) scans, magnetic resonance imaging, or X rays.

The treatment of choice is surgical removal. In the best situation, all of the tumor will be removed at an early stage before there is severe, permanent brain damage. If the entire tumor cannot be removed, radiation therapy may be administered to shrink the mass. Certain drugs may be used to reduce brain swelling. Chemotherapy also is showing more promise as a treatment for some brain tumors.

Cerebellar Tumors

More than 25 percent of all brain tumors in children arise in or adjacent to the cerebellum, which lies below the main brain mass and at the back of the head. The most common type is called an *astrocytoma*, which is a slow-growing tumor made up of a specific cell type. Surgical removal is the treatment of choice and often leads to a cure.

Medulloblastomas are a type of tumor that also arise near the cerebellum, but unlike an astrocytoma, these tumors are fast-growing and they cannot be completely removed by surgery. Radiation therapy and chemotherapy are the major treatments; about half the children with these tumors are alive and well after five years.

Other Tumors

Tumors attached to the brain's *fourth ventricle* (ependymomas) produce symptoms similar to those of an astrocytoma, but they are more difficult to remove. Radiation therapy can help, but even so, only a third of children with this type of tumor survive five years. Tumors arising in the *brain stem* can cause partial eye paralysis, with one eye becoming fixed; a change in gait; and even a change in whether the child is right- or left-handed. These tumors are inoperable, and radiation is the only treatment. Long-term survival is rare.

Spinal cord tumors are rare in children, and when they occur, they produce symptoms related to gait, posture, reflexes, bladder and bowel function, and sensory changes. Scoliosis, or a curved spine, as well as skin changes over the site of the tumor, also may occur. A test of the cerebrospinal fluid will confirm the presence of a spinal cord tumor. Early treatment is important to minimize lasting damage. Surgical removal of the tumor is the treatment of choice; radiation therapy also may be used. Such tumors usually respond well to treatment and the long-term outlook is good.

Although rare, other sites in which brain tumors can develop include the pineal gland, hypothalamus, cerebral hemispheres, and optic nerve. Symptoms depend upon the site and nature of the tumor. As with all central nervous system tumors, surgery, whenever possible, is the treatment of choice.

CEREBROVASCULAR DISEASES

As THEIR NAME implies, cerebrovascular diseases affect the brain's blood supply. Although most commonly associated with aging, these diseases are not unknown in children, with an incidence about half that of brain tumors.

Occlusive Cerebrovascular Diseases

In these disorders, the brain is deprived of blood and its essential supply of oxygen. If allowed to persist, these disorders can kill segments of brain tissue, or even cause death. Either the veins or the arteries may be involved. In *venous thrombosis,* which can be caused by injury, dehydration, or sickle-cell anemia, a vein that drains blood from the brain becomes blocked. In contrast, with *arterial thrombosis,* an artery is blocked, preventing blood from entering the brain. Both are emergencies requiring immediate treatment. Other cerebrovascular disorders include:

Cerebral Embolism. This occurs when an artery, most often the middle cerebral artery, is blocked. The blockage may be from a clot resulting from a broken bone or heart disease; it also may be caused by bacteria from an infection, a tumor, or air. Symptoms usually come on suddenly and include vomiting, headache, and paralysis.

Intracranial Hemorrhage. Injury is the most common cause of intracranial hemorrhage, or bleeding into the brain. Other causes include an abnormality of blood clotting; an aneurysm, a weakened segment of a blood vessel that balloons out and may rupture; a vascular malformation; an infection; or a tumor. Testing the cerebrospinal fluid will confirm the presence of blood; treatment involves finding the source of the bleeding and stopping it. The blood usually will be reabsorbed, but if a clot forms, it may have to be surgically removed.

Vascular Malformations. Sometimes there are tangles of blood vessels or other malformations resulting from congenital abnormalities. Some of these abnormal vessels may be weak and prone to rupture. Some can be treated surgically or radiologically, in which case the outlook is good.

INJURIES TO THE HEAD AND CENTRAL NERVOUS SYSTEM

As EVERY PARENT knows, the head seems to be a magnet for injury in children; indeed, 40 percent of all reported childhood trauma is to the head. Fortunately most injuries are mild, involving mostly bruises and cuts that heal without lasting damage. Still, all head injuries are potentially serious, and some are life-threatening. Since many injuries occur in motor vehicle accidents, young children and infants always should travel securely strapped into infant seats. Older children always should wear seat belts.

Scalp Injuries

These are among the most common of childhood head injuries. A scalp wound can be particularly startling because it often entails profuse bleeding. Still, most heal well. Obviously, any open scalp wound should be closed (stitched if necessary) and covered to prevent infection and further bleeding. Bumps and bruises usually disappear in a few days, although larger ones may take longer.

Craniocerebral Trauma

This category includes injuries that affect the skull and brain. The skull itself can withstand considerable force, especially in an older child whose "soft spot" has closed. Thus, if there is damage from a blow or fall, it is usually due to the motion and tearing of tissue within the brain itself. Minor bumps, cuts, and bruises can be dealt with at home, but any more serious head injury, especially in a baby or very young child, should be checked by a doctor. This is especially true if the child has lost consciousness or falls into a deep sleep after the injury (in fact, you should keep a child awake for several hours after a head injury, and over the next 24 hours, waken him or her every couple of hours just to make sure there are no evolving problems). Other symptoms that require prompt, even emergency medical attention, include vomiting, lethargy, visual changes, dizziness, difficulty moving, paralysis, or changes in speech, among others.

Concussion

A concussion is caused by a sudden head blow that results in a transient loss of consciousness, followed by full recovery. The concussion may be accompanied by vomiting, headache, apathy, impaired vision, and other symptoms. These complaints usually are transient and self-limiting. The child should be examined by a doctor and then monitored, at least for 24 hours. During that period the youngster should be wakened every two hours just to make sure he or she has not lapsed into unconsciousness. Hospitalization, however, usually is not needed, since the monitoring can be done at home.

Skull Fractures

Although unusual, skull fractures do occur among children. Since an infant's skull bone is not fully calcified and hard, fractures suffered in this age group are usually depression, or "pond" fractures, rather than linear cracks in the bone as seen in older children and adults. Usually no treatment beyond relief for the pain is required. Pond fractures usually do not require that the bones be elevated, or restored to their normal contour, unless the depression is deep.

There are, however, special situations that may require hospitalization and close observation. For example, if the cerebrospinal fluid leaks through a fracture into the ear or nose area, treatment with antibiotics and close observation is required to prevent meningitis. Sometimes a cyst will develop along the fracture line, causing the rift in bones to widen and the skull to erode. This can be detected by X rays, which should be done three months after the injury, to make sure the fracture is healing properly and that no cyst has formed. In most instances healing is complete in six months.

Cerebral Contusion and Laceration

A bruise or cut to the brain tissue itself may occur in a severe head injury. Prompt medical care, which often includes hospitalization, is required. Unconsciousness, if it occurs, may persist for days or even weeks, in which case life support and artificial feeding will be needed. The extent of recovery depends upon the nature of the injury; possible long-term consequences include seizures, memory loss, behavior problems, and movement disorders.

Extradural Hematoma

An extradural hematoma is a potentially serious head injury caused by bleeding into the space between the hard dura that surrounds the brain and the skull wall. A large clot, or hematoma, may form, pressing against the brain structures. Typically the child suffering this kind of injury will be knocked unconscious from the initial injury, and then will either waken only to relapse into unconsciousness, or will not wake and will progress directly into a coma. Left untreated, this kind of injury is invariably fatal, but most will survive if there is prompt surgery to remove the hematoma.

Spinal Cord Injuries

Spinal cord injuries are relatively rare in childhood, accounting for less than 5 percent of the serious injuries. Among babies, the most common cause of spinal cord injuries are difficult births; for example, a forceful breech delivery. Among older children, whiplash-type accidents and falls are the leading causes. Whenever a spinal cord injury is suspected, special care must be taken in moving or transporting the child—something that should be left to trained emergency medical personnel. The spinal cord, even in a young child, does not regenerate, so if it is severely injured, paralysis below the point of damage is irreversible.

Nerve Injuries

Peripheral nerve injuries, in which nerves serving specific body parts such as the arms, shoulders, legs, etc., are damaged, can lead to numbness, weakness, and varying degrees of paralysis. These are uncommon in childhood. *Cranial nerve injuries,* which can affect eye movement, facial muscle control, and sensory functions such as smell and hearing, rarely occur in an isolated situation. Instead they are usually part of larger head trauma.

SEIZURE DISORDERS

SEIZURES, OR CONVULSIONS as they are also called, are quite common among children. During a "grand mal" seizure, there is a sudden, violent contraction of a group of muscles, leading to uncontrolled twitching or other movements. A seizure is a result of abnormal activity or "firing" of the brain's nerve cells; children are more susceptible to seizures than adults because their central nervous systems are not fully developed. Seizures can occur in anyone, but are more common among the mentally retarded and children with cerebral palsy or other brain damage.

The seizure is usually accompanied by a loss of consciousness and bladder control. Although frightening to parents, a childhood seizure often is an isolated occurrence that passes quickly and is of no lasting significance. In other instances, it may be a sign of a serious underlying problem, such as a head injury, brain tumor, drug overdose, vascular malformation, or infection, such as meningitis. Not all seizures follow the same pattern. Some are subtle and involve no muscular contractions, but rather changes in the state of consciousness. (See box on the different types of seizures later in the chapter.)

There is a long list of possible causes of seizures; some of the more common are discussed below.

Febrile Seizures

Febrile seizures are among the most common seen in children—about 3 to 5 percent of all children will have one or more. They generally occur between the ages of six months and six years, and, as their name indicates, are related to fever. In some children, a very high fever is needed to provoke a seizure; in others even a low temperature of 101 degrees F. can lead to febrile seizures. For unknown reasons, these children seem to have a low seizure threshold. Typically the seizure will occur early in the illness, and often when the fever is in decline. Sometimes the seizure may actually precede a rash, as in roseola.

Generally febrile seizures, although alarming, are not serious if they last less than 15 minutes, or if a series of seizures lasts no more than 30 minutes. Prolonged seizures, however, can cause lasting brain damage.

Epilepsy

Epilepsy is the common term applied to a number of syndromes characterized by recurrent seizures. It is a result of abnormal electrical activity in the brain. In up to half of childhood seizure disorders and an even higher percentage in adults, there is no identifiable cause for the attacks. However, by studying the characteristic patterns on an electroencephalogram (EEG), the seizures can be categorized, and a physician can determine whether the child is, indeed, epileptic.

In general there are two major types of epileptic seizures, which can have either internal or external triggers: generalized seizures, which affect both motor function and consciousness, and partial, or *focal seizures*, which affect a specific sensory, motor, or psychological function.

Epilepsy in varying forms affects about 2 percent of the population, and the large majority (up to 90 percent according to some studies) have generalized seizures. About 55 percent of these patients have only generalized seizures, while the remaining also experience some type of partial seizure. In most cases, the cause of the seizures is unknown, but sometimes the epilepsy is related to an underlying disease. In such instances, treating that disease can often put an end to the seizures.

Epilepsy may begin at any age. Seizures suffered before two are usually due to metabolic disorders; injuries, including those suffered during birth; or congenital defects. (Epilepsy that begins in adulthood usually is due to brain injuries, tumors, or some other organic brain disease.)

At one time epilepsy carried considerable social stigma, and even today there is considerable misunderstanding about the disease. For example, there are still people who mistakenly assume that epilepsy is in some way related to mental retardation or defectiveness. This is not the case; there are any number of very intelligent and accomplished people who have epilepsy. While there may be some jobs that are unsafe for an epileptic whose seizures are poorly controlled, most are not handicapped by the disorder.

Up to 85 percent or more of people with epilepsy can either avoid seizures completely or greatly reduce their incidence by taking anticonvulsant drugs. Carbamazepine is the most popular anticonvulsant drug for both generalized or partial seizures. Phenobarbital and phenytoin also are used for both types. Some of these drugs can cause excessive drowsiness or lethargy; such side effects usually can be eliminated or minimized by adjusting the dosage or turning to some of the newer anticonvulsive agents. Since there is no single drug that works for all patients, finding the right regimen often requires months of trial-and-error until an appropriate dosage and combination of drugs are found. Even when seizures are brought under control, the medication should be continued, usually for four years, and in some cases even longer.

Many children outgrow the seizure disorders, especially the kind characterized by benign focal epilepsy or by "absence" or petit mal attacks. Those who do not outgrow the epilepsy often experience a decreased incidence of seizures with adolescence or adulthood. In any event, counseling may be important in helping both the parents and child cope with epilepsy. And it should be stressed that with drug therapy and understanding on the part of both the patient and those close to him or her, most people with epilepsy can lead quite normal lives. (See boxes on Types of Seizures, on the opposite page, and First Aid During a Seizure, on the page following.)

PAROXYSMAL (NONEPILEPTIC) DISORDERS

THIS IS A GROUP of varied neurological disorders that have no single common characteristic other than that they all involve paroxysmal attacks that are not epileptic in nature. Some of the more common include:

Breath-Holding Attacks

About 5 percent of children experience breath-holding attacks. Most are between the ages of two and three, and sometimes the disorder seems to run in the family. With *cyanotic breath-holding*, the child usually is reacting to being disciplined, denied something, or to some other slight. The attack usually begins with intense crying, and sometimes the child will declare his or her intention to stop breathing. Some youngsters will use the tactic as a threat to get their own way. The child will go rigid, curl up, and then lose muscle tone. The lips and fingertips may turn blue, but no matter how determined the child is to stop breathing, once he or she loses consciousness, breathing will automatically resume. Although the attacks are frightening, parents should remember that they are not dangerous, and they seldom last for more than a minute or so. Frequently after an attack of breath-holding, the youngster will want to go to sleep.

Pallid breath-holding attacks are somewhat different in that they occur without warning, usually in response to a painful, frightening, or other unex-

TYPES OF SEIZURES

Although all seizures represent a sudden disturbance of behavior, they take different forms.

Tonic-clonic (grand mal) seizure. This is the most common type of generalized seizure, and the one that most people visualize. Without warning, the child will lose consciousness and fall to the ground or floor. The arms and legs will be rigid for the first few seconds, and then begin to twitch. The child frequently loses bladder and sometimes bowel control. This type of seizure usually lasts for only a few minutes; the child will then regain consciousness, unaware of what has happened. Irritability, fatigue, and headache are common aftermaths; very often the youngster will fall into a deep sleep that will last for several hours. If the seizure is brief and not immediately followed by others, there is usually no lasting damage. Prolonged or rapidly recurrent seizures, however, can lead to brain damage and retardation.

Nonconvulsive ("absence" or petit mal) seizures. These are minor seizures in which there is a brief loss of awareness without actually losing consciousness. The child will suddenly become motionless and may appear to be daydreaming or staring vacantly into space. The episode usually lasts only a few seconds, and later the child will have no remembrance of anything out the ordinary happening. Sometimes the youngster may actually fall, and there may be a few minor muscle twitches or jerking.

This type of seizure occurs most often in children between the ages of four and twelve. Most children outgrow them, without lasting damage. Some youngsters, however, experience school problems because of them. Not uncommonly, a child may have 20 or more attacks in the course of a day. A teacher may mistake these attacks for daydreaming or inattention; they also can interfere with the learning process because suddenly the child is unaware of what is happening or being said.

Myoclonic seizures. The child will experience sudden, bilateral muscle jerking or twitching, but will remain conscious throughout the episode.

Photosensitive seizures. These are brought on by rapidly flashing lights (10 to 25 pulses per second). A TV or strobe light, or even the sunlight flickering through the leaves of a tree, can provoke a generalized convulsive seizure.

Atonic seizure. This is characterized by a loss of muscle tone and power, usually in the neck, trunk, or a limb. Without warning the affected part will suddenly go limp. There is a momentary loss of consciousness, and there is a danger that the child may be hurt falling.

Akinetic seizure. Movement is suddenly arrested, but without the loss of muscle tone seen in an atonic seizure. There is, however, a loss of consciousness.

Infantile spasms. These seizures occur mostly in babies, first appearing at about three months of age, and are characterized by a flexor spasm of the head and trunk. The spasms come in clusters, ranging from a few to hundreds per day. They seem to be aggravated by feeding, handling, and the transition from sleep to wakefulness. Very often (about 80 percent of the time) the child goes on to develop other forms of epilepsy and mental retardation.

Focal or partial seizures. These arise in only one part of the brain; they are often preceded by an aura or other preliminary symptoms. Focal seizures may spread within the brain and become secondarily generalized, with loss of consciousness.

Simple partial seizure. This seizure is characterized by a sudden spasm of a limb or facial muscle, which then may be paralyzed for a few minutes to hours following the attack. The child retains consciousness throughout the episode. The paralysis often can be avoided by massaging the limb or practicing a type of biofeedback. This type of focal seizure is often benign in childhood and disappears during the second decade of life.

Complex partial seizure. This is characterized by a change in mental status, such as hallucinations, altered consciousness, or strong fears or other emotions. This disorder is rare in children; when it occurs, the child may be aggressive and resist any type of restraint.

Unilateral seizures. These affect only one side of the body and are caused by damage to one hemisphere of the brain.

Miscellaneous seizures. These include gelastic (characterized by uncontrolled, inappropriate laughter), cursive (spontaneous running), and reflex seizures (precipitated by a specific stimulus).

pected event. In these, the child will suddenly lose consciousness. Again, breathing will automatically resume, and the aftermath is similar to what happens following cyanotic breath-holding.

Both types of attacks can occur as frequently as several times per week or as infrequently as one or two a year. The worst cases seem to take place when parents are most frightened by the child's actions. By the age of three or four, most children cease to engage in breath-holding. The best approach is a firm, but friendly one: "I'm sorry you are so upset, but you cannot————." The child will soon get the message that the breath-holding will not produce the desired results.

FIRST AID DURING A SEIZURE

Although a seizure, especially in a child, can be alarming to parents, most are brief and do not cause lasting damage. There are many misconceptions about what one should do to help a person having a seizure. The person should not be restrained, and contrary to popular belief, *nothing*—even a handkerchief or other soft object—should be forced into the person's mouth. This was once advised to prevent tongue biting—it is now recognized that it can do more harm than good. Specific steps that should be followed to help someone having a seizure include:

1. Lay the child on the side, especially if there is vomiting. This position will prevent choking.
2. Loosen clothing, especially around the neck.
3. Move furniture or other objects that may injure the person.
4. Place a pillow, rolled-up jacket, or some other object under the head.
5. If the seizure lasts more than five minutes, or is rapidly followed by other seizures, seek immediate medical attention.
6. Carefully observe all details of the seizure so you can later describe them to a doctor. After the child wakens, he or she may be somewhat disoriented, irritable and, frequently, very drowsy.
7. Any seizure, with the possible exception of those accompanying a fever (febrile seizures), warrants prompt medical investigation and further testing.

Syncopal Attacks

Syncope, what is commonly referred to as "fainting," can be triggered by a variety of circumstances —heat, suddenly standing up after a period of inactivity, a fright, hyperventilation (overbreathing), among others. Unless the fainting is linked to an underlying disorder, such as a congenital heart defect, children generally recover quickly and fully. If there is no obvious explanation for the fainting, or if the episodes recur, a doctor should be consulted.

Paroxysmal Disorders Involving Nausea

Cyclical Vomiting. In this disorder, the child is subject to recurrent paroxysmal vomiting that has no apparent cause. There usually is no underlying disease, although it may be related to epilepsy or migraine headaches. The disorder is relatively uncommon and is generally outgrown by age three or four.

Benign Paroxysmal Vertigo. This is another reasonably uncommon disorder that is seen mostly in children under the age of three. The child, who is otherwise normal, will be hit with sudden dizziness and nausea. During an attack, the youngster will close his or her eyes and grasp onto something in an effort to regain a sense of equilibrium. The attacks may occur as often as several times a week or as infrequently as every few months. An antinausea medication such as Dramamine may be prescribed to prevent the nausea, but this is usually recommended only if the attacks are frequent. The episodes usually taper off and disappear after a year or two.

Paroxysmal Torticollis. In this disorder, commonly referred to as "wry neck," the child will hold his or her head at a strange angle, usually to one side or the other. Vomiting may accompany the onset of the attack. An episode of wry neck may last from a few minutes to several weeks. There is no known cause for the disorder. In older children, biofeedback has been effective in helping some youngsters control or overcome the muscle contractions.

HEADACHES

MOST CHILDHOOD HEADACHES are not signs of serious underlying disease. Symptoms that indicate a headache may be linked to a serious problem are outlined in table 28.1.

Stress or Tension Headaches

As in adults, stress is a common cause of headaches. The arrival of a new baby, starting school, moving to a new home are common examples of the kinds of stress that may lead to recurrent headaches. The pain of a stress headache tends to be steady and dull, and is usually localized, such as in the temples, forehead, neck, or back of the head. If the child is asked: "Where does your head hurt?" he or she will usually point to one of these places. Resting in a darkened room, a gentle neck massage, or a warm bath often help. If these nonmedication approaches do not bring relief, a child's dose of aspirin or acetaminophen may be used.

Table 28.1 HEADACHE SYMPTOMS THAT NEED MEDICAL ATTENTION

- any headache accompanied by loss of consciousness, confusion, altered state of alertness, visual blurring, or other neurological symptoms
- a headache accompanied by a fever and stiff neck
- a recurrent headache in one area, such as an eye
- headaches that recur with increasing intensity
- a severe headache that comes on very suddenly or occurs on awakening

Migraine Headaches

Although migraine headaches are uncommon in children, they do occur, and as in adults, this type of vascular headache can be triggered by a wide variety of substances or circumstances. (See table 28.2, Common Migraine Triggering Factors.) Typically the pain is throbbing and located on one side of the head. In adults there are usually preliminary signs (the so-called *prodrome*) such as visual distortions, flashing lights, or loss of peripheral vision, to warn of an impending migraine. The visual warnings are unusual in children, but parents may note pallor, general malaise, increased irritability, or other symptoms just before a migraine hits.

The headache may be accompanied by vomiting. The actual pain of a migraine is caused by a swelling of the blood vessels in a particular area of the head or neck. Many children who suffer from migraines outgrow the problem with puberty; for others, the headaches may persist for life or return at some point during adulthood.

Treatment varies according to the severity of the problem and frequency of the headaches. Identifying and avoiding the triggering factors is one of the best approaches. For most children, resting in a darkened room until the attack passes will suffice.

Table 28.2 COMMON MIGRAINE TRIGGERING FACTORS

- certain foods or additives, especially chocolate, monosodium glutamate (MSG), caffeine, cheese, corn products, food dyes, and preservatives in cured meats, among others
- sudden changes in weather or temperature
- emotional upsets
- glaring lights
- strong odors
- cigarette smoke
- certain medications, especially those that may contain alcohol
- hormonal changes
- fatigue

Aspirin will often ward off the pain if it is taken during the prodrome period, before the migraine fully develops. There are medications, such as beta-blocking drugs, that are given to adults to prevent recurrent migraines, but their use in children is controversial.

SLEEP DISORDERS

SERIOUS SLEEP DISORDERS are unusual in children—the most common involve *somnambulism*, or sleepwalking, and *night terrors*.

Sleepwalking is seen mostly among boys, especially those between 5 and 12 years old. The episodes usually last 10 to 30 minutes, and often involve a series of complex, automatic actions. Not uncommonly, a child will go up and down stairs, open and close doors, and perform a number of other acts that are normally associated with being wide awake and fully conscious. In the morning, the child will have no memory of having been up and about the night before. Although sleepwalkers usually do not harm themselves, precautions should be taken to prevent falls or going outdoors.

Night terrors should not be confused with bad dreams or even nightmares, which are much milder than what is experienced during an episode of terrors. Typically the child will awake screaming and exhibiting intense fear. Sometimes it may take several minutes of shaking and loud talking to arouse the child out of the terror. The youngster will usually return to sleep with no memory of the terror. The problem occurs most often in children five to seven years old, and most outgrow it by the age of seven or eight.

Narcolepsy, or sleep attacks, entail a sudden, uncontrollable urge to sleep. The disorder is uncommon in children, and it should not be confused with the natural sleepiness that is common in babies and young children. However, young children may experience *hypnagogic phenomena*, which are particularly vivid visual or auditory illusions that are experienced just when falling asleep. They are sometimes described as particularly vivid dreams, but unlike ordinary dreams, the hypnagogic illusions occur during the initial stage of sleep, and not during the usual REM stage.

TICS

TICS, OR HABIT spasms, are relatively common, and although distracting, usually are not serious. Most tics are brief, repetitive muscular contractions.

Some of the most common are the nervous tics or twitching that develop around the eyes, mouth, or shoulders. At first a tic may be voluntarily controlled, but eventually it may become unconscious and beyond voluntary control. Invariably tics worsen when the person is upset or tired.

Typically a child may develop a tic at about age five or six, and most eventually outgrow it. An exception is *Tourette's disorder* (also called Tourette's syndrome), which is thought to have a metabolic basis. Tourette's disorder begins with tics, usually facial grimaces, blinking, or shoulder shrugging. As the disorder progresses, the tics increase in intensity, and the child also may begin making various verbal noises, such as barks, grunts, sniffing, or shouting. In about half of the cases, the person also utters curse words.

Many people mistakenly assume that Tourette's disorder is a psychological disease, especially if the person is one who utters strings of profanities at the most inappropriate times. This is not the case, however, and the discovery that most cases can be controlled by giving haloperidol (Haldol), a powerful antipsychotic drug, has demonstrated that the disease is essentially organic and not psychological. Since haloperidol can have numerous side effects, the smallest dose possible to control the tics and verbal utterances is given. Other tic disorders can be controlled with milder drugs, such as phenobarbital or clonazepam (Clonopin), a tranquilizer that is also a muscle relaxant. (For more information, see chapter 29, Psychiatric Disorders.)

GENETIC METABOLIC DISORDERS

ALTHOUGH MOST of these disorders are in themselves rare, when considered as a group they are a reasonably common cause of neurological symptoms. All involve some sort of metabolic deficiency, such as a missing enzyme, inability to absorb a particular vitamin, mineral, or nutrient. Most are progressive and can lead to permanent neurological and other damage. Many are fatal, but there are some that can be controlled through diet; while others respond to an infusion of the deficient substance. Disorders in this category include:

Phenylketonuria (PKU)

This is an inborn error in metabolism in which there is a deficiency of the enzyme needed to eliminate excess phenylalanine, an essential amino acid, from the body. As a result, the phenylalanine accumulates in the blood and, if not reversed, can lead to mental retardation, severe seizures, and other neurological problems. Newborn babies do not show signs of PKU, but the enzyme defect can be detected by screening babies for the defect shortly after birth. This is now mandatory in the United States. If the defect is detected, the baby is fed a diet that limits phenylalanine. This involves giving a milk substitute and a diet that provides enough protein for proper growth, but not enough to allow a buildup of phenylalanine. It is vital that treatment begin early, usually in the first few days of life, to prevent mental retardation. It is not known how long the protein-restricted diet must be followed; some experts think that it should be given for life, but others have found that it can be ended at about age five, when the myelin coating of the brain is complete.

Lipidoses

These are disorders of lipid, or fat metabolism. Most are genetic, and include Gaucher's disease, Tay-Sachs disease, Refsum's syndrome, van Bogaert's disease, and others. All are rare, and most are characterized by retarded development, progressive dementia, convulsions, paralysis, and other symptoms involving the nervous and other body systems. Most are fatal at an early age.

Miscellaneous Disorders

These include *mucopolysaccharidosis*, or MPS, a group of inherited diseases characterized by missing enzymes and excessive urinary secretion of a compound called glycosaminoglycan, an amino sugar. MPS is not apparent at birth, but as the baby grows, short stature, neurological problems, facial deformities, and other hallmarks of the disease become apparent. Treatment with enzyme infusions has been of limited value, but bone-marrow transplantation may be helpful.

Other genetic metabolic diseases involve abnormalities in lipid, carbohydrate, and copper metabolism. All have varying effects on growth, development, and neurological functioning.

NEUROMUSCULAR DISORDERS

IT IS THROUGH our neuromuscular system that the brain sends messages via the nerves to the muscles. The system is made up of: (1) *anterior horn cells* (nerve cells in the anterior horn part of the spinal cord), which transmit messages from the brain; (2) the peripheral nerves that carry these messages to the muscles; (3) the neuromuscular junction, the point where the message "jumps" from the nerve to the muscles; and (4) the muscles themselves. Neuromuscular disorders are diseases that can strike any part of this system.

Childhood Neuropathies

A neuropathy is a disorder that affects the nerves and their cells. There are many types of neuropathies; fortunately, most are not very common among children.

Anterior Horn Cell Disease. As the name implies, this disorder strikes at the nerve cells in the anterior horn portions of the spinal cord. By disrupting these cells, the disease leads to weakness, loss of muscle tone and muscle wasting, and absence of tendon reflexes. About 65 percent of cases arise in the first six months, beginning with a loss of head and trunk control and proceeding to general weakness. There is also a milder form, which usually strikes after the age of two and can last until adulthood. With this form, the afflicted person may retain the ability to sit, and some are even able to walk. Physical therapy and treatment of the scoliosis (curved spine) that accompanies the disease can be of help. Little can be done, however, for the more severe form.

Anterior horn cell disease is a genetic disorder. Parents who have one child afflicted with it have a 25 percent chance that other children also will be stricken. Genetic counseling is advisable for couples who have had a child with the disorder.

Peripheral Neuropathy. This disease strikes the peripheral nerves, causing weakness, numbness, and loss of sensation. Symptoms depend on the location of the affected nerves. They include a weak grip, footdrop, muscle wasting, tingling, and numbness, among others.

Various other diseases can mimic peripheral neuropathy, so diagnosis cannot be made on the basis of symptoms alone. Nerve conduction velocities, a technique to measure the electrical conductivity of a nerve, is the most accurate diagnostic test. If peripheral neuropathy is present, the electrical message traveling along the nerve will be slowed, whereas with disorders with similar symptoms, the electrical activity will be normal.

Peroneal Muscular Atrophy. This is the most common cause of chronic neuropathy in childhood. It is evident by the midteens (although some cases do not appear until later), and is characterized by footdrop. This causes an awkward gait, in which the knee is brought up high to avoid the toe being dragged, and the foot is then "slapped down." There is also muscle wasting. The atrophy can spread to the arms and hands, resulting in a loss of sensation. Most people with this disorder retain their ability to walk, however awkwardly, and it does not affect longevity.

Diseases of the Neuromuscular Junction

Disorders in this category affect the transmission of nerve messages to the muscles.

Myasthenia Gravis (MG). Myasthenia gravis can affect any age group, and although it is more common among adults, it also occurs among babies and young children. The disease is caused by a defect in the immune system, in which antibodies attack elements of neuromuscular transmission. About 12 percent of women with the disease can give birth to babies with a form of neonatal myasthenia, in which the mother's antibodies are transferred to the infant. The baby may have profound muscular weakness, but this usually lasts only a few weeks.

Congenital Myasthenia Gravis. This form is more severe; it is present from birth on and may progress rapidly. The disease affects any normal repetitive muscular activity, including respiration, and many of its young victims die of respiratory failure. It also causes difficulty in chewing, smiling, and eye movement. Some mild cases may cause symptoms only after exercising the affected muscles. The cause of myasthenia gravis is unknown in most cases, although some may be initiated by drugs or other illnesses. Congenital myasthenia gravis is inherited and is not associated with immune disturbances.

The disease varies greatly from person to person. In some the onset is sudden and the progression rapid; in others it comes on very slowly and may take years to worsen to the point that it is disabling. In about 25 percent of cases, there is a spontaneous remission. Treatment also varies. There are a number of drugs that may be tried, including corticosteroids and agents that inhibit the activity of certain enzymes. Removal of the thymus gland is another common treatment. A newer approach that has helped a number of patients involves plasmapheresis, in which the blood is put through a machine that "spins out" certain substances, and is then returned to the body.

Toxins. Certain toxins can attack the neuromuscular junction, leading to paralysis. For example, *botulism* produces a toxin that results in almost total, often fatal paralysis. Some ticks also produce a toxin that can cause paralysis. *Tick paralysis* usually can be reversed within hours or days of removing the tick, but it can be fatal if the tick is not detected or the disease is not treated promptly.

MYOPATHIES

MYOPATHIES ARE muscle diseases that are not caused by central nervous system disorders. They may be inherited or acquired, and many are progressive. Some are caused by infectious agents, nutritional deficiency, endocrine disorders, or toxic agents.

The most severe are the genetic dystrophies, which involve progressive muscle weakness.

Duchenne Muscular Dystrophy

This disease strikes only males, and usually starts before the age of four, and virtually always by the age of ten. The first manifestation is delayed ability to walk, and when walking the child will be clumsy, falling frequently and having great difficulty in rising from a lying position. The rate of progression varies, but most victims will be unable to walk by the age of 13. The disease becomes life-threatening when it progresses to the respiratory muscles and affects the heart muscle.

Although there is no specific treatment for Duchenne dystrophy, physical therapy and special equipment can be used to keep the child walking for as long as possible. Genetic counseling is advised for women who carry the gene, since there is a strong likelihood that her male children will be affected.

Other Dystrophies

Congenital dystrophy is present at birth and usually improves over time. *Emery-Dreifuss dystrophy* primarily affects the elbow, ankle, and neck muscles in males with the disease. *Limb-girdle dystrophy*, which is rare in children, affects the shoulder and pelvic muscles. There are miscellaneous other dystrophies that may affect specific body parts, such as the eyes or limbs, but these are very unusual in children.

Myotonia

Myotonia is a defect of muscle relaxation; after the muscles are tensed or contracted, they do not relax as quickly as they should.

Congenital Myotonia. This is most noticeable when a child is active after getting up from a nap or on a cold day. For example, a baby's eyes may remain shut even after awakening or stopping crying. The symptoms can be worked off by warming up and continuing to use the affected muscles. There are also drugs that can be taken to prevent the myotonia. These children usually have very large, well-developed muscles.

Myotonic Dystrophy. This is a slowly progressing disease that usually begins in adolescence, but it can also start shortly after birth. In the latter case, the baby may succumb to respiratory failure. Mental impairment, facial muscle abnormalities, and generalized muscle weakness and wasting are characteristics of the disease. The disease is inherited as a dominant trait and the mother almost always has the disease when the infant is affected.

Hypotonia

This term describes a reduction of muscle tone that may occur without muscle weakness. Examples include *Prader-Willi syndrome* or *floppy infant syndrome*. As the name implies, the baby will have poor muscle tone, and he or she is often hard to feed. In some instances the disorder is relatively benign, and the baby will improve with time. In others the hypotonia may improve, but the child may be mentally retarded.

In *periodic paralysis*, the trunk and limbs are struck with recurrent temporary flaccid paralysis. The attacks usually occur following a postexercise rest period or when the child is anxious. The youngster will be fine between attacks, which can last anywhere from a few minutes to days. Potassium salts given during an attack may help alleviate the symptoms and acetazolamide (Diamox) often prevents the attacks.

29 Psychiatric Disorders

David Shaffer, M.D.,
Gail A. Wasserman, Ph.D., and
Paul D. Trautman, M.D.

INTRODUCTION

THE PHYSICAL PROBLEMS of childhood have always been a major concern of those responsible for the well-being of the young, and most parents quickly learn the signs that precede illness in a child. Fortunately the common physical ailments of childhood are mostly short-lived and rarely progress to a chronic state.

Psychiatric disorders or emotional problems, on the other hand, may be more difficult to diagnose because the symptoms of a psychiatric problem often differ only in degree from normal behavior. Behavior, even in a disturbed child, may vary over time or with different situations. It can be a reaction to external events, or it may originate within the child. But when should a child's behavior be of concern?

Few children in today's society escape scrutiny by a knowledgeable individual. Pediatricians may observe behavior they consider to be outside the normal range, and may recommend further evaluation and testing. However, the typical visit to a pediatrician is brief and highly structured, so unless the parents raise a specific concern, the doctor may fail to detect a behavioral or emotional problem. Staff members at nurseries, preschools, or daycare centers may also note behavior that seems unusual, and they may suggest a referral for evaluation.

Parents may be the most likely to detect behavioral problems in their children because they have the advantage of seeing the child's behavior every day and can observe changes, however subtle. Since it is widely held that behavior problems are a reflection of inappropriate child rearing, parents may view asking for professional help as an admission of guilt and failure. Even though some will sense that something is wrong, many will be reluctant to admit a problem exists, although many psychological problems in young children are not necessarily the consequence of child rearing. In fact, parents of young children make a vital contribution to both the evaluation and treatment processes.

ASSESSMENT

AFTER REFERRAL has been made and before any treatment can begin, a formal evaluation, or assessment, is necessary. The assessment is most often performed by a child psychiatrist or a child psychologist. Differences in training and approach between psychiatrists and psychologists are discussed below. At the first visit many assessors prefer to see the parents without the child. At this time the assessor can ask questions that may not deal directly with the problems of the child but may have bearing on them. The presence of a very young child could be distracting to both the parents and the assessor; isolating the child in a strange waiting room would be distressing to him or her. At a subsequent visit, the child may be seen with or without the parents present. If, however, a single assessment visit is planned, parents and child will normally be present together.

An important aspect of the assessment is determining the nature of the problem. What made the parents decide to seek help at this time? How long has the problem been apparent? Did some stress precede the onset of the problem? It is most helpful to the clinician when parents provide concrete and detailed examples of the child's behavior, rather than generalizations. Once an appointment has been set, it may be helpful if parents start to keep notes listing specific problems or events. It is also useful if reports from the child's nursery school or daycare center are obtained in advance.

The clinician's encounter with the child can be upsetting to a youngster who is uncomfortable with strangers, especially if the child is separated from the parents. The clinician will often be skilled at distracting or settling the upset child. If separation proves too upsetting, the child can be evaluated with the parents present. For toddlers, assessment usually involves the use of objects that may not only be similar to the child's playthings at home, but may stimulate his or her curiosity about new toys as well.

Some clinicians find a visit to the home or school valuable. Relating to a small child in surroundings that are familiar to him or her can be less stressful and may offer insights into family interactions. The use of videotape recorders is another technique gaining acceptance.

Observation forms the greatest part of the assessment of an infant or young child beyond the information acquired from the parent. Evaluation may include observing the child with play materials, or it may include formal testing of intelligence or language competence.

After the formal evaluation has been completed and any test results evaluated, the clinician presents the parents with conclusions and recommendations for treating the child. At this time, the clinician can either conclude the relationship with the family, arrange referral, or provide the necessary treatment.

PROBLEM BEHAVIORS

THERE ARE MANY reasons a parent might seek professional help for his or her child. The most common types of problems are described below, with references to specific diagnoses; the latter are outlined at the end of the chapter. A discussion on sources of help and those practitioners who are qualified to treat problem behaviors is also included.

LANGUAGE DISORDERS

CHILDREN WITH language impairment often show behavior problems that lead parents to seek a psychiatrist's opinion. However, the problem starts earlier. The development of language begins with a newborn's earliest cries and continues throughout life. It involves auditory stimulation and hearing, mental processing, and the production of sounds and language. Auditory stimulation exposes the child to the sounds of the environment. Sounds received through the ears are transmitted via the nerves to the brain and "processed" through identification and interpretation. The interpretation, or comprehension, may be followed by language production or some other action.

Language is usually well developed before the age of four. For more information on language milestones, see chapters 9 through 12. Children who show no production of language by age two years should be referred for a thorough speech and hearing evaluation. The development of speech and language can be adversely affected by many factors, including hearing deficiencies, general mental development, and physical problems involving facial structure or musculature. Hearing can be tested in the youngest infant by observing startle response to noises such as door slamming or hand clapping that originate outside the infant's field of vision. If a question about hearing is raised by such simple procedures, specialized tests will normally be recommended.

Understanding of words always precedes their meaningful use, as illustrated by the young child who obeys an instruction before he or she attempts to issue one. Speaking requires motor skills, and with practice and reinforcement through auditory input, speaking skills grow. Physical abnormalities can affect the quality of the speech, making vocalizations unintelligible. The muscles must be able to control breathing and move the lips, tongue, and jaw to produce intelligible sounds.

Stuttering usually begins between the ages of two and seven, and its cause is often unknown. As the child becomes aware of the stuttering he may become anxious, and this anxiety may lead to more stuttering. In most cases, stuttering disappears spontaneously, although speech difficulties can reappear during times of stress.

The young child may be acquiring vocabulary on schedule and still show more subtle language problems. For example, the child may not use the words acquired for the purpose of informational and social communication. Even a preschooler should be able to use his or her language skills to describe thoughts and feelings, and should be able to relate simple events to a parent. Beyond this, children in this age range can be expected to engage in simple conversations, that is, to ask and answer questions, respond appropriately to other people's comments, and to ask follow-up questions. Language should, at least occasionally, take the form of dialogue rather than monologue.

For the child whose auditory functioning is normal but whose language development is not commensurate with his or her chronological age, a diagnosis of mental retardation may be made. When such a diagnosis is made, the child's language skills will often prove to be appropriate to mental age.

Pervasive developmental disorder is a rare condition in which young children fail to develop normal language and show unusual language patterns. They may repeat phrases they have heard (echolalia), use idiosyncratic utterances whose meaning is known only to family members, or show abnormal speech intonation.

For further discussion of specific disorders and diagnoses, see at the end of this chapter Chronic Motor or Vocal Tic Disorder, Developmental Articulation Disorder, Developmental Expressive Language Disorder, Developmental Receptive Language Disorder, Elective Mutism, Mental Retardation, Pervasive Developmental Disorder, Stuttering, Tourette's Disorder, and Transient Tic Disorder.

DISRUPTIVE BEHAVIOR

A COMMON PROBLEM in young children is socially disruptive behavior, which is often more distressing to others than to the disruptive children themselves. For example, such children may show excessive aggression toward others, overactivity, argumentativeness, or temper tantrums, or they may engage in stealing or truancy. Certainly these behaviors occur in all children to some degree, but the child who shows an extreme, in terms of the frequency or severity of such behavior, is considered to have a problem. All of these difficulties are more common in boys than in girls.

Disruptive behavior problems are broadly grouped into three overlapping problem areas. In one type, overactivity, easy distractibility, and inattentiveness cause problems for the child, especially in a structured setting such as a playgroup or nursery school. On the other hand, these problems may be noticed by parents in the home as early as the second year of life. Parents may observe excessive running or climbing, and the child may seem to be always "on the go." He or she may have difficulty following instructions and may shift rapidly from one incompleted activity to another. Impulsiveness may lead to accident-proneness. Many hyperactive children are also aggressive: they may be abusive to their playmates or show little regard for rules or the consequences that result from breaking them.

In a second subgroup, disruption takes the form of opposition—refusing to cooperate and responding with a firm "No!" Although negative replies are a normal element in establishing a sense of self in a young child, near-total unwillingness to agree is a cause for concern. These children tend to be negative, hostile, and defiant. They are often irritable and argumentative with adults, and frequently lose their temper, or swear. These problems may occur only at home, but often they are apparent in school as well. Peer relations may be normal.

Finally, in the third category are children who persistently violate the basic rights of others and major societal rules. These children often initiate physical aggressiveness, may be physically cruel to animals or to other people, or destroy other people's property. Stealing is common. The child's self-esteem is usually low, although he or she may project a "tough" image. These children also often show poor academic skills, hyperactivity, and inattentiveness.

One of the more effective treatments for disruptive behavior involves training the child's parents (and perhaps teachers) in new strategies for behavioral management. This involves establishing clear and consistent rules for the child. Parents also learn how to provide consistent positive consequences (rewards) for the child when he or she follows the rules and, alternatively, to establish sanctions for misbehavior (see chapter 12, Emotional and Intellectual Development).

Treatment for disruptive children can also involve medications that in adults function as stimulants. In children, these drugs increase attention and decrease hyperactivity and distractibility. Common medications for these problems include dextroamphetamine (Dexedrine) and methylphenidate (Ritalin). Tranquilizers such as chlorpromazine (Thorazine) and thioridazine (Mellaril) have also proven useful.

The prognosis for the disruptive child is mixed. Many will outgrow the problem, but some continue to show aggressive or irresponsible behavior into adulthood.

For further discussion on specific disorders, see at the end of this chapter Attention-Deficit Hyperactivity Disorder, Oppositional Defiant Disorder, and Conduct Disorder. (See also chapter 28, Neurological and Neuromuscular Disorders.)

ANXIETY AND EMOTIONAL DISORDERS

Fears

Fear is a normal, healthy reaction to many situations and may protect the individual from harm. Childhood fears are quite common and are usually situation- or object-oriented. Infants can become fearful when exposed to strangers or loud noises. By the age of two or three, a fear of animals, particularly those that are unfamiliar, may develop. Later on, fears of the dark and imaginary creatures are also normal.

Phobias

A phobia is an intense and unreasonable fear of specific objects or situations, such as dogs, insects, or elevators. Unreasonable fear of certain objects is quite common in both children and adults, but the additional appearance of strong avoidance behavior may cause difficulty for parent and child. A child who runs across the street or is unable to leave the house because of a fear of dogs is a danger to himself and disrupts the entire family's activity.

When simple reassurance is ineffective, behavior therapy may be required. This may take the form of gradual relaxation of the child in the presence of the feared object or situation.

Separation and Stranger Anxiety

A common type of anxiety in infants and young children concerns separation from the parent. At about seven months of age the average infant forms a specific attachment to another individual—his or her mother, in most cases—and also develops a fear of strangers. Once a bond has been established, situations that break it can trigger separation anxiety.

Stranger anxiety varies from child to child and depends on situational factors, such as whether or not the parent is present, how the stranger behaves, and whether the child has any familiarity with him or her. In most cases, a child will become less concerned about meeting strangers as he or she matures or is exposed to more people. Normally, separation anxiety is most common in the second year of life and decreases gradually after that.

If separation anxiety does not decrease with age, the child may not be able to attend nursery school or be left with a babysitter. Such children may follow the parent from room to room like a shadow, and may complain of nonspecific aches and pains (like a stomach ache) when separation is anticipated. They may also express fear about the well-being of family members. Refusal to sleep alone is common; nightmares may occur. Treatment usually follows the same procedures discussed previously under Phobias.

Other Anxiety Problems

Other children may show more general anxiety about a range of objects and situations, including new situations, the possibility of injury, inclusion in peer activities, and worries about past or future behavior. Such children may also be perfectionistic or may have nervous habits such as nail biting or hair pulling.

ALOOF, ASOCIAL BEHAVIOR

Social interaction begins very early in life. Certainly most infant social interactions occur with parents and siblings, although even infants and toddlers have the capacity to engage in simple social behavior with peers. As they mature and are exposed increasingly to peers in playgroup and nursery school settings, young children will show increasing friendliness to and interest in peers. At four or five years of age, youngsters focus on those close to their own age or younger, developing social skills in the process.

Young children who have difficulty relating to other children may be suffering from disturbed language development or from anxiety, as in the case of shy children. Some children may show avoidance of all unfamiliar people, but at the same time persist in their desire for interaction with familiar people. They may appear timid, socially withdrawn or embarrassed, or even mute in the presence of strangers. These problems are more common in girls than in boys.

Elective Mutism

Some children show persistent refusal to talk in one or more social situations. Most commonly the child will not speak at school, but will talk at home. This may lead to severe impairment in social and school functioning. The problem is rare and in most cases lasts for only a few weeks or months. Such behavior

may be the product of an overprotective parent who also exhibits socialization deficiencies. Elective mutism will usually be resolved with therapy, either for the child alone or, better still, for the family as a group.

Autistic Disorder (Pervasive Developmental Disorder)

An extreme, rare form of social withdrawal is autistic disorder, in which a child shows little or no interest in social interaction. Normal attachment to the mother does not occur at an appropriate age and communication skills are abnormal, limited, or nonexistent. These children are self-involved and do not receive the security from human contact that the average child does. The autistic child expresses little interest in imaginative play and instead spends long periods of time engaged in seemingly purposeless, repetitive actions. Treatment for the autistic child is designed to encourage normal development through constant reinforcement of learned skills.

For further discussion of specific disorders, see at the end of this chapter Avoidant Disorder of Childhood, Elective Mutism, and Pervasive Developmental Disorder.

CRYING, SADNESS, AND DEPRESSION

Behavioral studies have concluded that healthy babies have three different cries in their repertoire. A hunger cry is a rhythmic one that begins as a whimper and becomes progressively louder. A mad or angry cry is also rhythmic but is louder than the hunger cry. The third, a pain cry, begins as a loud shriek, is followed by a brief silence, and then continues as a loud wailing.

An infant's earliest cries are a reaction to discomfort, such as hunger or pain. Newborns as young as three weeks of age are also capable of a fourth type of cry, which is intended to draw attention. By the time infants reach their first birthday, they usually have learned that they can gain attention and affection by other means, such as a smile, a laugh, or outstretched arms.

An infant whose cries fail to produce a comforting response by a caregiver eventually stops crying. Crying also declines in infants whose cries are followed by a caring response. Consistency in the response to crying, therefore, would appear to bring about a decline in crying behavior. Parents must decide within the first year of life which child cries they want to respond to and which to ignore. For example, a child who falls needs immediate comforting, whereas brief crying at bedtime, seen as normal, may be ignored.

Infants or toddlers whose tearful, unhappy behavior is not relieved with normal attentive care may be depressed or anxious. Depression in infants and young children is unusual. The symptoms now recognized by mental health professionals are similar to those seen in adults, and include tearfulness, a sad appearance, loss of interest in once-pleasurable activities, lack of energy, sleep and appetite disturbance, and social withdrawal.

Depression is most likely to appear in those young children who have close relatives who have also suffered from depression.

Antidepressant medication may be helpful in treating depression in young children for whom other forms of treatment have failed. Consistent involvement of the parent is important in assessing and treating the depressed child.

For further discussion of specific disorders, see at the end of this chapter Dysthymia, Major Depressive Episode, Pervasive Developmental Disorder, and Separation Anxiety Disorder.

REPETITIVE BEHAVIOR

REPETITION IS a major component of the learning process. By practicing an action over and over, new activity is mastered. Sometimes repetition becomes an end in and of itself. Three types of repetitive behavior are discussed below.

In one type, a child who is severely understimulated because of mental retardation, sensory deficit, or parental neglect will attempt to provide stimulation for herself or himself. Typical of such self-stimulatory behavior are head banging, excessive rocking, or masturbation.

A second type of repetitive behavior is seen in tics. A tic is an involuntary, sudden, nonrhythmic movement or vocalization. Common tics include blinking, shoulder shrugging, and coughing. Tics may be transient or persistent. Tics are made worse by stress, such as that caused by the attention elicited by the tic itself. Anxiety-producing situations are likely to make tics worse, while tics diminish during sleep. Tics are common in close family members of children who have tics.

The third type of repetitive behavior is rituals, which are intentional and purposeful and are performed in accordance with certain self-imposed rules or in a stereotyped fashion. An example in young children is their having to hear the same story each night before bedtime or needing to have their toys arranged in the same order before going to school. Such rituals are very common in young children and are only a cause for concern if they interfere with normal social or family activities.

Tourette's Disorder

Tourette's disorder is a variant of tic disorder in which multiple motor and vocal tics occur. The motor tics usually involve the head, but the neck, torso and limbs also may be involved. The vocal tics include grunts, clicks, barks, or words, sometimes scatological ones. The specific symptoms and their severity may vary over time. The child may have a sense of inner tension that is relieved by ticking. Attention deficit disorder and obsessive-compulsive disorder may also be present. The causes of Tourette's disorder remain undetermined, but there is evidence for genetic inheritance. Tic disorders, and possibly also obsessive-compulsive disorder, are more common in close relatives than in those with Tourette's disorder in the general population.

Because of its many forms and degrees of severity, the prevalence of Tourette's disorder is difficult to establish. As many as one in 200 or 300 persons could have either the disorder or multiple tics resembling Tourette's. The disease is at least three times more common in males than females. It is sometimes misdiagnosed as epilepsy, or as other neurologically based movement disorders.

Family therapy, psychotherapy, and behavior modification have shown little value in relieving tics. Treatment for children with Tourette's disorder usually centers on medications. Haloperidol (Haldol) and clonidine (Catapres) are frequently prescribed, as are the phenothiazines, including trifluoroperazine (Stelazine) and chlorpromazine (Thorazine). The benefits of such medications must be weighed against their side effects, which include fatigue, intellectual dulling, and tardive dyskinesia, a rhythmic movement of the hands or face, or both. (For more information, see chapter 28, Neurological and Neuromuscular Disorders.)

ELIMINATION AND RETENTION DISORDERS

ACHIEVING URINARY and fecal continence is a developmental milestone in the life of a toddler. Because children do learn bladder and bowel control gradually, they are not considered to have enuresis or encopresis unless the problem continues beyond age five. Nevertheless, parents may wish to seek help with toilet training a younger child who is making slow progress in this area, or who seems particularly resistant to attempts at training. In the absence of a complicating medical condition, children usually achieve fecal continence before urinary continence and daytime control before nighttime dryness.

Enuresis

The precise cause of enuresis (bed-wetting) is not known. Genetic factors, abnormalities in bladder function, and inadequate toilet training may be contributing factors. Enuresis is not necessarily a symptom of psychiatric disturbance but about 20 percent of enuretic children have associated behavior problems such as anxiety and social withdrawal. Developmental speech problems are also more common in enuretic children. Their inability to achieve bladder control can prevent their participation in activities normal for their age, compounding their feelings of anxiety and withdrawal.

Treating an enuretic child requires several steps. An assessment of the problem by a physician is important to rule out possible urinary infections or anomalies that are not infrequently found with this condition.

The two most effective methods of treating bed-wetting are medication and behavior modification. Psychotherapy is rarely effective. Before beginning any treatment it is worthwhile attempting to get the child to chart the number of nights he or she is wet. Treatment is justified if the child wets more than four times in a two-week period. It is also important to reassure the child that he or she is not alone in suffering from this condition.

Medications reduce the enuresis, but wetting usually reappears soon after the medication is discontinued. Use of a bell apparatus, designed to wake a child at the first passage of urine, results in a cure in many cases. However, the treatment takes time, and it is normal for there to be no results in the first six weeks, with complete dryness achieved after three months. A child may become dry with this treatment but then relapse.

Encopresis

Encopresis involves soiling. It may take the form of either the repeated deposition of formed fecal matter in inappropriate places, or continuous soiling in which the child's underpants and pajamas are constantly soiled. Continuous soiling is more common and may follow an extended period of constipation, which distends the rectum and results in leakage of fecal fluid. Because of the odor, children with encopresis suffer from rejection by other school children, siblings, and even parents.

Treatment usually involves ensuring that any constipation is overcome soon after onset, and providing rewards for using the toilet in an appropriate way. As with enuresis, psychotherapy is rarely effective in treating encopresis.

SLEEPING DISORDERS

THE SLEEP PATTERNS of the typical newborn consist of cycles of 45 minutes to 2 hours of sleep that total as much as 18 hours each day. Gradually, the infant extends his or her waking and sleeping periods. By the time a child is between three and seven months of age, he or she is able to sleep through the night.

Certain types of sleep disturbances are more common in children than in adults, such as sleepwalking, sleep talking, and night terrors. In sleepwalking, which may or may not involve actual walking, a child suddenly sits up in bed and then may get up and walk around, perhaps appearing distressed. The next morning, there will be no recollection of the event. Sleep talking may accompany a dream and may or may not be recalled if the child is awakened. *Night terrors*, or *pavor nocturnus*, are marked by abrupt awakening and crying, which does not subside with attempts at comforting. The following morning, the child will be unable to recall the incident.

Regular sleep schedules and relaxing bedtime routines may help ease such disruptions of normal sleep patterns. If the daytime activities become affected by nighttime sleep disturbances or if the child fears the approach of bedtime, professional help should be sought.

For further discussion of specific disorders see at the end of this chapter Dream Anxiety Disorder, Major Depressive Episode, and Sleep Terror Disorder.

GENDER DISORDERS

THE DESIGNATION of a newborn as "boy" or "girl" takes place at the moment of birth, based on the external genitalia. From that moment on, culturally approved sex-role standards influence the child.

During the first three years of life, a child acquires a sex-role orientation, perceiving his or her masculinity or femininity. This is usually reinforced by a sex-role preference, characterized by a desire to adhere to society's standards and stereotypes for that sex. When the gender of an individual is obvious to others on the basis of behavior, that individual has adopted a sex role.

Establishing a sexual identity is a gradual process, during which problems are sometimes encountered. For a two-year-old, others can be sorted into males and females, but the child may be unsure of his or her own gender identity. Three-year-olds know their sexual identity and tend to prefer sex-typed toys and activities, but they still lack sex constancy. By the age of four or five, children understand that their parents would prefer their playing in sex-typed activities appropriate for them, but not until the age of six or seven do they realize that their gender is permanent.

The period between 18 months and three years is the critical time during which gender identity appears to be established. Children with congenital abnormalities of the genitalia that make them appear as a member of the opposite sex should be evaluated within this time so that sex reassignment can be performed surgically with fewer long-term complications than if surgery takes place later.

A child's awareness of his or her genitalia evolves as a general curiosity regarding the body. Some pleasure may be derived; infants have been observed manipulating their genitalia in the first year of life. Such behavior continues during early childhood, but usually by the time they are of school age, they understand that it is socially inappropriate, at least in public. When a child is preoccupied with excessive masturbation, the development of interpersonal skills can suffer.

The psychological effects of rape or other sexual abuse on a young child is a subject that is not fully understood. Some believe that in a very young child rape elicits a response identical to that resulting from any other injury; however, the effects of repeated sexual abuse pose a different, distinct set of problems still undergoing study.

For further discussion of specific disorders see at the end of this chapter Gender Identity Disorder of Childhood.

EATING DISORDERS

THE CONFLICTS between a child and his or her parents over food preferences is common and can continue into adolescence. Indeed, serious eating disorders such as anorexia nervosa and/or bulimia often first appear during adolescence. In younger children, overly selective eating habits may serve as a method of gaining attention or as a form of oppositional behavior. While most eating idiosyncrasies abate with maturity, there are two that can be life-threatening.

Rumination Disorder

In rumination disorder, the child eats and swallows, but then vomits the partially digested food to the mouth, to be expelled or chewed again. The odor emanating from the child's mouth can be most unpleasant, and, as a result, others may avoid the child. In extreme cases, fatal malnutrition can result. Behavior modification may help control the disorder.

Pica

Children have a habit of putting anything into their mouths. But eating specific nonnutritious substances, a behavior known as pica, is exhibited by some children to attract attention when they receive inadequate supervision or because they are understimulated. Children who are retarded or who suffer from sensory impairment (blindness, deafness) are particularly at risk. The dangers in pica are of choking and poisoning, especially if the child chews on painted surfaces. Pica usually disappears by the time a child reaches school age.

SOURCES OF HELP

THE FIELD of mental health has many qualified individuals capable of working with a child who has psychiatric problems. Descriptions of six types of mental health professionals are given here, including their training, type of practice, and suitability for treating a particular disorder. The professional category chosen depends on the diagnosis, the most appropriate method of resolving the problem, and intangibles that are always part of a health care decision. Recommendations by the child's pediatrician and the assessor should, of course, weigh heavily in any treatment decision.

Psychiatrists

Psychiatrists are medical doctors who have had special training in mental health problems. Their broad experience in problems with a physical cause makes them especially competent to undertake an initial diagnostic evaluation. They can legally prescribe medications, which are important in the treatment of some disorders. With additional training a psychiatrist can become a psychoanalyst, a practitioner of one specific form of treatment. Child psychiatrists have undergone two additional years of residency training that concentrates on the treatment of children.

Psychiatrists are licensed as medical doctors by the state in which they practice. The American Board of Psychiatry and Neurology accredits and issues certificates to those psychiatrists or child psychiatrists who complete an approved training program, have two years related work experience, and pass a written and oral examination. In order to maintain board certification, a psychiatrist must take continuing education programs.

Psychologists

Psychologists can choose a specific focus of work, research, testing, teaching, clinical training, or any combination for a concentration. Psychologists have either a doctorate of philosophy (Ph.D.) in psychology, or in educational psychology (Ed.D.), focusing on school, counseling, or educational psychology.

A clinical psychologist is required to complete a one-year supervised internship in clinical work on a full-time basis in order to obtain a doctorate degree. Licensing of psychologists is required in most states, and the licensing procedure may entail a written examination.

Psychologists are commonly involved in providing psychotherapy for children who have had a full evaluation. They practice a number of types of therapy, and may also participate in the evaluation process, providing detailed assessments of child intellectual and language abilities.

Social Workers

A social worker is usually employed in a clinic setting, hospital, family service agency, or private or group practice. With a bachelor's degree and a two-year graduate program an individual will earn an MSW or MSSW, a master's degree in social work. Of those who complete a master's degree, at least half are employed in clinical work.

Licensing requirements for social workers vary from state to state, with some jurisdictions requiring work experience or an examination or both for licensing. For certification by the Academy of Certified Social Workers (ASCW), a social worker must have obtained a master's degree, completed two years of supervised clinical experience, and passed a written examination. Doctorates in social work are also available.

Nurses

Although all nursing students receive some training in the psychiatric unit of a hospital, those who work one to two years after they have completed a four-year program to obtain a bachelor of science degree in nursing may earn a master's degree in psychiatric nursing. A registered nurse (R.N.) is licensed to work in the state in which he or she has passed an examination. Some psychiatric nurses work in hospitals and in schools and nursing homes. Others conduct individual, group, and family therapy programs in a private-practice setting.

Psychoanalysts

Psychoanalysts are those professionals who subscribe to the technique of psychoanalysis. Most psychoanalysts are psychiatrists, but others can be psychologists or lay nonprofessionals. All have been trained in the technique at a special training institute, a process that takes about four years to complete. Child psychoanalysis is a subspecialty for which no licensing requirements have been established.

Paraprofessionals

Although they have no training specifically designed for the jobs they perform, paraprofessionals, also known as mental health workers, psychiatric counselors, or mental health assistants, perform myriad tasks in a mental health setting. Some have undergraduate degrees in psychology and engage in counseling, usually in a clinic environment.

TREATMENT APPROACHES

SOME TREATMENT approaches are more suited to psychiatric work with children than others. For example, a very young child will usually not cooperate in extended discussions about his or her feelings while seated across a desk from a psychiatrist (assuming the child is capable of expressing his or her concerns). Parents usually work with the professional to bring about a change in a very young child.

Most toddlers are willing to take part in play therapy with the professional. Play can help the child understand the importance of limits and at the same time give the youngster a boost in self-confidence.

The assessment of the child's psychiatric problem may reveal a family dysfunction or a distorted relationship between the child and a family member, so treatment of more than one individual may be the best way of helping the youngster. Because the parents and siblings can affect the environment in the home, family counseling can increase the chances for a successful outcome for the child with the psychiatric disorder.

SPECIFIC DIAGNOSES

THE FOLLOWING are specific diagnoses for psychiatric illnesses found in children. Statistical information and details on symptoms are based on the *Diagnostic and Statistical Manual of Mental Disorders* (3rd edition, revised).

Attention-Deficit Hyperactivity Disorder

Symptoms

Inattention, impulsiveness, and hyperactivity that are developmentally inappropriate and persist for at least six months; in young children, gross motor overactivity and little interest in staying with one activity through its completion.

Prevalence

As many as 3 percent of children.

Age of onset

All cases appear before age seven; about half of all cases before age four.

Treatment recommendations

Medications: dextroamphetamine (Dexedrine), methylphenidate (Ritalin), chlorpromazine (Thorazine), thioridazine (Mellaril), and/or behavior modification.

Avoidant Disorder of Childhood

Symptoms

For at least six months, excessive avoidance of contact with strangers to the degree that social relations with peers are affected; occurs after normal stranger anxiety should have been relieved.

Prevalence

Not common.

Age of onset

At least 2½ years of age.

Treatment recommendations

Reassurance; presence of familiar adult when meeting strangers; mild tranquilizers.

Chronic Motor or Vocal Tic Disorder

Symptoms

Either motor tics or vocal tics but not both, occurring over a period of more than a year (see Tourette's disorder).

Prevalence

At least 0.5 per 1,000.

Age of onset

As early as one year of age.

Treatment recommendations

Medications: haloperidol (Haldol), clonidine (Catapres).

Conduct Disorder

Symptoms

Over at least a six-month period, persistent violations of either the rights of others, or of age-appropriate norms, including stealing, running away from home, lying, truancy, deliberate cruelty to animals or to people, fire setting, use of a weapon in fights, deliberate destruction of others' property; problems are more serious than in Oppositional Defiant Disorder.

Prevalence

Approximately 9 percent of males and 2 percent of females under the age of 18.

Age of onset

As early as four years.

Treatment recommendations

Advice on behavior management from behavior therapist. Family therapy. Medication for extremes of aggression.

Delirium

Symptoms

Fever, seizures, head injury, or exposure to toxic substances (such as poison) can lead to the following symptoms: reduced ability to concentrate; disorganized thought; hallucinations, delusions, sleep disturbances; disorientation; memory impairment.

Prevalence

Common in children.

Age of onset

May occur at any age.

Treatment recommendations

Correction of underlying cause.

Developmental Articulation Disorder

Symptoms

Despite age-appropriate initiation of speech, there is an inability to use developmentally expected speech sounds (e.g., failure to articulate *p*, *b*, and *t* by age three); speech and hearing normal; mental retardation or pervasive developmental disorder not present.

Prevalence

Approximately 10 percent of children eight years or younger.

Age of onset

Severe cases can appear by age three.

Treatment recommendations

Speech therapy.

Developmental Expressive Language Disorder

Symptoms

Marked impairment in the development of spoken language, which interferes significantly with activities of daily living; expressive language limitations may include limited size of vocabulary, simplified grammar, word substitutions, or generally slow rate of language development; not secondary to mental retardation, sensory deficit, or neurological difficulties.

Prevalence

3 to 10 percent in school-age children; unknown in younger children.

Age of onset

Severe forms are apparent before age three.

Treatment recommendations

Speech therapy.

Developmental Receptive Language Disorder

Symptoms

Difficulty in understanding spoken language and in discriminating differences between speech sounds, in the absence of general mental retardation, hearing impairment, or neurological disorder.

Prevalence

3 to 10 percent of school-age children.

Age of onset

Before age two in severe forms, otherwise usually noticed before age three.

Treatment recommendations

Special education.

Dream Anxiety Disorder (Nightmares)

Symptoms

Repeated awakenings following frightening dreams that the child is able to recall, most common in early morning; not secondary to known organic factors, including use of or withdrawal from medication known to be associated with nightmares; sleep terror disorder not present.

Prevalence

Less than 5 percent of total population.

Age of onset

Most commonly before age 10.

Treatment recommendations

Structured routines and schedules for bedtime and napping; change in parental response to child's awakening.

Dysthymia

Symptoms

Chronic depressed mood for at least one year; depressed mood need not occur every day but it appears more than half the time; can be associated with disturbances in eating, sleeping, energy level, and ability to concentrate; not secondary to major depressive episode.

Prevalence

Rare in children.

Age of onset

Can begin any time in childhood.

Elective Mutism

Symptoms

Persistent refusal to speak in one or more major social situations despite normal comprehension and normal, although sometimes delayed, language skills.

Prevalence

Rare.

Age of onset

Usually before age five.

Treatment recommendations

Behavior modification; family therapy.

Functional Encopresis

Symptoms

Involuntary or intentional passage of feces, soiling where inappropriate; occurs at least once a month for at least six months; neither structural abnormality nor physical illness is present.

Prevalence

Approximately 1 percent at age five.

Age of onset

Regarded as abnormal after age four.

Treatment recommendations

Behavior modification.

Functional Enuresis

Symptoms

Involuntary or intentional voiding of urine during the day or night at least twice a month; child must be at least five.

Prevalence

At age five, 7 percent of males and 3 percent of females.

Age of onset

Regarded as abnormal after age five.

Treatment recommendations

Behavior modification; family counseling; imipramine (Tofranil).

Gender Identity Disorder of Childhood

Symptoms

A child's persistent, strong concern over his or her assigned sex; desire to be of opposite sex or denial of assigned sex, with preference for clothing and activities usually associated with the opposite sex; disgust with or denial of anatomic structures that are specific to own sex; more profound than mere nonconformity to cultural stereotype (such as tomboyishness).

Prevalence

Uncommon.

Age of onset

In boys, before age four; comparable age of onset in girls, but less noticeable in girls because their sex roles are less rigidly defined.

Treatment recommendations

Behavior modification; family counseling.

Major Depressive Episode

Symptoms

In comparison to an earlier period of higher functioning, and in the absence of any physical causes, the child may show: depression, irritability, or loss of interest or pleasure in all or most activities for at least two weeks; disturbed appetite and sleep; weight loss or gain; decreased self-esteem; excessive guilt; suicidal thoughts or behavior.

Prevalence

Rare below age 12.

Age of onset

As early as infancy.

Treatment recommendations

Antidepressant medications such as imipramine (Tofranil); family counseling.

Mental Retardation

Symptoms

Significant delay of comparable magnitude in all areas of development as assessed by formal testing; interference with daily living skills such as feeding and dressing oneself.

Prevalence

Approximately 1 percent of the population.

Age of onset

Usually apparent by end of the first year, but may develop later following brain damage.

Treatment recommendations

Special education.

Oppositional Defiant Disorder

Symptoms

Child often loses temper and is easily annoyed; argues with or defies adults; is deliberately annoying and/or angry, spiteful or resentful; often blames others for his/her mistakes; curses; child does not meet criteria for Conduct Disorder; problems should have been apparent for at least six months and should not be secondary to some other disorder such as Dysthymia or Major Depressive Episode.

Prevalence

Unknown; more common in boys than in girls.

Age of onset

Typically by eight years, with possible precursors in early childhood.

Treatment recommendations

Family counseling; behavior modification with parent training.

Overanxious Disorder

Symptoms

Excessive or unrealistic anxiety; child is extremely self-conscious, worries about future events such as the possibility of injury or about meeting expectations; child needs reassurance about various concerns; may often be tense; has many physical complaints for which there is no medical basis (stomachache, headache, nausea); other nervous habits (nail biting, hair pulling) may be present; commonly in young children Separation Anxiety Disorder is also present; symptoms must be present for six months or longer; not secondary to a psychotic episode; anxiety should be unrelated to a recent clearly stressful event (such as parents' divorce).

Prevalence

Not uncommon; equally likely in boys and girls.

Age of onset

No information.

Treatment recommendations

Family counseling; behavior modification; medication with antianxiety drugs.

Pervasive Developmental Disorder

Symptoms

Problems in social interaction, communication skills, and in make-believe play; commonly there are associated problems in intellectual and language development.

Prevalence

10 to 15 per 10,000 children.

Age of onset

Usually before age three.

Treatment recommendations

Special education.

Pica

Symptoms

Persistent eating of nonfood, such as paint, cloth, string, or insects, for at least one month; diagnosis of mental retardation or autistic disorder inappropriate if pica is the sole problem.

Prevalence

Unknown.

Age of onset

Usually 12 to 24 months, may be earlier.

Treatment recommendations

Behavior modification; increased parental stimulation and supervision.

Reactive Attachment Disorder of Infancy/Early Childhood

Symptoms

Either persistent failure to initiate or respond to social interactions (as indicated by absence of reciprocal play, lack of vocal imitation, lack of social interest); or indiscriminate sociability, including excessive familiarity with relative strangers. At the same time, child's care is grossly pathogenic, as reflected by neglect or overly harsh punishment by the caregiver, or by repeated changes of primary caregiver; does not result from Mental Retardation, Pervasive Developmental Disorder or from a neurological abnormality (such as sensory impairment).

Prevalence

No information.

Age of onset

Before five years; as early as the first month of life.

Treatment recommendations

Alteration of the caregiving environment through family counseling, parent training, or, for extremes, foster care.

Rumination Disorder of Infancy

Symptoms

Repeated regurgitation of food followed by chewing and reswallowing or ejection from the mouth, lasting for a period of at least one month; congenital abnormalities of the digestive system are not present.

Prevalence

Very rare.

Age of onset

Three months to one year of age.

Treatment recommendations

Behavior modification; family counseling.

Separation Anxiety Disorder

Symptoms

Anxiety that can reach a state of panic over separation from person(s) to whom the child is attached; concern for safety for self and others; excessive fearfulness; symptoms persistent for at least two weeks.

Prevalence

Common.

Age of onset

As early as preschool age.

Treatment recommendations

Behavior modification; medications such as antidepressants.

Simple Phobia

Symptoms

Persistent and/or excessive fear of some specific object or event; exposure to the object or event prompts immediate anxiety, and exposure is generally avoided; avoidant behavior interferes with the child's normal routine or with expected social activities; not associated with a recent trauma or environmental stress.

Prevalence

Rather common, more common in girls than in boys.

Age of onset

Animal phobias generally begin at age two or later.

Treatment Recommendations

Most childhood phobias will remit without treatment.

Sleep Terror Disorder

Symptoms

Repeated instances of abrupt awakening, lasting one to ten minutes, usually in the early part of the night; the child is not able to be comforted; child may have a sense of terror but cannot recall his or her dream; child does not remember the episode the following morning; epilepsy not present.

Prevalence

1 to 4 percent of children.

Age of onset

Usually between four and twelve years of age.

Treatment recommendations

Medications: diazepam (Valium).

Stereotypy/Habit Disorder

Symptoms

Repetitive, voluntary nonfunctional behaviors such as rocking, scratching, or head-banging that cause physical injury or markedly disturb normal activities; problems are more serious and there is more disturbance of normal activities than with common thumbsucking or rocking in infants and very young children; Pervasive Developmental Disorder not present.

Prevalence

Unknown.

Age of onset

Early childhood, may intensify in adolescence.

Treatment recommendations

Behavior modification.

Stuttering

Symptoms

Frequent repetitions or prolongations of sounds or syllables; sometimes involves interjections; impairment of specific words or sounds.

Prevalence

Approximately 5 percent of children.

Age of onset

Usually between two and seven years of age.

Treatment recommendations

Speech therapy, including: fluency shaping; stuttering modification.

Tourette's Disorder

Symptoms

Multiple motor and vocal tics occurring with varying frequency, changing over time, and continuing for at least one year; no physical abnormality evident.

Prevalence

At least 0.5 per 1,000.

Age of onset

As early as one year of age, median onset seven years.

Treatment recommendations

Medications: haloperidol (Haldol), clonidine (Catapres), trifluoperazine (Stelazine), chlorpromazine (Thorazine); family counseling.

Transient Tic Disorder

Symptoms

Single or multiple motor and/or vocal tics that occur nearly every day for at least two weeks but no longer than 12 consecutive months.

Prevalence

Unknown.

Age of onset

As early as two years of age.

Treatment recommendations

By definition these are transient; only if they persist should medication be tried. (For more information see chronic tic disorder and Tourette's disorder in this chapter and tics in chapter 28, Neurological and Neuromuscular Disorders.)

30 Endocrine Disorders

Michael Novogroder, M.D.

FUNCTION OF THE ENDOCRINE SYSTEM

THE ENDOCRINE SYSTEM is a complex network of hormone-producing glands and glandular tissues affecting virtually every part of the body. (See figure 30.1, next page.) Hormones are the body's chemical messengers, which regulate all the body functions. They regulate metabolic processes governing energy production, growth, sexual reproduction, fluid and electrolyte balance, personality development, and stress responses. Acting in concert with the nervous system, with which the endocrine system is closely linked, it regulates homeostasis (the stability of all body functions at normal levels).

Although hormones travel throughout the body, they influence only those tissues that are responsive to them (target organs). Some hormones act only on a single target gland, while others, such as the sex hormones, have both specialized and general functions. Still others, such as growth hormone, have many effects on the body, including increasing bone growth. Many hormones work through complex feedback systems, enabling them to interact by either opposing or enhancing the functions of each other.

The speed of hormonal activity varies widely. Epinephrine (adrenaline), one of the major stress hormones, exerts immediate influence while insulin acts within minutes or hours. Thyroxine, a thyroid hormone, requires several days to produce measur-able results, and sex hormones can take weeks. And both sex and growth hormones regulate growth and development over several years.

The production and inhibition of hormones is regulated by a feedback mechanism, which is sensitive to the varying levels of the hormone. This feedback system may operate in three ways, the simplest and most common of which is a negative-feedback mode. In this case, the endocrine gland secretes a hormone that acts upon the target cell, which in turn produces a control substance that returns to the gland to inhibit further production of the hormone. In more complex feedback systems, there is an additional step. The hormone causes the target organ to release an enzyme that then activates the control substance, which, in turn, inhibits (or stimulates) further hormone secretion. There is also a positive-feedback system, whereby an adequate level of one hormone is necessary to stimulate secretion of another.

This feedback mechanism can be compared to a heating system. The *hypothalamus*, a part of the brain closely associated with the *pituitary gland*, acts as the thermostat to, in effect, set the level at which the gland should operate. If the setting of the thermostat is changed, there is a resultant increase or decrease in metabolic activity. Similarly, when the appropriate level has been reached, the thermostat automatically turns off until the level drops again, signaling the gland to start the process again.

Many endocrine functions are controlled by the

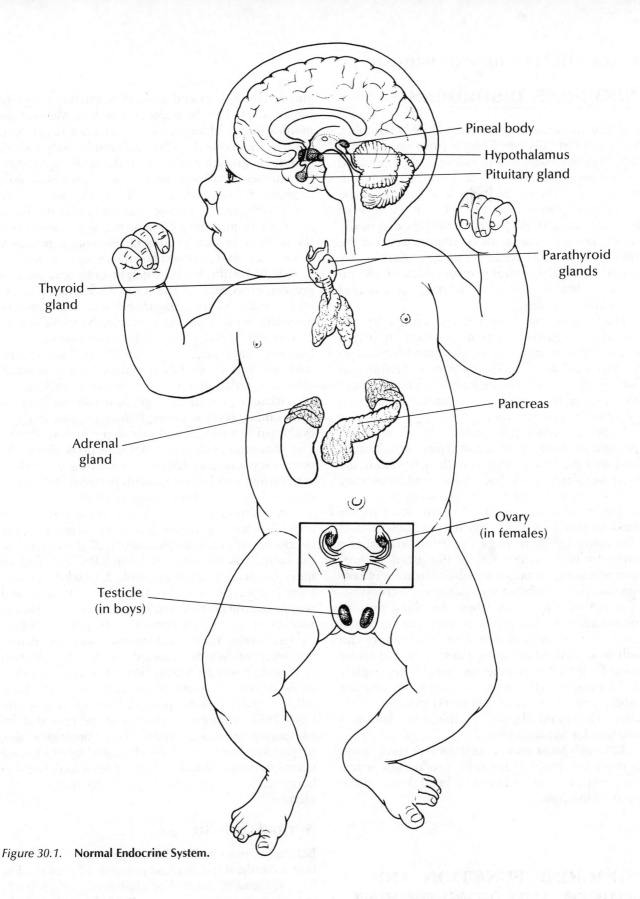

Pineal body

Hypothalamus

Pituitary gland

Parathyroid glands

Thyroid gland

Pancreas

Adrenal gland

Ovary (in females)

Testicle (in boys)

Figure 30.1. **Normal Endocrine System.**

hypothalamus, which lies at the base of the lower brain, and the pituitary, a tiny gland that is connected to the hypothalamus and is located in a bony cup at the base of the skull. The hypothalamus, which is controlled by the higher nerve centers, serves as a link between the endocrine and nervous systems. It directly controls the pituitary gland, and indirectly, through the pituitary, several others.

ENDOCRINE DISORDERS

ALTHOUGH THE ENDOCRINE SYSTEM is highly complex, involved in virtually every bodily function, and still not fully understood, it is so marvelously fine-tuned that serious endocrine disorders are relatively uncommon. But when something does go wrong, the intricate interplay of functions between the nervous and endocrine systems presents complex diagnostic puzzles. The physician must determine whether the problem is primary (within the gland), or secondary (somewhere in the central control system of the pituitary or brain), and what internal or external forces come into play.

Most endocrine disorders are caused by the overactivity (hyperfunction) or underactivity (hypofunction) of a gland, which upsets the body's delicate hormonal balance. The over- or underfunction of one gland often affects the function of another and may cause a wide variety of symptoms affecting many other organ systems.

Hyperfunction can be caused by an enlarged organ, an overgrowth of organ tissue, or a tumor, which may produce hormones itself or stimulate the endocrine gland to do so. These conditions may cause the organ to function independent of its control system, producing hormones without regard for metabolic needs. Or there may be some other defect in the control system. These conditions are usually treated by surgical removal of the gland or hormone-producing tumor or by administration of hormones and other substances to suppress secretions.

Hypofunction occurs when the gland fails to produce adequate hormones or when the hormonal control system malfunctions. Glandular failure can result from several causes: (1) destruction of tissue caused by infection or other disease; (2) genetically related enzyme deficiencies; (3) congenital absence of the gland or its removal; or (4) pituitary deficiency. Hormonal therapy is the most common treatment for hypofunction.

Although most endocrine disorders result from too much or too little hormone production, a few diseases are caused by hormone breakdown or impaired metabolism.

ENDOCRINE FUNCTION AND GROWTH AND DEVELOPMENT

IN INFANTS AND CHILDREN, growth-related problems are those seen most frequently by endocrinologists. Growth, a complex and continuous process that begins at conception and ends at maturity, is significantly affected by the endocrine system. Many of the maturational changes are hormone-dependent. Though endocrine disorders account for only a small number of growth problems in the total population, the number is still significant, and when a child fails to grow properly, doctors will consider whether or not this failure may be due to an endocrine problem.

Growth and development are dependent upon the activity of four groups of hormones: pituitary growth hormone, thyroid hormones, androgens, and estrogens. Insulin is also thought to be necessary to growth, especially in the fetus. Deficiencies or excesses of any of these hormones can cause growth disorders in children. For example, excessive insulin production by the fetus results in an oversize baby that may have many other problems. Lack of thyroid hormone in an infant causes failure to grow, mental retardation, and other serious disorders.

Because growth is a gradual process that involves many body systems, failure to grow must be evaluated in an organized way over a period of time. The physician will ask many questions about the pregnancy and conditions surrounding birth. Parents' growth-and-development patterns will be of interest as well as those of any siblings.

In addition to a complete medical history, the physician will be interested in all aspects of the child's growth and development. All those items in the baby book, such as when the baby first held up his or her head, first sat up, walked, or when the first tooth appeared will be important. Height and weight measurements will be taken over a period of months or years and compared to growth charts. Skeletal proportions, facial maturation, and dental development will be assessed and a determination of bone age will be made. (Bone age is determined by X raying the wrist where changes in the bone follow a fairly definite pattern from birth to maturity.) Other important clues will be provided by comparing the mental age to the chronological age, height, and bone age of the child and by evaluating sexual development. A variety of tests to determine hormone levels may be required to complete the picture.

Normal Growth

Before discussing disorders of growth, it is important to understand normal patterns of growth. The key indicator of normal or abnormal growth is the growth pattern or velocity. Growth tends to take place in spurts, so doctors generally assess the pattern of change over a period of time. If a child is growing a normal number of inches a year and follows a consistent pattern, then irrespective of where he or she falls on the growth chart—whether short, average, or tall—the indication is that probably all hormones are normal and there is no disease present that would cause abnormal growth. However, a change in this pattern may indicate problems. A baby that starts at the low end of the growth chart and suddenly spurts to the high end or vice versa may require investigation, even though he or she is still within a normal range.

Without question, the fastest growth occurs before birth, when in the course of 40 weeks the fetus grows from an egg the size of the head of a pin to an average length of about 20 inches and weight of about seven pounds. In the first year, the baby will add about another 10 inches, in the second, about 5 inches, in the third year about 2½ inches. Thereafter, growth levels off at roughly 2 to 2½ inches per year until the adolescent growth spurt.

The adult height of a person is determined in part by heredity, in part by environmental factors, and also by the age at which the child enters puberty. During puberty, sex hormones and other substances stimulate growth of the cartilage at the end of the long bones and calcium is deposited in the cartilage to form bone. When the growth potential is reached, all the cartilage has become calcified and the growth process stops. Those who enter puberty at a very early age begin the accelerated growth process when they are younger and therefore smaller. They have a smaller base upon which to build and are consequently apt to be somewhat shorter at maturity than those who begin puberty at a much later time.

Wide variations in growth patterns exist within the normal range. Children who have short parents will probably be short and in the low part of the normal range just as children with tall parents are apt to be tall and at the top of the normal range. However, in the Western world, parents seldom worry about children who are tall. It is children who are shorter than average who are brought to the doctor for consultation.

Normal but Unusual Growth Patterns

The most common cause of short stature is genetic. Genetic short stature is akin to starting a race a few minutes behind everybody else but running at the same speed. The difference is never made up, but normal progress is made along the course. Such a child is generally healthy and grows steadily along the same line on the growth chart, though this may be at the lower fifth or tenth percentile. If the child's height is recorded on a parental adjusted height chart that compares growth to that of the parents rather than to other children, the youngster usually falls into the 50th percentile.

This condition cannot be remedied with hormonal therapies. A few such children have been given growth hormone in an attempt to determine if such therapy can make a difference in the adult height, but it is too early to tell what effect, if any, such hormone therapy might have on children with genetic short stature.

Another variation of the normal growth pattern occurs when a child is much shorter than average throughout childhood, enters the pubertal growth spurt quite late, then proceeds to catch up with his or her peers. This is called constitutional delay in growth and development and it occurs about 10 times more frequently in boys than in girls. In such cases, the child's physiologic clock is set behind. Although the child may have a chronologic age of six, the physical age is two or three years younger. There is usually no abnormality; typically the parents will also have a history of delayed maturity. The bone age of such a child will be two or three years behind the chronologic age, and all stages of development and growth correlate with the bone age rather than the chronologic age.

This whole process can occur in reverse, and then the child is called a rapid maturer. Whether the process is that of delayed development or rapid maturity, these children have an excellent prognosis and no treatment is necessary unless the deviation from the norm causes the child serious emotional trauma, in which case some psychologic counseling may be warranted.

Abnormal Growth Patterns

Intrauterine Growth Retardation. In recent years there has been an increasing number of children with short stature resulting from intrauterine growth retardation. This is usually the result of a problem during pregnancy that slows fetal growth and causes the birth of a baby significantly smaller than average for the gestational age. The baby's maturity at birth determines how well the infant can function outside the uterus and is usually related to gestational age rather than size. Birth size depends on many factors such as inherited potential, nutrition, disease, and environment. The age of the mother is also a factor—an adolescent who has not completed her own growth is more likely to have an undersize baby.

Although in about 90 percent of undersize babies, the cause of their retarded fetal growth is unknown, there are a number of factors that do contribute to retarded growth at birth. These are summarized in table 30.1, next page.

The outlook for undersize babies varies. Those with intrinsic conditions such as chromosomal defects are usually small throughout life, whereas babies who encountered problems late in the pregnancy or who experienced uterine constraint,

Table 30.1 **FACTORS CONTRIBUTING TO RETARDED FETAL GROWTH**

Maternal Factors

1. Maternal nutrition: Poorly nourished mothers often bear babies that are small for gestational age.
2. Vascular disease in the mother: High blood pressure and toxemia may result in the birth of growth-retarded babies.
3. Infections: Rubella, toxoplasmosis, syphilis, and other infections may result in retarded fetal growth, often accompanied by other serious problems. Viral infections suffered in the first trimester of pregnancy have a greater potential for affecting the baby.
4. Multiple births: When two or more fetuses are contained within the uterus, there is sometimes inadequate room or nutrition for the fetuses to grow properly.
5. Maternal illness: Kidney and heart disease in the mother sometimes cause retarded fetal growth, but the mechanism is not understood.
6. Maternal age: Adolescent mothers are more apt to have undersize babies.

Fetal Factors

1. Chromosomal abnormalities: There are many possible chromosomal abnormalities; in several of them, e.g., Down's syndrome and Turner's syndrome, growth retardation is characteristic.
2. Genetic and nongenetic syndromes: Retarded fetal growth is one of several symptoms in a variety of conditions including impaired skeletal growth and dwarfing syndromes.
3. Placenta and umbilical-cord characteristics: A small or scarred placenta, a compressed umbilical cord (as one wrapped around the baby's leg), or a placental defect (such as the absence of an artery, compromising the flow of nutrients to the baby) may all cause retarded growth.

Environmental Factors

1. Drugs and medications: Mothers addicted to cocaine or heroin often produce undersize babies, as may mothers taking such prescription medications as warfarin (Coumadin) and phenytoin (Dilantin).
2. Alcohol: Alcoholic mothers often produce babies with fetal alcohol syndrome, a complex of symptoms that includes retarded growth. There is mounting evidence that even moderate social drinking during pregnancy may affect birth size.
3. Smoking: A substantial number of babies born to mothers who smoke are undersize.

such as twins, are likely to catch up within the first year of life.

Miscellaneous Growth Problems

Chondrodystrophies. These are characterized by abnormalities of the cartilage portion of the bones, causing short stature. Some of these disorders are inherited and others are not. In general the causes are unknown. Bone X rays usually show abnormalities and provide the information necessary to diagnose the underlying disorder.

Achondroplasia. "Dwarfism" is the common name for achondroplasia, one type of chondrodystrophy. Children with achondroplasia have normal trunk development with large heads and short arms and legs. Although there are some specific medical problems involved, most of them can be well managed and such children can grow up to lead normal lives and may produce normal offspring.

Chromosomal Defects. These account for some abnormal growth patterns. One such cause of short stature in girls is a defect called Turner's syndrome. In girls with this condition one of the X chromosomes is either misshapen or missing in many body cells. Because of this abnormality, such girls have underdeveloped ovaries and seldom reach a height of five feet. Replacing the missing ovarian hormones allows development of normal female body characteristics, but affected girls will remain infertile. There is recent evidence that growth hormone may increase growth potential in these girls.

Pathological Short Stature. Pathological, or disease-related, short stature occurs infrequently, but it is the most serious cause of short stature. Less than 15 percent of children with growth deficiencies fall into this broad category, and among these, many will not be affected until after the fifth year because their conditions are not necessarily present from birth.

Diseases that contribute to short stature include nutritional, endocrine-metabolic, renal, and cardiac disorders. Examples of nutritional disturbances causing short stature are caloric deficiency, malabsorption syndromes, chronic inflammatory bowel disease, and zinc deficiency. The more common endocrine disorders causing short stature are discussed below.

PITUITARY DISORDERS

THE PITUITARY, acting under the control of the hypothalamus, produces a variety of hormones that control functions of other glands. The front, or anterior, portion of the pituitary gland produces hormones regulating growth and other endocrine functions. The rear, or posterior, portion also produces hormones, but they do not directly affect growth. As mentioned above, the pituitary releases its hormones under the direction of the hypothalamus.

Growth hormone (GH) is the pituitary hormone most directly promoting growth. Other pituitary hormones affecting growth through their effect on other glands include:

- *Thyroid Stimulating Hormone* (TSH)—causing secretion of thyroid hormone by the thyroid gland.
- *Adrenocorticotropic Hormone* (ACTH)—causing the adrenal gland to produce cortisol and other hormones.
- *Luteinizing Hormone* (LH)—causing the testes to secrete male hormones in men and the ovaries to produce estrogen and progesterone in women.
- *Follicle Stimulating Hormone* (FSH)—causing the testicular tubules to produce sperm in men and the ovarian follicles to produce eggs and estrogen in women. (See table 30.2.)
- *Vasopressin*—controlling water output through the kidney.
- *Oxytocin*—causing uterine contractions.

Hypopituitarism.   When the pituitary gland is impaired, one or more of its hormones may be deficient. Most commonly, however, it is growth hormone that is insufficient. In most cases no cause can be found, although sometimes the problem results from damage to the pituitary gland before, during, or after birth.

Panhypopituitarism.   Tumors of the hypothalamus or pituitary or both often lead to failure to secrete some or all hormones (panhypopituitarism). This can also be caused when the gland is destroyed through head injury, infection, or surgery.

Growth hormone deficiency may occur at any time during infancy or childhood. The major symptom is a marked slowing of the growth rate. Some children continue to show regular but slow gain in height with normal weight gain, resulting in an overweight child. Body proportions remain normal but facial structure is immature and the child usually looks younger than his or her chronological age. Mental development is usually normal.

Diagnosis is made by special blood tests to determine the level of GH in the blood. These tests may be done on an outpatient basis or in the hospital, but usually several different tests are performed to be sure that growth hormone is deficient.

Treatment will depend upon the cause of the deficiency. Replacement of the growth hormone is the most desirable treatment for hypopituitarism of unknown cause. Until recently the only growth hormone available was from human pituitary glands and was limited in supply, quite expensive, and potentially dangerous. However, a synthetic growth hormone has now been approved by the FDA, and though expensive, there is no longer a problem of supply. Children receiving GH replacement therapy may experience a dramatic change in the first year, after which there is usually a tapering off of rapid growth. Normal height is often achieved, and sexual maturity will take place at the expected time.

When other hormone deficiencies occur, replacement therapy is also given. If a tumor is causing hypopituitarism, surgery and radiation therapy may be required.

Diabetes Insipidus.   This disorder is caused by a lack of *antidiuretic hormone (ADH)*. As a result, the kidneys secrete excessive amounts of water. It should not be confused with the more common disorder, diabetes mellitus, sometimes called juvenile diabetes or sugar diabetes. The primary symptoms are excessive thirst and urination. Treatment is replacement of ADH either by injection or nasal spray.

A reverse condition in which too much ADH is produced, causing a decrease in urine secretion and dilution of the blood, can be caused by malfunction of the hypothalamus or by certain diseases. To correct this problem the underlying cause must be identified and treated.

THYROID DISORDERS

THYROID DISORDERS are among the most common endocrine problems encountered in newborns. Located in the neck on either side of the windpipe, the thyroid gland secretes hormones that affect, by their presence or absence, virtually all metabolic processes. Too much thyroid hormone causes metabolism to speed up; too little slows everything down. Either condition may be accompanied by goiter, an enlargement of the thyroid gland.

Unlike other endocrine glands, the thyroid requires an outside substance, iodine, to produce its hormone thyroxine. At one time, iodine deficiency accounted for most thyroid disease. Today, however, iodine is readily available in the normal diet in North America and is seldom a factor in thyroid problems.

Hypothyroidism.   This condition can be present at birth or develop anytime thereafter. When a baby is born with an underactive thyroid it may be the

Table 30.2 **MAJOR ENDOCRINE GLANDS AND THEIR FUNCTIONS**

Gland	Hormones	Target Area	Action
Pituitary Anterior lobe	GH (growth hormone, somatotropin)	Bones, soft tissue	Promotes protein anabolism; bone, and soft-tissue growth; promotes fat mobilization and catabolism
	TSH (thyroid-stimulating hormone)	Thyroid	Promotes secretory activity
	FSH (follicle-stimulating hormone)	Ovaries, seminiferous tubules	Promotes development of ovarian follicle and seminiferous tubules; estrogen secretion; sperm maturation
	LH (luteinizing hormone) ICSH (interstitial cell-stimulating hormone in male)	Graffian follicle, interstitial cells (testes)	Promotes ovulation and formation of corpus luteum; secretion of estrogen and progesterone; secretion of testosterone
	Prolactin (luteotropic hormone)	Corpus luteum, breasts	Maintains corpus luteum and secretion of progesterone during pregnancy; stimulates milk secretion
	ACTH (adrenocorticotropic hormone)	Adrenal cortex	Stimulates secretion of glucocorticoids
	MSH (melanocyte-stimulting hormone)	Skin	Promotes skin pigmentation
Pituitary Posterior lobe	ADH (antidiuretic hormone, vasopressin)	Distal tubules of kidneys	Enhances reabsorption of water
	Oxytocin	Uterus, breasts	Stimulates uterine contraction; milk ejection into breast ducts
Thyroid	Thyroid hormones (thyroxine, triiodothyronine)	Widespread	Controls growth rate of body cells; regulates metabolic rate; promotes gluconeogenesis and fat mobilization; influences exchange of water, electrolytes, and protein
	Calcitonin	Skeleton	Promotes calcium and phosphorus metabolism
Parathyroids	PTH (parathyroid hormone)	Bone, kidneys, gastrointestinal tract	Promotes calcium reabsorption and excretion of phosphorus; bone calcification
Adrenal gland Cortex	Mineralocorticoids (aldosterone)	Primarily kidneys	Maintains fluid/electrolyte balance; reabsorbs sodium; excretes potassium
	Glucocorticoids (cortisol)	Widespread	Promotes fat, protein, and carbohydrate metabolism; mobilizes body response to stress; promotes gluconeogenesis; suppresses inflammation
	Sex hormones (androgens, estrogens, progesterone)	Gonads	Influences secondary sex characteristics; bone development; development of reproductive organs

Table 30.2 **MAJOR ENDOCRINE GLANDS AND THEIR FUNCTIONS** (continued)

Gland	Hormones	Target Area	Action
Adrenal Gland Medulla	Epinephrine, norepinephrine	Widespread	Produces vasoconstriction with increased blood pressure; increases blood sugar via glycolysis; stimulates ACTH production; activates sweat glands; inhibits gastrointestinal action
Pancreas	Insulin	Widespread	Promotes glucose transport into cells (decreased blood glucose); increases glucose utilization and glycogenesis; promotes lipogenesis and protein synthesis
	Glucagon	Widespread	Acts as antagonist to insulin, increasing blood glucose concentration via glycogenolysis
Gonads Ovaries	Estrogens	Widespread	Promotes development of secondary sex characteristics and sexual function; promotes protein anabolism and epiphyseal closure of bones; breast development; stimulates water and sodium reabsorption in kidney tubules
	Progesterone	Uterus, breasts	Prepares for and maintains pregnancy; inhibits myometrial contractions; promotes development of mammary gland secretory tissue; aids salt and water retention in endometrium
Testes	Testosterone	Widespread	Promotes development of secondary sex characteristics and normal sexual function; promotes epiphyseal closure; increases protein anabolism for growth

result of a missing or underdeveloped gland, enzyme deficiency, iodine deficiency, or an underactive pituitary gland. Such babies may have been born later than usual, weigh more than average, feed poorly, have newborn jaundice, sleep a lot, or be constipated. However, fewer than 5 percent of newborns with hypothyroidism have noticeable symptoms in the first few weeks of life. Fortunately most states now require newborn screening for thyroid hormone so that diagnosis can be made quickly and treatment begun promptly. Early diagnosis is critical in order to avoid cretinism, a severe form of mental retardation. Replacement of the missing hormone, which must be continued throughout life, leads to quick recovery of growth. If begun early enough, all but the most severely affected children should develop normally and lead a normal life.

Hypothyroidism that appears after the newborn period is most often related to Hashimoto's thyroiditis, a disorder described below. It can also be caused by arrested growth of the thyroid gland or partial removal of the gland by surgery. The symptoms (i.e., tiredness, muscle aches, constipation, and weight gain) often appear gradually and may be attributed to other causes. As with congenital hypothyroidism, treatment is by replacement of thyroid hormone.

Hashimoto's Thyroiditis. This disorder is thought to be an autoimmunity problem, resulting in damage to the host thyroid gland. Children usually have no symptoms other than goiter. Many will experience a resolution of the disease after a few years, but some will continue to have goiter, and a few will develop hypothyroidism. Because it is important to detect hypothyroidism in its early stages, children with Hashimoto's thyroiditis should be checked annually for signs of this disorder. If detected, it is easily treated by replacement therapy.

Goiter. Enlargement of the thyroid gland is much more common among adolescents than among infants or young children, and it appears 10 times more frequently in girls than in boys. Though goiter has several possible causes, the most common in North America are the autoimmune thyroid diseases, Hashimoto's thyroiditis or Graves' disease. A few children are born with goiter, and others develop the condition because of an error in synthesis of thyroid hormones. The underlying cause of goiter will determine which treatment will be used: replacement therapy, antithyroid therapy, antibiotic treatment, or surgery.

Graves' Disease. Overactive thyroid is called Graves' disease; in newborns it is extremely rare, usually appearing in infants born to mothers with hyperthyroidism. Such infants are frequently premature and may be asymptomatic for a few days. However, they will soon develop rapid heartbeat and respiratory distress, and if not treated promptly they may suffer mental impairment or even death. Older children who develop the disease usually have an enlarged thyroid gland (goiter), and symptoms include weight loss, fatigue, insomnia, muscle weakness, and bulging eyes. There is no therapy for the underlying immunological abnormality. This condition is treated in three ways: by giving drugs that inhibit production of thyroid hormone, by removing part of the thyroid gland, or by radioiodine therapy.

PARATHYROID DISORDERS

THE PARATHYROID GLANDS are located behind the thyroid gland, two on either side. *Parathyroid hormone (PTH)*, along with vitamin D, maintains stable levels of calcium and phosphorus in the blood. Vitamin D is obtained through exposure to sunlight and through certain foods such as milk and fish.

A deficiency in vitamin D, which can be caused by insufficient intake or improper utilization by the liver or kidneys, results in rickets, a condition in which the bones are not properly mineralized and therefore become soft and bowed. A deficiency in PTH leads to low serum calcium, which can cause convulsions and other symptoms.

Hypocalcemia. Low serum calcium levels in the newborn are usually due to a problem in utero or a difficult birth. When levels drop after the baby is a few days old, the cause is usually a formula containing too much phosphorus. (The phosphorus binds with the calcium, preventing its absorption by the body.) Other causes include magnesium or PTH deficiencies. Unless there is the total absence or a malformation of the parathyroid glands, most parathyroid deficiencies are temporary, lasting only a few weeks or months. Treatment involves changing the formula and perhaps giving calcium and vitamin D supplements.

Acquired hypocalcemia (appearing after the newborn period) is generally due to an underactive parathyroid, usually caused by an autoimmune disorder in which the body's immune system mounts a reaction against itself. Treatment is with lifelong vitamin D supplements. (Vitamin D is given because there is no replacement hormone for PTH.) Because vitamin D can be toxic if given in too high doses, children must be closely monitored when they are getting extra exposure to the sun to be sure that they are not given an overdose. Symptoms of overdose are bed-wetting, constipation, and lethargy.

Some children get hypocalcemia when the parathyroid hormone is present but ineffective (pseudo-hypoparathyroidism). The classic signs of this disorder are short stature, round face, short forth and fifth fingers, and some degree of mental retardation. Treatment is the same as that for acquired hypocalcemia.

Hypercalcemia. Increased PTH production is usually caused by some other disorder, such as chronic kidney failure, intestinal malabsorption of calcium, and rickets. Children who are immobilized for long period of time through fractures or surgery may also develop high levels of calcium in the blood. Primary hyperparathyroidism, which begins during fetal life, is due to hyperplasia or other tissue growth. The symptoms include loss of appetite, constipation, vomiting, listlessness, and poor kidney function. If the cause of excess calcium is primary hyperparathyroidism, a portion of the parathyroid tissue is removed. In other cases, treatment is directed at the underlying cause. If the basic cause is irreversible, drug therapy and diet modification may be used.

ADRENAL DISORDERS

THE ADRENALS are triangular glands that rest atop each kidney. Each has two parts—the cortex, or outer layer, and the medulla, or inner core. The medulla, which secretes catecholamines, such as epinephrine (adrenaline) and norepinephrine, is not essential to maintain life because catecholamines are produced by many other body tissues. Conversely, the cortex, producing the steroid hormones such as aldosterone and cortisone, is the only source of these hormones, which are essential to many body functions. While the other adrenal hormones are under the control of the pituitary hormone ACTH or the sympathetic nervous system, aldosterone production is controlled by renin, an enzyme produced by the kidneys. Specific disorders related to adrenal insufficiency include the following:

Cushing's Syndrome. This condition is characterized by chronic excessive production of cortisol. Although there are four categories of this disorder, the cause in children under seven years of age is usually an adrenal tumor. (If the cause is excessive ACTH secretion, it is called Cushing's disease, a condition rarely found in very young children.) The primary feature is an accumulation of fat on the face, neck, and trunk, hypertension, and a decrease in growth velocity. (This is one of the rare instances when growth retardation is caused by excessive production of a hormone.) Signs of virilization may occur due to the androgen production of tumors.

Treatment of Cushing's syndrome is surgical removal of the tumor. Medication may also be used to decrease the production of cortisol. If the tumor is malignant, chemotherapy may be employed as well.

Cushing's symptoms may also be caused by chronic steroid therapy for asthma, juvenile rheumatoid arthritis, and other diseases. In such cases, treatment must be reevaluated.

Congenital Adrenal Hyperplasia. This is a family of inherited disorders. Each disorder results from a deficiency of one of the various enzymes necessary for cortisol synthesis. In the most common type of disorder, the resulting deficiency in cortisol causes the pituitary to secrete increased ACTH, which in turn causes an oversecretion of androgens.

The developing fetus, then, is exposed to an excess of androgens. As a result, babies who are genetically female may be born with external genitalia that range from mildly ambiguous to completely masculine. The uterus and fallopian tubes are not affected. Boys generally do not have genital abnormalities at birth, but may have a large penis and excessive pigmentation of the scrotal skin and nipples.

These abnormalities of sexual differentiation are often in combination with excessive salt secretion. After birth, the continued exposure to excessive androgens causes untreated boys and girls to exhibit the following symptoms of premature puberty: rapid growth, advanced bone age, progressive penile

or clitoral enlargement, and early appearance of facial, axillary, and pubic hair. The rapid advancement of bone age will result in short stature for untreated children. If treatment is started early in life, normal puberty and sexual maturation can usually be expected.

Treatment for boys is hormone therapy to restore the proper balance. In genetic females with ambiguous or virilized genitalia, appropriate sex assignment and surgical correction must be made in addition to providing hormone therapy. Reconstructive surgery, often done in stages during the first two years of life, provides good results and usually does not interfere with normal sexual activity or satisfaction.

When adrenal hyperplasia appears after infancy (late onset), the symptoms and treatment are the same, but milder, as for congenital adrenal hyperplasia, with the exception that girls will not have totally virilized genitalia.

Addison's Disease. When the adrenal gland is damaged by infection or other destructive process, the result is chronic insufficiency of adrenal hormones known as Addison's disease. The most common cause is an autoimmune disorder that may be accompanied by diseases of other endocrine glands (hypoparathyroidism and diabetes) or nonendocrine organs (pernicious anemia). It is these syndromes that most often appear early in life.

Children with Addison's disease grow progressively weaker. They lose weight, have a variety of gastrointestinal symptoms, cardiovascular problems, and a darkening of the skin. The inability to overcome even a minor infection may precipitate extreme weakness, shock, and death. The disease is treated by replacement of the missing cortisol and with oral administration of Florinef, an aldosterone substitute.

DISORDERS RELATED TO GONADS

BABIES OFTEN are born with somewhat enlarged genitalia and breast tissue. Although first-time parents are apt to be concerned that this is abnormal, the suggested sexual characteristics usually are related to the mother's necessarily high hormonal levels during pregnancy. As the baby's hormonal levels return to normal, the genitalia and breasts take on the sexually immature appearance that persists until the onset of puberty.

In unusual instances, babies and young children will have disorders related to sexual development that may be caused by an excess or deficiency of hormones produced by the gonads (testis or ovary) or of hormones produced by the pituitary that regulate gonadal function. They may also result from chromosomal abnormalities. Although relatively rare, abnormalities in sexual development cause particular concern in parents. In fact, these abnormalities are no different from any other anatomical disorders, and parents who adopt an objective approach to the diagnosis, amelioration, and/or correction of such conditions will enhance the opportunities for their children to lead normal lives.

Ambiguous Genitalia.

The infant born with ambiguous genitalia requires prompt evaluation to discover the cause and to establish gender assignment as soon as possible. Sexual ambiguity in a newborn may be caused by virilization of a genetic female (for example, congenital adrenal hyperplasia, discussed above), undervirilization of a genetic male (for example, testicular feminization), or a combination of gonadal and chromosomal abnormalities (for example, true hermaphroditism).

In complete testicular feminization, the genetic male's genitalia are entirely female, the uterus is rudimentary or not present, and the vagina ends in a blind pouch. In these children the hormone testosterone is present in normal or elevated levels, but the body cannot utilize it, and male characteristics such as penile growth cannot occur. The testes are located within the abdomen or in the groin area. These children grow and develop normally as girls until puberty, when they fail to menstruate. Physically they have normal breast development, but no axillary or pubic hair. Often the disorder is not diagnosed until this time, or when what was thought to be a hernia is found on examination to be a testis.

Incomplete testicular feminization is similar, except that the external genitalia are abnormal with an enlarged clitoris and partially fused labia and scrotum. Virilization occurs at puberty. All youngsters with complete testicular feminization and most with incomplete feminization are reared as girls and have a female psychosocial orientation. Some who have incomplete feminization are reared as boys and others adopt a male orientation at puberty.

Because there is a predisposition to gonadal cancer in this group, removal of the gonads either before or after puberty is recommended. Replacement estrogen-progesterone therapy is given afterward.

True Hermaphroditism.

In true hermaphroditism the baby has both ovarian and testicular tissue. There may be a separate testis and separate ovary, or tissue may be combined as an ovotestis. The gonads may be found within the abdomen or anywhere along the testicular pathway. A uterus is usually present, and there is often later breast development and menstruation. Ambiguous genitalia are common, as are hernias in the groin and undescended testicles. The ability to produce sperm is rare.

Sex assignment is made on the basis of appearance of external genitalia and capabilities for a normal adult sexual life. Surgical correction is made where appropriate, usually before the child is two years old, and hormone therapy is given when appropriate. Gonads are frequently removed as a precaution against gonadal cancer.

Precocious Puberty.

True sexual precocity, a condition that occurs when the hypothalamic pituitary axis is activated prematurely, occurs five to seven times more frequently in girls than in boys. It may arise from a variety of causes, though in girls an underlying pathologic change is seldom present. In some children the cause is familial, but more frequently (especially in boys) there is a central-nervous-system (brain) abnormality. These include congenital anomalies, changes due to inflammation or trauma to the brain, and various tumors of the brain. Primary hypothyroidism is another, albeit unusual, cause.

Pubertal development beginning before the age of eight in girls and 9½ in boys is considered to be precocious puberty. There are three major reasons for concern upon the advent of early puberty. First, it is undesirable for a very young child to have to deal with the physical and emotional changes of adolescence. Second, if the condition is untreated and puberty is allowed to progress, the child will grow excessively for a time but will stop growing when puberty ends, with consequent short stature. Third, the cause of precocious puberty may be a tumor requiring immediate treatment.

The signs of puberty are the same whether they occur at the normal chronological age or in the preschool child. Treatment will depend upon the cause of onset. If a tumor is causing early onset, then that will be treated. If the tumor cannot be treated or if the cause is not clear, effective therapy is problematic. In the past, a variety of drug therapies have been tried with the goal of decreasing the secretion of *gonadotropins*, the pituitary hormones that stimulate the sex glands. There have been unpleasant side effects, however, and little effect upon growth and bone maturation is achieved.

The most promising treatment is the use of long-acting drugs called LHRH analogs. These drugs cause the levels of gonadotropin secretion to return to prepubertal levels and pubertal development regresses. When treatment is discontinued, hormonal levels and reproductive function return to normal. Eventual adult height is very much dependent on the age of onset of LHRH analogs.

PANCREATIC DISORDERS

THE PANCREAS, located behind the stomach, contains specialized cells in the *islets of Langerhans* that produce and secrete several hormones. The beta cells produce *insulin*, and the alpha cells produce *glucagon*. Normally these two hormones regulate the amount of glucose in the blood.

Diabetes Mellitus. Almost all carbohydrates and 50 to 60 percent of proteins are converted into glucose, which is used as fuel by most of the body cells. Diabetes mellitus is a condition in which there is either a lack of insulin or an inability of the body to use it, so that glucose levels are not properly regulated. When the body cannot utilize its glucose, it starts to burn its own fat and muscle, a potentially dangerous situation because it can allow *ketones* and other acidic by-products to accumulate in the blood. If untreated, this can lead to coma and death. However, although there is no cure for diabetes, it can be controlled well enough in most cases to allow the child to live a normal, productive life.

According to a recent classification system, there are two major forms of diabetes. Type I diabetes mellitus, or insulin dependent diabetes, is characterized by a lack of insulin production and a tendency to develop ketosis, or increased body acid. This type is sometimes referred to as juvenile diabetes since the overwhelming number of children with diabetes have this form. People with Type I diabetes form antibodies to various parts of the islet cells (the pancreatic cells that produce insulin) and have certain HLA antigens (chromosomal markers presently being used to match donors for transplantation).

Type II diabetes, also called adult onset diabetes, is usually present in older people and is strongly associated with obesity. Unlike Type I, insulin levels are usually normal or elevated. Therefore, except during illness, stress, or conditions of poor control, these people do not require insulin. On the rare occasions when Type II diabetes appears in children, it is usually in obese children. Weight reduction is the primary treatment.

In the Western world, Type I diabetes occurs in approximately one in 500 children with the prevalence peaking in the mid-teens. Every year there are approximately 16 new cases of diabetes per 100,000 children. Although it is an autoimmune disease, virral infections are thought to trigger the disease process. This may explain the increased incidence of diabetes in winter months.

Because early diagnosis prevents potential serious metabolic complications and allows for easier control, it is important that parents understand the disease process and recognize the symptoms. When insulin production is decreased, the blood sugar level is increased. This increased sugar "spills" out into the urine, forcing the kidneys to produce large volumes of urine. To compensate, the child will become very thirsty and drink excessively. Because the body cannot metabolize food normally, the child will also eat excessively but will lose weight. In an effort to supply energy, the body will also break down fats and produce an increased amount of acid.

Thus, the newly diabetic child will drink, eat, and urinate excessively, will lose weight, and may experience a recurrence of bed-wetting. Parents should notify the doctor if these symptoms persist for more than a few days.

Initially the child will be hospitalized in order to correct the metabolic abnormalities, and, more important, to educate the child and the parents on how to care for a diabetic.

Overall, the major goals of diabetic therapy are to ensure normal glucose control and normal physical growth and psychological development. It is hoped that careful control of the child's blood sugar will help delay or significantly lessen the incidence of diabetic complications. However, normal growth and psychological development are equally important.

Daily glucose stabilization is accomplished by controlling three factors: diet, exercise, and insulin.

Diet. The diabetic diet restricts the amount of concentrated sweets, although there are times when these are allowed. However, the major components of carbohydrates, proteins, and fats are similar to those of a diet for all children. Approximately 50 percent of the daily calories should be carbohydrates, 30 percent fat, and 20 percent protein. The total daily calories are divided among three meals and three snacks to provide for a more even distribution of food over the day. Foods with complex carbohydrates, high fiber content, and polyunsaturated fats are emphasized, while cholesterol intake is limited. A system of food exchanges is employed to allow for individual tastes and preferences.

Exercise. In general, the diabetic child is never restricted from participating in any sport. In fact, exercise can only be helpful in maintaining normal blood-sugar levels and lowering lipid levels. The timing and placement of insulin injections and adjustment of the diet can assure that the exercise will not be harmful. Encouragement of normal daily exercise not only helps the child medically, but assists in his or her physical and mental development.

Insulin. There are three types of insulin: regular, or rapid-acting; NPH or lente, intermediate-acting; and (rarely used) ultralente, the very long-acting insulin. These are derived from animals (either pigs or cows) or are synthesized in the laboratory (recombinant DNA).

Depending on the child's metabolic state, either one or two injections a day are used. Usually each injection is a mixture of the rapid and intermediate insulin. Other variations of insulin administration include more frequent injections each day, or use of an insulin pump that delivers a constant insulin infusion. The specific instructions are tailored for each individual child.

A major breakthrough in daily care is the use of home blood glucose monitoring. Kits and machines are now available that allow the child or family to measure the blood glucose level at home. The frequency of testing is determined by the physician. In many cases monitoring of glucose in the blood has replaced the testing of urine glucose levels.

Overall management. The use of multiple injections and home glucose monitoring have made possible both better diabetic control and less restriction on the child's daily activity. This is significant because maintaining a normal daily schedule is of prime importance when planning a child's insulin administration, diet, and exercise program.

Routine physician visits will assure normal physical growth and development. In addition to the daily blood glucose monitoring, the doctor will have blood tests done in the laboratory that can help in evaluating the long-term diabetic control. These include measurement of hemoglobin, hemoglobin A_1C, cholesterol, and triglycerides. Dietitians and psychologists can also assist in assuring complete care.

To the new diabetic and family members alike, the complex factors in diabetes management seem overwhelming at first. However, experience has shown that within two months a family with adequate education and training can become comfortable with the entire treatment process. The greater the knowledge acquired, the fuller and more independent is life for the diabetic child. The probability of reduced incidence of diabetic complications with improved control is a strong motivator. And ongoing research in islet cell transplants and implantable devices promise improved and easier control in the future.

Hypoglycemia. Infantile hypoglycemia may occur in the following situations: (1) children born to diabetic mothers; (2) severe stress during birth; (3) infants small for gestational age; (4) inborn errors of metabolism such as glycogen storage disease or galactosemia; (5) ingestion of drugs such as aspirin or alcohol; (6) endocrine dysfunctions such as adrenal insufficiency; and (7) pancreatic hyperplasia or tumor. Symptoms include apathy, turning blue, pallor, hypothermia, twitching, jitteriness, convulsions, and coma. Regardless of the cause, immediate treatment is necessary, either with glucose by mouth or with dextrose intravenously. Sometimes hormone replacement therapy may be necessary, and where a tumor is involved, removal is required.

Low blood glucose levels are fairly common in juvenile diabetes. This can be brought on by giving too much insulin, skipping a meal, or physical activity without proper food intake. This is often referred to as insulin reaction and its initial symptoms are hunger, weakness, lack of energy, or irritability. This reaction is easily avoided by eating a simple sugar. If a large and sudden drop in the blood glucose level occurs, sweating, dizziness, nausea, vomiting, and rapid pulse ensue. Prompt diagnosis and treatment are necessary to prevent coma or brain damage. Treatment consists of giving glucose immediately (an injection of glucogon if the child is unconscious or uncooperative), followed in a few minutes by a meal of carbohydrate and protein.

SUMMING UP

THE ENDOCRINE SYSTEM comprises a highly complex system of glands that enables the body to adapt and respond to its internal and external environments. Its intricate network of feedback mechanisms and chemical and neural signals keeps the system in balance. Though most endocrine disorders are rare, diabetes and thyroid disorders are relatively common. Whenever an endocrine abnormality occurs, it can cause a vast array of symptoms affecting all organ systems and even psychological responses. Continuing biotechnological advances make diagnoses increasingly accurate and the development of new and more effective therapies are a regular occurrence. Most endocrine problems can be treated either by replacing deficient hormones or curtailing the overproduction of others.

31 Allergies

William J. Davis, M.D.

INTRODUCTION

VISITS TO THE pediatrician by children with allergy symptoms constitute the greatest number of office encounters, with the exception of those for the common cold. Various studies have indicated that at least one in five children has some type of allergic problem, ranging from itchy, troublesome skin problems to rhinitis or bronchial asthma. In the United States, allergy is the leading cause of acute and chronic disease among children and adults. It causes children to miss more days from school than any other illness. Indeed, the National Institute of Allergy and Infectious Diseases indicates that 35 to 40 million Americans have allergies (see table 31.1, next page); 7 million children have hayfever, and more than 2 million children suffer from atopic dermatitis or eczema.

An allergy is an altered or abnormal response of the immune system to a foreign substance, called an allergen or antigen, that is ordinarily harmless. To the body, the world is a hostile environment, teeming with bacteria, viruses, and other invader substances. These outsiders crave the body as an ideal place to live, grow, and multiply. It is only through the body's vigilant defense network—the immune system—that we are protected.*

For children with allergies, however, the immune system can be too sensitive, responding to foreign substances that are inert and normally harmless—such as pollen, house dust, or animal dander—or ones that are even normally beneficial, such as foods or drugs. Instead of ignoring these substances, the immune system reacts to them, provoking inflammation, irritation, and many other forms of distress and discomfort in particularly sensitive sites—the skin, nose, eyes, throat, lungs, and digestive system.

Allergic problems have plagued mankind from the beginning of recorded time. Documented allergic reactions occurred in ancient Egypt and in other early civilizations. The Austrian pediatrician

---

* Portions of this chapter originally appeared in *The Columbia University College of Physicians and Surgeons Complete Home Medical Guide*, copyright © 1985 by G. S. Sharpe Communications and The College of Physicians and Surgeons of Columbia University.

Table 31.1 **ALLERGY PROBLEMS IN CHILDHOOD**

Problems	Onset	Duration/Comments
Allergic Skin Conditions		
1. Eczema or Atopic Dermatitis	Birth to 2 years, may occur later	Sometimes ends by 2 or 3; often continues to puberty until offending agent is removed
2. Contact Dermatitis	Any age	Usually ends quickly with acute allergic problem
3. Hives and Angioedema	Any age	May be chronic
Allergic Rhinitis	1–2 years (dog, cat, dust)	Until offender is removed
	4–8 years (pollen, mold)	Throughout childhood
Food Allergy	Birth to 1 year (milk, soy, egg, wheat, grains)	Until excluded from diet
	Any age (milk, soy, egg, wheat, nuts, peanuts, fish, shellfish, citrus)	Until excluded from diet
Asthma		
1. Allergy triggered	Birth to any age (food, pollen, mold)	Until substance is removed or child treated
2. Nonallergy triggered	3–6 months to any age (virus, pollutants, irritants, exercise)	Until problem avoided or treated
Drug Allergies	Throughout childhood	Until agent identified and avoided
Insect Allergies	Later childhood (8 years and older)	Can be lifelong; avoidance of sting or specific treatment

Clemens von Pirquet coined the term *allergy* in 1906 from the Greek *allos* ("change in the original state"), referring to the fact that for some people an encounter with an otherwise harmless substance produces an altered sensitivity. (See box on Common Allergy Terms.) Repeated contact or additional, repetitive exposures leads to a "hypersensitive" response and allergic disease.

The child with allergic parents or other relatives has a greater potential to be allergic than one with no such family history. With one allergic parent the newborn has a 25 to 35 percent chance of allergy and with two allergic parents the chances escalate to 50 to 60 percent. Still, allergies may occur in children with no immediate family history of them, a phenomenon that undoubtedly represents genetic mutation or spontaneous changes in genes inherited from the parents. Although potential for allergy is inherited, specific allergic problems are not. The acquisition of such specific problems depends upon the variety and repetition of exposures to foreign substances throughout the child's life.

THE ROLE OF THE IMMUNE SYSTEM

To UNDERSTAND ALLERGIES, one must first understand the immune system, whose misdirected response causes allergic reactions. The job of the immune system is to search for, recognize, and destroy germs and other dangerous invaders of the body, known as antigens. It does this by producing antibodies or special molecules to match and counteract each antigen.

The organs of the immune system are located throughout the body and are called lymphoid organs. These include the bone marrow, the thymus, the lymph nodes, and the spleen. *Lymph nodes* are small bean-shaped structures found in the neck, armpits, groin, and abdomen. They contain specialized compartments that house *B cells* and *T cells* and are filled with scavenger cells called macrophages. Here antigens stimulate antibody production.

The key soldiers of the immune system are the

COMMON ALLERGY TERMS

Allergy (hypersensitivity): An overzealous reaction to otherwise harmless antigens, resulting in allergic symptoms.

Allergen (antigen): Any foreign substance that causes specific antibodies (IgE) to be formed and can trigger an immune response. In allergic children this includes pollens, molds, dust, animal danders, foods, and drugs.

Antibody: A unique protein substance manufactured by blood plasma cells in response to a foreign antigen or allergen. In allergic reactions, the antibody is Immunoglobulin E (IgE). Other immunoglobulins, such as IgA, IgD, IgG, and IgM, protect against bacteria and viruses.

Antigen-antibody interaction: The keystone of the allergic reaction. This combination of specific antibody (IgE) and antigen takes place on the surface of specialized cells called mast cells and results in the release of chemicals (mediators) responsible for allergic symptoms.

Mast cell: A cell in body tissues that is coated with more than 100,000 IgE allergic antibodies and that releases packets of chemical mediators following allergen-IgE interaction.

Mediators: Chemicals released from mast cells in an allergic reaction that are responsible for allergic symptoms. Mediators include histamine, leukotrienes, and kinins.

Mold spores: A type of fungus living on decaying matter. Spores are microscopic parts of the mold plant that float in air currents. They are often found outdoors, in attics, and in basements.

Pollen: Microscopic grains of plant protein material used for reproduction. Trees, grasses, and weeds produce millions of light, dry, airborne granules each day.

lymphocytes, the white blood cells manufactured by the millions in the bone marrow. The lymphocytes produce antibodies specific to each unwanted antigen. Circulating in the bloodstream, the antibodies attack the antigen, or protect the body's cells from invasion by the antigen, or make the invader palatable to roaming macrophage cells. Antibody-producing lymphocytes or plasma cells are called B cells. Scientists have discovered that some lymphocytes can attack antigens directly. These are processed by the *thymus,* a lymph gland in the chest, and are called T cells. T-cell immunity is called cell-mediated, while antibody immunity is known as humoral.

Allergic symptoms and problems can develop in infancy and throughout childhood and adolescence, into early adult life. It is unusual to develop allergies after age 40.

Children with allergies may be treated by primary-care physicians or specialists such as otolaryngologists (ENTs) or allergists. An allergist is a physician who has had at least two years of formal training in a certified allergy-immunology training program beyond primary specialty training and has been certified by the American Board of Allergy and Immunology. A pediatric allergist is a board-certified pediatrician who has received advanced training in allergy and has been additionally certified by the American Board of Allergy and Immunology.

Whenever lymphocytes are activated, some of them become "memory" cells. Then the next time a person encounters the same antigen that earlier turned the lymphocytes on, the immune system "remembers" it and is primed to destroy it immediately. This is acquired immunity. Another way to acquire immunity is through immunization. Vaccines contain bits of an antigen that has been altered in some way so that it doesn't provoke a full-blown disease, but rather a weak immune response. This leaves a few memory cells standing guard to mount a quick, full-scale response should an invasion by the natural antigen occur.

The only natural immunity humans have lasts for a few months after birth. Babies are born with approximately the same antibodies their mothers have, but these soon die out. A very small number of children are born not only lacking natural immunity but also the ability to acquire immunity. Some of these immunodeficient patients may live for years in germ-free rooms or "bubbles"; a few have been successfully treated with bone-marrow transplants.

Transient immune deficiencies can develop in the wake of diseases like leukemia and multiple myeloma, and even common viral infections. Certain drugs, radiation, stress, and malnutrition can also cause temporary, but nevertheless dangerously compromising, immunodeficiency.

The immune system produces five main kinds of antibodies, but the principal one that participates in allergic reactions is *immunoglobulin* E (IgE). Every individual has different IgE antibodies, and each allergic substance stimulates production of its own specific IgE. An IgE antibody made to respond to ragweed pollen, for example, will react only against ragweed and not oak tree or bluegrass pollen.

Among people with allergies, the IgE antibodies

to specific allergens exist by the millions, attached to either a type of circulating white blood cell (basophil) or to the so-called mast cells lining the respiratory tract, the gastrointestinal tract, and the skin.

When the antibodies encounter the allergen they are programmed against, they immediately signal the *basophils* or *mast cells* to unleash *histamine* and other potent "mediating" chemicals into the surrounding tissue. It is these chemicals—mainly histamine—that cause the familiar allergic reactions. Histamine released in the nose, eyes, and sinuses, for example, stimulates sneezing, a runny nose, and itchy eyes; released in the lungs it causes narrowing and swelling of the lining of the airways and the secretion of thick mucus; in the skin, rashes and hives; and in the digestive system, stomach cramps and diarrhea.

The intensity of the reaction is directly related to the amount of histamine and other chemical mediators flooding the tissues. This in turn depends on the person's state of health and genetic makeup, or more specifically, on his total level of IgE. Scientists believe a single major gene determines an individual's IgE concentrations.

ALLERGIC SYMPTOMS IN CHILDREN

Most children will at some time develop any of a variety of problems or symptoms that may be allergic. Allergic symptoms are quite specific and are often chronic or long-lasting. Common ones and the organs they affect are:

Skin—Typically a rash appears that is almost always itchy. The rash may consist of spots that are raised, flat, red, white, hivelike, or raw and oozing.

Nose—The most troublesome area for allergic problems, the nose can be plagued by sneezing (often repetitive), itching, nasal congestion or stuffiness, and runniness (rhinorrhea). Often it is difficult to distinguish between a cold and an allergy, but in general, nasal discharge in allergies is thin, clear, and watery in appearance, in contrast to the colored, thickened mucus of a cold.

Eyes—Itching and tearing, with reddened conjunctiva (white of eye), is common. Often there is swelling of the lids and the area around the eye. (See figure 31.1 for characteristic signs.)

Mouth—Symptoms include itching of the palate and the back of throat and postnasal drip, which often precipitates a variety of throat-clearing sounds and maneuvers.

Ears—"Clogged" ears may make sound seem far away. Fluid accumulation in the middle ear results in decreased acuity or the inability to hear parents, teachers, or television sets.

Chest—A frequent cough, especially a spasmodic, dry one, may accompany shortness of breath, rapid breathing, "tightness" of the chest, and wheezing.

Gastrointestinal tract—Symptoms such as nausea, vomiting, cramps, loose stools, or diarrhea may all be part of an allergic problem.

Evaluating Childhood Allergies

Most allergic problems originate in childhood. Sneezing, wheezing, scratching, itching, and a host of other annoying symptoms eventually stimulate parents to take their child to their pediatrician for evaluation. *Every* child with suspected chronic or recurrent allergic problems (rhinitis, asthma, skin rash) deserves at least one consultation with an allergist.

Symptoms and signs of allergies in children often differ considerably from those in adults, which may be confusing to parents. Asthma, for example, frequently presents itself as a cough in infants and young children, rather than wheezing, as it would appear in older children and adults. What is more, because respiratory infections are so common in infants, the cough may be attributed to infection rather than allergy and the proper treatment not given. The same is true of skin eruptions, which are so frequent in young babies that parents often pass them off as temporary and localized irritations rather than a condition that requires medical attention.

Even when an allergy is suspected, the cause may prove to be elusive. Sometimes a child will react almost immediately to a particular food such as eggs, milk, or peanuts, and it is not necessary to look any further for clues. Another child will break out in hives or another rash, or develop uncontrollable sneezing for no obvious reason.

The allergist will do three things—take a medical history, do a physical examination, and perform various pertinent laboratory and allergy tests.

Interviewing the patient, or history-taking as physicians call it, is one of the most sophisticated and important investigation techniques in medicine today. It has no substitute. The patient must have adequate time to explain all of his or her symptoms and the doctor must take the time to ask probing questions in order to define the medical problem as specifically as possible. In an allergy evaluation, the questions asked and information obtained contrib-

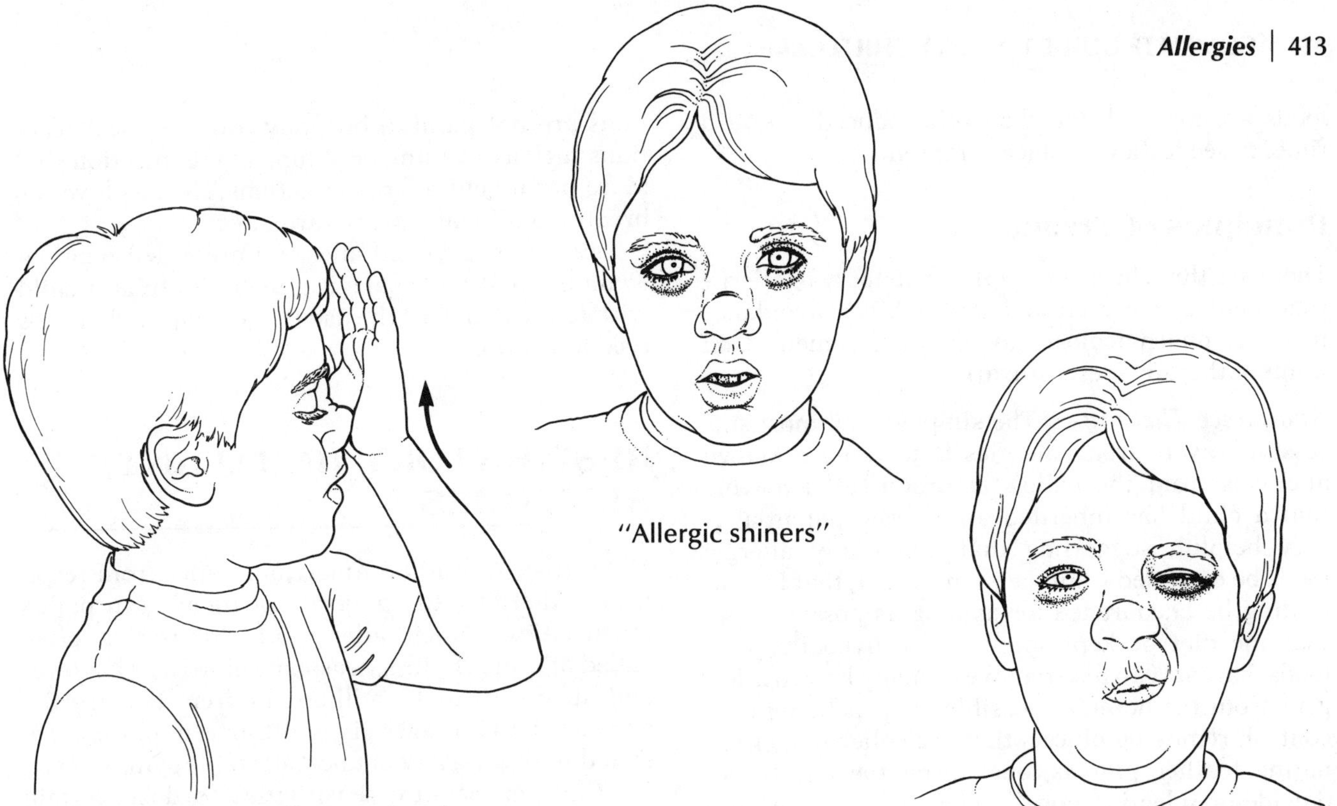

"Allergic shiners"

"Allergic salute"

"Allergic wink"

Figure 31.1. **Signs of Allergies.**

ute roughly 80 percent to the solution. The questions will cover these areas:

- the chief complaint
- any present illness
- past medical problems
- family medical history
- environment history (whether pets are kept at home, what trees are in the yard, etc.)
- food history (everything eaten or drunk for meals and snacks)
- social and emotional condition, current and past

Ideally both parents should be present with the child and should be prepared to give extensive information. Specifically, parents should think about the following points:

- when did the problem start?
- how long has it lasted?
- what circumstances are related to the problem?
- what are the symptoms and how long do they last?
- what sort of treatment has been given and with what success?

The physical examination will include a close look at the skin, eyes, nose, ears, lungs, and abdo-men. Diagnostic tests may include blood counts, nasal smears, X rays, pulmonary function tests, and various cultures to test for the presence of infectious agents such as bacteria.

Specific allergy tests may include skin tests, lab tests such as the radioallergosorbent test (RAST), and bronchial challenge.

Skin tests may be performed by the scratch, prick, or intracutaneous technique. In a skin test the doctor introduces a tiny amount of the suspected allergen into the skin. If the child is allergic to that substance, a local reaction in the form of a wheal (hive) with surrounding redness will appear within a few minutes. Skin testing is extremely reliable in identifying airborne allergens such as pollen, dust, and molds, as well as stinging insect allergies. It is not as reliable in pinpointing food allergies. Skin testing is not often employed in children under three years old.

A positive skin test, however, is not always proof that an allergen is going to cause a problem when encountered in a child's daily life. Conversely, a negative skin test does not always mean that the substance will never cause an allergic problem. Skin test results must be interpreted cautiously and in conjunction with the child's medical history. For foods, doctors prefer to have a parent keep a diet diary or put a child on an elimination diet, where foods are avoided and then reintroduced one at a time, to see if they produce symptoms.

Principles of Treatment

There are three basic principles that apply to allergy treatment of children and adults alike: avoidance therapy, pharmacologic (drug) management, and immunotherapy (desensitization).

Avoidance Therapy. The simplest and most successful way to treat allergies is to remove known allergens from the child's environment. Knowing that a child has inherited an allergic potential is very helpful, suggesting that potentially allergic foods be excluded from the infant's diet, that breastfeeding be encouraged for as long as possible, and that the diet be kept simple, with hypoallergenic foods. Parents can also remove as many known allergens from the home as possible, by practicing dust control, removing objects that are collectors, eliminating feather pillows, quartering the family pet outside or selecting nonallergenic pets, discontinuing scented cosmetics, and eliminating cigarette smoke.

Pharmacologic Management. If elimination or avoidance is not possible, it may be necessary for the doctor to prescribe medications to control symptoms and improve allergic problems for the child. The doctor will choose the medicines that are most effective for the child based upon the type of allergy, its severity, the child's tolerance, potential side effects, and parental philosophy concerning medications. Parents should always discuss their concerns about drugs with the doctor and receive an adequate explanation of what to expect before a plan is implemented.

Some commonly prescribed drugs are antihistamines and decongestants. Other agents include bronchodilators for asthma, cortisone and other steroids, and inhaled prophylactic or preventive medications such as cromolyn sodium. (Various drug therapies are discussed specifically under each condition.)

Immunotheraphy. Injections (allergy "shots") are used in conjunction with avoidance and medications to treat allergies. Through frequent injections of increasing doses of the allergen that is causing the child's problem, he or she becomes desensitized. These injections are primarily used for patients with respiratory symptoms caused by allergic rhinitis and asthma.

The goal of such therapy is eventually to eliminate or reduce the allergy symptoms and problems and to reduce the need for medication. The injections are not painful, but may produce local reactions such as swelling or itching at the injection site. More prominent allergic reactions, such as hives or breathing difficulties, are rare.

Effective modified allergens are now becoming available that will make it possible to treat a child with fewer than half the usual injections and far less risk of reactions.

RESPIRATORY (INHALANT) ALLERGIES

MORE THAN 20 million Americans suffer from respiratory allergies, the majority of them from pollen sensitivities. Pollen allergy in children is often called allergic rhinitis, seasonal rhinitis, or hayfever and affects 10 to 12 million children. It generally appears between ages six and thirteen and is associated with a variety of uncomfortable symptoms.

Children acquire sensitivities to dust, certain molds, and animal dander even before problems with seasonal rhinitis. In this case the frequent, early-on contact with these allergens in the genetically programmed child results in allergy problems as early as age two, and quite regularly in the three- to six-year-old.

Pollen

To reproduce by cross-pollination, plants make male germ cells called pollen. Those produced by flowers and taxied from one plant to another by bees are relatively large, waxy, and generally harmless to people. But the tiny, light, dry pollens thrown off in prodigious quantities by weeds, grasses, and trees—and carried on wind currents for up to 400 miles—are nasty pests to the estimated 20 million Americans with hayfever (as well as to most asthma victims). When these people breathe in airborne pollen, it combines with IgE antibodies and provokes mast cells to release histamine, which in turn causes inflammation and swelling of the fragile lining of the nose, sinuses, eyelids, and surface layer of the eyes (conjunctiva). The result: a watery nasal discharge, violent sneezing, runny eyes, nasal congestion, and an itching sensation in the nose and throat and on the roof of the mouth. Some ultrasensitive people sneeze 10 to 50 times in a row several times a day, becoming so exhausted they cannot work.

Pollen allergy is seasonal, following the cycles of nature according to local geography. Trees generally shed pollen in the spring, grasses in the early summer, and ragweed—the chief irritant east of the Rocky Mountains—in the late summer. In warm, southern states this means eight or nine months of pollen exposure a year.

After ragweed, the most significant sources of allergic weed pollen are sagebrush, redroot pigweed, careless weed, spiny amaranth, Russian thistle or tumbleweed, burning bush, and English plantain. Next to weeds in producing troublesome pollen are grasses, most notably timothy, redtop, Bermuda, orchard, sweet vernal, rye, and some bluegrasses. As for trees, almost every popular variety is a culprit, including elm, maple, oak, ash, birch, poplar, pecan, cottonwood, and mountain cedar.

Most airborne pollen is so small it is invisible—no bigger around than the width of a hair. It can enter houses through tiny cracks, screens, even window air-conditioners. One plant can generate a million pollen grains, and counts as low as 20 (grains per cubic meter of air) can provoke allergic reactions. Counts drop on rainy days and soar on hot, sunny, windy days.

Pollen counts announced on radio stations or printed in newspapers, while they may be accurate for the exact time and spot when they were taken, are practically meaningless. The amount of pollen in the air varies mile to mile and hour to hour, depending on local vegetation, wind direction and velocity, and other weather conditions. And different sampling methods produce different counts. Reports based on samples from a local network of pollen-counting stations may be more accurate.

Molds

These simple microscopic fungi abound in the environment, living in the soil and on food, plants, leather, dead leaves, and other organic matter. Though they can be destructive, causing food to spoil or clothes to mildew, they are also beneficial, speeding decay of garbage and fallen trees, helping to make cheese, and fertilizing gardens. One of the best known molds is in fact a lifesaver—penicillin, which grows on bread.

Molds reproduce by developing and shedding spores, or seeds, and these spores can cause hayfeverlike symptoms in susceptible children (strictly speaking, hayfever refers only to pollen allergy). Like pollen, mold spores are borne by the wind and predominate in the summer and early fall. But molds thrive year-round in warm climates, causing allergy at least nine months a year in most of the South and Southwest. Indoors, they also shed spores year-round, living in damp cellars, mattresses, stuffed furniture, stuffed animals, fibers, wood, and even wallpaper. Generally speaking, though, it requires exposure to dry soil or composting debris and such activities as cutting grass, harvesting crops, or walking through tall vegetation to provoke an allergic reaction.

Most mold allergy is caused by the spores of *Alternaria* and *Hormodendrum* (claudosporium), which flourish in the Midwest and grow least in dry regions. The usual indoor offenders are *Aspergillus*, *Penicillium*, *Mucor*, and *Rhizopus*.

It is impossible to avoid mold spores completely, but exposure can be minimized. Old, moldy, or mildewed books, furniture, and bedding should be discarded, and damp basements should be dried with dehumidifiers. Visible mold growths on basement and bathroom walls should be attacked with disinfectant sprays or liquids. Moldproof paint can be used in place of wallpaper, and synthetic materials should be used for furniture and bedding. Humidifiers and cold water vaporizers can also be sources and should be avoided unless kept scrupulously clean.

Animal Dander

Dander, or the scales shed from the skin, hair, and feathers of birds and animals, is a significant source of year-round allergy. In most cases, anyone allergic to pollen or molds is or will become sensitive to dander. This creates a wrenching dilemma for cat, dog, and bird lovers, because allergists say the only acceptable pets for the dander-sensitive are fish and reptiles.

Unfortunately, bathing dogs frequently does not help enough to matter. Down-stuffed pillows, quilts, and coats should also be kept out of the child's environment. For some dander-susceptible children, wool is also a problem; they should avoid clothing, bedding, or carpeting made with significant amounts of it.

Dust

Although house dust harbors pollen, mold spores, and animal dander, its principal allergen is thought to be mites, microscopic spiderlike insects found throughout the world. Mites live only during the warm months but reactions of those allergic to them are usually worse in winter. This may be because after summer the mites die and disintegrate into fragments, which can reach the respiratory tract more easily than intact mites.

Dust also contains disintegrated stuffing materials from pillows, mattresses, toys, and furniture, as well as bits of fibers from draperies, blankets, and carpets. The breakdown of these materials from prolonged use seems to make them irritants to children with allergic rhinitis, hayfever, and asthma.

Miscellaneous Irritants

There are scores of other substances that exacerbate allergic reactions once they enter the respiratory tract. These include smoke, mists, and fumes from commercial and industrial activities; insecticides, fumigants, and spray paints; smoke from pipes, cigars, and cigarettes; cosmetic powder and baby powder; and some powdered laundry detergents. Children allergic to pollen, mold spores, and dust are more than likely sensitive to one or more of these irritants, whereas those who have none of the major inhalant allergies are probably not bothered. No one with any inhalant allergy should smoke or spend much time in an environment contaminated with tobacco smoke.

Diagnosing Respiratory Allergies

Pinpointing specific allergies—sufferers usually have more than one—is no simple task. Furthermore, allergies have become a "wastebasket diagnosis"; without evidence, diverse, vague symptoms may be attributed to all kinds of allergies.

Careful notation of the time of an allergic reaction is the best starting point on the path to a correct diagnosis. For example, if a child has respiratory symptoms at the same time each year, then certain pollens or molds, depending upon geography, are suspect. Or if symptoms flare only when visiting certain people's homes, then an animal allergy could be at work. For these reasons, the physician may ask a parent to keep a diary of the child's reactions.

The next step will probably be a *skin test*, in which tiny amounts of suspected allergens are applied to the skin and the reaction is observed. Usually 6 to 12 substances are tested at the same time, each injected separately into the uppermost layer of the upper arm skin. Within 10 to 20 minutes, if any of the substances are allergenic, they will cause a pale bump, like a hive or mosquito bite, surrounded by an angry red halo (*erythema*). The bigger and more ragged-edged the bump, the greater the degree of allergic reaction, but not always. Young children ages three to six with obvious histories suggestive of a specific indoor problem (pet, dust) may require fewer tests. It is of no value to do large numbers of tests in young children whose limited exposure to allergens could result in but a few sensitivities.

Unfortunately, skin tests are far from foolproof. Not all substances to which a person shows an allergic reaction on a test will actually produce symptoms in the course of natural exposure. (This "false positive" result plagues many medical tests.) And if too much of the allergen is injected, almost anyone will seem to be allergic to it. Moreover, a few people react to the very solvent used to prepare the test solution, or just to the injection itself.

Nor are skin tests always 100 percent safe. In very rare cases, even the tiny amount of allergen being tested can trigger a systemic reaction by the entire body, rather than just a local reaction at the injection site. Unless a drug called epinephrine is administered promptly, the reaction may result in sneezing, hives, wheezing, and, very rarely, even in shock.

Because of the problems of the skin test, scientists have been searching for an alternative, but nothing superior or even equal to it has turned up. The best new diagnostic technique is a simple blood test called *radioallergosorbent test (RAST)* that determines how much of a specific kind of IgE antibody the patient carries. But the blood sample must be sent off to a special laboratory and fewer allergenic substances can be tested than with skin challenges. RAST is also less sensitive, but it is safer. Research on it is continuing.

Treatment and Control of Respiratory Allergies

If the specific causes for the respiratory allergy can be pinpointed, then the treatment is fairly simple: avoidance of the allergen. In most cases, however, causes are multiple, and treatment must be nonspecific.

The first and most important rule is avoidance of all inhalants that are proven allergens. During the pollen season, children with obvious discomfort should be kept indoors until midmorning, since pollen is released very early in the morning. Even though pollen does not become airborne at night, windows should not be left wide open. Cut flowers should not be brought into a house with an allergic child. Vacations should be planned with a thought to areas where pollen counts are low.

Making a house mold- and dust-free is sometimes difficult, but such allergens can be decreased significantly by frequent cleaning of rooms where the child spends most of his or her time, especially the bedroom. The room should be rather spartan, with no upholstered furniture, carpeting, venetian blinds, bookshelves, or stuffed animals. Bunk beds and canopy beds should be avoided, and mattresses, box springs, and pillows enclosed in allergen-proof coverings. The entire room should be damp-dusted daily.

In the rest of the house, frequent damp-dusting is also advised, along with weekly washing of scatter rugs and furniture covers. If the allergic child does the cleaning, he or she should wear a disposable surgical mask covering the mouth and nose. Disinfectant cleaners will help to remove mold from appliances in the home; mildewed rugs, bedding, clothing, and other material should be discarded at once.

All dust collectors should be removed from the rooms where the child spends time and, throughout the house, shades and wooden shutters are preferable to drapes.

Ideally the house should have a centralized system that heats, humidifies, cools, and filters the air throughout. The level of dust can be further reduced by attaching various air purifiers to the central unit. If a central unit is not available, room humidifiers and air conditioners are helpful, but humidifiers must be kept free of molds and air conditioner filters should be changed weekly. There are also portable air-purifying machines that can be used in the bedroom, but allergy sufferers should be aware of exaggerated claims for these appliances. On the other hand, an electrostatic precipitator or HEPA filter (a machine that removes pollen and dust from the air) is an advantage in homes where dust and mold still accumulate even after meticulous cleaning. Such an appliance, although expensive, will soon pay for itself in the comfort of the child.

No respiratory allergy can be cured, but its miseries can be greatly lessened. The first line of attack is avoiding the allergen as much as possible through the routines suggested above. If controlling the environment is not feasible, antihistamines and decongestants might adequately lessen the symptoms. Antihistamines are more effective when given prophylactically or at the first sign of an attack; some are sold over the counter, but the more potent ones can be obtained only with a prescription. (See table 31.2, next page.) The more effective they are, though, the greater their chances of causing drowsiness, dry mouth, and blurred vision.

Newer antihistamines terfenadine (Seldane) and astemizole (Hismanal) are effective in older children without producing drowsiness or impairment in school performance or even in the ability of a teenager to drive an automobile. There are also effective nasal sprays. Cromolyn (Nasalcrom) prevents the mast cells in the nose from releasing histamine. The nasal steroids—beclomethasone (Beconase and Vancenase) and flunisolide (Nasalide) are antiinflammatory agents that chemically resemble hormones. These drugs can be dramatically effective but they should not be used at high doses or for very long periods because of the possibility of mild atrophy (thinning) of the nasal membrane.

For long-term alleviation, there are "allergy shots," a form of immunotherapy or desensitization that involves the periodic injection of small amounts of the confirmed allergens over the course of several years. Simply put, the injections make the immune system more tolerant of the allergen. Instead of producing the troublesome IgE antibodies, the body makes a protective blocking antibody that combines with the allergen to block the release of histamine and other bothersome chemicals.

Each offending allergen has its own preparation, but several allergens can be combined in one shot. Weekly dosages begin very small and are gradually increased, but not to the point where they actually provoke allergic symptoms. It can take anywhere from 12 weeks (in the case of ragweed allergy) to two or three years to attain a maximum dose of immunization. After that, maintenance shots are given every two to six weeks, sometimes for many years. Timing is important for seasonal pollen and mold allergies. Shots should be planned so that the maximum dosage will be reached by hayfever season.

Allergy shots work well for many people—six million Americans alone get them—but they have several drawbacks. For one thing, they are inconvenient and expensive, requiring repeated visits to a physician over an indefinite period. The visits can be long since many doctors ask patients to remain in the office for up to 20 minutes after the shots to observe the reaction (in very rare instances, generalized reactions can occur).

Another drawback is that for some people allergy shots simply do not work. A program of allergy shots for a child should be carefully and frequently evaluated. If injections do not produce obvious improvement—less need for antihistamines, fewer specific symptoms, fewer trips to the hospital for emergency care—the usefulness of the program should be questioned.

ASTHMA

MORE THAN 10 million Americans, 4 to 5 million of them children under 16, have or have had asthma during their lives. In fact in some areas of the country asthma seems to affect from 5 to 10 percent of school-age children. All asthma appears to be familial, involving each generation. An exact genetic inheritance has not been elucidated, although it is suspected. In children, asthma frequently develops following a serious respiratory infection, usually a viral one. In infants, a bout of bronchiolitis may predispose the child to subsequent asthma, and the second and third episodes of respiratory distress may be asthma, rather than repeat episodes of bronchiolitis. Treatment is usually given on a year-round basis.

Table 31.2 **ANTIHISTAMINES**

Chemical Group	Generic Name	Common Brand Name	Available Forms	Comments
Ethanolamines	Diphenhydramine	Benedryl	Liquid, capsule	Very effective, but potent sedative, don't take for school
	Clemastine	Tavist	Liquid, tablet	Less drowsiness, longer duration of action
	Carbinoxamine	Rondec	Liquid, tablet, S-R*	Less drowsiness, longer duration of action
Ethylenediamines	Tripelennamine	Pyribenzamine (PBZ)	Liquid, tablets S-R*	Drowsiness and possible GI upset
	Pyrilamine	in Rynatan in Triaminic	Liquid, tablets	Drowsiness and possible GI upset
Piperazines	Hydroxazine	Atarax, Vistaril	Liquid, tablets, capsules	Used mainly for skin problems, itching, hives, causes drowsiness
	Meclizine	Antivert, Bonine	Tablets	Mild agent used for dizziness and motion sickness
Piperidines	Cyproheptadine	Periactin	Liquid, tablets	Mainly for skin problems, hives
	Azatadine	Optimine	Tablets	Effective for allergic rhinitis, less drowsiness
Phenothiazines	Promethazine	Phenergan	Liquid, tablets	Very sedative, do not take for school
	Methdilazine	Tacaryl	Liquid, tablets	Somewhat less sedation than with Phenergan

The following are over-the-counter drugs that were formerly available only by prescription. They are relatively potent.

Chemical Group	Generic Name	Common Brand Name	Available Forms	Comments
Alkylamines	Bromphenarimine	Dimetane	Liquid, tablet, S-R*	Effective with little sedation
	Chlorphenarimine	Chlor-Trimeton Allerest ARM Dristan Contac	Liquid, tablet, S-R* tablet or capsule	Effective with little sedation
	Triprolidine	in Actifed	Liquid, tablet	More sedation, but effective
New—peripheral H₁ Antagonist	Terfenadine Astemizole	Seldane Hismanal	Tablet Tablet	Effective with no sedation or central nervous system side effects

* Sustained-release tablet

Distressing in children are recent trends showing that asthma is causing more sick days, more days missed from school, more emergency treatments, and more hospitalizations, as well as an increased number of deaths. These problems are often greater in inner-city children of low socioeconomic status. In early childhood, more boys than girls have asthma, but the numbers begin to even out in the later teen years. Many younger children show improvement around age six, when airways begin to widen, and many "outgrow" their asthma after puberty.

Asthma is a chronic, reversible obstructive disease of the bronchial tubes, which supply air to the lungs. During an asthma attack, these bronchials exhibit a hypersensitive response to certain triggers. The muscle surrounding the tube goes into spasm, constricting the tubes. This is followed by stimulation of the mucous glands, producing clogged airways, and irritation and inflammation of the lining of the bronchials, which further contributes to the narrowing.

A child suffering an asthma attack will experience a variety of symptoms, including coughing, shortness of breath, tightness in the chest, wheezing, apprehension, restlessness, fright, and fatigue.

Asthma problems can be mild or severe, rare, infrequent, or chronic. Asthma may be triggered by a variety of allergic and nonallergic stimuli. Nonallergic triggers, which are more common, include: viral infections; tobacco smoke; polluted air; irritants such as paint, insecticides, perfume, hair sprays, and strong odors; weather changes, especially cold air; and exercise. Allergic triggers include pollens, inhalants, danders, foods, and dust. In individuals with very hyperactive airways, even laughing, crying, coughing, or rapid breathing will result in asthma.

Exercise-induced asthma is the major problem for the school-age child, as running is a major trigger of the hyperreactive airway. This problem can often be managed prophylactically with before-exercise drug treatment.

Accumulating medical evidence about asthma mechanisms suggests that chronic inflammation of the bronchioles acts as a stimulus for hyperactivity, or "twitchiness" of the airway. Greater understanding of these mechanisms through research should lead to more effective control of the problem. The development of a preventive approach is critical to successful management.

Controlling Allergen-Induced Asthma

The same basic principles of control—avoidance, drugs, and immunotherapy—that apply to allergic rhinitis apply to asthma as well. The first step in controlling allergen-induced asthma is the removal of offending allergens: from feather pillows to (sad as it may be) the family cat or dog, if the pet is the cause of the problem. Dust control and avoidance of irritants in the house are important. (For specific measures, see the section above on treatment and control of respiratory allergies.) Air conditioning may be helpful, as may air-filtration systems when pollens and molds are causes of asthma.

Pharmacologic management of asthma is discussed in detail in chapter 22, Childhood Respiratory Disorders. It should be pointed out here that cromolyn sodium (Intal), known to be effective in controlling allergic asthma attacks by inhibiting mediator release from mast cells, has been demonstrated to be an effective prophylactic agent for preventing asthma attacks in the first place.

Immunotherapy is effective in asthma, as it is in allergic rhinitis, and information found in chapter 22 is applicable here, too.

To track his or her progress, the child with asthma should have regular, objective pulmonary function monitoring, through a combination of laboratory tests and a simple peak flow monitor that can be used at home.

Goals of Asthma Management for Children

The primary goal in treating asthmatic children is to maintain as normal a life-style as possible, one that allows the child to participate in normal daily activities and sports with few, if any, restrictions. This goal is best achieved through educating the child and family to understand, accept, and manage asthma.

Successful management means gaining maximum control of symptoms with a minimum number of the safest medications, preventing acute episodes that require emergency treatment, reducing the number and frequency of hospitalizations, relieving airway obstruction, and normalizing pulmonary function. These in turn promote normal growth and development, reduce school absenteeism, and improve long-term prognosis. These goals should be regularly reviewed and management changed or modified to meet them. (Also see chapter 22, Childhood Respiratory Disorders.)

SKIN ALLERGIES

THE LARGEST organ of the human body—the skin—is much abused in childhood by scrapes, scratches, cuts, and bruises. But the condition that causes the greatest distress is allergy. Skin allergies can be divided into three types: atopic dermatitis, allergic contact dermatitis, and urticaria (hives).

Atopic Dermatitis (Eczema)

Principally a disorder of infancy and childhood, atopic dermatitis is characterized by extreme itching; persistent, frantic scratching; and thickening of the skin. Although the specific cause of eczema remains unknown, all patients have a highly sensitive skin susceptible to dermatitis. They also suffer from abnormal sweating, decreased skin-oil production, and a low itch threshold; things like heat, abrasions, and psychological tension can set them to scratching.

Up to 3 percent of infants develop eczema. Most come from families prone to allergy and suffer from other allergic disorders such as hayfever and asthma. Children usually outgrow the disorder by age six, with delayed improvement setting in at puberty.

The eczematoid rash is usually found on the cheeks, ears, and neck in infancy and the inner creases of the elbows and knees of toddlers, but it may involve the entire body, sparing virtually no area. The skin rash of eczema is characterized by its acute and chronic appearance:

Acute stage—redness, swelling of skin, scratched areas, weeping, oozing surface areas.
Chronic stage—dry, irritated, thickened, scaling leathery appearance.

Successful treatment depends on breaking the itch-scratch-itch cycle. General treatment measures for children include increasing relative humidity in the home, avoiding contact with allergens, wearing cotton clothing, controlling the diet (in cases of a causal food allergy) and avoiding emotional upsets. More specific measures are directed at control of itching, skin lubrication, and treatment of inflamed skin.

When itching is controlled, skin lesions tend to heal on their own. Antihistamines most effective for itch control are hydroxyzine (Atarax, Vistaril), diphenhydramine (Benadryl), and cyproheptadine (Periactin). In difficult cases, a physician will prescribe a dosage level that promotes sedation.

Regular lubrication of the skin is paramount in the management of atopic dermatitis. Moisturizers, lubricants, and emollients help to retain water within the superficial layers of the skin. Such over-the-counter preparations as Aquaphor, Eucerin, Keri Lotion, Lubriderm, and Compound 15 work quite effectively. Bathing requires the use of bland, neutral soaps such as Dove, Basis, Neutrogena, or Lowilla. For children who cannot tolerate baths, Cetaphil, a fat-free skin cleanser, is available.

Inflammatory reactions of the skin require aggressive use of topical cortisone preparations. These preparations (creams, gels, and ointments) vary in their potency and should only be used under the direction of a physician. Milder agents are required for "thin-skinned" areas of face, neck, and groin, while stronger agents may be used elsewhere.

Contact Dermatitis

This is an inflammation of the skin caused by an irritant, such as a strong acid or alkali, or by an allergy. In contrast to respiratory allergy, contact dermatitis is a delayed-type hypersensitivity produced by the T cells and not by IgE antibody. In infants, the most common cause is urine that produces a rash on the buttocks and in the anal area. This is an irritant, not an allergic reaction. In older children, the most common cause is exposure to poison ivy, poison oak, and poison sumac. Other problem sources for children include soaps and detergents, dyes and chemicals in furniture and toys, household paints, polishes, and sprays.

Plants.   About half of all children are allergic to poison ivy, poison oak, and poison sumac, with reactions ranging from slight to severe. The offending agent in all three plants is an oily resin called *urushiol* that can be picked up directly by accidental rubbing or indirectly by touching clothing or pets that have come in contact with it. It takes only a tiny amount to provoke a reaction. But urushiol must actually be touched to cause a problem; it's a myth that a rash can result from just being near poison ivy. Also contrary to popular belief, neither washing nor scratching the rash and blisters will spread the outbreak; there is no urushiol in the blister fluid.

It usually takes one or two days for the skin to begin reacting to poison ivy, but in the highly sensitive it may start within as little as four hours. At first the exposed skin becomes red and then bumps and blisters arise, usually accompanied by itching and swelling. The rash peaks at about five days and will disappear within one or two weeks even without treatment. Outbreaks rarely occur on the scalp, palms, or soles. Scratching the blisters risks introducing bacteria into the open sores, causing secondary infection.

The desert plant heliotrope, characterized by bluish-purple flowers on a stem that coils into the shape of a fiddle neck, can also cause contact dermatitis. Skin rashes are usually confined to the ankles and legs of children walking through desert landscapes in the Southwest. The leaf and the pollen of the ragweed is another, though infrequent, cause of skin rashes; both contain a resin that dissolves in the natural oil of the skin. Other plants associated with skin rashes are sagebrush, wormwood, daisies, tulips, and chrysanthemums. A few children even have reactions to handling such foods as oranges, limes, mangoes, celery, carrots, and potatoes.

If the offending oils from poison ivy and the other plants can be washed off within five minutes of contact, a reaction may well be prevented. Washing after that won't be protective, but it at least will contain the area of involvement. Not only the exposed skin but also clothes should be washed with strong laundry soap and water as soon as possible. Rubbing alcohol should be avoided, as it tends to make the rash worse.

Itching can be relieved with calamine lotion, a poultice of baking soda or Epsom salts, or an over-the-counter ointment containing hydrocortisone. Severe cases, or outbreaks on the face or genitals, may require prescription cortisone ointments, antihistamines, and in some cases oral cortisone.

There is no practical way to desensitize the average person to poison ivy and its relatives, so avoidance is essential. Poison oak is more shrublike than poison ivy and its leaves are shaped something like those of oak trees. It grows mainly on the West Coast and in the Southeast. Poison sumac, which favors swampy habitats, is a small five-foot tree that produces telltale clusters of green berries. Harmless sumacs have red, upright berry clusters.

Cosmetics. Cosmetics in general are quite safe, and the proportion of users who develop allergic reactions is small. For susceptible children, the most common allergens are hair dye, eye shadow and eye makeup, lipstick, and nail polish. Less frequently, antiperspirants, perfumes, and colognes cause reactions.

Because the skin reaction—usually rash and inflammation—can be mistaken for other dermatologic conditions, many doctors will do patch tests. These involve applying suspected allergens to the skin, covering them, and waiting two days to see if a reaction occurs. Patch tests are the best single means of confirming a cosmetic as an allergen.

When allergy is suspected or confirmed, the use of cosmetics made with "hypoallergenic" ingredients is an alternative. A list of firms that make truly nonallergenic cosmetics is available without charge from the Asthma and Allergy Foundation of America in Washington, D.C.

Chemicals and Metals. Formaldehyde, chlorine, phenol or carbolic acid, the various forms of alcohol, and other chemicals, as well as metals such as chrome, nickel, mercury, and beryllium can cause skin reactions among those who have developed a sensitivity to them after years of low-level exposure.

Most often, the rash—accompanied by itching and swelling—will break out within 24 to 48 hours of contact with the irritant material. It will then build in severity for up to a week and gradually go away. Certain allergens, such as film developers and rubber chemicals, can cause hives (urticaria) instead of the classic red rash and blisters.

Most allergy-generating exposure to chemicals and metals occurs in certain industrial occupations, but because the substances are used in many household products—ranging from furniture to insecticides and antifreeze to nylon—sensitivity can build up in the home as well. Of all the offending chemicals, formaldehyde is by far the most ubiquitous. A highly active compound that exists in nature as a gas, it has little odor but can cause a burning sensation in the eyes and mucous membranes. It is found in foam insulation, particle board or wallboard (used in construction and in nearly all furniture), rugs, carpets, permanent-press clothing, waxes, dyes, polishes, plaster, and paper. A by-product of gasoline combustion, it also exists as a pollutant in the atmosphere.

Not surprisingly, specific chemical and metal allergens can be difficult or even impossible to pin down. The physician will have to ask detailed questions about work and leisure activities and do careful examinations of the rash so as not to mistake it for other skin disorders. The best means of confirming a suspected allergen is with a patch test. A tiny amount of the allergen is placed on the skin and left covered for two days to see if a reaction occurs.

The treatment for all types of contact dermatitis—essentially the same as that for poison ivy (see section above on plants)—can only somewhat alleviate the symptoms, so the best strategy is avoidance. In the case of formaldehyde, this may not be feasible, but at least protective steps can be taken. New permanent-press clothing should be washed several times before use; products made with particle board should be coated with a sealant, and homes insulated with formaldehyde foam should be avoided.

Drugs. Aspirin and ampicillin often cause skin rashes, but these are not usually true allergic reactions. Agents that provoke actual contact dermatitis because of an allergic response are novocaine and other local anesthetics, penicillin, neomycin, streptomycin, and the sulfa drugs.

Urticaria and Angioedema

Urticaria (hives) is a rash consisting of wheals or blotches that itch and sometimes burn. Angioedema is a more diffuse swelling that may affect the hands, feet, eyelids, lips, genitals, and mucous membranes. In evaluating these conditions, a detailed history and a two- to four-week diary are crucial. Treatment can be with antihistamines, epinephrine, terbutaline, cimetidine, cromolyn, and rarely, oral cortisone.

Antihistamines, particularly hydroxyzine (Atarax or Vistaril) and diphenhydramine (Benadryl) should be used first in managing hives and angioedema. Most episodes will be acute and self-limited and will respond with a few doses of medication. Some problems become chronic (exist for more than six weeks) and require continuous antihistamine therapy.

Severe, generalized hives or *angioedema* should be treated by epinephrine (Adrenalin) injection, which will produce relief rapidly. Continued treatment with antihistamines is often necessary.

Difficult cases of urticaria or angioedema unresponsive to antihistamines may require treatment with oral corticosteroids such as Prednisone or Medrol. These powerful antiinflammatory medications have significant undesirable effects and should be reserved for cases that fail to respond to milder drugs.

A rare hereditary form of hives, called *hereditary angioedema (HAE)*, exists as a disorder of a blood protein that is part of the immune system. It causes nonitchy swelling and often includes cramping abdominal pain and diarrhea. The condition can be dangerous if the throat swells (laryngeal edema). Treatment is with specialized hormones.

FOOD ALLERGIES

PROBABLY MORE misguided apprehension and misinformation surround food allergies than any other type of allergic disease. The result is that many people think they are sensitive to certain foods when in fact they are not.

A common source of confusion is that a bad reaction to food can be caused by factors other than allergy: contamination by a toxin-producing bacteria, irritable bowel syndrome, stress, an inability to digest a particular substance, such as lactose in milk or gluten in wheat (called food intolerance). Some people can even talk themselves into allergiclike reactions. Another cause of misdiagnosis: popular books that blame foods for conditions they couldn't cause—fatigue, nervousness, painful menstrual cramps, and bed-wetting, to mention only some.

Food intolerance and food allergy are often confused but are quite distinct: those with intolerance lack certain enzymes needed for digestion, while those with allergy have an antibody response. The enzyme lactase, for example, helps digest one of the sugars in milk, and when it is absent the undigested milk fraction causes abdominal cramps and diarrhea—clearly not an allergic reaction. Most peoples of the world, except those from Northern Europe or descended from Northern Europeans or other pastoralists, cannot (except as infants) tolerate cow's milk or any product, including baby formula, to which milk or milk solids have been added. (Many lactose-intolerant people can, however, consume hard cheeses and cultured dairy products like yogurt and sour cream, in which much of the lactose is predigested.) A blood test can confirm lactose intolerance.

Another common intolerance is for the glutamate in the food additive monosodium glutamate (MSG). Susceptible children experience dizziness, sweating, ringing in the ears, and a feeling of faintness shortly after eating MSG-laden foods. Because so many Chinese dishes call for MSG, the reaction is sometimes called "Chinese restaurant syndrome."

Some children have a mild intolerance to vegetables—especially peas and broccoli, which cause intestinal gas. Others experience indigestion and diarrhea when they consume mushrooms.

A true food allergy produces a set of specific allergic symptoms, and this relationship can be repeatedly demonstrated. Classic symptoms are abdominal pain, diarrhea, nausea or vomiting, cramps, hives, eczema, swelling of the eyes, lips, face, and tongue, and occasionally, hayfeverlike reactions. Foods most often incriminated include cow's milk, eggs, nuts, fish or shellfish, chocolate, wheat, corn, berries, peas, beans, and gum arabic, a thickener used in processed foods.

A few foods provoke a reaction almost as soon as they are put in the mouth and thus are easy to identify and eliminate from the diet. Most, though, are difficult to pinpoint, not only because of their delayed reaction but because some provoke reactions only at certain times or in certain quantities or with a certain frequency of consumption. Degree of cooking also modifies the allergic response, and additives—mainly vegetable gum thickeners and yellow food dye No. 5—can sometimes be the culprits rather than the food itself.

Diagnosing Food Allergies

Doctors will usually begin their detective work in tracking down food allergens by taking a detailed history of the child's diet and its relationship to the complaints. One of the first and easiest steps for a parent is to keep a detailed record of what and when the child eats and drinks (including snacks), and what happens.

Another method of diagnosis is an elimination program, which should be undertaken *only under a doctor's supervision*. In general these programs require avoiding all but a few foods. After a week or so the abandoned items are added back to the diet one by one. Or if certain foods are suspected, they are eliminated for at least a week and then added back one at a time in excess quantity to see if a reaction occurs. On one such program, a child is given nothing but the two foods that rarely produce allergic reactions—lamb and rice. After 10 days, one food or food group is added every few days. When the allergy-causing food appears in the diet, the symptoms will appear again.

Skin and blood tests have limited value in testing for food allergies, because most extracts used in testing are prepared from the food in its raw or fresh state; yet patients with positive test results eat it in cooked form, which may so alter the allergen that it will not produce an allergic reaction. Conversely, a negative skin test, also to the food itself, may belie the fact that the sensitizing allergen may be a breakdown product of the digestion of the food. A child may, as a result of an erroneous skin or blood test, be put on an unnecessary avoidance diet, which may lead to long-lasting food phobias as well as harmful effects on growth and development.

One valuable but complicated way to confirm a food as an allergen is for the doctor to challenge the patient with the food in a "double-blind" fashion in which neither the doctor nor the child knows whether the suspect item has really been administered (a nurse or other third party keeps track of things). This is done by making a dried preparation of the food and enclosing it in opaque capsules. If the child reacts to capsules with the test food but not the blanks—and does so more than once—this confirms that the food is allergenic.

Common Food Allergens

Almost all foods are capable of producing an allergic reaction. What follows is a brief overview of the most common foods that have been found to cause allergic reactions in children.

Cow's Milk. This is believed by many doctors to be the most common food allergen, and the culprit seems to be a protein called *lactalbumin*, to which infants become easily sensitized. Because infants are slow in producing the antibody (IgA) that normally blocks absorption of this and other milk proteins, the allergenic proteins are free to be absorbed from the intestinal tract into the body where they produce allergies. The trend today toward breast-feeding is beneficial because mother's milk is extraordinarily rich in IgA and can protect a baby from absorbing harmful milk allergens during the first three months of life.

Eggs. Allergies usually develop to the *albumin* in egg white rather than to the fatty yolk. Egg allergy is sometimes associated with an allergy to chicken and other poultry. Eggs are a difficult food to avoid because they appear in so many different foods as well as in vaccines used in young children.

Cereals. Wheat and corn are the most frequent offenders in this group and are used in so many ways in so many different foods that complete elimination is difficult. Barley and rice, on the other hand, rarely cause problems and hence are often the first cereals offered to infants.

Nuts. These usually can be easily identified in foods, except when they are ingredients in baked goods and ice cream in powdered or crumb form. Nut sensitivity is not as common as other food sensitivities, but when it does occur, it is generally very acute, producing asthma, swelling, and severe skin reactions.

Fruits. Fruits with seeds are usually the more allergenic. Symptoms generally occur more often after eating raw fruit than cooked, canned, or preserved varieties.

Vegetables. The most common offenders are the legumes (beans, peas, peanuts), and tomatoes. As with fruits, a child may be allergic to the raw versions and not the cooked. Soybean, a member of the legume family, has recently been used extensively as a milk substitute for children who are intolerant to milk. Because of this, doctors are beginning to notice a significant increase in allergy to soybean.

Fish and Seafood. These may produce immediate and sometimes violent reactions. Sometimes even the odor of cooking will bring on the allergic reaction. Group reactions are common, and children who are proven allergic to one fish (reaction usually occurs the second time the fish is eaten) may react to other members of the fish family, even those they have never eaten before.

Spices and Condiments. Children tend not to like highly spiced foods, which explains the infrequent appearance of allergies to this group of foods. But when symptoms do appear, they are often very severe. Mustard is the most powerful allergen in this group.

Vegetable Gums. These ingredients, not foods in the strict sense, are used in many foods to add bulk and thickness. They are found in fillings of candies, creamed cheese, whipped creams, cake icings, toothpaste, commercial potato salad, gelatin desserts, wheat cakes, cupcakes, and chewing gums.

Managing Food Allergies

If a food produces an immediate and severe reaction in a child, it should never, under any circumstances, be included in the diet. If the reaction is delayed and mild, the food may be eliminated for six months and then reintroduced into the diet in very small amounts.

When food is prepared at home it is easier to control food elimination, but this doesn't mean that a child with food allergies can never eat in a restaurant. A request to the kitchen should bring forth an exact listing of ingredients; reasonable preparation changes can be requested, too. When in doubt, it is best to stick to the simplest items on the menu.

Symptomatic treatment should be given whenever appropriate. For example, gastrointestinal symptoms such as vomiting, diarrhea, and abdominal pain, which often accompany food allergy, should be treated as though they occurred in a nonallergic child. (See chapter 23, Gastrointestinal Disorders.)

The early feeding of solid foods to infants, with their immature digestive systems, invites absorption of food in an undigested state and probably increases the likelihood for allergic reactions. After four to six months, new foods may be introduced one at a time to see if a specific food causes an allergic reaction. In families where there is a history of allergy, foods that commonly cause allergic reactions should be delayed until the child is a year old or older.

Sometimes, despite the best efforts of both the doctor and the parents, the cause of a suspected food allergy cannot be found. In such cases the doctor may prescribe antihistamines or other drugs to relieve the symptoms. No drug is curative or preventive. Attempts to produce tolerance to foods by allergy shots have been unsuccessful. Fortunately, many food allergies disappear as the child grows older.

DRUG ALLERGIES

WHILE ANYONE can develop a drug allergy, children are less vulnerable because they are less likely to have the exposure necessary to acquire sensitization. Still, about 20 percent of children are allergic to drugs.

There is a difference between drug intolerance and drug sensitization. The child who is intolerant of a drug expresses reactions often associated with that drug (drug-specific), but to a much greater degree. The child may even show signs of a toxic reaction to the drug, as though he or she had taken an overdose. On the other hand, a true drug-sensitization reaction results in symptoms that are identical regardless of the drug. The allergic drug reaction is not dose related and can be caused by minute doses.

Drug allergies can show up in almost any organ of the body. The most frequently encountered reactions are: systemic (respiratory distress, serum-sickness-like reaction, fever, swelling of the throat); skin (dermatitis, skin eruptions, eczema); blood (anemia, coagulation defects); gastrointestinal (nausea, vomiting, diarrhea, gastritis, peptic ulceration); and neurological (dizziness, psychosis).

Almost any drug is capable of causing an allergic reaction, but penicillin—including relatives like ampicillin—is the major offender. Other medications children are sensitive to include the sulfa drugs, anticonvulsants, insulin, local anesthetics, and contrast dyes used in X-ray studies. As for over-the-counter medicines, aspirin is one of the most common drug offenders. Even the most minute dose of aspirin in a highly sensitive child can be dangerous, especially if the child has asthma.

Because drugs are so important in modern medicine, children with known allergies are sometimes successfully induced to tolerate them. The drug is given in slowly increasing doses until therapeutic levels are reached. In some patients, the immune system comes to tolerate the drug permanently. Another strategy is to give antihistamines and steroids before and along with the drug, thereby countering the allergic reaction.

In the case of penicillin, skin testing can predict sensitivity in nearly all patients. Skin testing can also forewarn of allergy to insulin, but for almost all other drugs, it is ineffective or dangerous.

Experience, then, is the only means of uncovering sensitivity to most drugs. In this kind of discovery process, the doctor relies strongly on the parents' accurate and detailed recall about the drug the child has taken—when, where, how much, the length of time before symptoms appeared, and what other medications were in use at the time. Parents will often fail to report the concurrent use of nose-drops, laxatives, cold remedies, and other products purchased off the drugstore shelf because they don't consider them to be "drugs." Once a child is confirmed to be allergic to one or more drugs, this information must be passed on to any new doctor during the initial visit.

INSECT ALLERGIES

FOR MOST CHILDREN, an insect sting is a mildly uncomfortable event. But for those allergic to insects, it can cause a serious and even dangerous reaction. Their skin breaks out in hives, their eyes itch, chest and throat feel constricted, a dry cough comes on, and there is often nausea, abdominal pain, vomiting, and dizziness.

Children are subject to more stings but, fortunately, do not experience the very severe sensitivity that one sees in adults. Therefore, loss of consciousness or shock in a child who has been stung is very rare.

Unfortunately there is no way to know in advance which children will have an allergic reaction to an insect sting. Presence of other allergies is not a clue, because allergy to insects may exist in those who have no other allergies.

An allergic reaction to an insect is not to the insect per se, only to its venom. Toxic components of the venom cause the irritating local reactions that everyone gets. It is the venom's other chemicals, those that provoke the release of histamine, which in turn provokes allergic responses. In the United States, only a few stinging insects—honeybees, bumblebees, wasps, hornets, yellow jackets, and fire ants—cause the serious allergic reactions. Of these six, reactions to the yellow jacket and the honeybee are the most common. Mild reactions can be caused by biting flies, mosquitoes, ticks, and a few spiders.

A reaction to an insect sting can be immediate or delayed. In most cases, the sooner the reaction starts the more severe it will be. Systemic responses usually begin in 10 to 20 minutes. Delayed reactions can occur several hours to several days later, producing a form of serum sickness—painful joints, fever, hives, and swollen lymph glands. Both immediate and delayed reactions can occur in the same person following a single sting.

Diagnosis. If the offending insect is not available, the doctor may be able to identify the culprit by asking about its appearance, mode of movement, and the time of day and the place where the sting occurred. Some insects leave telltale mouthparts or a stinger in the skin, while others, such as the fire ant, make characteristic patterns of multiple bites. (See box on The Sting.) Unfortunately, although most children are "sure" about the insect that stung them, they are seldom correct. All stinging insects are bees to some, wasps to others, and hornets to still others. It is always helpful if the insect can be caught and brought to the doctor.

A diagnosis can often be confirmed with a skin test, but the test cannot be given until a few weeks after the sting, by which time the body has replenished its supply of IgE antibodies used up during the allergic reaction. The arm is the usual site for the test because a tourniquet can be applied to impede absorption of the tiny venom sample if the patient reacts too strongly to it.

The radioallergosorbent test (RAST) may also be used. A blood sample is taken and sent to a lab where it is exposed to a specially prepared venom from the suspected insect. The test reveals whether the patient produces an IgE antibody in response to the venom.

Treatment. The first goal of treatment is to keep the amount of venom in the blood as low as possible. Honeybees leave their stinger in the skin, so it should be removed immediately. If the sting is on

THE STING

Venom is generally believed to contain a number of proteins that act as allergens to cause an allergic response in sensitive individuals. Some children are allergic to one insect, others are sensitive to two or more. Most often, however, a child who is allergic to one insect will be similarly allergic to others. The following are some common insects a child might encounter outdoors:

Honeybee. This is the most common of the stinging insects, but only the female stings. She has a squat, hairy body, with bright yellow or black markings. Her stings are easy to identify because she usually leaves her barb-shaped stinger in the skin (loss of the stinger is fatal to the bee). A soft, white bulb-shaped sac contains the venom and is attached to the embedded stinger. The stinger and the venom will be driven farther into the victim's skin by muscle contractions of the sac, even after the bee flies away to die. The stinger should be flicked or scraped off, rather than plucked; attempts to grasp it between the fingers may drive it even farther into the skin.

Wasp. A narrow pinched waist identifies this insect. Most are hairless and are black, brown, or dark red. The sting is quite similar to the honeybee's, with one exception: the stinger is not barbed. That means that the wasp, not injured by the sting, may continue stinging the same person in other places, or go on to another victim.

Hornet. The black-and-yellow striped body of this insect is easy to identify; its sting is just like the sting of the wasp.

Yellow-Jacket. This insect may be mistaken for a hornet, but it is smaller. It is especially attracted to sweet foods and is often found at picnics. The sting is like that of the wasp or hornet.

Fire Ant. This insect has a volatile temper and a well-developed abdominal stinger. When angered, the fire ant will attach to the skin and bite with strong jaws. The ant then turns in a circle, inflicting multiple stings that feel similar to bee stings. Fire ants are found only in the southern United States. Travelers should be wary of them.

the arm or leg, a tourniquet should be applied above it and loosened briefly every 10 minutes so that circulation is not impaired. A cold pack will help reduce pain and swelling.

A serious response should be treated as an emergency. A double dose of antihistamine will decrease the severity of the reaction, but *the most effective treatment is an injection of epinephrine (Adrenalin).* In acute shock or airway closure, intravenous fluids, oxygen, and a surgical opening in the windpipe (tracheotomy) may be necessary. Steroids, which act more slowly than epinephrine, may be given for persistent swelling and hives.

For children with a known serious insect allergy, physicians recommend two precautionary measures. First, the child should wear a Medic Alert identification bracelet or tag or have some other visible form of information stating the specific allergy. Second, on any family outing, parents should carry an emergency kit (available only by prescription) containing epinephrine in a syringe ready for injection, antihistamine tablets, a tourniquet, and alcohol swabs. The kit is not intended to replace medical help, but to buy precious time to get the victim to a hospital emergency room. A preloaded, spring-propelled Epi-pen injection can be successfully self-administered by most children after adequate demonstration.

Prevention. Just as allergy shots can be used to help build up tolerance to pollens and other respiratory allergens, children with known allergies to insects can obtain protection via periodic injections. Extracts of the offending insect's venom are used and, at first, the weekly shots are very weak. Gradually the strength of the extract builds until the child can tolerate what might be a normal exposure to a sting or bite. Once the maintenance dose is reached, it is given at four- to six-week intervals throughout the year. The maintenance shots must be continued indefinitely; if they are stopped, the child returns to the same level of risk as before he or she started.

Avoidance. Susceptible children should be made as unattractive to insects as possible. To bees, brown or black clothing is provocative, whereas white is not. Scented soaps, perfumes, suntan lotions, and other cosmetics should not be used on or around children out of doors. Recent studies indicate that treatment may be successfully discontinued in some children after several years with continued immunity.

Another preventive strategy is to avoid loose-fitting clothes that would allow the insect to get between the garment and the skin. And as little skin should be bared as possible, despite the warm weather; thus, closed shoes are preferable to sandals.

Picnics are a bad idea because they attract yellow jackets and ants. Garbage cans should be kept clean, sprayed with an insecticide, and tightly closed. Trees laden with ripe fruit should be avoided, and allergic children should not be allowed to work in a garden or on a lawn. When susceptible children are in a car, windows should be kept closed if reasonable. They should be trained not to panic, flail their arms, or make sudden movements, but to remain calm if a stinging insect lands on their body.

ANAPHYLAXIS

CHILDREN are not usually subject to the violent allergic reaction known as anaphylaxis, but it can be dangerous or fatal if it does occur. The main reaction is a constriction or narrowing of the airways and the blood vessels, resulting in difficult breathing, rapid pulse, a fall in blood pressure, and even cardiovascular collapse and shock.

Anaphylaxis can result from reactions to drugs, such as penicillin, insulin, aspirin, and contrast materials used in X rays; horse serum (now rarely used); insect stings; and certain foods. Even everyday respiratory allergens like pollen can sometimes provoke reactions that suddenly escalate into anaphylaxis. If a child is known to have severe reactions to any of the above allergens or to insect stings, an *Epi-pen* or emergency kit containing epinephrine should always be kept in the house and brought along on outings.

The therapy for anaphylaxis is an immediate injection of epinephrine, which opens up the airways and blood vessels. Other medications may be used to aid breathing or increase the blood pressure; these include antihistamines, oxygen, steroids, and aminophylline. These treatments are only available in a hospital emergency room. Anaphylactic shock is a critical medical emergency in which just a few minutes' delay in getting treatment can be fatal.

32 Childhood Skin Disorders

Fred Bomback, M.D.

INTRODUCTION

"Baby's skin" is often cited as the paragon of a lovely, clear, soft, dewy complexion. But this image doesn't always fit reality. An infant's skin is subject to a number of the same disorders as adults' skin, as well as to others unique to infancy and early childhood. A baby's skin is just the first stage in a journey that winds through childhood, adolescence, adulthood, and for females, pregnancy and menopause. Parents can't change genetics or the future destiny of their child's skin, but it is possible to give baby's skin a smooth start in life.

From the temperature- and humidity-controlled, protected and sterile environment of the uterus, a newborn emerges into the cooler, dryer, less protected, and unsterile environment of the world. The skin has some adjustments to make! From the moment of birth and throughout a human's lifetime, skin is in a continuous state of change, evolving from the "new" skin of infancy to the "old" skin of adulthood.

A baby's skin does differ from adult skin. An infant's skin is more sensitive and reactive because it is thinner, less hairy, more permeable and absorbent. It is more prone to infection because it does

427

not yet have protective surface bacteria, or "flora." Nor has it developed its full working complement of sweat or sebaceous (oil) glands.

TRANSIENT SKIN CONDITIONS OF THE NEWBORN

THE "BIRTHDAY SUIT"—the skin for the first few hours and days of life—comes into the world with some preexisting characteristics, the result of accommodations to life in the amniotic fluid and in the womb.

Vernix Caseosa

At birth, the skin is covered by a slightly greasy white material known as the *vernix caseosa*. It is formed by secretions from the sebaceous glands as well as materials derived from the natural decomposition of the outermost layers of skin (the epidermis) while in the womb. The vernix forms a moistureproof seal against the amniotic fluid so that the developing infant's skin does not get waterlogged. Some of this coating is wiped off right after delivery to make the baby look more presentable to the parents. This hasty swabbing may leave the skin looking red and blotchy, but the skin color soon evens out. Any remaining vernix should be left on the skin to wear off naturally, usually with successive changes of clothing and routine cleansings.

Scratches and Bruises

These result from the "labor" of birth. These marks are all common skin disturbances in the newborn, arising from a stressful trip through the birth canal. Bruising may occur if forceps are used to facilitate delivery. These conditions are temporary and clear up within the first few days or weeks.

Hair

A newborn's body may also be completely or partially covered by soft, downy hair. This hair develops in the uterus and helps repel amniotic fluid, protecting the skin. This hair is usually shed just prior to birth, but fuzzy patches may remain, noticeably on the back and shoulders, especially if the baby is premature. Similarly, some infants are born with a full head of hair, while others are not. Soon after delivery, both body and scalp hair are usually shed and will be replaced in time with permanent hair.

Peeling

In the first weeks after birth, after the vernix has disappeared, an infant's skin may start to peel, especially on the hands and feet, around the wrists and ankles. Sometimes the skin will crack. Since an infant's skin is very sensitive to ingredients commonly found in lotions (such as fragrances or preservatives), try to avoid their use. However, if peeling areas become red and irritated, petroleum jelly, baby oil, or unscented (often sold as hypoallergenic) moisturizing lotions can help prevent further drying.

Cutis Marmorata

This is skin mottling and is a normal response to chilling. It appears as a bluish-purplish reticulated pattern on the trunk, arms, legs, hands, and feet and disappears on warming. No treatment is indicated as this patterning has no clinical significance. A far rarer condition is the so-called harlequin color change. In this condition an infant lying on its side reddens on one half of the body and whitens on the other. Appearances of this color change are sudden and unpredictable, may last from 30 seconds to two minutes, and may continue for as long as the first two to three weeks of life. They are of no medical concern.

Milia

This appears as tiny white raised dots on the cheeks, nose, chin, and forehead of the newborn. These are caused by extra oil-gland activity due to the influence of the mother's hormones before birth. When these tiny oil glands become stimulated, they plug up easily, forming the bumps. Do not attempt to remove or "pop" them—they will clear up of their own accord within three to four weeks.

Sebaceous Gland Overgrowth (Hyperplasia)

This is another example of maternal hormones exerting an influence after birth. These tiny flesh-colored to yellow papules, or elevated lesions, occur on the nose, cheeks and upper lip. They result from high levels of androgen hormones, which stimulate oil glands in the baby's skin. They also clear up of their own accord as the baby's hormone levels adjust to life outside the uterus.

Erythema Toxicum Neonatorum

This is a common body rash that can crop up any time from birth onward. Contrary to its name, it is not toxic; it occurs when newborn skin is exposed to the environment outside the womb. It consists of flat, red, blotchy patches with minute white or whitish yellow centers. Resembling pimples or flea bites, they erupt mainly on the trunk and face, but also on arms and legs. The lesions fade, without medical treatment, in a matter of hours or days, only to appear on another area of the skin. The tendency is for this rash to disappear in one to two weeks.

Moles and Birthmarks

Other skin markers that appear at birth or develop soon after birth are birthmarks and moles. The most common are:

Salmon Patch. This appears as a flat red or pink patch on the nape of the neck or the eyelids or in the middle of the forehead. Ninety-five percent fade within the first year of life. They are also known as "stork bites" or "angel kisses" and are found in about 40 percent of all newborns. They are due to the persistence of tiny fetal capillaries in the dermis layer of skin.

Mongolian Spots. These are temporary, rounded blotches of blue, black, or slate-colored pigment and are most commonly found at the base of the spine or on the buttocks. They are most frequent in Asian, American Indian, and black newborns. Most disappear by late childhood.

Strawberry or Capillary Hemangiomas. These are birthmarks that generally appear in the first two to five weeks of life. They resemble berries—round or oval in shape, red to purple in color, raised and somewhat lumpy. The most common sites of involvement are the face, neck, scalp, or shoulders. Often solitary, a hemangioma may grow rapidly for several months after its initial appearance. These skin markers may remain and enlarge on the surface of the skin, as a "superficial" type of hemangioma, or they may extend into the tissue beneath the skin surface, becoming a deeper "cavernous" type. The vast majority of hemangiomas disappear without any appreciable trace by about the age of seven or eight years. Of course, during this period of time, the noticeable appearance of the mark may be cause for concern and comment on the part of the parents, relatives, and passersby. Also, its size may increase before it starts to recede. Generally, no treatment is indicated save for the healing passage of time. However, if the birthmark is large and threatens to obstruct or interfere with normal functioning of the mouth, eye, or nose, medical or surgical treatment may be recommended to remove or minimize the mark.

Nevus Flammeus. Often referred to as port wine stain, this is another vascular birthmark. It appears at birth as a reddish or slightly violet discoloration, usually on the face. Sometimes it will cover up to one whole side of the face. On other parts of the body, however, it usually is less extensive. Microscopic examination will show dilated blood vessels in the skin. The color intensifies with crying, which can be alarming to parents. Unfortunately these birthmarks do not resolve themselves with time and the darker the stain, the more likely it is to persist and become thicker. However, the lighter the color, the more apt it is to fade. Traditional treatment methods—excision, tattooing, cryosurgery, and dermabrasion—have proved largely unsatisfactory. Newer treatments with the argon laser, which is selectively absorbed by the red pigment present in the stain, have resulted in lightening of these birthmarks. Skin-tone opaque makeup, such as Lydia O'Leary's Covermark, may be effective in masking the birthmark.

Moles. Also called *pigmented nevi*, these are black or brown lesions that can be dark or light, flat or elevated, large or small, hair-bearing or smooth, numerous or not. They may be seen at birth, but the vast majority appear in infancy, childhood, or adolescence. They are very common in adults (30 being an average number) and even though many adults call them "birthmarks," because they believe they were born with them, such is usually not the case. There is really nothing to do for moles, unless they are unsightly due to their color, size, or location. Moles are often removed from an area of skin that is frequently subject to repeated trauma. Moles are generally nonmalignant growths, but in rare instances malignancies can arise from them. It is important to keep visual track of the child's moles, noting any changes. Moles should be inspected by a physician (and possibly removed) if:

- They are present at birth, especially when they are large.
- They suddenly enlarge.
- Their pigment suddenly spreads or changes.
- They begin to bleed or become sore (ulcerate).

SKIN INFLAMMATIONS

MANY SKIN PROBLEMS crop up in the first few weeks after birth, through no fault on the part of the parents. But parents can help to prevent or speed the healing and resolution of these conditions. One of

DEALING WITH ECZEMA

- Bathe baby less often; and bathe only the areas of the body that really need it. "Topping and tailing" —sponging head and diaper area—every few days is a good way to minimize excess exposure to water and soap, which can dehydrate and irritate skin.
- If the baby is bathed daily, keep baths short (five minutes maximum) and use only lukewarm to cool water.
- Use mild cleansing products. Anything that is a soap is actually very drying. Ivory soap, for example, is "mild" in the sense that it is pure soap, but it is not mild in the dermatologic sense. Better choices for a baby with eczema include moisturizing soaps, such as Dove or products such as Basis, Lowila, or Neutrogena.
- Use a mild lotion, such as Cetaphil, as a spot cleanser instead of soap and water—just massage it on and gently wipe it off.
- Moisturize right after bathing, while skin is still wet, to maximize the amount of water held next to the skin. You'll also use less moisturizer and thus save money.

- Moisturize between baths—simply moisten hands, pat water on the child's skin, then apply lotion.
- Use plain, nonmedicated moisturizing skin lotions as a simple, inexpensive way to calm irritated skin. If the condition does not improve, topical steroid medications may be used in conjunction with skin lubrication. The most common of these are the nonprescription 0.5 percent hydrocortisone creams, which soothe, reduce itching, and ease redness.
- Humidify the air with a vaporizer or humidifier. Dry air due to climate or indoor air cooling or heating can dry the skin.
- Avoid troublesome clothing fabrics such as wool or scratchy upholstery or carpets—these can set off the itch response.
- Dress the child in all cotton if possible and wash clothing in nondetergent suds with no fabric softeners or bleach.
- Ask the pediatrician about using antihistamines at bedtime, which may alleviate the incessant itch and allow the child a good night's sleep.

the biggest groups of skin conditions are inflammations, or more technically, eczemas or dematoses.

Neither *eczema* nor *dermatitis* is a specific disease, but rather they are umbrella terms for certain types of skin reactions. Both simply mean "inflammation of the skin." Skin inflammations may be classified as acute, chronic, or subacute, and the skin reaction may vary from oozing sore patches to dry scaly patches.

Atopic Dermatitis (Eczema)

This was once defined as an itch that rashes rather than a rash that itches because one of the primary problems is dry itchy skin that, when irritated or scratched, leads to a rash. The underlying problem is very sensitive, dry skin, and much of the skin reaction that a child gets is secondary to the scratching and rubbing. In addition, broken skin is an invitation to bacterial invasion.

This form of eczema or dermatitis usually runs in families. In fact a family history of atopic disease (asthma, hayfever, eczema) is present in 60 to 70 percent of patients. It is generally not due to being allergic to anything specific, but rather due to having skin with a genetic predisposition to being highly reactive. Atopic skin is also predisposed to other dermatoses, such as hand dermatitis or dry skin dermatitis, which are discussed later in this chapter. The most common areas of involvement in the infantile stage are the cheeks, forehead, scalp, arms, and legs. Its appearance varies from red, oozing, blistering lesions with crusts to thick scaly

patches with well-defined margins. Since a baby does not develop the muscular coordination necessary to scratch until around two or three months of age, most atopic dermatitis is not obvious until this time. The tendency to atopic skin cannot be cured, but it can be controlled. Preventive skin-care measures are aimed at keeping the skin moist and irritation-free and treating the inflammation. (See box on Dealing with Eczema.)

Cautions on Cortisone

Many parents have heard (and rightly so) that steroids can cause permanent changes to the skin, such as scarring, thinning, or *telangiectasis* (broken blood vessels). Certain areas of the skin—the thin skin of the genitalia and the face—are more likely to undergo these changes. However, a competent pediatrician generally uses the mildest concentration possible and uses it for only a short time—just to get the inflammation and eruption under control— with a subsequent return to the lubrication program. With this conservative approach, the risk of any permanent skin changes is almost nil.

Many parents are already familiar with the very mild hydrocortisone cream—0.5 percent—that is available without a prescription. Stronger preparations—1 percent or 2.5 percent—require prescriptions, but are still considered mild. In fact, recent research has revealed that most of the skin changes listed earlier were associated with cortisone preparations containing fluorine, which is not present in hydrocortisone.

Contact Dermatitis

Remember, dermatitis and eczema mean the same thing—"inflammation of the skin." Contact dermatitis has two major forms: *primary irritant dermatitis*, caused by direct skin contact with some irritating chemical, physical, biologic agent or substance, and *allergic contact dermatitis*, caused by an acquired reaction, or allergy, to some irritating chemical, physical, biological substance. The latter form is regarded as a delayed hypersensitivity reaction of the skin to the offending agent.

The most familiar forms of allergic contact dermatitis are those in response to exposure from the so-called "poison plants"—poison oak, poison ivy, and poison sumac. Nickel, a metal commonly found in earrings, watch bands, and belt buckles, is also a common allergen. No one is born allergic to these substances, but an allergy is acquired, in those susceptible, through repeated exposures. Affected areas of skin develop blisters, red swollen patches, scaling, crusting and/or oozing.

Preventive measures include avoiding soaps that further dry irritated skin and skipping vigorous rubbing and scrubbing of the skin. Substitute hypoallergenic soaps or cleansers for ordinary soap. To quell the itching urge, apply cool wet compresses and bathe in lukewarm water to coolish water. Aveeno, a bath preparation containing oatmeal, is soothing to add to bathwater for its antiitching effects.

Diaper Rash

This is the most common form of primary irritant dermatitis. At first, irritation takes the form of red, dry, chafed skin. Untreated, this can progress to an irritation involving blisters, pimples, and oozing sores. Not surprisingly, the most common sites for this eruption are the areas covered by diapers—the buttocks, genitals, anal area, thighs, and lower abdomen. The most common cause is prolonged contact with wet or soiled diapers. Other possible causes or contributing factors include inadequate rinsing of detergents or other laundry products from diapers or soap residue on the skin due to inadequate rinsing after bathing/cleansing. The use of fragranced fabric softeners, certain baby oils and ointments, and rubber or plastic diaper covers has also been incriminated. The old idea that diaper rash was an irritation caused by the breakdown of urine into ammonia that irritated skin is currently not considered a central cause, even though the rash is often accompanied by the sharp odor of ammonia. Most cases arise after three to four weeks of life and tend to go away in a few weeks or months.

Treatments and prevention tips are outlined in the box on preventing diaper rash, top of the next page.

Baby Powder

Baby powder has been a traditional part of an infant's layette—supposedly to keep skin dry and to prevent diaper dermatitis. But there is evidence that suggests the need for a break with this tradition. Recent studies suggest that talcum powder is unhealthy for both babies and their parents. Tumors known as *granulomas* may be caused by powder coming into contact with broken or abraded skin. Inhalation of the talc may be associated with lung damage. In extreme cases, aspiration of talc can be fatal. In addition, powders are not terribly helpful for diaper rash and similar skin inflammations. Occlusive creams are more effective in protecting skin from further irritation.

A less harmful alternative to talcum powder is cornstarch powder. If inhaled, it is basically harmless. And the old medical adage that yeast can metabolize the cornstarch and so flourish has never been shown to be clinically significant.

Intertrigo

This is dermatitis in skin folds, appearing as rash around the neck, behind the ears, in the bends of arms, knees, groin, inner thighs, armpits, and in the diaper area. In these skin folds, trapped heat, perspiration, and friction between opposing skin surfaces give rise to the characteristic skin redness and "weeping" or oozing of this irritant dermatitis. The inflammation lowers the skin's resistance to secondary fungal, yeast, or bacterial infections. Some self-help techniques are listed in the box on Tips to Counter Intertrigo, next page, bottom left.

SCALP CONDITIONS

Cradle Cap

This is the common name for *"seborrheic dermatitis,"* an inflammation that occurs in the oily areas of the body—the scalp, face, ears. Cradle cap is a yellowish, crusted collection of shedding skin caught around scalp hairs. In infants, residual vernix may also be involved. Cradle cap is caused by overactive oil glands in the scalp. Under the influence of maternal hormones, these oil glands are stimulated to work overtime. A reticence on the part of the new parent to wash the scalp thoroughly for fear of dam-

TIPS ON PREVENTING DIAPER RASH

- Change diapers frequently, as soon as they become wet or soiled.
- Keep the diaper area on the child clean. Wash with a mild soap, rinse thoroughly, and dry thoroughly—especially the skin folds.
- Apply a protective ointment, such as Desitin Ointment, Diaparene PeriAnal, zinc oxide, Balmex, A & D Ointment, or Vaseline to keep skin protected from moisture while under wraps.
- Dusting the diaper area may also keep skin dry. Use cornstarch powder only.
- Avoid rubber or heavy plastic diaper covers—these prevent the evaporation of moisture and perspiration and add to the dampness problem. Substitute wool or cotton diaper covers.
- Switch to a mild laundry detergent, such as Dreft or Ivory Snow, and double rinse diapers to ensure all residual detergent is removed. Avoid using fabric softener or dryer softener sheets—these may irritate baby's skin.
- Allow the baby several hours "au naturel" each day. The exposure to sun and air will encourage healing.

- If red pimplelike bumps appear along with the red skin of diaper dermatitis, the yeast candida may be present. Apply miconazole nitrate cream (available over the counter in drugstores as Micatin Antifungal Cream) sparingly to these areas. Your pediatrician may also suggest a thin application of a 0.5 percent hydrocortisone cream. In addition, other topical antiyeast agents with or without hydrocortisone work equally well.
- Diaper dermatitis may also have a bacterial cause. If the diaper area becomes populated with blisters filled with a cloudy fluid or that leave shallow red sores, a doctor should be consulted. These are classic signs of impetigo, a bacterial skin invasion of streptococcal or staphylococcal germs. This condition needs treatment with topical antibiotics and/or oral antibiotics to clear it.
- Be patient and consistent in clear-up efforts. The tendency to have this dermatitis will fade with time.

TIPS TO COUNTER INTERTRIGO

- Ease irritated skin by keeping affected areas clean, washing with mild soap (or an antibacterial soap) and lukewarm water several times a day. Pat areas dry—don't rub.
- Ask the pediatrician about applying 0.5 percent hydrocortisone cream sparingly after each cleansing, to soothe inflammation.
- Be on the lookout for the pimples that may signal a yeast infection. If a yeast infection is suspected, apply Micatin at the time of cleansing. Antiyeast creams may also be applied at the same time hydrocortisone cream is applied.
- If no improvement occurs after a week or if the rash begins to involve larger areas of skin (not just skin folds), consult your pediatrician.

DEALING WITH CRADLE CAP

- Use a mild dandruff shampoo two or three times a week. Good safe shampoos for baby are Head and Shoulders, Sebulex, or T-Gel.
- Lather shampoo well but gently. Leave on scalp for four to five minutes to allow the active ingredients to work. Loosen scales by rubbing gently with a washcloth. Rinse well.
- Keep up this shampooing regimen until the scalp clears.
- For very flaky cradle cap, apply some mineral oil to the scaly patches one hour before shampooing. The oil loosens the flakes for easier removal. Follow with a dandruff shampoo treatment.

aging the "soft spots" or fontanels is also a contributing factor. Rest assured that the soft spots are quite tough, resistant to puncture, and will withstand shampooing. Some tips to get a handle on cradle cap are outlined in the box, above right.

Hair Loss

The major causes of hair loss in children are most commonly temporary conditions that do not result in permanent baldness.

Alopecia Areata. This usually affects only localized areas of the scalp, resulting in patchy hair loss. *Alopecia universalis* results in the loss of all body hair and *alopecia totalis* results in the loss of all scalp hair.

In *alopecia areata,* characteristic "exclamation point" hairs—so named because they have a tapered shaft and a clublike bulb—are found at the margins of the bald areas. This condition usually resolves itself—the hair simply regrows in one to three months, leaving no sign of baldness. The cause of alopecia areata is not known, although it may be associated with various autoimmune disorders, and in adults its onset has been linked to emotional stress.

Telogen Effluvium. In infants, the resynchronization of hair follicles after birth can cause all hairs to enter into the same shedding mode or phase. Normally hairs are in one of two phases—an anagen, or growth phase and a telogen, or resting stage. When hair follicles are in the resting stage, they fall out to make way for new hair. When the majority of scalp hairs enter into the telogen phase, shedding results in diffuse thinning of hair. This may be due to changing hormone levels. Before birth, the fetus has a high level of sex hormones, which promote hair growth. When these levels fall after birth, the hair goes into a resting phase and falls out. Interestingly, the same phenomenon happens to the mother. Most new mothers experience a marked shedding of hair after giving birth. Normal hair growth is resumed after a few months. Telogen effluvium can also occur well after birth, several months after a bad illness, especially one involving a high fever.

Traumatic Alopecia. This is hair loss caused by mechanical trauma—rubbing, friction, vigorous brushing, or the continuous pulling from overly tight braids, cornrows, or ponytails can cause hair thinning and loss. It is most commonly noticed on the front hairlines and temples.

Trichotillomania. This is the habitual tendency of pulling, plucking, or twisting scalp hairs, which eventually results in breakage of hairs near the scalp and thus areas of baldness. Bald areas are usually irregularly shaped, not round as in alopecia areata. Trichotillomania may also involve eyelashes, eyebrows, body hair, and pubic hair. It is seen in children as young as four or five years of age.

As with all forms of alopecia, the best treatment for trichotillomania is gentle hair care, avoiding undue or vigorous manipulation, styling, or harsh chemicals. Because trichotillomania is a habit, professional help may be needed to alter it. However, it is not usually indicative of serious psychiatric problems.

Ringworm or Tinea Capitis

As the name implies, ringworm is a round, ringlike lesion of the scalp caused by a fungal infection of the hair shafts. Most commonly the causative fungus comes from an infected puppy or kitten or from another person with ringworm. It presents itself in one of three ways:

- As a reddish, slightly elevated round/oval ring (sometimes just an arc) with an area of broken hairs and balding. This is the noninflammatory type, which clears up without scarring.

- As round, pustular scaly patches with boils (called "kerion"). These red lumps are tender to the touch, at least one quarter inch in diameter (perhaps larger), and develop a white, pus-filled center in a few days. This inflammatory type of ringworm, commonly seen in black children, may be associated wtih some residual scarring and hair loss, but if treated properly, it usually resolves without residue.

- As noticeable dry, crusty scalp flaking (dandrufflike) in a child who has outgrown the tendency to seborrheic dermatitis (cradle cap).

Ringworm is contagious. The child with ringworm should avoid close contact with others until the problem is cleared up. Avoid sharing beds, sheets, towels, and clothing, and limit playing with other children. Topical therapy is insufficient to treat tinea capitis. All patients should receive an oral agent (griseofulvin) usually for one to two months.

Head Lice or Pediculosis Capitis

The medical term for head lice is pediculosis capitis, the most common type of lice infestation found in children. The other two types of lice—body lice and crab lice—are found more generally in adults. Any form of lice causes severe itching; scratching can break the skin, leaving it vulnerable to a secondary infection by bacteria. An examination of an itchy scalp reveals lice that look like black to gray-brown dots and are easily missed by the untrained eye. Far more easy to spot are the *nits* (lice eggs), which appear as elongated whitish specks that are firmly attached to the side of a hair shaft, about ½ inch from the scalp skin. At first glance they may look like dandruff, but they cannot be shaken off hairs like dandruff flakes. The best place to look for nits is in warm areas of the scalp—right over the ears or on the back of the head.

Lice are transmitted by direct contact with another contaminated person or via indirect contact with contaminated objects—combs, brushes, bedding, towels, furniture, clothing—used by someone who has lice. Lice are human parasites—they do not come from animals. They are rarely seen in infants, but the incidence rises among children in daycare centers or attending school for the first time. Interestingly, lice are not seen very often among blacks—the texture of their hair does not seem to be as attracting or hospitable to lice. Blacks do however have a much higher incidence of fungal infections of the scalp, such as ringworm.

Treatment is aimed at killing live lice as well as the nits. Currently there are many effective shampoos and lotions, some of which are over-the-counter preparations containing pyrethrin (RID, A-Zoo, R & S). The most commonly used prescription preparations are lindane (Kwell) and Nix. The most recent data indicate that the nonprescription preparations are almost as effective as the prescription ones and that of the prescription items, Nix is probably the best.

All family members should be examined and treated to prevent the spread or reinfection of previously treated individuals. Treatment should be conducted according to package directions and repeated one week later. The initial treatment (if properly done) kills the lice and some nits, while the second treatment will kill the hatching nits. Many parents are unnerved by the persistence of nits even after a second treatment and assume that lice are still present and thus keep treating. Repeated dosages or "super doses"—treating two successive days—are ineffective and superfluous.

Nits, dead or alive, are difficult to remove. Some preparations come with a lice comb to aid in the removal of nits. Combing should be done daily between first and second treatment, and after the second treatment. Another trick to remove nits: make a solution of white vinegar diluted one to one with water and apply to scalp, thoroughly wetting hair. Cover head with a shower cap for 30 minutes, comb dripping hair with a "lice comb," and then shampoo with mild shampoo. The solution seems to loosen the gluelike hold nits have on the hair shaft. This procedure may be repeated daily for a few days.

To treat possibly contaminated objects:

- Wash sheets, clothes, towels in the washing machine on the hottest setting and dry for at least 20 minutes on the hottest setting of the dryer. Or dry-clean all such items.
- Cleanse combs and brushes with a medicated shampoo, soak in Lysol, or wash with hot water and rubbing alcohol. How scrupulous should you be about other possibly contaminated objects? Since lice cannot survive more than a few days without a blood meal, once they are off the human body for that time, they die. So if something is not cleaned or is overlooked for several days, there's no real need to decontaminate it.

CONDITIONS OF THE EXTREMITIES

ARMS, LEGS, hands, and feet are not immune to skin difficulties.

Hand and Foot Dermatitis

Most dermatoses of the hands and feet start as dry skin. This dryness may lead to skin cracking and eventually the red, scaly, itching, and sometimes infected skin of dermatitis or eczema. Dermatitis of the hands affects primarily the backs of hands—palm skin is thicker, "moisturized" by many sweat glands, and so doesn't have the same vulnerability to dryness as the thinner skin on the back of the hand. This dermatitis occurs frequently in children with atopic dermatitis, but it also occurs as a result of exposure to harsh chemicals and environmental conditions or as a result of a contact allergy. Moisturizers and hydrocortizone cream (0.5 percent) keep the skin moist and supple so that it heals faster.

Dermatitis on the tops of feet is also usually a matter of simple skin dryness. However, another possible cause is a contact allergy due to chemicals present in footwear—dyes, glues, rubber, shoe and sock fabric. One clue that it is contact allergy—red areas will assume the pattern of the shoe or irritating material. For contact dermatitis, apply hydrocortisone cream several times daily to affected areas. Switch shoes; put on absorbent socks to insulate feet from direct contact with shoes. Change shoes and socks frequently to prevent perspiration buildup. Perspiration causes chemicals to leach out of shoes and onto skin.

Dyshidrotic Eczema/Pompholyx

This is a skin inflammation that affects the palms of the hands and occasionally the soles of the feet. The first signs are small fluid-filled blisters that form deep in the skin of the palm or sole; so deep that they are perceived as itchy or painful bumps. The blisters break down to become red, itchy, scaly patches. Most likely, these conditions are the result of overactive sweat glands, although the exact cause is unknown. This inflammation is frequently associated with excessive perspiration (hyperhidrosis) and seems to be more prevalent in hot weather. Treatment includes the use of moisturizers and hydrocortisone cream or ointment. Avoiding overheating of hands and feet is recommended to prevent stimulating sweat glands, thus provoking problems.

Athlete's Foot

Tinea pedia or athlete's foot is a fungal infection of the skin of the foot. Not every itchy rash on feet is athlete's foot—it is rare for a young child to have athlete's foot. Instead, it may be one of the foot eczemas such as "sweaty sock dermatitis," an irritation caused or aggravated by heat, perspiration, wet socks, and hot shoes. Scaly soles may be the hallmark of atopic skin. However, even if the parent mistakenly applies an antifungal medication to a dermatitis not of fungal origin, it may clear it up. The reason—these preparations have cream bases and are very moisturizing—just what the dermatitis needs. The best treatment is probably skin lubrication, with topical cortisone if needed.

Winter Dermatitis

As the name suggests, climatic factors play a role in this itchy, scaly inflammation. It usually worsens in winter due to dry air with little humidity and improves in hot humid weather. To treat, keep skin moist with moisturizers, cut back all unnecessary bathing/washing and use a room humidifier to raise indoor humidity.

Warts

Warts, or *verrucae*, are benign growths of the skin, caused by a virus. When the wart virus comes into contact with susceptible skin, it infects the epidermal cells and produces the bump or growth known as a wart. Warts are contagious—to some people more than to others. But close contact with warts should be avoided by everyone. Scratching or picking at warts can spread them—sometimes to the area under and around fingernails, a very difficult place to treat. Some of the most common wart varieties:

> *Verruca vulgaris*, or the common wart, is most commonly seen on the sides of the fingers. It can be a single skin-colored bump or a cluster of them with an elevated rough dry surface.
> *Verruca plana*, or the flat wart, is skin-colored or light brown, flat or slightly elevated and smooth. It occurs on the face and back of hands, arms, and legs. It is small and occurs in groups.
> *Verruca plantaris*, or plantar warts, grow on the soles of the feet and can be painful and disabling.

Treatment options are many and depend on the type of wart, location, and associated symptoms. Most warts can be left untreated and will spontaneously regress. Wart treatment is not always successful. The different treatment modalities range from topical preparations, to freezing, burning, or surgical removal. Sometimes combinations of therapy and repetitive treatments are necessary.

Molluscum Contagiosum

Also known as "water warts," these are also caused by a virus and transmitted through close bodily contact or via clothing or towels. These flesh-colored, waxy-looking bumps have a central white core or dimple, which differentiates them from warts. Most of the time molluscum crops up in clusters, but it can appear as single bumps on the trunk, face, and arms. They can be seen as early as nine or ten months of age. These growths occasionally develop in the scratched areas of those children with atopic dermatitis. There is a good spontaneous remission rate, so treatment may not be necessary. One complicating factor is that molluscum spreads on an individual by autoinoculation. That means if the lesion is scratched, the child can spread the virus to other areas of skin. The lesions usually spontaneously resolve in three to six months. If not, they are easily removed with gentle destructive treatments (light liquid-nitrogen therapy, picking out the core with a needle or curette) or a topical blistering agent called cantharidin.

GENERALIZED CONDITIONS OF THE TRUNK

Psoriasis

Psoriasis is characterized by an overgrowth of skin, so that red scaly patches are produced instead of normal skin. It is distinguished from patchy dermatitis in that it consists of well-demarcated lesions with a silvery, shiny scale. It also erupts in a symmetrical pattern—that is, both buttocks, both knees, or both sides of the scalp are affected. The exact cause is unknown although there seems to be a hereditary tendency. Psoriasis may skip generations and it is variable in terms of extent, course, and appearance. It is most commonly found on the scalp, knees, and elbows, but it can involve any part of the body, even the fingernails. The disease comes and goes, returning when there is some sort of trauma or injury to the skin. Even overdryness can cause the scaly patches to reappear. Psoriasis is uncommon in children; it may be confused with eczema. It probably is best treated by a dermatologist because of its chronicity.

Pityriasis Rosea

This is a relatively common skin rash in children as well as young adults. *Pityriasis* means "scaling"; *rosea* means "pink" or "rose-colored." At first, in about half the patients, a "herald patch"—a large, reddish raised spot—that may resemble a ringworm infection is the only sign of this condition. The patch then begins to fade and more oval spots appear. These spots become more numerous and seem to grow together, producing a generalized eruption of red to salmon-colored patches. It lasts four to six weeks and is confined to the trunk and upper extremities, taking on a characteristic "Christmas tree" pattern. In children, it is common to have unusual variations of the disease, such as lesions on the face and/or larger, irregular patches on the body. Pityriasis rosea is not contagious and recurrences are very rare. It may or may not be itchy.

Avoiding the use of drying soaps and keeping the skin cool bring temporary relief of itching. Calamine lotion dabbed on patches may be too drying and actually increase itchiness. To soothe mild itching, try a bath with Aveeno (a colloidal oatmeal preparation) or Argo starch in a tub containing six to eight inches of lukewarm water. For more severe itching, antihistamines or steroid creams or pills may be prescribed. While its exact cause is unknown, a viral agent is suspected.

Tinea Corporis

This is a ringworm infection of the body. Just like ringworm of the scalp, it is caused by close contact with an infected puppy or kitten, another child with ringworm, or contaminated soil. It is highly contagious and immediate treatment should be begun to limit the extent of the infection. If the diagnosis is accurate and infected areas are limited, ringworm can be successfully treated at home using an over-the-counter antifungal medication. Some effective ones that can be purchased without prescription include tolnaftate or miconazole nitrate.

Nummular Dermatitis

This is another condition that parents as well as doctors often confuse with ringworm. It is probably a variant of atopic dermatitis/eczema and is characterized by a coin-shaped eruption, usually appearing on the buttocks, legs, backs of the hands, or forearms. The red, crusty lesions may itch. Hydrocortisone cream may be prescribed to soothe the itch. Keep the skin from becoming overly dry by shortening bathing times, using lukewarm water, and using mild soaps and plenty of bland moisturizers.

Miliaria or Prickly Heat

Commonly known as heat rash or prickly heat, miliaria results from overheating. Many first-time mothers bundle up their babies, summer and winter. Well padded and insulated by "baby fat," infants generate plenty of heat. When their skin gets too hot, it perspires, yet the perspiration is unable to evaporate due to layers of clothing. This gives rise to the angry red bumps of heat rash. Look for it in the extra-warm areas of the skin—in skin folds, around the neck, behind the ears, under the arms, behind the knees, and in the diaper area.

The treatment is easy—keep baby cooler: in a cooler room, in lighter-weight clothing. Most of the rash will clear up with this lowering of temperature and exposure to cooler air. Any areas that do not clear will benefit from a gentle washing with cool water and mild soap a few times daily. Dry thoroughly and dust lightly with cornstarch, if desired.

Urticaria or Hives

Urticaria, or hives, are notable for their rapid sudden onset. Baby's skin is clear one moment, then blossoms with red, itchy, swollen bumps or welts. Hives are a sign of an allergic reaction to some food, medication, airborne inhalant, or a generalized reaction to stress, hot or cool temperatures, fever, or an infectious agent.

Parents should note that in children, hives are often associated with a viral or bacterial infection. It is not uncommon for a child to have a streptococcus bacterial infection in the throat (a strep throat) without any throat soreness, yet develop hives.

In general, hives erupt within a few hours of exposure to the offending substance. The eruption is usually transient, lasting 12 to 24 hours. They are clinically classified as acute (sudden onset, never to recur), recurring (sudden episodes that repeat themselves at varying intervals), or chronic (seemingly constant). In the case of acute and recurring types, long-term treatment involves isolating, eliminating, and avoiding the trigger factors if possible—food, drink, medication, eyedrops, nosedrops, toothpaste, candy, mouthwash, environment, activities, etc.—to prevent future outbreaks. For the short term, cool compresses, bathtub soaks, and lotions are helpful to alleviate itching and swelling. For moderate to severe cases, an oral antihistamine that eases itching and swelling may be recommended. Benadryl and Chlor-Trimeton are effective antihistamines that do not require a prescription. Even so, give according to package directions—these are powerful drugs. Aspirin can make any case of hives worse, so avoid it. For chronic cases, a consultation with a dermatologist or allergist is in order. Be patient—it is often difficult to find the exact cause, and more than one factor may trigger attacks. In some cases the cause is never found.

Impetigo

The hallmark of this bacterial skin infection is rapidly spreading, superficial, oozy, red crusty sores, or blisters that break down to form such sores. In infants and children, it may occur as a complication of a preexisting skin problem (such as diaper dermatitis). The causitive bacteria—streptococci and staphylococci—need to get a foothold in already compromised skin in order to flourish. Infants' and children's skin is not as resistant as adult skin and thus may be more vulnerable. Impetigo spreads rapidly and is contagious. Bedding, towels, clothing, and other personal articles that come into contact with infected skin are potential carriers of the germs and should be kept separate.

Impetigo can cause ugly sores but scarring is rare. It is most effectively treated with prescription oral antibiotics, such as erythromycin, a cephalosporin (such as Keflex), or antistaphylococcal penicillins and a regimen of good personal hygiene—lots of soap and water. It is not necessary to use an antibacterial soap (such as Hibiclens Antimicrobial Skin Cleanser, PhisoHex, or Betadine Skin Cleanser) to clean skin with impetigo, although certainly this will do no harm. A bland soap is fine. For mild cases involving a single lesion, soap and water followed by application of a topical antibacterial ointment or cream (Bacitracin, Neosporin Ointment, or Betadine Ointment) may be all that is needed to clear it up. If secondary lesions develop, then oral antibiotics are necessary. A new topical antibiotic, Bactroban, can often clear up impetigo without the use of oral antibiotics and may be worth a try in mild cases.

Scabies

This is a skin infestation by a mite known as *Sarcoptes scabiei*. Female mites tunnel under the top layer of skin and lay eggs in the shallow burrows. This causes itching and red shallow blisters, most commonly around the wrists, ankles, legs, nipples, underarms, pubic area, lower abdomen, and back. It is not uncommon for scabies to set up housekeeping in the face, neck, and scalp in young children. This condition is highly contagious and is transmitted through close skin-to-skin contact with another infected individual. Unlike a lice infestation, no eggs are visible. The prime symptom is itching, which gets worse at night when the child is warm in bed and the mite more active. Diagnosis is made by scraping burrows and examining under the microscope for evidence of mites or eggs. In many cases, however, the burrows are difficult to find and the diagnosis is based on clinical signs.

Treatment consists of an application of gamma benzene hexachloride (Kwell lotion or cream), after a shower or bath. Scrubbing affected areas well while in the bath or shower is often recommended. Recently animal studies have raised some furor by showing that extended contact on warm moist skin (conditions that would exist after bathing) with this active ingredient resulted in elevated blood levels of the chemical. However, the current feeling is that this is highly unlikely when skin is cool and dry. Take a shower and wait until the skin is dry and cool (at least room temperature) before applying. Leave on for six to eight hours (in severe cases in older children, twelve hours) and wash off. A second application is usually unnecessary, but may be repeated a week later. Apply any scabies-fighting preparation everywhere—even where there is no visible evidence of itching or burrowing, because it may take several days for symptoms to appear in newly colonized areas.

It is not unusual for itching to continue for up to two weeks even after effective treatment. However, this itching is not due to any active infestation. The mistake parents make here is to assume that the mites are still present and treat the skin again. Repeated treatments may penetrate the traumatized skin and get into the blood. The medication is irritating to skin. Instead of re-treating the child for scabies, soothe the itch with hydrocortisone cream (0.5–1 percent). If, however, itching persists after a month, reexamination is called for because of the possibilities of reinfestation or incorrect diagnosis.

Erythema Chronica Migrans

This is the ringlike rash associated with Lyme disease, a condition transmitted by the bite of a deer tick. Three to 20 days after being bitten by a tick, a red pimple appears at the bite site (usually the thigh, buttocks, or trunk) and later expands to a large, ringlike rash. Sometimes the center of the ring clears and in this state is mistaken by parents for ringworm. The fact that the tick is small and the bite not particularly painful is another complicating factor—the child may not remember being bitten. However, medical treatment is necessary. Complications may develop in other organ systems—arthritis in the joints, especially in the knees, as well as neurologic and cardiac abnormalities.

Symptoms associated with this rash may include chills, fever, headache, fatigue, backache, stiff neck, nausea, vomiting, and sore throat. The presence of the rash, incidence in the spring and summer (when deer tick populations flourish), and occurrence in an area endemic to deer (and deer ticks) all point strongly to a diagnosis of Lyme disease. Tetracycline is the drug of choice in children above age eight, followed by penicillin or erythromycin.

PIGMENT CONDITIONS

FROM BIRTH, the pigment *melanin* gives skin its basic color. The two main variants of pigmentation are hyperpigmentation (too much pigment) and hypo-

PREVENTING SUNBURN

Young children are more susceptible to the damaging effects of sun exposure than adults. A bad sunburn can be very dangerous for a small infant. Studies have found that the risk for melanoma, the deadliest form of skin cancer, doubles or triples when a child is seriously sunburned before age 10. For this reason alone, preventing sunburn in young children is essential. The risk for skin cancer is greatest in fair-skinned children who have blond or red hair, freckles, and light-colored eyes. These are individuals who always burn and never tan. Other factors that increase the risk of an individual developing skin cancer are:

- A family history of skin cancer.
- Multiple or atypical moles, called dysplastic nevi. These are moles that have irregular borders and are multicolored within a single mole. They tend to be larger than pencil erasers, and numerous (an individual may have over 100).
- A genetic disease, for example, albinism, that increases the individual's intolerance to sunlight.
- Living in areas, such as the south or southwest, where the sun is intense.

To prevent sunburn in a child

- Protect the child's skin with clothing, hats, carriage hoods, and umbrella/canopy attachments to strollers.
- Avoid exposing children to the sun during peak hours (between 10 A.M. and 2 P.M. in most areas).
- Always use a sunscreen to filter out the damaging rays of the sun (see below).
- Apply sunscreen to all exposed areas of the skin. Reapply frequently during sun exposure, at least every two hours. Always reapply after swimming, even if the preparation indicates this is not necessary. Friction and perspiration can also remove sunscreen from the skin.
- For very fair-skinned children, especially redheads, apply an opaque total sunblock, such as zinc oxide, to such easily burned areas as the nose and lips. If the child rubs it off, you will spot it readily and can reapply it.

- Don't be fooled by cloud cover. Overcast weather can result in a burn because the invisible ultraviolet rays filter through even though the clouds block the sun.
- Be aware of reflected light. Glare from snow, water, cement, or sand can bound up under an umbrella or hat and cause burning. Even if the child is shaded, apply a sunscreen to counteract reflections.
- Take special care at higher altitudes: radiation increases the higher you go above sea level because the protective atmosphere thins.

Choose a sunscreen carefully

- Sunscreens are labeled with a number from 2 to 15 known as the sun protection factor or SPF, an indication of the relative strength of the product. The higher the SPF, the more ultraviolet radiation is blocked from the skin. Children, even offspring of parents who tan easily, should use an SPF of 15.
- Waterproof sunscreens are practical for use at the pool or beach. They are formulated to remain on the skin for 80 minutes in the water. Water-resistant sunscreens remain on the skin for 40 minutes in the water.
- A child's skin may be sensitive to adult-formula sunscreens. The active ingredient in many sunscreens, PABA, is a potent sensitizer. Look at the label for the less sensitizing but just as protective PABA esters and benzophenones. Test a prospective sunscreen by applying a small amount on the child's inner forearm or the back. If no rash or redness develops within two to three days, the sunscreen is safe to apply to the rest of the child's skin.
- Consult your doctor before using sunscreen on an infant younger than six months old. Studies by the Food and Drug Administration have found that babies of this age have varying abilities to metabolize and excrete sunscreens.

pigmentation (too little pigment), either of which can be caused by disease or the environment.

Vitiligo or White Spots

Vitiligo is a condition characterized by a gradual loss of pigment. While the exact cause is unknown, it is known that it results from a loss of pigment-producing cells, melanocytes, in the skin. The decrease shows up as irregular areas of stark white patches with well-demarcated borders. These patches are of varying size and shape and are most commonly found on exposed areas of the skin, such as the face, the neck, the backs of the hands, and the tops of feet, but they can occur anywhere on the body. There is no cure for this condition and its course is progressive, though there may be extended periods when the depigmented patches remain stable. Current treatment consists of taking special pills (psoralens) and exposing affected skin to sunlight to repigment areas. When the pigment failure involves only small patches of skin, the use of a cover-up makeup is recommended.

Sun Exposure

Tanning, with its requisite extended exposure to the sun's ultraviolet radiation, has come under fire of late for its connection with certain forms of skin cancer. This is particularly relevant for children, not only because a child's skin is more vulnerable, but because sun damage is cumulative. A study found that the average child from ages one to eighteen years receives three times more ultraviolet exposure than the average adult and that blocking this radiation would reduce the risk of basal-cell and squamous-cell carcinomas by 78 percent. Another study has linked blistering or painful sunburns suffered under the age of 20 years with a doubled risk of malignant melanoma, a particularly virulent form of skin cancer. The message is clear—children need to be sunproofed. (See box on Preventing Sunburn, preceding page.)

33 Childhood Dentistry

Martin J. Davis, D.D.S.

INTRODUCTION

EVEN BEFORE A BABY IS BORN, his or her future dental health is influenced by such factors as diet, exposure to certain medications, and other factors. A baby's first or "primary" teeth actually begin to form before birth, starting during the sixth week of pregnancy. These teeth begin to erupt into the infant's mouth at about six or seven months of age. The permanent teeth generally do not begin to appear until approximately age six.

EARLY DENTAL DEVELOPMENT

IT IS NOT KNOWN how much the mother's diet during pregnancy affects the development and strength of her child's teeth. Nonetheless, it can be said that a good diet, including sources of calcium, phosphorous, and vitamins D, C, A, and B, is necessary for the development of the baby's teeth. Furthermore, a good prenatal diet means a healthier baby; healthy babies have better dental health as well. Research suggests that ingestion by the pregnant woman of fluoride—a substance that protects against tooth decay—will benefit the baby's teeth. If a woman lives in an area with fluoridated water (she can call her local water department to check), her fetus probably receives beneficial amounts of fluoride. If there is no fluoride in her drinking water, her doctor may suggest that she take a small daily dose of fluoride during her pregnancy.

The first *primary teeth* to erupt are most often the two lower front teeth, known as the central incisors (*incisors* are the four front teeth in each arch), followed by the top front teeth. A few babies may get their teeth as early as three months or as late as one year. At 12 months, most babies will have eight teeth—four above and four below. A few months later, the four first *molars*—two up and two down—should erupt. Then come the primary first molars, leaving a space for the next teeth, the pointed *"eyeteeth,"* or canines. Finally, by age two to two and a half, the primary second molars complete the set of twenty primary teeth.

Many parents look upon teething as a significant milestone and some worry that something is amiss if the baby seems to lag behind others in getting that first tooth. Actually, a parent need not be concerned about late onset of teeth, as long as the primary teeth begin to erupt by 12 months of age. Early onset of teeth does not signify intelligence or maturity. Nor does late onset mean the child is "slow" or will have better or stronger teeth. Early or late eruption of teeth may be hereditary—in one family the children teethe early, in another they teethe late. If, however, a tooth is already present at birth or soon afterward, or if no tooth has appeared by age 12 months, a pediatric dentist or pediatrician should be consulted, as these occasionally may be

440

signs of a health problem or systemic disease. Teething is not recognized as a true cause of fever, diaper rash, diarrhea, or other problems. In fact, attributing such problems to teething could result in the overlooking of a serious illness.

Many parents make the mistake of thinking that the primary teeth are of little or no importance. After all, the permanent teeth *do* replace them. But a child needs those baby teeth for good speech development, for chewing and eating, and for a good appearance. Furthermore, when baby teeth become infected, the whole body can become ill and the infection potentially can be damaging to the permanent teeth developing underneath. A child with a cavity is in pain, and the cavity can affect how a child eats, sleeps, and copes with life experiences. Another item to consider: early loss of primary teeth due to decay can lead to orthodontic problems. Other teeth will drift or erupt into the space left open by the missing tooth, and the permanent tooth will have no room to come in. Missing teeth also interfere with speech development and may hurt a child's self-image. Even at the age of three, the child may realize that he or she is missing teeth and may feel self-conscious.

Some parents complain if their children's baby teeth are less than perfect looking. At first eruption the teeth may be crooked or turned sideways and there may be spaces between them (which is normal). Slight irregularities are not unusual. Only when these teeth continue to have poor position after complete eruption should there be serious concern. Preventive and interceptive orthodontics may be suggested for baby teeth, although some early problems may correct themselves as a result of the natural pushing of the tongue and lips against the teeth. These forces work to align the primary teeth during eruption.

More unusual dental conditions are *twinning* and *fusion* of teeth. Twinning occurs when two teeth grow from one tooth bud; fusion, when two separate teeth grow together as one. Neither occurrence has to be a problem. Both the function and appearance of these teeth can be improved. There is no indication that the permanent teeth will develop along the same lines as the primary teeth. Only when a primary tooth is absent or injured by decay or trauma is it possible that the permanent tooth will also be absent or damaged.

The second or *"permanent"* teeth begin to erupt at about age six. Mild teething discomfort may accompany their arrival, but is rarely as bothersome as when the baby teeth erupt. Usually, the first permanent tooth is the first permanent or *"six-year"* molar. It does not replace any baby teeth, but comes in behind the primary molars. The first primary

teeth to be lost are often the lower two central incisors. Over the next four years, the rest of the permanent teeth will replace the primary teeth as they fall out. Upper eyeteeth, however, can appear as late as age 12, and the second molars may come anytime between ages 11 and 14. The third molars or *"wisdom teeth"* are due between ages 16 and 20. They are the teeth most likely to have eruption problems, especially if they become blocked, or impacted, and require removal.

In all, the average adult has 32 permanent teeth. The permanent teeth are more yellow than the primary teeth, a change that alarms some parents but that is perfectly normal. Permanent teeth are also much larger than baby teeth and may seem out of proportion to the child's face. With time and maturity, the teeth will appear more appropriately sized.

Sometimes the second teeth will come in before the baby teeth are lost, forming a double row of teeth. The dentist will examine the child and frequently may decide to remove the baby teeth if they do not fall out by themselves. This allows the second teeth to move forward into their proper positions. If this move does not occur naturally after removal of the baby teeth, the dentist may decide to move the teeth forward by simple mechanical means.

COMMON PROBLEMS

Teething

Discomfort due to the eruption of the primary teeth may be mild, moderate, or substantial, depending on the individual child, his or her particular teeth and gums, and the level of pain the child is able to tolerate. The pain a baby feels is caused by the pressure and the sharp edge of the tooth cutting into the gums. A child who is teething may drool excessively and bite on fingers or other handy objects. He or she may act cranky during the day or have trouble sleeping at night. Some children teethe for months before the tooth actually appears. Others may teethe only for a few days and a few show no signs of teething problems at all—the tooth simply appears one day.

To help ease any discomfort, parents should provide the baby with safe, chewable toys. Rubber teething rings, especially when chilled, are the safest and usually the most satisfying to the teething child. Or the parent may offer a frozen bagel or biscuit. Rubbing the gums also helps. Parents should beware of plastic toys that are sharp or easily breakable; these can be dangerous for a child to chew.

The old advice that alcohol on the gums will help teething problems has not been proven. Alcohol may be dangerous for a young child; besides, it does not soak through the skin and really has no effect on the discomfort felt by the baby. Topical pain relievers for teething babies help temporarily, but the effect soon wears off; some of these have caustic chemicals and are better not used. Acetaminophen, a nonaspirin pain reliever, may be suggested by the pediatrician or pediatric dentist if the child is having trouble sleeping at night.

Occasionally a tooth may push so hard against the gums as it works to emerge that it causes a blood blister or *"eruption hematoma,"* a purple or blackish-blue area in the gums that appears some time before the tooth does. Normally, this is nothing to worry about and will disappear on its own. If it is large enough to prevent chewing, the blister may need to be lanced, but this is unusual.

A child who seems to suffer severe teething difficulties should be seen by a pediatrician or pediatric dentist. The cutting of teeth is a normal process and should not cause undue pain. If it does, it may be a sign of another problem unrelated to teething. Also, illnesses such as diarrhea, fevers, and colds warrant a pediatrician's attention and should not be attributed to teething.

Tooth Decay

Dental caries are still the most common problem healthy children face. Tooth decay results from acid and plaque on the teeth. *Plaque* is the sticky film of bacteria that forms on the teeth and provides the perfect environment for the development of acids that dissolve the enamel of the teeth, eventually causing pain and infection in the gums and teeth. Primary teeth decay the same way permanent teeth do. Parents should not make the mistake of assuming that first teeth are in any way immune to dental decay. Many children get cavities before the age of two, usually as a result of frequently eating sugary foods and neglecting proper dental hygiene. The young child is totally dependent on the parents for dental care and cleaning of the teeth. The parent must be responsible for consistent care of a child's teeth. Occasional brushing, for example, while better than none, is not good enough—acid-producing plaque reforms on the teeth every 24 hours. (See the section on good dental habits.)

A child with a cavity should see a dentist immediately. Parents should suspect a cavity if the child experiences pain while eating cold or sweet foods, complains of a toothache, or wakes during the night with pain in the tooth. The earlier a cavity is treated, the easier and less traumatic for the child. The dentist will probably use xylocaine to anesthetize the nerve or pulp and then remove the decay and restore the tooth. Xylocaine has very few side effects and wears off after about 90 minutes. Be-

cause it causes numbness, though, a parent should take care that the child does not bite his or her own lip or tongue immediately after the treatment.

Bottle Mouth or Nursing Caries

When a child goes to sleep sucking a bottle, the results can be disastrous. Rampant decay of the teeth can develop. It is always a good rule that unless a child is actively feeding, the bottle should be removed. Otherwise the milk or formula or juice that is in the bottle will "pool" in the mouth and the teeth will be bathed in sugary liquid. Asleep, a child does not swallow often enough to wash these liquids away, and saliva, which protects the teeth, is reduced during sleep. The sugary liquid begins to change to acid and breaks down the enamel of the teeth, eventually causing nursing-bottle syndrome —total decay of the front and even the back teeth. Often the problem is so severe that teeth cannot be saved and must be pulled.

Some babies fall asleep better if they have something to suck on. Letting a child have a pacifier to suck on is far better than using a bottle. If a bottle is necessary, it should contain nothing but plain water.

If a child has nursing-bottle mouth it must be treated right away. Dental caries is an infection that can only worsen. Neglect of cavities results in pain, infection of the gums, premature loss of teeth, and potential problems for the permanent dentition.

Bleeding Gums

A child should not experience bleeding gums. Should this happen, a pediatrician should be consulted right away, because this may be the first sign of serious disease.

Crowded Teeth

Crowding of the primary or permanent teeth may occur, for example, if a child inherits large teeth from one parent and a small jaw from the other. Crowding may indicate the need for orthodontic work either now or when the child is older. Certain severe problems are actually best treated in the three- to six-year-old. Crowding may also occur if teeth are shifting places due to premature loss of a baby tooth. Space maintainers may be used to hold a place for the permanent tooth. Habits such as thumb- or lip-sucking beyond age six may cause orthodontic problems.

Buck Teeth

Upper teeth that protrude are usually inherited. Sometimes, however, buck teeth are caused by finger- or thumb-sucking habits that go on too long or by unusual swallowing patterns. Parents should not worry about lip- or thumb-sucking unless it continues past age six. Most children will give up the thumb by themselves before then. Often orthodontic work will be suggested to correct protruding teeth and protect them from traumatic injury.

Canker Sores

Canker sores are painful ulcers that occur on the insides of cheeks, roof of mouth, lips, and tongue. Sometimes only one or two ulcers may occur. Other times a child may suffer from sores throughout the mouth. The first occurrence of these lesions may be severe and is known as acute primary herpes; it lasts 10 to 14 days and little can be done to hasten its departure, although treatment can lessen the discomfort. The major concerns are the accompanying fever and the fact that, due to discomfort, the child may refuse to eat or drink anything. The parent should try having the child drink through a straw and should offer plenty of soothing liquids. Foods that are salty, acidic, or hard to chew should be avoided in favor of bland, soft foods and ice cream. Oral hygiene should be maintained as best possible.

The first time a child experiences a mouth infection such as this is the worst. Later in life, the child will probably only have an occasional canker sore instead of a complete outbreak. The condition is contagious; parents and other siblings should wash their hands carefully after contact and not share foods with the child until the condition disappears. If the fever is high, if the child will not eat or drink, or if the condition is severe, the pediatrician must be consulted.

Stained Teeth

Some children develop stains on their teeth. The teeth may occasionally come in discolored, or stains may be caused by bacterial or iron supplements. A dentist can usually clean these spots off with a rotary instrument or improve the appearance of the teeth by bonding a plastic "veneer" or covering onto the tooth. Tetracycline, a useful antibiotic for adults, can also stain the teeth and should not be given to young children.

GOOD DENTAL HABITS

As soon as the first baby tooth comes in, the parents are responsible for keeping it clean. The most important times to clean the teeth are before bed at night and in the morning, although it is even better if teeth can be cleaned after meals. To remove plaque, a parent may use a soft toothbrush (manual or electric) or a piece of gauze or a clean washcloth. If a toothbrush is used, the parent should be sure that the bristles are soft and that the brush head is child-size, meaning that it is smaller and will fit more comfortably in the child's mouth. Electric toothbrushes are fine, although they are not in any way superior to a manual brush. The parent is responsible for using these items to keep a child's teeth clean until the child is old enough to really handle the job alone—usually by age six, when coordination is adequate to reach all of the surfaces of the teeth.

Once a week, the parent should use a small flashlight to look into the child's mouth, check to see that the teeth and gums look healthy, count the child's teeth, and note any new eruptions. (See box on Dental Hygiene, next page.)

PREVENTIVE DENTISTRY

Fluoride and sealants have swept the dental world and changed the nation's dental health for the better. Fluoride is now in the drinking water of about 50 percent of communities across the country and is proven safe and beneficial. There is significantly less tooth decay in areas with fluoridated water. Parents should contact the local water department to find out if a particular area has fluoride in the water. If there is none, a fluoride supplement should be prescribed for the child. (Breastfed children also need a supplement as fluoride probably does not pass through the milk in adequate amounts.)

Some vitamin preparations have fluoride in them. Fluoride drops are also available. Children should also be using a "pea-size" portion of fluoridated toothpaste when cleaning their teeth and, by age five or six, a fluoride rinse may be recommended, even in areas with fluoridated water. Fluoride protects the smooth surfaces of the teeth but is *not* effective in protecting the grooves and pits of the biting or "occlusal" surfaces. Until 1960, 75 percent of cavities formed in between teeth, on the smooth surfaces. The use of fluoride has greatly reduced the number of cavities there. Today, more than 50 percent of cavities occur on the biting surfaces, but new preventive treatments may reduce this.

Sealants are now being used to protect the biting surfaces of the teeth against decay. Sealants are ultra-thin layers of liquid plastic that flow into the fissures of the teeth, harden, and help seal out decay.

DENTAL HYGIENE

Hold the toothbrush at a 45-degree angle and move it in small circles to clean the teeth. Pay particular attention to where the tooth meets the gums, as bacteria tend to proliferate there. Do not neglect the back teeth and the insides of the front and back teeth. Use a scrubbing motion to remove plaque on the chewing surfaces. Use a little fluoride toothpaste on the brush since this has an "outside" effect of increasing the strength of the enamel. Toothbrushes should be replaced every three to four months.

For the very young child, a piece of gauze or a wet washcloth is often easier to use than a brush. Sit down on the floor with the child's head in your lap. Wet a two-inch-square piece of gauze or use the end of a clean washcloth and wrap it around your finger. Gently polish the teeth. Don't forget to do the insides of the teeth and the back teeth as well. To make it easier to reach these spots, you can ask the child to

"open wide like an alligator." Cleaning the teeth can be made as much fun and pleasurable as bath time is. By about one year of age, the gauze or washcloth should be replaced by a toothbrush.

If the teeth are touching or close together, the parent must also use dental floss; the brush cannot get between these teeth. Gently pass the floss through the teeth once a day. Use about 18 inches of floss, wrapping the ends around your middle fingers. Hold the floss tightly and use your fingers to gently guide the floss between the child's teeth. Move the floss gently under the gum line. Be careful not to use too much force and not to snap the floss into place, as this can harm delicate tissue. Scrape the floss up and down the side of the tooth and then remove. Repeat the process anywhere teeth are especially close together.

Bacteria and food are kept from getting into the grooves of the back teeth. These crevices cannot be reached with brushing, nor does fluoride work as successfully on such surfaces. The sealant process does not work as well on baby teeth as on the permanent teeth, especially the molars, but in high-risk cases it may be used on a young child's primary molars.

Dental researchers are now working on a vaccine against cavities. A complex community of bacteria work together to cause caries, making the discovery of a single vaccine unlikely, but scientists remain hopeful.

THE FIRST VISIT TO THE DENTIST

VISITING THE DENTIST should be a positive experience for a child. Much depends on how calm the parent remains and how positively the parent looks upon the experience. Most children should see a pediatric dentist, or pedodontist, just as they see a pediatrician. A pediatric dentist is trained not only in dentistry, but also in child behavior. These specialists have been taught how to make a visit to the dentist a pleasurable experience for the young. Their offices are set up for handling their young patients, whereas some regular dentists may not want to see children as patients. A parent who wishes to take a child to his or her own dentist should call first to

make sure this is appropriate. Often the dentist will have the parent bring the child along to observe the parent's visit.

A child should make the first visit to the dentist when he or she is between 12 and 18 months of age, although many pediatric dentists want to screen all infants at about the time the first teeth are erupting (at approximately six months). The important thing is never to wait until the child experiences pain. The child should see the dentist first in a nonthreatening situation, when all teeth are fine and healthy. At the first visit, the dentist will probably concentrate on discussing diet and teeth cleaning or oral-hygiene procedures. The dentist will also check for any irregularities of the teeth or jaws and will discuss good and bad dental habits with the parent and child. It is also possible that the dentist will clean the child's teeth and apply fluoride. The first visit will probably take no more than 15 minutes. After this, the child should return every six months or at intervals recommended by the dentist. Regular visits like this will help the child to feel more at ease with the dentist and will give the dentist the opportunity to be sure that teeth and jaw development are proceeding normally.

X rays may be used by the dentist as a diagnostic tool during one or more of the visits. If no problems are noted during the examination, the first X ray, to check for proper development of the permanent teeth under the primary teeth, will often not occur until age 4 or 5. Another full series should be done at age 12 and again at age 18. In between, the occasional bite-wing X ray may be used. Parents can feel secure that the X ray process is safe because the amount of radiation in a dental X ray is only 1/1000th of that in a chest X ray, for example—or equal to the health risk of breathing New York City air for two days!

Whenever visiting the dentist, the parent should be sure to act relaxed and calm. Overexplaining the visit to the child or saying "It won't hurt" may actually make the child more wary of the visit. A matter-of-fact, "We're going to see the dentist who is going to count and clean your teeth," will be much less threatening.

DIET AND NUTRITION

PARENTS SHOULD try to regulate between-meal snacks and should be especially careful to avoid frequently giving a child sweet, sticky foods such as caramel. Healthful snacks, such as cheese, vegetables, and crackers, should be served instead. Parents should read package labels and be wary of foods touted as "healthy foods," such as granola bars and certain breakfast cereals, which actually may be high in sugar. Some cereals are so high in sugar that the child may be eating a half teaspoon of sugar for every teaspoon of cereal. Dried fruits seem like a wonderful idea, but they are very sticky and contain concentrated sugar. Fresh fruits are much better. Raisins should be given in limited quantities—they are not good for the teeth because they are high in sugar and tend to stick to the teeth, promoting caries.

Children who eat something sugary by itself or at frequent intervals subject their teeth to more sugar than children who eat a sugary food along with another food. The other foods can actually help to remove the sweets and provide a buffer to neutralize the acids forming in the mouth from the sugar.

Babies need no sugary snacks and parents should never dip a pacifier into honey. For healthy teeth, they do need calcium, phosphorous, and vita-mins C and D. These vitamins and minerals are found in breastmilk and in formula, but a doctor may prescribe a vitamin supplement as well.

FIRST AID

IF A BABY TOOTH is knocked out, there is, unfortunately, no hope for saving it. A dentist should still be seen, however, to determine how the space left by the missing tooth can be maintained and to determine if other teeth were damaged in their roots or elsewhere.

A permanent tooth that is knocked out may actually have a good chance of survival *if* it is rapidly replanted in its gum socket. Rinse the tooth with water and put it back into the socket immediately. Have the child hold it in place by biting on gauze or a washcloth until you reach the dentist. If you cannot get the tooth back into its socket, place it in some cold milk (or ice-water if you have no milk) and transport it to the dentist as quickly as possible. The dentist will splint the tooth back into place, where it will usually rejoin and heal just the way a cut would somewhere else on the body. A root canal is also usually needed within a few days; this is a relatively simple and painless procedure for the child. Remember: time is of the essence. The longer the tooth is out of the mouth, the less the chance of tooth survival.

Although saving the tooth is important, remember that any dental injury is a head injury; a child who acts disoriented or dazed should be rushed to the emergency room of a nearby hospital *first.*

A chipped tooth can be restored by bonding, using an artificial substance to replace the lost part of the tooth.

A bad cut in the mouth should always be looked at by a pediatric dentist or a pediatrician. There are many different bacteria in the mouth and a tetanus shot may be needed if the child has not had one.

34 Medical Emergencies and First-Aid Procedures

Fred Agre, M.D.

INTRODUCTION

HANDLING AN INFANT'S or small child's medical problems can be frightening. A parent or caregiver is confronted with the thorny task of ascertaining which conditions or symptoms are life-threatening and warrant immediate medical attention, and which ones can be handled at home. Determining what constitutes a medical emergency is difficult enough when the victim is an adult, but the problem is compounded in a young child. Because infants and most small children are unable to explain where they hurt or how bad they are feeling, parents and those caring for them must assess the severity of the problem by interpreting what are often confusing and conflicting symptoms.

When an accident occurs or some other need for immediate medical attention arises, parents are faced with many questions. What warrants a trip to the emergency room? How and when should paramedics or an ambulance be called? What can be handled at home using basic first-aid procedures? When should the pediatrician be called—immediately, within an hour, or after a few days? With basic knowledge, adults caring for young children will be able to make decisions that help ensure and maintain a child's safety and health. And they will be able to do so with confidence that the measure chosen for the situation is correct.

Medical problems can be divided into three categories—emergency, near-emergency, and nonemergency. (See table 34.1.) An emergency is any life-threatening situation in which immediate action must be taken; a near-emergency is a serious situation that requires prompt medical attention; and a nonemergency, in many cases, can be treated

Table 34.1 **PEDIATRIC EMERGENCIES, NEAR-EMERGENCIES, AND NONEMERGENCIES**

Body Part/System	Emergencies (3–60 minutes)	Near-Emergencies (1–12 hours)	Nonemergencies (12–48 hours)
Heart	Ventricular tachycardia	Atrial tachycardia	
Lungs/Respiratory System	Epiglottitis Airway obstruction/choking Near-drowning/drowning	Status asthmaticus Croup with respiratory distress Pneumonia with difficulty breathing	Pneumonia without difficulty breathing Cold with fever Croup with mild distress
Nervous System	Persistant convulsions Meningitis Head injury w/progressive signs and symptoms	Stupor Coma Reye's syndrome	
Circulatory System	Hemorrhage Shock Anaphylaxis	Laceration with intermittent bleeding Nosebleeds	Minor bleeding—cuts
Gastrointestinal System	Intussusception Vomiting large amounts of blood	Persistent pain Persistent vomiting Persistent diarrhea Incarcerated hernia Passing large amounts of blood rectally	Colic
Eyes	Lacerations of the globe Blunt trauma with hemorrhage	Corneal abrasions Caustic injuries	Conjunctivitis Sties Blocked tear ducts
Skeletal System	Head, neck, or back injury	Compound fractures Fractures Dislocations	Soft tissue injuries (muscles, tendons, etc.)
Skin	Severe burns Animal bites (on the face or with marked break of skin)	Chemical or electrical burns Animal bites (moderate break of skin)	Minor burns Sunburns Hives Stings Animal bites (slight break of skin)
Nonspecific	Poisoning	Fever greater than 104 degrees F.	Fever less than 104 degrees F.

with basic first-aid measures and may or may not necessitate a medical consultation. Which category a medical problem falls into depends on the amount of time there is to seek medical attention. In an emergency, medical aid must be received within 3 to 60 minutes; in a near-emergency, within 1 to 12 hours; in a nonemergency, 12 to 48 hours, if needed.

The goal of this chapter is to give parents and those caring for small children the knowledge necessary to separate true emergencies from near-emergencies and nonemergencies and to know what to do, whom to call, and how quickly to act. But no book can or should be a substitute for basic hands-on training. Such training in first-aid procedures is recommended for every parent or caretaker of children. Training programs are available in many communities through the Red Cross, in adult- or continuing-education classes, from local chapters of YMCA/YWCA, and at some health clubs.

THE EMERGENCY ROOM

A TRIP TO an emergency room (ER), because it is usually necessary and not voluntary, is accompanied by worry and anxiety. Knowing how the emergency room (or emergency department as it is often called now) of a hospital operates, what the steps are from registration to discharge, and what to expect will help ease some of the tension. (See box on What to Expect at the Emergency Room.)

WHAT TO EXPECT AT THE EMERGENCY ROOM

- Be prepared to tell your story clearly and frequently. You will be seen by several members of an emergency-room staff before you leave. Mention any current medications, allergies, and history of illnesses and injuries.
- Be patient. Treating emergencies takes time. Patients are treated in one sitting, from start to finish.
- Bring along an insurance card or information or be prepared to pay cash. Bring money for filling prescriptions.
- Ask the name of the person who is caring for the child. She or he will most likely be able to answer questions about your child's condition and progress.
- Expect to accompany the child into the treatment area, but don't be surprised if you are asked to leave. Usually relatives and friends are not allowed into this area. Try to stay to provide support to the child unless this compromises the child's care, or you are unable to tolerate the events.
- Realize that at any time another patient's case could take precedence over yours.
- Don't expect privacy in the treatment area. Emergency-room patients need to be observed by the staff in addition to being monitored by equipment.

An emergency room consists of a reception or waiting room and one or more treatment areas, in which small cubicles are partitioned by doors or curtains or both. Patients entering the emergency room should go directly to the reception or information desk to announce their arrival and problem. It is here that patients are prioritized according to a special system called triage.

The Triage System. In order to handle the large number of people whose symptoms vary from minor to severe, patients are seen in order of need, not in order of arrival. Most departments sort cases according to the triage system—a term used during World War I for classifying battlefield casualties according to treatment requirements.

In a hospital emergency department, a medical staff member will assess the patient's condition immediately and designate him or her as an emergency, near-emergency, or nonemergency. (Alternatively, these categories may be called "emergent," "urgent," or "nonurgent.") Emergencies are those whose lives are in immediate danger; near-emergencies are those whose illnesses or injuries may become a threat to life within 1 to 12 hours; nonemergencies are those whose conditions are not life-threatening or dangerous but do require treatment within a day or so. If classified as an emergency, the patient will be taken immediately into the treatment area. Near-emergencies and nonemergencies will be asked to register and wait. For tips on what to expect and take to an emergency room, see the accompanying box.

GETTING TO THE EMERGENCY ROOM

Calling 911

The 911 number, or its local equivalent, should be used only for true emergencies, such as when the child cannot be moved due to injuries or when the child's condition is worsening. A police operator answers 911 calls and transfers them to an emergency medical service where a skilled technician will handle the call. By asking questions, the technician assesses the severity of the situation, what type of life-support vehicle to send, and what special equipment to place aboard. He or she is trained to verify quickly and efficiently patient information—age, sex, immediate problem, any pertinent medical history, present location (with cross street), the name of the party calling, and the telephone number from which the call is being made.

Is an Ambulance Really Necessary?

For the majority of pediatric emergencies, driving the child to the emergency room is recommended over calling an ambulance because of the time it saves. An ambulance will take a certain amount of time to get to the house (or scene of the accident) and then additional time to retrace its route back to the hospital. Children are readily transported—they can usually be picked up, carried to the car, and driven to the emergency room. Parents of small children should know the fastest route to a local emergency room. A practice run should be made to familiarize yourself with the roads, to avoid losing precious minutes to a wrong turn in the event of an emergency. (If no car is available, call a neighbor to drive.)

Even in many cases of suspected neck, head, or spinal injuries, the body can be supported evenly and the spine and neck can be kept in alignment and immobilized by placing the child on a board or other makeshift stretcher.

WHEN TO CALL THE DOCTOR

WHEN TO CALL the doctor depends in large part on whether the situation is an emergency or not. In true emergencies, a call to the doctor may seem superfluous—the child must go directly to the hospital. However, it is always a good idea to call the doctor if reasonable. Sometimes, as in the case of poisoning, the doctor or the Poison Control Center may recommend immediate treatment at home first. If the doctor can't be reached, time should not be spent waiting for a return call. Instead the adult should take the child to the emergency room and leave a message with the doctor's service, stating to which hospital they are going (or being taken) and the reason for the trip.

As a precaution, parents should keep the number of the local emergency room among a list of numbers close to the telephone. If the child's doctor cannot be reached, a call can be made to the emergency room to help assess how critical the situation is. Calling the emergency room in an emergency will also help prepare the staff.

In near-emergencies, it is wise to call the pediatrician, as he or she can help the parent decide if the youngster should be seen immediately at the local emergency room or at the doctor's office. In addition, the doctor may suggest ways to make the child more comfortable until he or she can be examined.

For nonemergencies, the doctor should be called for consultation when a parent is uncertain what course of action to take. No one should take unnecessary risks or put off telephoning the doctor for fear of being considered overreactive. A parent who isn't sure should ask for help.

TALKING TO THE DOCTOR

TO ASSESS AND TREAT the illness or injury quickly and correctly, the doctor (either private physician or emergency-room staff) needs accurate information. To facilitate this and to ensure that nothing is forgotten or mistaken, it is helpful to take notes on the following:

- What the child was doing at the time of injury or onset of the illness.
- The onset of the symptoms.
- Order of occurrence of the symptoms.
- Severity of the symptoms (for example, the exact temperature if the child has a fever).
- Status of the symptoms: whether they are getting worse, staying the same, or getting better.
- Any known medical problems, chronic diseases, routine medications, or allergies the child has.
- The first-aid steps, if any, that were administered and the child's response to them.
- The replies or suggestions from the doctor.

FEVER

AN ABNORMAL RISE in body temperature is not an illness, but a symptom, usually signaling the presence of an infection. In and of itself, fever is harmless or may be beneficial, but it can make a child (and parent) miserable. Fever is not brain-damaging even when it is as high as 106 or 107 degrees F. However, the underlying disease that causes the fever, encephalitis, for example, may pose a threat.

Most parents suspect a fever when their child's head feels warmer than usual. The best area to feel for fever is the trunk or abdomen, not the head. The body should be felt using the back of the hand, not the palm, because the skin there is thinner than that of the palm, and therefore is more sensitive to temperature changes.

Most parents are accurate in detecting the presence of fever simply by feeling their youngsters. However, the younger the child, the less reliable this method is. Babies have a large surface area in relation to their body mass and warm and cool rapidly at the skin surface.

The only certain way to ascertain if a child has a fever is to take his or her temperature at one of three sites: in the rectum (the rectal temperature), in the mouth (the oral temperature), or in the armpit (the axillary temperature). For infants and toddlers, the most reliable method is rectally. It is difficult to obtain an accurate reading orally from a child who cannot hold the thermometer in the proper position under the tongue. If the child is uncooperative during attempts to take a rectal reading, try measuring the axillary temperature. To do so, place the mercury end of a thermometer high up in the armpit and hold the child's arm down against his or her body.

Timing is key in determining the presence of a fever. For a rectal reading, the thermometer should be left in place for three minutes, for an oral reading, three to five minutes, and for an axillary reading, nine minutes. The object is not to get an exact reading, but a range to establish the fact that the child has a fever.

In pediatrics a rectal temperature of:
100 degrees F. or less is considered normal.
100–102 degrees F. is low-grade fever.
102–104 degrees F. is elevated fever.
104 degrees F. or more is high fever.

Fevers, unless the child has symptoms indicating that he or she is seriously ill, can be treated at home, usually with aspirin or acetaminophen. A fever that persists for several days should also be brought to a doctor's attention. For more information on how to treat a child who has a fever, see the accompanying box below.

TREATING A CHILD WITH FEVER

- Dress the child in light clothing to prevent heat retention and permit cooling. Do not overdress.
- Do not use fever strips or other seemingly convenient methods of measuring temperature. They are unreliable and can be expensive. Use a standard mercury thermometer.
- Use the correct thermometer. Don't use an oral thermometer to take a rectal reading (the bulb end of a rectal thermometer is thicker and blunter, and less likely to break). However, if necessary, a rectal thermometer can be used to take an oral reading. Make sure it is clean (wash with cold water and soap before and after taking a reading) and keep it in the mouth for longer than usual.
- Do not convert readings. Generally, a rectal reading is one degree higher than an oral reading and as much as two degrees higher than an axillary reading. Be sure to specify to the doctor which reading—rectal, oral, axillary—was taken.
- Do not rely solely on sponging. Sponging or bathing the infant or child with tepid water lowers temperature a bit sooner (and may give the parent the feeling of helping the child) but its emphasis in practical terms is not greater than oral medications, such as aspirin or acetaminophen. Although these medications don't act quite as quickly as sponging, their effect lasts hours longer.

PEDIATRIC EMERGENCIES, NEAR-EMERGENCIES, AND NONEMERGENCIES

Cardiac Emergencies

Atrial and Ventricular Tachycardia. These are rare pediatric conditions that are marked by abnormal heartbeats (arrhythmia). External signs may include weak rapid pulse with or without labored or rapid breathing, clammy or mottled skin, listlessness, nausea, vomiting, agitation, or irritation. Arrhythmias may degenerate to the point where the heart does not contract properly and therefore does not pump blood adequately. When the heart arrests, or stops beating, breathing will also cease rapidly. A child with a weak or racing pulse should be taken to the emergency room immediately. *If you cannot find a pulse, begin cardiopulmonary resuscitation as instructed below and opposite in figures 34.1–34.5.*

Cardiopulmonary Resuscitation (CPR).

1. *Check for lack of responsiveness and a pulse.* Get close to the child and tap his or her shoulder or loudly call his or her name. If unconscious, the child will not move, moan, or cry; his or her legs and arms may be limp. Check the *brachial pulse* located on the inside of the arm, midway between the elbow and armpit. (The pulse of the carotid, or neck artery, in a child may be hard to locate.)

2. *Position the child.* Place the child on his or her back, preferably on a flat, hard, sturdy surface such as a table or the floor.

3. *Open the airway.* Gently place one hand on the forehead, with the other hand cradling the neck. With one hand, tip the head back, and lift the neck up with the other. This action opens the breathing airway. Bend over and place your cheek next to the nose and mouth to check for breathing—you will either feel it, hear it, or see the chest and abdomen rising or falling. If you discover the child is breathing, maintain the open airway, *but do not start rescue breathing.*

4. *If you detect no breathing, begin rescue breathing.* Seal the nose with your fingers and the mouth with your mouth. Give 4 quick, gentle breath puffs. Remember, a child's lung capacity is smaller than yours. Too much air can distend the stomach and result in vomiting.

5. *Check for a pulse.* If there is no pulse, continue rescue breathing, 1 breath every 3–4 seconds. If there is no pulse, begin chest compressions.

6. *Initiate chest compressions.* Place your index and middle fingers on the middle of the breastbone, and press down gently, compressing the area no more than ½ to 1 inch. Compressions should be done in groups of 5 every 3 seconds; count aloud to keep track. After the fifth compression, give 1 gentle breath.

7. *Summon help.* After 4 cycles of compression and breathing or just breathing, get medical help. If you are

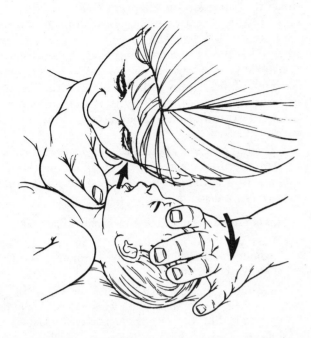

Figure 34.1. **To open a child's airway place your hand that is closest on the child's forehead and tilt back gently while lifting the chin with one or two fingers of the other hand.**

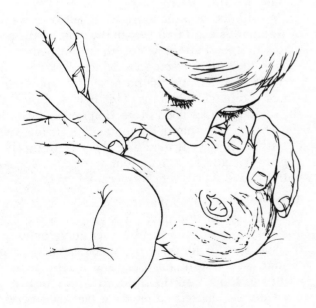

Figure 34.2. **The mouth-to-mouth and nose seal on an infant.**

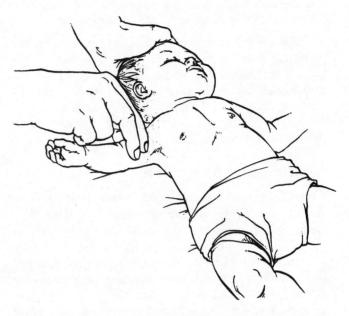

Figure 34.3. **Check the pulse on the inside of the upper arm.**

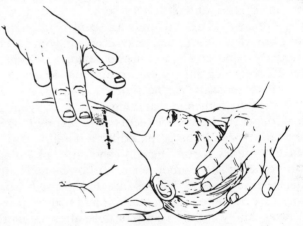

Figure 34.4. **Place index, third and fourth fingers between an infant's nipples and in the middle of the breastbone for chest compressions.**

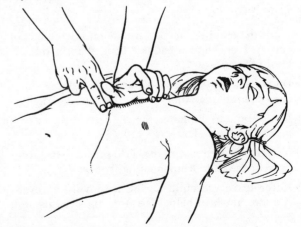

Figure 34.5. **For chest compressions on a child over 1 year, use the heel of one hand on the breastbone 2 fingers' breadth above its tip.**

alone, call out until someone comes to your aid. Continue breathing and, if necessary, compressing.

For cardiopulmonary resuscitation (CPR) truly to be effective, it must be performed properly. Improper technique can lead to internal-organ injury and worse, failure to save the child. In addition to reading about CPR, parents should learn the techniques by taking hands-on training programs and periodic refresher courses.

Neurologic Emergencies

Convulsions or Seizures That Won't Stop or That Are Persistently Recurrent (Status Ellipticus). Seizures result from abnormal electrical activity in the brain. This abnormal activity can be caused by a fever, an injury to the brain or head, disturbances in body chemistry or water balance, as well as by other serious illnesses, or the cause may be unknown. A seizure is frightening to watch—the child generally loses consciousness, falls to the ground, becomes stiff, and starts to jerk or twitch in a rhythmic way. The child may lose control of bladder and bowel function, and may drool or vomit. (For more information about causes of seizures, see chapter 28, Neurological and Neuromuscular Disorders.)

Most seizures last no more than five minutes, although to someone watching they may seem to last longer. If the seizure seems to be lasting longer, the family should be prepared for a possible trip to the emergency room. The child should be in a place where he or she cannot harm him or herself until the seizure passes. The seizure has passed when there are no more jerking motions and body stiffness relaxes. Many children sleep or doze after a seizure. After a seizure, the child's pediatrician should be called or the child taken to the emergency room to determine the cause of the episode. *During convulsions do the following:*

- Place the child on his or her side on a wide bed or a carpeted or blanket-padded floor that is relatively clear of furniture.

- Do not attempt to restrain the child, unless he or she risks self-inflicted injury.

- Do not put anything into the child's mouth, for example a spoon, towel, etc.

- If vomiting occurs, turn the child's head to one side, to prevent the child from inhaling the vomitus.

- Never leave the child during a convulsion, even to summon medical help. Wait until the convulsion has ended.

Convulsions caused by high fevers, known as febrile convulsions, are common in infants and young children. Controlling the fever is thought to help re-

duce the number of seizures. Before rushing the child to the doctor or emergency room, it is important to try to lower the fever. Even if the fever is lowered and no further seizures occur, seek medical consultation. In rare cases convulsions concurrent with a high fever may indicate meningitis. The presence or absence of meningitis is determined by a physical examination and spinal tap (lumbar puncture).

During a febrile illness, the fever may be reduced by using tepid compresses or by sponging the child in a bathtub with cool, not cold, water. *The following measures are also advised:*

- Do not use alcohol as the fumes may prove toxic.

- Dress the child in light clothing to permit cooling without causing chills. Cotton clothing cools faster than synthetics or blends.

- Give medications such as aspirin or acetaminophen every four hours. Medication works more slowly than sponging, but the fever-reducing effect lasts hours longer.

Head Injury or Trauma with Progressive Neurologic Symptoms. Most blows to the head are not serious. But if after a child sustains a head injury and certain symptoms increase in severity, he or she should be taken to an emergency room immediately. These include progression from such states as dizziness to confusion (reduced awareness of environment, slowed cognitive abilities) to stupor (lethargy and a state of unawareness which can only be broken through vigorous, repeated stimuli, such as a pin prick) to coma (complete unresponsiveness even to painful stimulation).

Most knocks to the fontanels (the two soft spots on an infant's skull that eventually close as the bone plates of the skull grow together) are benign. Although the anterior soft spot, which closes between 12 to 18 months, and the posterior soft spot, which closes within a few months of birth, look vulnerable, the scalp provides good protection for the brain tissue. On the other hand, if a fontanel protrudes (with or without injury), it should be checked promptly by a pediatrician. This symptom is often associated with meningitis or other intracranial events.

Meningitis. This inflammation and infection of the membranes that cover the surface of the brain and spinal cord is marked by fever and a bulging of the soft spot or fontanel in infants; and by severe headache, confusion, nausea, and a stiff neck (inability to touch chin to chest) in children. It is almost always caused either by a bacterial or viral agent.

Viral meningitis is less life-threatening than bacterial forms. Confirmation of the presence and type of meningitis is made using a test called the spinal tap or lumbar puncture in which a needle is inserted between two of the bony vertebrae of the back and a small amount of fluid is withdrawn for laboratory analysis. This procedure is not dangerous or harmful to the child. Many children recover without complications, but some are left with muscle weakness, hearing loss, partial paralysis, seizures, and delayed development.

Respiratory Emergencies

Near-Drowning. Death from drowning results from suffocation when an individual has been immersed in water. Near-drowning involves similar immersion with the difference that the victim survives. A body of water need not be especially large or deep to be deadly to infants and small children—bathtubs, sinks, baby bath basins, buckets, or toilets are potential sites for tragedy. Suffocation, or the lack of oxygen to body tissues, first results in disturbance in heart function. The heart may cease pumping altogether or pump erratically and ineffectively. Lung function ceases promptly after heart cessation. Other damage—swelling of brain tissue and circulatory failure (known medically as shock)—can have permanent effects. *When you are confronted with a near-drowning, follow these steps:*

1. *Remove the child from the water.* Lie the child on his or her back on a flat, solid surface. If the child is not breathing, initiate rescue breathing (see previous cardiopulmonary resuscitation [CPR] instructions).

2. *Check for a pulse.* If there is no pulse, begin CPR immediately.

3. *Get help.* If someone is with you, he or she should call the paramedics or drive you to the emergency room. If you are alone, continue CPR while periodically shouting for help.

4. *Don't stop your CPR efforts unless a paramedic or someone certified in CPR can take over for you.* Once CPR is initiated, it must be continued.

5. *Go to the hospital.* Any victim of near-drowning should be assessed medically. Let the emergency-room staff know if the accident occurred in salt or fresh water—it may influence the type of aftercare. Complications of near-drowning include heart attack, respiratory dysfunction (due to the accumulation of water in the lungs), and salt and fluid imbalance.

Croup That Doesn't Improve with Steaming. Croup is not a specific disease but a group of symptoms that arise in connection with a viral or bacterial infection, and cause a swelling of the upper airway. It is marked by a difficulty in inhaling, noisy breathing with a distinctive croaking sound (known as stridor), and a harsh barking cough. It is most

commonly ameliorated by the child's breathing steam generated by a hot tub or shower for 20 to 30 minutes. (In order to allow sufficient steam to build up, the bathroom door should be closed.)

If symptoms continue or worsen despite the steam treatment, or the child shows signs of insufficient oxygenation of tissues, such as blue lips or nails (known as cyanosis), a trip to the emergency room is mandatory. In the hospital, moist-air therapy is given with a face mask or oxygen tent. Sometimes medication to open the airways is given.

Epiglottitis is a particularly severe form of croup, caused by bacteria, that can cause a child's throat to swell and close. When this happens, an artificial means of respiration—either a nasal breathing tube or a surgically created airway—is necessary. Epiglottitis is characterized by a voice change, a sudden onset of high fever, drooling, and an inability to lie flat. This is an emergency and the doctor should be notified immediately and the child should go directly to the emergency room.

Pneumonia with Labored Breathing. A child with pneumonia (an infection or inflammation of the lungs of viral or bacterial origin), and not just a bad cold, will have congestion, and a cough and fever that worsens rapidly. Breathing may be troubled and rapid. Abnormal movements of the chest, known as retractions, may also occur. If these symptoms are present, the child should be taken to the local emergency room after a telephone consultation (if possible) with the pediatrician. A chest X ray will confirm the diagnosis as well as provide possible clues as to the type and severity of the pneumonia. Difficulty breathing will be ameliorated by the use of oxygen tents and/or other breathing treatments.

Airway Obstruction/Choking. Complete or partial blockage of the airway is an emergency and results from the aspiration (inhalation) of food or objects, for example, a button or a toy. In a partial blockage, the child will make sounds (choking, gagging, retching, crying, coughing) because some air is getting into and out of the lungs. In this case, it is often better to leave the child alone, but under observation, to expel the material or object.

In a complete blockage, the child makes no sound and may become unresponsive. In this situation, the child should not be transported to the emergency room. Instead, immediately, call an ambulance or the paramedics. *If there is a complete blockage of the airway do the following while waiting for help to arrive:*

1. Turn the child face down over your knees or lap, with the head slightly lower than the chest. Support the head with your hand on his or her jaw.

2. Using the heel of your other hand, rapidly administer 3 to 4 sharp blows to the back between the shoulder blades.

3. Turn the youngster on his or her back, your hand supporting the neck and head, and give 3 to 4 quick upward chest jabs. In infants, use your middle and index fingers; for children, use the heel of your hand. For both, perform this over the lowest part of the breastbone.

Alternate back blows with chest thrusts. Try either or both methods for about 1 minute—4 or 5 times, waiting 15 seconds between attempts. If neither works to dislodge the obstructing object, have someone call the paramedics or drive you to the hospital as you continue these efforts.

Do not try to dislodge an object with your fingers; this may wedge it more firmly in the airway. But if the object is visible and it seems that it can be scooped up and out without reaching deeply, then do so. While doing so, do not lay the child on his or her back, because any retrieval attempts made from this position may push the object back into the throat. Lay the child on his or her stomach on a hard flat surface such as a kitchen table or counter, and from a crouching position remove the object.

Neurologic Near-Emergencies

Stupor and Coma. A loss of consciousness that lasts days is technically not an emergency because its onset is gradual and steady, not sudden. It is, however, a near-emergency, demanding prompt medical attention.

Reye's Syndrome. This is an uncommon nonspecific illness that usually arises as a complication of a viral disease, most frequently chicken pox or influenza. While the exact cause of this condition is not known, there is a statistical association (but no cause-and-effect link) between the syndrome and the use of aspirin during a bout of the flu or chicken pox. Because of this, these illnesses should not be treated with aspirin. Instead, the aspirin substitute, acetaminophen, should be given. The more recent aspirin substitute, ibuprofen, is not recommended for children under the age of 12.

The illness mainly affects the brain and liver. It can cause severe brain swelling, resulting in an increase in pressure on the brain, and can cause damage to the liver. In its mildest form, Reye's syndrome causes nausea and vomiting; in more serious forms it may bring on stupor and coma. Typically the child afflicted with Reye's syndrome is thought to be recovered from the flu or chicken pox, when he or she becomes ill and is usually sleepy, with persistent vomiting and changed mental status. If you suspect Reye's syndrome, notify your physician immediately. How early a diagnosis is made and how soon treatment is initiated can affect the degree of brain swelling and influence the recovery from this disease.

Respiratory Near-Emergencies

Asthma That Doesn't Improve (Status Asthmaticus). Asthma, a disease of partial, reversible blockage of the smaller airways of the lungs, bronchi, and bronchioles, cannot be cured, but it can be controlled. Attacks are thought to be precipitated by allergy and respiratory infection.

If the youngster has been diagnosed as having asthma, a home treatment regime, including medication, will be prescribed. In the event that the usual treatment does not alleviate symptoms—wheezing, shortness of breath, a feeling of tightness in the chest—the doctor should be called for advice and evaluation. He or she may suggest going to the emergency room for help.

Teachers, babysitters, or daycare-attendants of a child with asthma should be informed, so that they will be prepared to seek medical attention if appropriate.

Nonspecific Cardiorespiratory Emergencies

Anaphylaxis. This is an overwhelming allergic reaction that may be caused by the sting from an insect, ingestion of a prescribed drug (most commonly penicillin), food, plants, and inhaled substances. Anaphylaxis is a natural protective mechanism that overresponded. The overresponse produces symptoms of general itching, blotchiness, redness, or welts (or "hives") on the skin, difficulty breathing, wheezing, coughing, voice change (indicating swelling around the larynx), dizziness, lightheadedness, generalized weakness, severe vomiting and/or diarrhea, faint pulse, sweating, and falling blood pressure.

In most cases, for anaphylaxis to occur the child must have prior exposure to the substance. Unfortunately, the previous exposure may be unknown or may have gone unrecognized because no initial reaction occurred, and therefore the anaphylactic reaction is unanticipated. Since any episode of anaphylaxis carries with it the risk of possible cardiac and respiratory arrest, medical attention should be sought immediately so the child can be treated. If the child's doctor is unavailable, the child should be taken without delay to the emergency room, by ambulance if possible. If necessary, CPR can be administered en route.

Circulatory Emergencies

Hemorrhage. Bleeding that won't stop or that continues for more than half an hour can result in a loss of blood volume that can lead to shock or circulatory collapse. Whether major or minor, all bleeding is managed the same way: by applying pressure with a dry cloth.

To treat hemorrhaging:

• Stop the bleeding where you can see it by applying enough pressure to stop the flow.

• Do not use anything wet. A dry cloth forms a clot better and faster. When the cloth becomes saturated, don't replace it; cover it with another dry cloth. If a clean dry cloth is not available, use the following substitutes: disposable diapers, sanitary napkins, paper towels, your hand.

• Do not apply pressure points and tourniquets. Leave these measures to the professionally trained.

• Elevate the affected part to reduce the blood flow.

Shock. The symptoms of shock include weak pulse, clammy, mottled, or cold skin or both, weakness, light-headedness, and labored or rapid breathing that results from blood loss. Blood supply can be reduced by heart failure, lack of blood volume (caused by severe bleeding), or faulty blood-vessel function (due to various diseases). When blood supply declines rapidly, the body attempts to redirect blood flow to vital organs, thus causing the primary superficial symptoms. However, shock can progress to respiratory or heart failure and death. If a child exhibits the symptoms of shock, he or she should be kept quiet, lying down with feet elevated, and lightly covered to conserve body heat. If needed, CPR should be administered, and the child should be transported immediately to the emergency room.

Bleeding Nonemergencies

Minor Bleeding. As stated in the section on hemorrhage, all bleeding is treated in the same way: by applying pressure with a dry cloth or paper towel to the site. Tourniquets and other indirect pressure techniques require real expertise to be used effectively and correctly. For basic first-aid purposes, minor bleeding can be stopped by applying pressure at the site of the bleeding.

Nosebleeds. The most common cause of nosebleeds in children is picking, which injures the lining of the nose. The lining is very rich in blood vessels and bleeds readily. Certain circumstances—a cold or excessively dry air—can make the lining of the nose more vulnerable to injury. Although it may look like more because it is combined with nasal mucus, blood loss from a nosebleed is usually very minor. In the event of a nosebleed, a child should sit upright and pinch the nostrils firmly shut for 10 to 15 minutes. The child should not be put in a prone position, as this increases the flow of blood to the head. After this time, the bleeding should be checked to see if it has stopped. If it has not, pressure should be reapplied for another 10 minutes. If after 30 minutes the bleeding has not stopped, the doctor should be called for advice. After the bleeding has stopped, a child should not be allowed to blow or pick his nose in order to prevent recurrence.

Nonspecific Emergencies

Poisoning. This is the unintentional or intentional ingestion or inhalation of or contact with a dangerous substance, for example, a caustic household cleanser or chemical, household plant, medication, cosmetic, aerosol product, paint, etc. Even seemingly harmless substances, such as alcohol, can be toxic to toddlers in certain quantities. Because of the dangers, all toxic items should be stored out of sight and reach of children. When you are in doubt about whether a child has been poisoned, it is better to assume that he or she has and to take the appropriate action. Symptoms of poisoning include sudden vomiting, diarrhea, or choking, without other signs of distress or illness, such as fever, cough, drooling, abrupt behavior changes (lethargy, irritability, excitability), sudden perspiration, and flushing. If poisoning is suspected, look for the evidence: an open or spilled container, traces of the substance in the child's breath, face, or clothing. It is important to locate the container to gauge how much the child has taken and to get further instructions. Many products contain information on whether or not to induce vomiting. If it is recommended to induce vomiting, do so immediately. Use syrup of ipecac according to label directions or irritate the back of the child's throat with the back end of any utensil. Do not use fingers, as they could be seriously bitten.

If you suspect poisoning, call the family doctor, the local emergency room, or the local Poison Control Center for instruction. Be prepared to relay the following:

• The type of poison.

• How much was taken.

• How long ago it was taken.

• Whether the child is showing any adverse signs and what those signs are.

• The child's age and weight.

• What steps you have taken and what response has been elicited.

If instructed to go to the emergency room, be sure to take the suspected poison and its container along. Watch for signs of shock, breathing difficulty, or other serious symptoms, such as convulsions, and report these to any medical personnel.

Gastrointestinal/Abdominal Emergencies

Vomiting of Blood (Hematemesis). Vomiting of small amounts of blood (half a cup or less) is not a cause for excessive concern, except in the case of infants and toddlers. It can be caused by irritation, infection, or blood swallowed from a nosebleed. If more than half a cup of blood is vomited, the physician should be notified and a trip to the emergency room may be required.

Passing Excessive Amounts of Blood Rectally. Passing less than half a cup of blood from the rectum (except with infants and toddlers) is not an emergency. A small amount of blood that streaks the stool is not urgent. This is usually the result of an internal or external fissure caused by constipation. A blood clot that is passed from the rectum in an infant or toddler warrants promptly notifying a doctor.

Abdominal Emergencies

Persistent Pain. When a youngster suffers from abdominal pain, parents most often suspect appendicitis, the inflammation and infection of the appendix, a fingerlike extension of the large intestine. There are, however, many causes of abdominal pain, including overeating, constipation, and the flu. Appendicitis starts gradually and cannot be distinguished from other causes of moderate pain in this area. With appendicitis, the pain does not disappear and worsens after two to three hours. It usually begins as a generalized abdominal pain around the navel, and only later becomes concentrated on the right side of the abdomen. *Warning signals of appendicitis are:* failure of the pain to abate, lack of appetite, tenderness of the area to the touch, nausea, vomiting, fever, and progression of pain.

If the doctor cannot be reached or if he or she advises, take the child to the emergency room. If appendicitis is suspected, the child may be admitted to the hospital and the appendix surgically removed. When possible the appendix should be removed before it ruptures (which can result in peritonitis, a very serious condition in which the abdominal lining becomes inflamed and infected). Studies suggest that the appendix will rupture if untreated (not surgically removed) in about 36 hours.

In infants and young children, any abdominal pain that persists longer than two hours warrants a call to a physician.

Persistent Vomiting. Vomiting, or the forceful ejection of the contents of the stomach, is common in infants and children. It can signal a dietary indiscretion, a cold or flu, or a more serious illness or injury. Vomiting that occurs for several hours or that is strangely colored—green, brown, "coffee ground," or red—is a near-emergency, as it may represent a bowel blockage, severe inflammation, or appendicitis. Persistent vomiting, with or without diarrhea, can lead to a loss of body fluids or dehydration, a situation that warrants prompt medical attention. Signs of dehydration include markedly reduced urine output, dry mouth, listlessness, greater than usual thirst, doughy skin, and sunken eyes.

Persistent Diarrhea. Persistent diarrhea, the passing of watery bowel movements, can result in dehydration. When the infant or child has diarrhea, more water than usual is passed out from the body with the stools; the frequency and constancy of the stools account for the amount of fluid lost. If watery stools persist, prompt medical attention should be sought.

Diarrhea that contains large amounts of mucus or blood also merits punctual medical attention. Certain foods and substances, such as Kool Aid, beets, Jell-O, food coloring, and certain medications, can look like blood in the stool. Vomiting or the presence of a high fever or both accompanied by diarrhea should also be medically evaluated.

Incarcerated Hernia. A hernia occurs when a portion of any abdominal organ (usually the intestine) slips between a weak point in the band of muscle in the groin. From the outside, a hernia appears as a sudden lump that may be tender. It usually occurs in the groin area, but it can cause a swelling in the testicle or labia. In most cases, the hernia rides up and down, in and out of the gap in the abdominal wall, but if it becomes trapped permanently outside the muscle "girdle," it becomes incarcerated. The incarceration may prevent normal passage of the bowel contents, and is known as an obstruction. In serious cases, a loss of blood to the herniated section of the bowel can cause the tissue to die, leading to complications such as infection and gangrene. An incarcerated hernia requires prompt medical attention. If the incarceration cannot be restored to normal, surgery is required.

Abdominal Nonemergencies

Colic. A daily recurring pattern of irritability and crying known as colic usually occurs in infants three months old or younger but can last longer. The spells can last up to 12 hours. The causes of colic are unknown but are variously ascribed to milk allergies, immaturity of the gastrointestinal tract, gas, sensitivity to a disruptive noisy environment, poor feeding techniques, parental anxiety, or individual temperament. It is rarely attributed to a serious physiological condition. Once any coexisting physical conditions are ruled out, there is little medical treatment known to relieve colic. Patience and perseverance are required and tested. Happily most children outgrow it within a few months.

During a spell of colic, the infant may draw up his or her legs close to the body, the abdomen may appear distended, and gas may be passed. At-home measures—rhythmical movement, such as rocking or riding in a car, and continual monotonous sounds may bring some relief, as may being carried in a soft baby carrier (such as a Snugli).

Eye Emergencies

Laceration of the Globe. A laceration or cut of the eyeball may appear as a thin line. The youngster will experience light sensitivity and blurred vision. The child should keep the eye closed and medical attention should be promptly sought.

Blunt Trauma. Any injury that results from a direct blow to the eye, for instance, from a ball or a fist, should be promptly evaluated by a physician (preferably an ophthalmologist). Even though no damage is apparent, there may be bleeding which results in damaging pressure in the eye.

Hyphemia. Hyphemia or trapped blood in the iris (the pigmented portion of the eye), usually results from blunt trauma—a blow or a bump—and warrants a trip to the emergency room. Pressure from the accumulation of blood can result in permanent loss of vision.

Eye Nonemergencies

Conjunctivitis. Commonly called "pink eye," conjunctivitis is an inflammation of the thin mucosal layer lining the eyelids. It is caused by an allergy or a viral or bacterial infection and is characterized by generalized redness, usually in both eyes, itching, burning, swelling, tearing, and pus formation. The pus may cause the eyelids to stick together. In children, conjunctivitis usually accompanies or follows a cold. A doctor can recommend treatment. Most cases can be easily treated at home with antibacterial drops or ointment but these should not be used without the doctor's guidance.

Sties. Pimples that form under the eyelid in an eyelash follicle are called sties. The cause is usually the staphylococcus or "staph" germ. Many pediatricians recommend frequent warm compresses to ease any discomfort and to bring the sty "to a head" to drain accumulated pus. To prepare a warm compress, moisten a clean, lint-free towel in warm water, wring it out, and hold it against the affected area for about 10 minutes. Warm compresses may be applied as frequently as needed. The doctor may or may not prescribe an antibiotic for use along with the compresses.

Blocked Tear Ducts. When a duct becomes completely or partially blocked, tears cannot drain properly and the retained fluid can be invaded by bacteria. This is a common occurrence in the first few weeks of life. Symptoms include a white or yellow discharge in the corner of one or both eyes, or increased tearing in the eye with discharge or both. Most of the time the condition resolves itself, but if it is a continuing problem or increases in severity, it should be brought to the doctor's attention at the next routine visit. Occasionally a tear duct may need to be surgically widened, between 9 to 15 months of age.

Skeletal Emergencies

Head, Neck, or Back Injuries. The skull, neck, and backbone act as armor, protecting the organs of the central nervous system, the brain, and the spinal cord. Injury to these bony structures can affect the ability to move, speak, or breathe. If an injury to the head, neck, or back is suspected, do not move the child unless it is to prevent further injury. If the child is not breathing, begin CPR and have someone call paramedics or an ambulance. If emergency personnel are not available, immobilize the child on a board with pillows and blankets, keeping the neck in alignment with the rest of the backbone (to minimize further movement or injury of the head, neck, or back) and transport him or her to the emergency room. Try to calm the child so that he or she lies as quietly as possible.

Compound Fractures. These are breaks in the bone in which a portion of the bone protrudes through the skin. When this happens, the bone is exposed to dirt, debris, and bacteria, increasing the risk of infection. The bone should be cleansed and then covered with a clean cloth or piece of sterile gauze to protect it from exposure. As soon as the situation is stabilized, the child should be taken to the emergency room.

Skeletal Nonemergencies

Fractures. These are breaks in the bone. A bone may be broken completely (known as a "simple" fracture) or it may be incompletely broken (called a "greenstick" fracture). Incomplete fractures are common in children, due to the pliability of their bones. When a child fractures a bone, a parent will usually notice a swelling or stiffness that occurs immediately and does not resolve itself in a day or two, or an obvious deformity (part of the bone juts out). The child will often complain of pain. A physician's evaluation and examination (which includes X rays) are necessary to determine the type and extent of the injury.

The only urgency involved with a fracture is that the child get relief from the pain associated with the injury sooner rather than later. The doctor should be called. If the doctor is unavailable, the child should be taken to the emergency room for treatment, which may include putting the bone back in alignment, known as "reducing" a fracture.

If you suspect a child has a fracture:

- Immobilize the affected bone. A temporary splint can be made from a pillow, a piece of wood, or a rolled-up newspaper or magazine. Tape or tie the affected body part to the splint—this will immediately relieve some of the pain.

- Keep the arm or leg elevated to minimize swelling that causes pain.

- Apply an ice pack to the affected area. Use a commercially available ice pack or make one by filling a plastic bag with ice and wrapping it in a towel. Apply to the injured area. Icing, by reducing swelling, helps to reduce pain.

- Don't allow the child to use or place weight on the affected area until it has been examined by a doctor.

Dislocations.   When a bone slips from its proper alignment in a joint, pain, as well as the potential damage or stretching of the ligaments, muscles, or joints involved can occur. Signs of dislocations are similar to those of a fracture—pain, swelling, tenderness, or stiffness, or any combination of these symptoms, of the affected area. Ice packs, immobilization, and elevation may make the child more comfortable. Consult the doctor for the next appropriate step. If no doctor is available, go to the emergency room.

If a child has a dislocation:

- Consult the doctor even if the joint has slipped back into alignment. An injury to the joint, ligament, or muscles may have occurred.

- The child should not immediately resume normal activities. A period of rest, determined by the doctor, is needed to allow healing.

Skin Emergencies

Severe Burns.   The heat from a burn continues to penetrate the skin, damaging nerves, hair follicles, blood vessels, and sweat glands for up to 25 minutes, resulting in pain after the initial contact. This progressive damage is known as thermal injury. For this reason, it is important to cool the skin temperature through immersion in cool water or the use of cool compresses.

The following types of burns should receive immediate medical examination because there is a risk of loss of body fluids, infection, scarring, nerve damage, shock, or potential serious disability:

- Burns on the face, hands, feet, or genitals.

- Third-degree burns. The skin appears white or charred. These destroy all layers of skin.

- Second-degree burns. These cause blistering and injure the layers of skin beneath the surface.

In the emergency room, the patient will probably be connected to an IV (intravenous infusion), a preliminary step to counteract loss of body fluid and prevent shock. Pain medication may also be administered via the IV. If the child has not been immunized against tetanus, he or she will most likely be given a tetanus inoculation.

When a child is seriously burned, follow these steps:

- Immerse the burn in cold water to halt the progress of thermal injury and help relieve pain.

- Do not remove any clothing or debris from the burned area.

- Don't apply any ointment or over-the-counter pain medications (recognizable by the suffix -caine). These do not help and may impede the healing process.

- Don't apply butter, toothpaste, or other "home remedies."

Electrical or Chemical Burns.   Skin damage caused by accidental contact with an electrical wire or caustic chemicals is deceptive, and may not look as bad as it is. In any case, such burns need medical evaluation. When the doctor is unavailable, the child should be taken to the emergency room. For a chemical burn, the affected area should be flushed with cool water from a garden hose, a shower, tub, or buckets of water for at least 5 to 10 minutes. Do not direct a strong stream of water on the affected area, as this may cause pain and further injury.

Skin Nonemergencies

Minor Burns.   An accidental contact with a hot object or liquid, steam, flame, or prolonged exposure to the sun can result in a minor, first-degree burn. With these burns, only the top layer of skin has been injured. Healing almost always leaves no scars. Immersion in cold water can halt the potentially damaging (or at least painful) thermal injury progression.

Cool running water from the tap or a cold pack (ice cubes in a plastic bag) should be applied to the burn until the pain subsides. The longer the source of cold can be held to the burn, the better. Although this may be difficult to accomplish on a wiggling, protesting, crying child, it should be done. (For other ways to deal with a minor burn, see the accompanying box; for sunburns, see box on Preventing Sunburns in chapter 32.)

TREATING A MINOR BURN

- Don't cover the burn with a paper towel or terrycloth towel. These may adhere to the injured area and cause more damage when peeled off.
- Don't apply butter, grease, ointments, or other creams. These are not recommended first-aid treatment for any burns.
- Use basic wound hygiene techniques. Once a mild burn is cooled, clean the area with tepid water and a mild soap. First-degree burns need not be covered, except for personal comfort.
- Don't be overly concerned if a burn takes a long time to heal. Even if kept infection-free, a minor burn may take a month to heal completely.

Hives or Urticaria. These are red, raised welts that may occur anywhere on the body. They are generally caused by an allergy to food, medicines, or other items that are ingested or inhaled, or that come in contact with the skin. They may occur as a response to cold, heat, or stress. A mild case of hives will disappear in several hours. If another outbreak occurs, it means the child is still reacting to the al-

lergen. A doctor should be consulted as to the need for testing or treatment.

Insect Stings. The sting from a bee or hornet rarely causes anaphylaxis, or a severe generalized reaction. A sting that results in swelling both locally (around the site of the sting) as well as a larger area that is contiguous with the sting site is not a generalized reaction and will virtually never progress to anaphylaxis.

For stings causing a local reaction only, apply an ice pack immediately to reduce the swelling and pain. Over-the-counter antihistamines do not relieve pain, but they may help the itching associated with the sting.

Animal Bites. The greatest risk from an animal bite is infection, not tetanus or rabies. The wound should be washed carefully with soap and water and the doctor called for advice. If the bite comes from an otherwise healthy pet, this basic hygiene will suffice. If the child has received a primary series of tetanus shots and the injury is minor, a booster may not be needed; however, a more severe wound may warrant a booster. High-risk wounds for tetanus include rip-and-tear bites or a dirty wound—one that occurred in a farm or zoo setting, where animal waste, manure piles, or compost heaps are present.

Animal bites on the face, with broken skin, and those with marked skin disruption require immediate attention. Bites with moderate skin disruption also require notification of a doctor but may not require a doctor's intervention. Bites with slight or minor breaks of the skin require cleansing, but do not warrant notification of a doctor.

Rabies is very rare in domestic animals. Currently most rabies is carried by bats and skunks. If the child has been bitten by a wild animal, the local Department of Public Health should be called to find out if there is rabies in the area. The Department of Public Health issues updates every three months on the occurrence of rabies and denotes certain counties as "endemic to rabies." This classification will determine whether you should seek medical treatment for rabies.

Appendix A
Poison Control Centers

ALABAMA

Birmingham
Children's Hospital of Alabama
  Poison Center
1600 Seventh Avenue, S.
Birmingham, AL 35233
Within AL: (800) 292-6678
Outside AL: (205) 939-9201

Tuscaloosa
Alabama Poison Center
809 University Boulevard, E.
Tuscaloosa, AL 35401
(205) 345-0600
(800) 462-0800

ALASKA

Fairbanks
Fairbanks Poison Center
Fairbanks Memorial Hospital
1650 Cowles
Fairbanks, AK 99701
(907) 456-7182

ARIZONA

Phoenix
Central Arizona Region Poison
  Management Center
St. Luke's Medical Center
1800 E. Van Buren
Phoenix, AZ 85006
(602) 253-3334

Tucson
Arizona Poison and Drug Information
  Center
Health Sciences Center, Room 3204K
1501 Campbell Hall
Tucson, AZ 85725
Within AZ: (800) 362-0101
Outside AZ: (602) 626-6016

ARKANSAS

Little Rock
Arkansas Poison & Drug Information
  Center
University of Arkansas College of
  Pharmacy
4301 W. Markham, Slot 522
Little Rock, AR 72205
(501) 666-5532
(800) 482-8948

CALIFORNIA

Fresno
Fresno Regional Poison Control
  Center
Fresno Community Hospital
P.O. Box 1232
Fresno, CA 93715
(209) 445-1222

Los Angeles
Los Angeles County Medical
  Association
Regional Poison Center
1925 Wilshire Boulevard
Los Angeles, CA 90057
(213) 664-2121
(213) 484-5151

Orange
Regional Poison Control
  University of California Irvine
  Medical Center
101 The City Drive, S.
Route 71
Orange City, CA 92668
(714) 634-5988

Richmond
Chevron Poison Information Center
15299 San Pablo Avenue
P.O. Box 4054
Richmond, CA 94804
(415) 233-3737
(415) 233-3738

Sacramento
Regional Poison Control Center
University of California at Davis
  Medical Center
2315 Stockton Boulevard
Sacramento, CA 95817
(916) 453-3692

San Diego
San Diego Regional Poison Center
University of California at San
  Diego Medical Center
225 Dickinson Street
San Diego, CA 92013
(619) 294-6000

San Francisco
San Francisco Bay Area Poison
  Center
San Francisco General Hospital
1001 Potrero Avenue
San Francisco, CA 94110
(415) 476-6600
(800) 233-3360

San Jose
Central Coast Counties Regional
  Poison Center
Santa Clara Valley Medical Center
751 S. Bascom Avenue
San Jose, CA 95128
(408) 299-5112, 5113, 5114
(800) 662-9886, 9887

Santa Rosa
Sonoma County Poison Center
3325 Chanate Road
Santa Rosa, CA 95404

COLORADO

Denver
Rocky Mountain Poison Center
645 Bannock Street
Denver, CO 80204
(303) 629-1123

CONNECTICUT

Farmington
Connecticut Poison Control Center
University of Connecticut Health
  Center
Farmington, CT 06032
(203) 674-3456

DISTRICT OF COLUMBIA

Washington
National Capital Poison Center
Georgetown University Hospital
3800 Reservoir Road, N.W.
Washington, DC 20007
(202) 625-3333

FLORIDA

Inverness
Citrus County Poison Control
Citrus Memorial Hospital
502 S. Highland Boulevard
Inverness, FL 32650
(904) 726-2800

Jacksonville
St. Vincent's Medical Center
1800 Barrs Street
Jacksonville, FL 32204
(904) 387-7500
(904) 387-7499

Tampa
Tampa Bay Regional Poison
  Control Center, Inc.
Tampa General Hospital
P.O. Box 18582
Tampa, FL 33679
(813) 253-4444
(800) 282-3171

Winterhaven
Winterhaven Hospital Poison
  Control Center
200 Avenue F, N.E.
Winterhaven, FL 33880
(813) 299-9701

GEORGIA

Atlanta
Georgia Poison Control Center
80 Butler Street S.E.
Box 26066
Atlanta, GA 30335
(404) 589-4400

Savannah
Savannah Regional EMS Poison
  Center
Memorial Medical Center, Inc.
Emergency Department
P.O. Box 23089
Savannah, GA 31403
(912) 355-5228

HAWAII

Honolulu
Kapiolani–Children's Medical
  Center
1319 Punahou Street
Honolulu, HI 96826
From within the Islands:
  (808) 941-4411
From outside the Islands:
  (800) 362-3585

IDAHO

Boise
Idaho Poison Center
1055 N. Curtis Road
Boise, ID 83706
(208) 378-2707
(800) 632-8000

Pocatello
Idaho Regional
   Poison Control Center and
   Drug Information Center
755 Hospital Way, Suite F2
Pocatello, ID 83201
(208) 234-0777
(800) 632-9490

ILLINOIS

Chicago
Chicago Poison Control Center
1753 W. Congress Parkway
Chicago, IL 60612
Within Chicago and northeastern
   IL: (800) 942-5969
All other areas: (312) 942-5969

Normal
Brokaw Hospital Poison Center
Virginia at Franklin
Normal, IL 61761
(309) 454-1400

Peoria
Peoria Poison Center
St. Francis Medical Center
530 N.E. Glen Oak Avenue
Peoria, IL 61632
Within IL: (800) 332-5330
Outside IL: (309) 655-2334

Springfield
Poison Resource Center
St. John's Hospital
800 E. Carpenter
Springfield, IL
(800) 252-2022
(217) 544-6464, Ext. 4608

Urbana
National Animal Poison Control
   Center
University of Illinois Department of
   Veterinary Biosciences
2001 S. Lincoln Avenue, 1220 VMBSB
Urbana, IL 61801
(217) 333-3611

INDIANA

Indianapolis
Indiana Poison Center
Wishard Memorial Hospital
1001 W. Tenth Street
Indianapolis, IN 46202
Within IN: (800) 382-9097
Outside IN: (317) 630-7351

IOWA

Des Moines
Variety Club Drug and Poison
   Information Center
1200 Pleasant Street
Des Moines, IA 50309
(515) 283-6254
(515) 283-6534

Sioux City
Marian Health Center
801 5th Street
Sioux City, IA 51104
(712) 258-6424
(712) 279-2066

St. Luke's Poison Center
St. Luke's Regional Medical Center
2720 Stone Park Boulevard
Sioux City, IA 51104
Within Iowa: (800) 352-2222
From Nebraska and South Dakota:
   (800) 831-1111

KANSAS

Kansas City
Mid America Poison Center
Kansas University Medical Center,
   Department of Pharmacology
39th and Rainbow Boulevard
Kansas City, KS 66103
(913) 588-6633
(800) 332-6633

Topeka
Stormont Vail Regional Medical
   Center
1500 S.W. 10th
Topeka, KS 66606
(913) 354-6100

KENTUCKY

Ft. Thomas
Northern Kentucky Poison
   Information Center
St. Luke Hospital
85 N. Grand Avenue
Ft. Thomas, KY 41075
(606) 572-3215

Louisville
Kentucky Poison Control Center of
   Kosair Children's Hospital
P.O. Box 35070
Louisville, KY 40232
Within KY: (800) 722-5725
Outside KY: (502) 589-8222

LOUISIANA

Shreveport
Louisiana Regional Poison Center
Louisiana State University Medical
   Center
P.O. Box 33932
Shreveport, LA 71130
(318) 425-1524
(800) 535-0525

MAINE

Portland
Maine Poison Control Center
Maine Medical Center
22 Bramhall Street
Portland, ME 04102
Within ME: (800) 442-6305
Outside ME: (207) 871-2381

MARYLAND

Baltimore
Maryland Poison Center
University of Maryland Pharmacy
   School
20 N. Pine Street
Baltimore, MD 21201
Within MD: (800) 492-2414
Outside MD: (301) 528-7701

MASSACHUSETTS

Boston
Massachusetts Poison Control
   System
300 Longwood Avenue
Boston, MA 02115
(617) 232-2120
(800) 682-9211

MICHIGAN

Adrian
Bixby Hospital Poison Center
Emma L. Bixby Hospital
818 Riverside Avenue
Adrian, MI 49221
(517) 263-2412

Ann Arbor
University of Michigan Poison
   Center
Emergency Services B1C255
1500 E. Medical Center Drive
Ann Arbor, MI 48109
(313) 764-7667
(313) 963-6666

Detroit
Poison Control Center
Children's Hospital of Michigan
3901 Beaubien Boulevard
Detroit, MI 48201
Outside metropolitan Detroit only:
   (800) 462-6642
All of MI: (800) 572-1655

Grand Rapids
Blodgett Regional Poison Center
1840 Wealthy Street, S.W.
Grand Rapids, MI 49506
Within MI: (800) 632-2727
Outside MI: (800) 442-4571;
   616 area WATS

Kalamazoo
Bronson Poison Information Center
252 E. Lovell Street
Kalamazoo, MI 49007
(800) 442-4112 616 area WATS only
(616) 383-6409

Midwest Poison Center
1521 Gull Road
Kalamazoo, MI 49002
(616) 383-7070
(800) 632-4177

Saginaw
Saginaw Regional Poison Center
1447 N. Harrison
Saginaw, MI 48602
(517) 755-1111

MINNESOTA

Minneapolis
Hennepin Regional Poison Center
701 Park Avenue
Minneapolis, MN 55415
(612) 347-3141

Rochester
St. Mary's Hospital Poison Center
1216 Second Street, S.W.
Rochester, MN 55902
Within MN: (800) 222-1222

St. Paul
Minnesota Regional Poison Center
640 Jackson Street
St. Paul, MN 55101
(612) 221-2113

MISSISSIPPI

Jackson
University of Mississippi Medical
   Center
2500 N. State Street
Jackson, MS 39216
(601) 354-7660

MISSOURI

Kansas City
Poison Control Center
Children's Mercy Hospital
24th at Gillham Road
Kansas City, MO 64108
(816) 234-3000

St. Louis
Regional Poison Center
Cardinal Glennon Children's
   Hospital
1465 S. Grand Boulevard
St. Louis, MO 63104
Within MO: (800) 392-9111
Outside MO: (314) 772-5200

NEBRASKA

Omaha
Mid-Plains Poison Center
Children's Memorial Hospital
8301 Dodge Street
Omaha, NE 68114
Within NE: (800) 390-5400
From surrounding states:
   (800) 642-9999

NEVADA

Reno
St. Mary's Hospital Poison Control
Center
235 W. 6th Street
Reno, NV 89520
(702) 789-3013

NEW HAMPSHIRE

Hanover
New Hampshire Poison Center
Dartmouth-Hitchcock Medical
Center
Hanover, NH 03756
Within NH: (800) 562-8236

NEW JERSEY

Berlin
West Jersey Poison Center
White Horse Pike at Townsend
Avenue
Berlin, NJ 08009
(609) 768-6060

Newark
New Jersey Poison Information and
Education Systems
201 Lyons Avenue
Newark, NJ 07112
Within NJ: (800) 962-1253
Outside NJ: (201) 926-4987

Phillipsburg
Warren Hospital Poison Control
Center
185 Roseberry Sstreet
Phillipsburg, NJ 08865
(201) 859-6768

NEW MEXICO

Albuquerque
New Mexico Poison & Drug
Information Center
University of New Mexico
Albuquerque, NM 87131
Within NM: (800) 432-6866
Outside NM: (505) 843-2551

NEW YORK

Albany
Bureau of Child Health
New York State Department of
Health
Corning Tower Building
Room 878, Empire State Plaza
Albany, NY 12237
(518) 474-2162

Buffalo
Western New York Poison Control
Center
Children's Hospital of Buffalo
219 Bryant Street
Buffalo, NY 14222
(716) 878-7654

East Meadow
Nassau County Medical Center's
Long Island Regional Poison
Control Center
2201 Hempstead Turnpike
East Meadow, NY 11554
(516) 542-2323; 2324; 2325

New York City
New York City Region Poison
Control Center
455 First Avenue, Room 123
New York, NY 10016
(212) 764-7667
(800) 255-0658

Nyack
Hudson Valley Poison Center
Nyack Hospital
N. Midland Avenue
Nyack, NY 10920
(914) 353-1000

Rochester
Life Line Finger Lakes
Regional Poison Control
Center
University of Rochester Medical
Center
P.O. Box 321
Rochester, NY 14642
(716) 275-5151

NORTH CAROLINA

Charlotte
Mercy Hospital Poison Center
2001 Vall Avenue
Charlotte, NC 28207
(704) 379-5827

Durham
Duke Regional Poison Control
Center
Erwin Road, Box 3007
Durham, NC 27710
Within NC: (800) 672-1697
Outside NC: (919) 684-4050

NORTH DAKOTA

Fargo
North Dakota Poison Center
St. Luke's Hospital
Fifth Street and Mills Avenue
Fargo, ND 58122
Within ND: (800) 732-2200
Outside ND: (701) 280-5575

OHIO

Akron
Akron Regional Poison Center
281 Locust Street
Akron, OH 44308
Within OH: (800) 362-9922
Outside OH: (216) 379-8562

Canton
Stark County Poison Control Center
1320 Timken Mercy Drive N.W.
Canton, OH 44708
(216) 489-1310
(800) 722-8662

Cincinnati
S.W. Ohio Regional Poison Control
System and Cincinnati Drug and
Poison Information Center
231 Bethesda Avenue ML #144
Cincinnati, OH 45267
(513) 872-5111, 5112, 5113
(800) 872-5111

Cleveland
Greater Cleveland Poison Control
Center
2101 Adelbert Road
Cleveland, OH 44106
(216) 231-4455

Columbus
Central Ohio Poison Center
700 Children's Drive
Columbus, OH 43205
(614) 228-1325
(800) 682-7625

Dayton
W. Ohio Regional Poison and Drug
Information Center
One Children's Plaza
Dayton, OH 45404
(513) 222-2227
(800) 762-0727

Youngstown
Mahoning Valley Poison Center
St. Elizabeth Hospital Medical
Center
1044 Belmont Avenue
Youngstown, OH 44501
(216) 746-2222
(216) 746-5510

OREGON

Portland
Oregon Poison Control and Drug
Information Center
3181 S.W. Sam Jackson Park Road
Portland, OR 97201
Within OR: (800) 452-7165
Outside OR: (503) 224-8968

PENNSYLVANIA

Allentown
Lehigh Valley Poison Center
The Allentown Hospital
17th and Chow Streets
Allentown, PA 18102
(215) 433-2311
(215) 778-2696

Altoona
Keystone Regional Poison Center
Mercy Hospital
2500 Seventh Avenue
Altoona, PA 16603
(814) 949-4197
(814) 946-3711

Danville
Susquehanna Poison Center
P.O. Box 273-A
Danville, PA 17821
(717) 275-6116
(717) 271-6116

Erie
Northwestern Poison Center
St. Vincent Health Center
232 W. 25th Street
Erie, PA 16544
(814) 452-3232

Poison Control Center
Hamot Medical Center
201 State Street
Erie, PA 16550
(814) 870-6111

Hershey
Capital Area Poison Center
Milton Hershey Medical Center
Pennsylvania State University
P.O. Box 850
Hershey, PA 17033
(717) 531-6111

Philadelphia
Delaware Valley Regional
Poison Control Program
One Children's Center
34th and Civic Center Boulevard
Philadelphia, PA 19104
(215) 386-2100

Pittsburgh
Pittsburgh Poison Center
One Children's Place
3705 Fifth Avenue at DeSoto Street
Pittsburgh, PA 15213
(412) 681-6669

Williamsport
The Williamsport Hospital
Poison Control Center
777 Rural Avenue
Williamsport, PA 17701
(717) 321-2000

RHODE ISLAND

Providence
Rhode Island Poison Center
593 Eddy Street
Providence, RI 02902
(401) 227-5272
(401) 227-8062

SOUTH DAKOTA

Aberdeen
St. Luke's Hospital
Poison Center
305 S. State Street
Aberdeen, SD 57104
(605) 225-2131

Rapid City
Rapid City Regional Poison Control
Center
353 Fairmont Boulevard
P.O. Box 6000
Rapid City, SD 57709
(605) 341-3333

Sioux Falls
McKennan Poison Center
800 E. 21st Street
Sioux Falls, SD 57117
Within SD: (800) 952-0123
In IA, MN, NE: (800) 843-9595

TENNESSEE

Memphis
Southern Poison Center
848 Adams Avenue
Memphis, TN 38103
(901) 528-6048

TEXAS

Conroe
Medical Center Hospital Poison
  Center
P.O. Box 1538
Conroe, TX 77305
(409) 539-7700

Dallas
North Central Texas Poison Center
Parkland Hospital
P.O Box 35926
Dallas, TX 75235
(214) 920-2400
(800) 441-0040

El Paso
El Paso Poison Control Center
R. E. Thomas General Hospital
4815 Alameda Avenue
El Paso, TX 79905
(915) 533-1244

Galveston
Texas State Poison Center
University of Texas Medical Branch
Galveston, TX 77550
(713) 654-1701
(409) 765-1420
(512) 478-4490

Tyler
East Texas Poison Center
  Medical Center Hospital
Box 6400
Tyler, TX 75711
(214) 597-0351

UTAH

Salt Lake City
Intermountain Regional Poison
  Control Center
50 N. Medical Drive
Salt Lake City, UT 84132
(801) 581-2151
(800) 662-0062

VERMONT

Burlington
Vermont Poison Center
Medical Center of Vermont
Colchester Avenue
Burlington, VT 05401
(802) 658-3456

VIRGINIA

Charlottesville
Blue Ridge Poison Center
University of Virginia Medical
  Center
Box 484
Charlottesville, VA 22908
(804) 924-5543

Hampton
Peninsula Poison Center
3120 Victoria Boulevard
Hampton, VA 23669
(804) 722-1131

Norfolk
Tidewater Poison Center
DePaul Hospital
150 Kingsley Lane
Norfolk, VA 23505
(804) 489-5288
(800) 552-6337

Richmond
Central Virginia Poison Center
MCV Station
Box 522
Richmond, VA 23298
(804) 786-9133, 2222

Roanoke
Southwest Virginia Poison Center
P.O. Box 13367
Roanoke, VA 24033
(701) 981-7336

WASHINGTON

Seattle
Seattle Poison Center
Children's Orthopedic Hospital
P.O. Box C5371
Seattle, WA 98105
Within WA: (800) 732-6985
Outside WA: (206) 526-2121

Spokane
Spokane Poison Center
Deaconess Medical Center
W. 800 Fifth Avenue
Spokane, WA 99210
In Washington: (800) 572-5842
In surrounding states: (800) 541-5624

Yakima
Central Washington Poison Center
2811 Tieton Drive
Yakima, WA 98902
(509) 248-4400
(800) 572-9176

WEST VIRGINIA

Charleston
West Virginia Poison Center
3110 MacCorkie Avenue, S.E.
Charleston, WV 25304
(304) 348-4211
(800) 642-3625
(Statewide)

Parkersburg
St. Joseph's Hospital Center
19th and Murdoch Avenue
Parkersburg, WV 26101
(304) 424-4222

WISCONSIN

Eau Claire
Eau Claire Poison Center
Luther Hospital
1221 Whipple Street
Eau Claire, WI 54702
(915) 533-1244

Green Bay
Green Bay Poison Center
P.O. Box 13508
Green Bay, WI 53407
(414) 433-8100

La Crosse
La Crosse Area Poison Center
700 W. Avenue, S.
La Crosse, WI 54601
(608) 784-3971

Madison
University of Wisconsin Hospital
Regional Poison Center
600 Highland Avenue
Madison, WI 53792
(608) 262-3702

Milwaukee
Milwaukee Poison Center
1700 W. Wisconsin Avenue
Milwaukee, WI 53233
(414) 931-4114

Appendix B
Useful Resources

Most voluntary health agencies and some professional associations can provide information and educational materials and, in some cases, referrals to board-certified specialists or special clinics. Although only the national offices of these organizations are listed below, many of them have local chapters, which can be found in the white pages of the phone directory. It is generally better to contact the local chapter first.

ALLERGY AND ASTHMA

American Allergy Association
Box 7273
Menlo Park, CA 94025
(415) 322-1663

American Lung Association
Box 596-COL
New York, NY 10001
(212) 245-8000

Some local chapters will make referrals and give lists of special programs for children with asthma.

Asthma and Allergy Foundation
Suite 305
1717 Massachusetts Avenue NW
Washington, DC 20036
(202) 265-0265
(800) 7 ASTHMA

ARTHRITIS

National Arthritis Foundation
1314 Spring Street NW
Atlanta, GA 30309
(404) 822-7100

AUTISM

National Society for Children and Adults with Autism
Suite 1017
1234 Massachusetts Avenue NW
Washington, DC 20005
(202) 783-0125

BIRTH DEFECTS

March of Dimes/Birth Defects Foundation
1275 Mamaroneck Avenue
White Plains, NY 10605
(914) 428-7100

Can make referrals to local genetics clinics as well as clinics that handle high-risk pregnancy and those that treat children with birth defects.

CANCER

American Cancer Society
1599 Clifton Road NE
Atlanta, GA 30329
(404) 892-0026

Some local chapters will make referrals.

CEREBRAL PALSY

United Cerebral Palsy Associations
66 East 34th Street
New York, NY 10016
(212) 481-6300

The professional services department will make referrals to centers for diagnosis, treatment, and therapy.

CYSTIC FIBROSIS

Cystic Fibrosis Foundation
Suite 111
1655 Tullie Circle
Atlanta, GA 30329
(404) 325-6973

Local chapters make referrals.

DIABETES

Juvenile Diabetes Foundation International
23 East 26th Street
New York, NY 10010
(212) 889-7575

EPILEPSY

Epilepsy Foundation of America
Suite 406
4351 Garden City Drive
Landover, MD
(301) 456-3700

GENETIC DISEASES

National Genetics Foundation
555 West 57th Street
New York, NY 10019
(212) 586-5800

Referral services for individuals interested in genetic diseases or genetic counseling.

GROWTH DISORDERS

Human Growth Foundation
Montgomery Building
4720 Montgomery Lane
Bethesda, MD 20814
(301) 656-7540

HEARING AND SPEECH

National Association for Hearing and Speech Action
10801 Rockville Pike
Rockville, MD 20852
(800) 638-8255

Referrals to speech pathologists and otolaryngologists.

HEART DISEASE/DEFECTS

American Heart Association
7320 Greenville Avenue
Dallas, TX 75231
(214) 373-6300

AHA does not make referrals, but local chapters can identify area hospitals that have pediatric cardiology departments.

HEMOPHILIA

National Hemophilia Foundation
Room 406, Soho Building
110 Greene Street
New York, NY 10012
(212) 219-8180

LEUKEMIA

Leukemia Society of America, Inc.
733 Third Avenue
New York, NY 10017
(212) 573-8484

Some referrals, as well as lists of comprehensive cancers, major hospitals dealing with cancer.

MENTAL HEALTH

American Academy of Child and Adolescent Psychiatry
3615 Wisconsin Avenue NW
Washington, DC 20016

American Psychological Association
1200 17th Street NW
Washington, DC 20036

National Center for Clinical Infant Programs
733 Fifteenth Street NW Suite 912
Washington, DC 20005

National Consortium for Child Mental Health Services
3615 Wisconsin Avenue NW
Washington, DC 20016

National Mental Health Association
1021 Prince Street
Arlington, VA 22314

One to One (advocacy for the mentally retarded)
c/o Cantor, Fitzgerald, Inc.
One World Trade Center, 105th floor
New York, NY 10048

Society for Pediatric Psychology
c/o Dr. Dennis Harper
Department of Pediatrics, College of Medicine
University of Iowa Hospital and Clinic
University of Iowa
Iowa City, IA 52242

MUSCULAR DYSTROPHY

Muscular Dystrophy Associations of America, Inc.
810 Seventh Avenue
New York, NY 10019
(212) 586-0808

Referrals to a system of local clinics throughout the country that provide diagnosis and treatment.

PLASTIC SURGERY

American Society of Plastic and Reconstructive Surgeons
233 North Michigan Avenue
Chicago, IL 60601
(800) 635-0635

Will send a list of 10 plastic surgeons in your geographical area who specialize in the type of plastic surgery you need.

SICKLE-CELL ANEMIA

National Sickle Disease Program
Division of Blood Diseases and Resources
National Heart, Lung and Blood Institute
Room 504, Federal Building
7550 Wisconsin Avenue
Bethesda, MD 20892
(301) 496-6931

Staff doctors will make referrals when possible.

SKIN DISEASES

American Academy of Dermatology
P.O. Box 3116
Evanston, IL 60204-3116
(312) 869-3954

SPINA BIFIDA

Spina Bifida Association of America
Suite 540
1700 Rockville Pike
Rockville, MD 20852
(800) 621-3141

Referrals to specialists, where to go for AFP testing.

STOMACH AND INTESTINAL DISORDERS

American Digestive Disease Society
7720 Wisconsin Avenue
Bethesda, MD 20814
(301) 652-9293

Physician referrals (and other services) available to members ($30 annual fee).

UROLOGY

American Urological Association
1120 North Charles Street
Baltimore, MD 21201
(301) 727-1100

Requests for information handled by personalized letter response (send letter to attn: Mr. Richard Hannigan).

VISION

National Society to Prevent Blindness
79 Madison Avenue
New York, NY 10016
(212) 684-3505

Referrals to various hospitals or low-vision clinics and to local affiliates who are aware of services in their area.

Appendix C
Medical Record Keeping

Child's Health Record

Birth History

Name _____ Sex _____

Date of birth _____ Day of week _____ Time _____

Place of birth _____
                    City   County   State

Birth certif. no. _____

Hospital _____

Address _____

Obstetrician _____

Address _____

Pediatrician _____

Address _____

Weight at birth _____ Length _____ Gestational age _____

Blood type _____ Rh factor _____

Color of eyes _____ Color of hair _____

Pregnancy _____ Normal _____ Complications
                                   (List below)

Delivery _____ Normal _____ Complications
                                   (List below)

Newborn   Complications
period_____ Normal _____   (List below)

Birth defects/complications, if any _____

_____

_____

_____

_____

Mother's maiden name _____

Mother's birthplace _____ Date of birth _____

Father's name _____

Father's birthplace _____ Date of birth _____

Family History

_____ Allergies _____ Asthma _____ Heart disease

_____ High blood pressure _____ Diabetes

Other _____

_____

_____

_____

_____

_____

Mother's date of birth _____

Health status _____

_____

_____

_____

Father's date of birth _____

Health status _____

_____

_____

_____

Sisters and brothers	Year of birth	Health status
1.		
2.		
3.		
4.		

Screening Tests

Year test recommended		1	2	3	4	5
Tine	Date					
	Result					
Hct	Date					
	Result					
Urine	Date					
	Result					
Lead	Date					
	Result					
B.P.	Date					
	Result					
Sight	Date					
	Result					
Sickle	Date		Hearing	Date		
	Result			Result		
Other	Date					
	Result					

Medical History

Past serious illnesses _____

_____

_____

_____

_____

Hospitalizations _____

_____

_____

_____

_____

Allergies _____

_____

_____

_____

_____

Reasons for Special Care

Problem	Age of onset	Plans/ Therapy

_____

_____

_____

_____

_____

_____

_____

_____

_____

_____

_____

_____

_____

_____

_____

_____

_____

_____

Date history recorded _____

Name _____
(please print)

(medical record continued next page)

Immunizations (dates)

Age:	2 mos	4 mos	6 mos	18 mos	5 yrs
Diptheria Pertussis Tetanus					
Signature					

	2 mos	4 mos	6 mos	18 mos	5 yrs
Oral Polio Vaccine					
Signature					

Measles Mumps Rubella		Other	
Signature		Signature	

Health Care Visits

Date	Place	Diagnosis	Lab Tests/Plan/Medication	Provider's name and telephone number

Glossary

Abruptio placentae Partial or complete separation of the placenta from the uterine wall.

Absence seizure See **Nonconvulsive seizure.**

Accessory lobe A portion of the lung that is cut off from the bronchial system.

Achondroplasia An inherited disorder in which the long bones of the arms and legs are stunted in growth, resulting in dwarfism.

Acute bacterial pyelonephritis Infection and inflammation of the kidney caused by bacteria.

Acute cerebral ataxia A disorder characterized by gradual loss of balance over several days, often following a viral infection.

Acute interstitial nephritis Inflammation of the spaces between the glomeruli and renal tubules, caused by an allergic reaction to drugs secreted through the kidneys.

Acute postinfectious glomerulonephritis Inflammation of the glomeruli between one and three weeks after an infection, caused by antibodies against the infectious organism.

Acute viral encephalitis Inflammation of the brain caused by viral infection. The brain cells themselves may be affected, or the myelin sheaths covering nerve fibers in the brain may be destroyed in an autoimmune reaction.

Acyclovir An antiviral drug effective against herpes infections.

Addison's disease A disorder caused by insufficient secretion of aldosterone and cortisol from the adrenal glands, resulting in a variety of serious symptoms.

Adenoiditis Inflammation of the adenoids, which are masses of lymphatic tissue on the upper rear wall of the throat.

Adrenal glands Endocrine glands that are situated just above the kidneys and which secrete important hormones. Among the hormones secreted are epinephrine (adrenaline), which affects heart rate and blood circulation and is instrumental in the body's response to physical stress, and cortisone, a natural antiinflammatory.

Adrenocorticotropic hormone (ACTH) A pituitary hormone that causes the adrenal gland to produce cortisone and other hormones.

Agammaglobulinemia A rare, inherited immunodeficiency disease in which the body is unable to produce antibodies properly.

Aganglionic megacolon A condition in which a part of the large intestine is undeveloped, impeding the passage of stool. Also called **Hirschprung's disease.**

Agenesis A congenital defect in which one or more organs or parts of organs fail to develop in the fetus.

AIDS (autoimmune deficiency syndrome) An incurable, invariably fatal disease in which the causative **HIV (human immunodeficiency virus)** organism attacks the body's immune system. The HIV organism is spread by direct contact with blood, semen, and other body fluids. The virus can be passed to an unborn baby if the mother is infected with it.

Akinetic seizure A type of epileptic seizure in which sudden paralysis occurs without loss of muscle tone but with loss of consciousness.

Albinism Inherited partial or total absence of pigment in the skin, hair, and eyes.

Albumin A protein found in animals, plants, and egg whites; the presence of albumin in the urine may indicate kidney disease.

Aldosterone A hormone produced by the adrenal glands that regulates salt uptake by the kidney.

Allergic contact dermatitis Skin inflammation caused by an acquired sensitivity, or allergy, to a substance that has come into contact with the skin.

Allergy A hypersensitivity or exaggerated reaction to certain substances or conditions, such as sunlight. Manifestations of allergies include rashes, coldlike symptoms, headaches, gastrointestinal symptoms, and asthma.

Alopecia Loss of hair. Patterns include **alopecia areata,** or hair loss from localized areas of the scalp; **alopecia totalis,** or loss of all scalp hair, **alopecia universalis,** or loss of all body hair; and **traumatic alopecia,** or hair loss resulting from mechanical trauma, such as vigorous brushing.

Alpha-fetoprotein A substance normally found in fetal blood. Higher than normal amounts in maternal circulation may indicate presence of neural tube defects in the fetus.

Alveoli The microscopic air sacs in the lungs through which oxygen and carbon dioxide are exchanged.

Amblyopia Loss of vision in a crossed or otherwise misaligned eye.

Amnion The bag of waters in which the fetus and amniotic fluid are contained during pregnancy.

Amniotic fluid Fluid contained within the amniotic sac.

Amylase A digestive enzyme in saliva that breaks down starches.

Anagen Growth phase in hair life cycle.

Anal fissure A small tear in the lining of the anus caused by passing a large or hard stool.

Analgesic A medication that reduces pain.

Anaphylactoid purpura See **Henoch-Schoenlein purpura.**

Anaphylaxis A severe allergic reaction, rare in children, in which the airways and blood vessels contract, causing blood pressure to fall and sometimes leading to cardiovascular collapse.

Androgens Hormones, such as testosterone and aldosterone, which are produced in the testes and are responsible for male characteristics. They are also produced normally in small amounts in females.

Anemia A deficiency in hemoglobin, in the number of red blood cells, or in total blood volume. Anemia is usually a symptom of an underlying disorder.

Anencephaly Congenital absence of portions of the brain and spinal cord.

Aneurysm Localized abnormal dilation of a blood vessel.

Angioedema Diffuse swelling of skin or mucous membranes, usually as part of an allergic reaction.

Angiotensin An artery-constricting substance formed by the body in response to release of renin by the kidneys.

Ankylosing spondylitis Arthritis of the spine that may lead to ossification, and resulting stiffness, of the vertebral joints.

Anterior chamber The area of the eye behind the cornea.

Anterior horn cell disease An inherited disorder in which function of the anterior horn cells is disrupted, causing weakness and muscle wasting.

Anterior horn cells Large nerve cells in the anterior horn (front) of the brain and spinal cord.

Antibiotic-associated colitis Abdominal cramps, diarrhea, and bright red blood in the stool of a child taking antibiotics.

Antibody The components of the immune system that eliminate or counteract foreign substances in the body.

Anticholinergic Blocking impulses of the parasympathetic nervous system, which controls many involuntary functions. Anticholinergic drugs may help dry up nasal and sinus secretions.

Antidiuretic hormone (ADH) A hormone formed in the hypothalamus that acts to conserve water in the body.

Lack of ADH causes **nephrogenic diabetes insipidus.**

Antigen A substance, usually a protein found in bacteria viruses or foreign tissue, that stimulates production of antibodies.

Antigen-antibody interaction The keystone of the allergic reaction. A specific antibody (IgE; see **Immunoglobins**) and antigen combine on the surface of specialized cells called **mast cells,** resulting in the release of chemicals (mediators) responsible for allergic symptoms.

Antihistamines Drugs used to treat allergic reactions by reducing mucus secretion and sneezing.

Antipyretic A medication that lowers fever.

Antitussive A medication that suppresses coughing.

Antrum A partially or completely closed chamber.

Aorta The body's largest artery, which carries blood from the left ventricle of the heart and distributes it to all parts of the body.

Aortic stenosis Narrowing of the valve between the left ventricle of the heart and the aorta.

Apgar score A uniform system for rating the well-being of an infant at birth. Heart rate, respiration, muscle tone, reflexes, and color are each rated on a scale from 0 to 2, usually at one, five, and ten minutes after birth. These ratings are totaled to determine the Apgar score.

Aphasia Absence or impairment of ability to communicate through speech, writing, or signs because of brain dysfunction. **Developmental aphasia** is an inability to learn language because of an abnormality in the part of the brain that processes auditory information.

Apnea The absence of breathing.

Appendicitis An inflammation of the appendix that results in severe pain on the lower right side, fever, and nausea or vomiting. Appendicitis calls for immediate medical attention, usually requiring removal of the appendix.

Appendix testis An appendage on the upper portion of the testes.

Appendix testis torsion Twisting of the appendix testis, causing pain similar to that of testicular torsion.

Aqueous humor The fluid in the anterior part of the eyeball.

Argon laser A laser using the inert gas argon, which is selectively absorbed by red skin pigment, making it useful for removal of certain birthmarks.

Arrhythmia Any deviation from the regular heartbeat rhythm. Also called **dysrhythmia.**

Arteriole A tiny artery that joins another artery to the capillaries.

Arthritis Inflammation of a joint as a result of infection or an autoimmune response. **Infectious arthritis** may be caused by bacteria, viruses, or fungi.

Arthrogryposis multiplex congenita A congenital syndrome in which several joints are immobile and incompletely developed. May be caused by restricted fetal movement in the uterus.

Ascariasis Roundworms. Intestinal parasites passed through ingestion of contaminated feces deposited in the soil.

Aseptic meningitis Inflammation of the membranes of

the spinal cord or brain, caused by infection with various agents, usually viruses. Ordinarily aseptic meningitis runs a short course and occurs in late summer or early fall.

Asphyxia Suffocation due to lack of oxygen or overabundance of carbon dioxide.

Asthma A chronic, reversible disorder of the respiratory system due to bronchial spasm that results in breathing difficulties. Asthma may be triggered by allergy, infection, chemical irritants, tobacco smoke, weather changes, or exercise.

Astigmatism Irregularity in the shape of the cornea leading to blurred vision.

Astrocytoma A slow-growing tumor of the cerebellum, made up of cells called astrocytes.

Atelectasis Collapsed lung.

Atherosclerosis Formation of fatty substances (plaque) on the inner walls of the arteries, causing obstruction in the flow of blood.

Athlete's foot See **Tinea pedia.**

Atonic seizure A type or epileptic seizure in which a sudden loss of muscle tone occurs in one area of the body, along with a brief loss of consciousness.

Atopic Reacting to a specific agent with symptoms of hypersensitivity, such as skin redness, sneezing, and watering eyes.

Atopic dermatitis A rash that occurs when dry, scaly skin is scratched and rubbed. It usually develops around two to three months of age and runs in families. The rash may be either acute (red, weeping, scratched) or chronic (dry, scaly, leathery) in appearance.

Atresia Congenital absence or closure of a normal opening or tube in the body.

Atria The two upper chambers of the heart whose function is to collect blood.

Atrial septal defect A congenital heart defect in which an opening in the wall between the atria causes blood to pool in the right side of the heart.

Atrial tachycardia Rapid heart rate, usually between 160 and 220 beats per minute, arising from the atria.

Atrioventricular canal defect A congenital heart defect in which there is a hole in the center of the heart, where the atrial septum and ventricular septum intersect. Additionally, only one valve, instead of two, separates the upper and lower chambers of the heart. Also called **endocardial cushion defect** or **atrioventricular septal defect.**

Attention deficit disorders Disorders of infancy and childhood characterized by inappropriate attention span and impulsive and hyperactive behavior. Also called **hyperactive child syndrome** and **minimal brain damage or dysfunction.**

Audiometry Testing of hearing using sounds of different frequencies and volumes transmitted via earphones in a soundproof booth.

Auricle Earlobe.

Auscultation A method of examining the body by listening, usually through a stethoscope.

Autism A cognitive disorder of childhood characterized by self-absorption, solitary behavior, inability to relate, late development of speech, and a tendency to engage in ritualized, repetitive movements.

Autoimmune disease Any disease in which the body manufactures antibodies against itself. The body regards its own tissue as a foreign body and acts accordingly to eliminate it.

Autoinoculation A secondary infection arising from an already present disease.

Autosomes The numbered chromosomes; all chromosomes besides the X and Y, or sex chromosomes.

Avoidance therapy Controlling allergies by eliminating known allergens from the environment.

Avoidant disorder of childhood Excessive avoidance of contact with strangers beginning after age 30 months.

Babinski sign Upward arching of the big toe when the sole of the foot is stroked. This response often indicates a neurological disorder.

Bacterial arthritis Joint inflammation caused by bacterial infection after organisms gain entry to the bloodstream via a skin infection or wound.

Balanitis Infection beneath the foreskin of the penis.

Balloon angioplasty A surgical procedure in which a balloon is inserted through a catheter that is passed through an artery to a narrowed coronary artery or aorta, where the balloon is inflated to expand the artery.

Balloon atrial septostomy A procedure in which a balloon is inserted up an artery through a catheter to the aorta to relieve the symptoms that occur when the pulmonary artery and aorta are congenitally reversed in position, a defect that causes constriction of the aorta.

Barium A chalky contrast material administered either orally or as an enema before X rays of the digestive system.

Basal cell A cell in the deepest layer of the epithelium.

Basophil A type of granulocyte. See **Granulocyte.**

B cells Antibody-producing lymphocytes. See **Lymphocyte.**

BCG vaccine A tuberculosis vaccine used in developing countries where the disease is common.

Benign paroxysmal vertigo A disorder marked by sudden attacks of dizziness and vertigo.

Berger's disease Inflammation of the glomeruli, often associated with respiratory illness. Also called **IgA nephritis.**

Biliary atresia Congenital obstruction or absence of the ducts between the liver and the gallbladder.

Bilirubin A bile pigment produced by the breakdown of red blood cells and chemically changed in the liver to an excretable form. Buildup of bilirubin often causes jaundice, especially in newborns.

Biofeedback A behavior-modification therapy by which a patient is taught to control involuntary body functions such as blood pressure.

Biopsy The examination of a small sample of tissue, taken from a patient's body, usually to determine if a growth is cancerous.

Biotinidase deficiency A congenital metabolic disorder that renders the body unable to utilize vitamin B.

Blast   An immature cell, especially any type of immature blood cell.

Blepharitis   Infection of the edges of the eyelids.

Blood groups   Grouping of hereditary factors in the blood. The four major groupings are **O, A, B, and AB.** It is essential to determine if a donor's and recipient's blood types are compatible before a transfusion is administered.

Blood pressure   The force exerted by the blood against the arterial walls. A sphygmomanometer measures both the systolic pressure (when the heart is at maximum contraction) and the diastolic pressure (when the heart is resting between beats).

Blount's disease   A rare growth disorder causing severe bowlegs and occurring in West Indian populations.

Boil   A round, painful, pus-filled bacterial infection of a hair follicle, usually caused by staphylococci bacteria. Also called a **furuncle.**

Bolus   A mass of chewed food prepared to be swallowed, or a rounded or concentrated dose of medicine for oral or intravenous administration.

Bone age   A measurement of a child's maturation made by taking an X ray of the wrist.

Bone conduction aid   A hearing aid that bypasses the inner ear, transmitting sound via a vibrating pad placed over the bone structure surrounding the ear.

Bone marrow   The soft substance present in bone cavities. Red marrow is responsible for red blood cell production. Yellow marrow is marrow that is no longer involved in making blood cells.

Bone marrow transplantation   A leukemia treatment in which donor bone marrow is used to replace diseased marrow. In **autologous bone marrow transplantation,** the patient uses his own marrow, which was harvested during remission.

Botulism   A severe form of food poisoning from a toxin produced by the bacterium *Clostridium botulinum.* Botulism can cause total paralysis.

Bougie   A thin, flexible instrument used for dilating organs.

Brachial pulse   The pulse point on the inside of the arm between the elbow and the armpit.

Bradycardia   Slow heartbeat.

Brain abscess   A focal infection or localized buildup of pus in an area of the brain caused by disintegration of tissue. Common types include **epidural,** located between the dura and the skull, and **subdural,** located beneath the dura.

Brain stem   The part of the brain that connects the cerebral hemispheres with the spinal cord.

Brainstorm auditory-evoked response (BAER)   A hearing test that measures brain waves produced in response to sound, via electrodes placed on the scalp.

Breath-holding   A paroxysmal disorder usually affecting children between ages two and three. In **apnotic breath-holding,** which often occurs in response to frustration or anger, the child holds his breath until his extremities and lips turn blue and he loses consciousness. In **pallid breath-holding,** the child, without warning, loses consciousness, usually in response to fear or surprise.

Breath hydrogen test   A test to diagnose or confirm carbohydrate malabsorption. After the patient ingests a specific carbohydrate, measures are taken of the amount of hydrogen expelled in the breath. Elevated hydrogen means the carbohydrate is being digested in the large intestine and so confirms malabsorption.

Bronchi   The two tubes branching off at the lower portion of the trachea.

Bronchiestasis   Persistent dilation of the bronchi because of chronic infection and inflammation of the airway walls.

Bronchioles   Subdivisions of the bronchi that lead to the alveoli in the lungs.

Bronchiolitis   Inflammation of the bronchioles.

Bronchitis   Inflammation of the bronchi.

Bronchoconstriction   Narrowing of the bronchi.

Bronchopneumonia   Viral pneumonia characterized by patchy inflammation in the lower part of the lungs.

Bronchopulmonary dysplasia (BPD)   Lung damage resulting from treatment of respiratory distress syndrome, particularly ventilation under high pressure.

Bronchoscopy   Examination and sometimes biopsy of the lower trachea and bronchi using an endoscope that is passed through the mouth and trachea.

Bronchospasm   Spasm of the bronchus, one of the manifestations of asthma.

Brudzinski sign   Spontaneous flexion of the hip when the neck is flexed. Occurs in meningitis.

BUN (blood urea nitrogen)   Nitrogen, in the form of urea, in the blood. Elevated levels indicate decreased kidney function.

Candidiasis   An infection caused by the *Candida albicans* fungus. Also called **moniliasis.**

Canker sore   An ulcerlike sore on the mucous membrane of the mouth or lip.

Capillary   Minute, thin-walled blood vessel in a network that facilitates the exchange of substances between the surrounding tissues and the blood.

Capillary hemangioma   Raised, lumpy, red to purple birthmark consisting of small, closely packed capillaries. The birthmark appears in the first two to five weeks of life and usually disappears spontaneously in early childhood.

Carcinoma   The type of cancer that originates in the epithelial cells located in glands, skin, and mucous membranes.

Cardiac catheterization   Examination of the blood vessels of the heart by injecting radiopaque substances so that any disorder or abnormality shows up on X ray film. The record of pictures is called an angiogram.

Caries   Tooth or bone decay.

Cartilage   The white, elastic tissue located in joints, the nose, and the outer ear. In infancy, certain parts of the skeleton are composed of cartilage that, over time, turns into bone.

Casts   Fibrous material that has collected in body cavities and hardened to their shape.

Catecholamines   Biologically active substances that affect the cardiovascular and nervous systems, the metabolic rate, temperature, and smooth muscle.

Cautery   The application of caustic chemicals or electrically heated devices for the purpose of eliminating infected, unwanted, or dead tissue.

Cecum   The first portion of the large intestine below the entrance of the ileum.

Celiac disease   A malabsorptive disease in which the small intestine, for unknown reasons, is damaged by foods containing gluten, especially wheat products. Also called **gluten enteropathy.**

Cellulitis   Inflammation spreading from the skin to the underlying connective tissue, often caused by staphylococcus bacteria.

Central line   Thin tubing inserted into a deep vein for intravenous feeding.

Centrifuge   A laboratory device that spins test tubes containing blood, urine, or other liquids at high speed to cause heavy particles to fall to the bottom of the tube while lighter ones float to the top.

Cerebellum   The part of the brain lying beneath and behind the **cerebrum,** responsible for muscle control and coordination of voluntary movements.

Cerebral palsy   Nonspecific term for several syndromes characterized by motor disturbances and caused, most often, by birth or neonatal injuries. Types, which may overlap, include **dyskinetic cerebral palsy,** which is marked by involuntary movements of the face, neck, and extremities, and **ataxic cerebral palsy,** marked by a wide gait and difficulty turning. Some degree of spasticity is almost always present as well.

Cerebrum   The largest part of the brain. The two sides of the cerebrum are called **cerebral hemispheres.**

Cervical adenitis   An infection of the skin and lymph nodes, especially in the neck, usually caused by streptococcal or staphylococcal bacteria but sometimes caused by mycobacterium.

Chalazion   A painless, round lump in the eyelid caused by blockage of a small gland.

Chelation therapy   Treatment of a toxic condition such as lead poisoning using an agent that chemically encloses the toxin and renders it inactive.

Chicken pox   An infectious, highly contagious disease caused by the varicella zoster virus. Symptoms include fever, malaise, and a red rash that evolves into tiny blisters that break and crust within a week.

Child maltreatment   Physical, sexual, or emotional abuse or neglect by the person or persons responsible for a child's well-being.

Childhood demyelinating disease   A rare, progressive childhood condition similar to multiple sclerosis in adults, in which the myelin sheaths that cover nerves are destroyed for unknown reasons. The disease often follows chronic viral infection. Early symptoms include visual disturbances and loss of sensation.

Chlamydia   Microorganisms that cause a variety of disorders, particularly inflammation of the urethra and cervix. Chlamydia can be sexually transmitted and passed from mother to fetus.

Choanal atresia   A congenital obstruction at the back of the nose that impedes breathing.

Cholesteatoma   A cystlike growth that may form in several areas of the body, but most commonly develops in the middle ear and may erode adjacent bones.

Cholesterol   A crystalline fatlike substance found in the brain, nerves, liver, blood, cell membranes, and bile. It is synthesized in the liver and is essential in the production of sex hormones, nerve function, and a number of other vital processes. Excessive consumption of dietary cholesterol (found only in animal products, particularly organ meats and dairy products) is believed to contribute to heart disease.

Chondrodystrophies   A class of growth disorders characterized by short stature and caused by abnormalities in the cartilage.

Chondrosarcoma   A malignant tumor derived from cartilage cells.

Chordee   Congenital downward curve of the penis.

Choroid   The layer of blood vessels that nourishes the retina.

Choroiditis   Infection of the choroid, often caused by *Toxoplasma gondii,* the parasite that causes toxoplasmosis.

Christmas disease   Hemophilia B. The less common form of hemophilia, in which clotting factor IX, rather than factor VIII, is missing.

Chromosome   Any one of the rod-shaped bodies in the nucleus of a cell, which carries hereditary information.

Chronic motor or vocal tic disorder   Motor or vocal tics occurring for more than a year, with onset as early as one year of age.

Cilia   Moving, hairlike projections along the lining of the bronchi and other epithelial cell layers throughout the body.

Circumcision   Surgical removal of the foreskin covering the end of the penis.

Clavicle   Collarbone.

Cleft lip   A congenital separation of the upper lip that may be associated with cleft palate. Also called **harelip.**

Cleft palate   Congenital defect of the mouth in which the palate bones fail to fuse and result in a groove in the roof of the mouth.

Clubfoot   A congenital abnormality of the foot caused by faulty development of the soft tissue of the instep. **True clubfoot** is a rigid twisting and pointing of the foot that requires surgical correction. **Postural clubfoot** is flexible and more easily corrected.

Clumsy child syndrome   A syndrome marked by impairment of both fine and gross motor skills in children.

Coagulation factors   Proteins in plasma that, with platelets, promote blood coagulation. Also called **clotting factors.**

Coarctation   Compression of vessel walls.

Coccidioidomycosis   A fungal disease, usually respiratory, caused by inhaling dust infected with the *Coccidioid immitis* fungus. It occurs mainly in the southwestern United States.

Cochlea   A snail-shaped structure covered with tiny hairs in the inner ear. The hairs perceive sound vibrations and send signals along the auditory nerves to the brain.

Colic   Spasmodic pain in the abdomen. Also, the name given to cyclic evening crying bouts that seem to occur without cause in some infants.

Colitis Inflammation of the large intestine characterized by bowel spasms, diarrhea, and constipation. Ulcerative colitis is a more serious form of the disease, characterized by open sores in the lining of the colon and the passage of blood- and mucus-streaked stools.

Collagen The major protein of connective tissue, cartilage, and bone.

Colloidal A term for substances in solutions that resist filtering and separation.

Colon Large intestine extending from the small intestine to the rectum. Undigested food that is not absorbed by the body passes from the small intestine into the colon; water is extracted from the waste and it is eventually eliminated from the body as a bowel movement.

Colonoscopy Endoscopic examination of the large intestine.

Colostomy Surgical procedure to create an artificial anus in the abdominal wall.

Complete blood count (CBC) A blood test in which the number of each type of blood cell is counted and cells are examined microscopically for abnormalities.

Complete testicular feminization See **Testicular feminization, complete.**

Computerized tomographic scan (CT scan) An image of a thin cross-section of a part of the body made with an X ray beam that is transformed by a computer into a picture on a screen. CT scans can detect tumors, cysts, abscesses, and calcium deposits, and be used to look into an organ or part of the body, including the brain.

Concealed penis A normal-size penis that is hidden by fat or anchored by skin that is too tight following circumcision.

Concussion Injury resulting from a severe blow or shock to the head.

Conductive hearing loss Loss of hearing due to faulty transmission of sound waves from the outer ear to the cochlea.

Conductive hearing test A test of hearing using earphones that transmit sounds through the bones of the head.

Cone cells Specialized retinal cells that receive color stimuli.

Congenital Present at or before birth.

Congenital adrenal hyperplasia A group of inherited disorders caused by deficiency of different enzymes needed for cortisol synthesis.

Congenital dystrophy A myopathy (muscle disease) that is present at birth and usually improves over time.

Congenital myotonia An inherited disorder apparent in infancy and characterized by muscle spasms brought on by movement.

Congestive heart failure A condition in which weakened heart muscles are unable to pump strongly enough to maintain normal blood circulation. As a result, blood backs up in the lungs and veins leading to the heart. Often accompanied by accumulation of fluid in various parts of the body.

Conjunctiva The transparent membrane lining the front of the eyeball and eyelid.

Conjunctivitis Inflammation of the conjunctiva.

Connective tissue The framework that supports the body, consisting of various types of tissue, including fat, fibrous, elastic, cartilaginous, and bone.

Constitutional delay in growth and development Physical development lagging a few years behind chronological age.

Contact dermatitis Skin inflammation caused by an irritant or allergy and produced by activity of certain immune cells called T cells rather than by the IgE antibody, which is involved in most allergic reactions.

Continuous positive airway pressure (CPAP) A technique for maintaining slight lung inflation to prevent collapse of the alveoli, particularly in infants with respiratory distress syndrome.

Contractures Shortened muscle fibers that cause joints to be abnormally bent or extended.

Contralateral routing of signals (CROS) aid A hearing aid for people with hearing loss in only one ear. The CROS aid sends sounds that would normally hit the deaf ear into the functioning ear.

Cooley's anemia See **Thalassemia.**

Cornea The transparent membrane that protects the outer surface of the eye.

Cortisol A principal hormone produced by the adrenal gland and closely related to cortisone.

Cortisone Hormone preparation that acts as an antiinflammatory agent and is used in treating various diseases.

Cradle cap See **Seborrheic dermatitis.**

Creatine A substance that, when combined with phosphate, supplies energy for muscle contraction.

Creatinine A substance found in the urine and blood, produced by the metabolism of creatine.

Cretinism Severe form of retardation and arrested physical development caused by congenital deficiency of thyroid hormone.

Crohn's disease A chronic inflammatory disease of the ileum. Symptoms, including diarrhea, weight loss, and abdominal pain, often occur sporadically, interspersed with periods of remission.

Croup A generic term for a number of respiratory conditions, all marked by stridor and a barking cough. May be **viral,** accompanied by low-grade fever following an initial upper respiratory infection; **spasmodic,** occurring in brief, repeated episodes; **diphtheritic,** associated with diphtheria; or **acute epiglottitis,** a severe form caused by *H. influenzae* type B in which the inflamed epiglottis may block off the trachea entirely.

Cryoprecipitate Frozen blood products, especially clotting factors, derived from numerous donors and used to treat hemophilia.

Cryoprobe A device that applies cold to tissues, often used in surgery.

Cryosurgery Surgery using instruments that decrease temperature.

Cryptorchid testes See **Undescended testes.**

Cryptosporidium An intestinal parasite that causes chronic diarrhea in people with AIDS.

CT scan See **Computerized tomographic scan.**

Curette A sharp loop, ring, or scooplike instrument used to scrape the inside of a cavity.

Cursive seizure A type of epileptic seizure marked by spontaneous running.

Cushing's disease Cushing's syndrome caused by excessive ACTH secretion.

Cushing's syndrome A condition caused by chronic, excessive cortisol production and characterized by hypertension, fat deposits on the face and neck, and slowed growth. May develop as a result of long-term steroid treatment, but in children under seven the cause is usually an adrenal tumor.

Cut-down An incision made under local anesthetic to place a central line in a deep vein for intravenous feeding.

Cutis marmorata Bluish-purple mottling of the skin caused by exposure to cold.

Cyanosis A condition in which tissue takes on a bluish tinge due to lack of oxygen.

Cyclical vomiting An uncommon paroxysmal disorder in which episodes of vomiting occur without apparent cause.

Cyst An abnormal cavity or sac enclosing a fluid, gas, or semisolid substance.

Cystic fibrosis A hereditary respiratory disease occurring in early childhood. It is characterized by the buildup of mucus in the lungs and other abnormalities affecting the exocrine system (glands that secrete directly into their target organs, such as the sweat glands).

Cytogenic stage The earliest period in embryonic development, during which chemicals are organized into cells and different types of cells are made.

Cytomegalovirus A relative of the herpes simplex virus that can cause a moderate to severe flu-like illness, or that may cause no symptoms initially but reappear later in life. Infants whose mothers are infected with cytomegalovirus during pregnancy may suffer severe complications, including brain damage, microcephaly (see **Microcephaly**), and liver and spleen damage.

Decongestant A medication that shrinks swollen mucous membranes.

Deep hypothermia Dramatic lowering of body temperature, which slows blood flow, thus permitting heart surgery. This technique is sometimes used in heart surgery on infants below one year of age.

Delirium Mental confusion and excitement, marked by disorientation, aimless movement, and incoherent speech. May be caused by fever, shock, exhaustion, anxiety, or drug overdose.

Dementia Impairment of memory and loss of developmental skills, even though alertness remains.

Dental bonding Use of an artificial substance to repair a chipped tooth.

Dental fusion A dental condition in which two separate teeth are fused and grow together.

Dental sealant A very thin layer of liquid plastic that hardens on the chewing surfaces of teeth and keeps out bacteria and food.

Dental twinning Two primary teeth growing from one tooth bud.

Depression An organic disease characterized by profound feelings of sadness, discouragement, and worthlessness not necessarily explained by life's events. Symptoms include sleep disturbance, appetite disruption, loss of interest in pleasurable activities, withdrawal, fatigue. May be classified as a **major depressive episode** if symptoms persist for two weeks or more.

Dermabrasion An operative procedure using sandpaper, wire brushes, or other abrasive materials to remove skin lesions.

Dermatitis Skin inflammation.

Developmental articulation disorder Inability to use speech sounds that should be acquired by a given age.

Developmental coordination disorder Impaired development of motor skills requiring coordination.

Developmental expressive language disorder Difficulty understanding speech because of inaccurate sound interpretation.

Deviated septum A crooked septum, usually referring to the nasal septum.

Diabetes mellitus A chronic condition characterized by an overabundance of blood sugar due to insufficient insulin production by the pancreas or inability of the body to utilize insulin. Diabetes is classified as **Type 1,** or **juvenile diabetes,** most common in children, and **Type 2,** or **adult onset diabetes,** which mainly affects adults. In Type 1 diabetes, antibodies to the islet cells of the pancreas prevent sufficient insulin production. In Type 2 diabetes, insulin levels are normal, but the insulin cannot be utilized.

Dialysate A solution used in hemodialysis machines to regulate chemicals, fluid, and wastes in the blood.

Dialysis A technique for separation of waste products or toxins from the bloodstream. Used in cases of kidney failure and overdose. Types include: **hemodialysis,** which is performed two to three times a week using a dialysis machine to filter the blood, which flows through a surgically created fistula or shunt connecting an artery and a vein; **intermittent peritoneal dialysis,** which is a short-term measure in which dialysis solution is infused into the capillary bed of the peritoneum to filter the blood; **continuous ambulatory peritoneal dialysis (CAPD),** which uses the same technique as intermittent peritoneal dialysis, only at less frequent intervals; and **continuous cycling peritoneal dialysis,** which is a variation of CAPD in which the infusion and draining take place during sleep.

Diaphragm The large muscle between the chest and the abdomen.

Diaphragmatic hernia Protrusion of the intestines into the chest cavity through the diaphragm.

Diastole The interval in between heartbeats during which the heart relaxes. The diastolic reading obtained in blood pressure measurement is the lower number.

Diphtheria An infectious disease caused by *Corynebacterium diphtheriae* bacilli and marked by the formation of a false membrane in the mouth and throat.

Disaccharidase deficiency A malabsorptive disorder in which the chemical reaction that breaks down certain sugars is blocked.

Dislocation   Slippage of a bone from proper alignment in a joint.

Diuretic   Any substance that increases the flow of urine and excretion of body fluid.

DNA (deoxyribonucleic acid)   The fundamental component of all living matter, which controls and transmits the hereditary genetic code.

Dominant inheritance   The pattern of genetic inheritance in which a gene will produce a trait even when inherited from only one parent.

Doppler echocardiography   An ultrasound test that measures blood flow in the heart.

Down's syndrome   A congenital condition that may include mental retardation and physical malformations caused by abnormal chromosomal distribution. Formerly called mongolism.

DPT   The diphtheria, pertussis, and tetanus immunizations, which are given to infants at two, four, and six months of age.

Dream anxiety disorder   Episodes of awakening after frightening dreams and recalling the content of the dreams.

Duchenne muscular dystrophy   An inherited myopathy (muscle disease) that appears only in males, with symptoms beginning early in life and progressing at varying rates. Boys with the disease often lose the ability to walk by age 13, and survival past the late teens is unusual.

Ductus arteriosus   A fetal blood vessel connecting the left pulmonary artery with the aorta, thus bypassing the lungs.

Duodenoscopy   Endoscopic examination of the duodenum.

Duodenum   The portion of the small intestine closest to the stomach.

Duplication of kidney   Congenital abnormality in which there are two compartments in the renal pelvis, each connected to a separate ureter.

Dura   The outermost layer of fibrous membrane covering the brain and spinal cord.

Dyshidrotic eczema   Skin inflammation characterized by tiny, fluid-filled blisters on the palms of the hands and, occasionally, the soles of the feet and thought to be caused by sweat gland dysfunction.

Dyslexia   An impaired ability to interpret written language.

Dysplasia   Abnormal tissue development.

Dyspnea   Difficulty breathing.

Echocardiography   The use of ultrasound waves in the detection and diagnosis of abnormalities of the heart. The results are called an echocardiogram.

Echolalia   A language disorder in which a child repeats the words of others involuntarily.

Eclampsia   A sudden convulsive attack caused by toxemia during pregnancy.

Ectopic ureter   A congenital malformation in which the ureter is improperly connected to the bladder, sometimes opening into the vagina or urethra.

Eczema   Inflammation of the skin, producing an itchy, scaly rash.

Edema   Swelling of body tissue caused by a buildup of fluid.

Elective mutism   A child's refusal to speak in certain social situations despite normal understanding and language development.

Electrocardiography (ECG, EKG)   A diagnostic procedure in which electrodes are placed on body surfaces for the purpose of detecting and tracing electrical impulses from the heart.

Electroencephalography (EEG)   A diagnostic procedure in which the electrical impulses of the brain are traced and recorded through electrodes attached to the head.

Electrolytes   Salts in the blood, tissue fluids, and cells.

Electrostatic precipitator   A machine that filters pollen and dust out of the air.

Embolism   Obstruction of a blood vessel by a solid body called an embolus. Common emboli include blood clots, fat globules, and air bubbles.

Emery-Dreifuss dystrophy   A myopathy (muscle disorder) that causes weakness mainly in the elbow, ankle, and neck.

Encephalitis   Inflammation of the brain due to viral infection, lead poisoning, or other causes.

Encephalocele   Protrusion of the membranes covering the brain through a fissure in the unfused skull bones of an infant.

Encopresis   Repeated deposition of feces in inappropriate places. May be **retentive** (characterized by a continual release of fecal matter) or **nonretentive** (characterized by deposition of formed stools in inappropriate places). **Functional encopresis** is nonretentive encopresis beginning after age four and occurring at least once a month for at least six months.

Endocardial cushion defect   See **Atrioventricular canal defect.**

Endocarditis   Inflammation of the lining of the heart, usually involving only the valves, and most often caused by staphylococcus or streptococcus bacterial infection.

Endocrine system   The physiological network of ductless glands that secrete hormones into the bloodstream to control the digestive and reproductive systems, growth, metabolism, and other processes.

Endoscopy   Diagnostic procedure using an illuminating optical instrument to examine a body cavity or internal organ.

Endotracheal tube   A tube inserted into the trachea to provide an airway.

End stage renal disease   Loss of 90–95 percent of kidney function.

Enuresis   Urinary incontinence. **Functional enuresis** occurs at least twice a month, between ages five and six.

Eosinophil   A type of granulocyte. See **Granulocyte.**

Ependymal membrane   The membrane that lines the ventricles of the brain.

Epididymitis   Bacterial infection of the vas deferens.

Epiglottis   The flap of cartilage that covers the larnyx during swallowing and aids in directing food to the esophagus.

Epiglottitis   Inflammation of the epiglottis, which may be severe enough to block the trachea entirely.

Epilepsy   A disease of the nervous system characterized by convulsive seizures as a result of an imbalance in the electrical activity of the brain.

Epinephrine The hormone produced by the medulla (inner core) of the adrenal glands. It is secreted in stressful situations in order to increase the body's capacity to respond or to speed up bodily processes.

Epi-pen A spring-propelled device for self-administration of a preloaded dose of epinephrine for treatment of severe allergic reactions to insect stings.

Epispadias Congenital misplacement of the urethral opening in males, with the opening on top of the penis.

Epistaxis Nosebleed.

Epithelium The nonvascular layer of cells covering the skin as well as other parts of the body, including the mucous membranes.

Epstein-Barr virus A relative of the herpes virus that causes infectious mononucleosis.

ERCP (endoscopic retrograde choledoco pancreatoscopy) An endoscopic examination in which contrast material is injected through a small tube inserted into the pancreatic or bile duct so that X rays of those structures can be taken.

Eruption hematoma A purple or dark blue area appearing on the gum where a tooth is about to erupt.

Erysipelas A severe infectious skin disease caused by a streptococcal organism and characterized by swelling and redness.

Erythema Reddening of the skin due to dilation of the capillaries beneath the skin.

Erythema chronica migrans The ringlike rash associated with Lyme disease, occurring three to twenty days after a bite from a certain species of tick infected with disease-causing bacteria.

Erythema marginatum A rash with a lacy or wavy pattern that sometimes occurs in rheumatic fever.

Erythema toxicum neonatorum A skin eruption of red, blotchy patches mainly on the trunk or face that occurs when newborn skin is exposed to the environment outside the womb.

Erythrocytes Red blood cells.

Escherichia coli (E. coli) A group of bacteria normally present in the lower intestinal tract, certain forms of which cause urinary tract infections and diarrhea, particularly traveler's diarrhea.

Esophageal atresia Congenital failure of the esophagus to join the stomach.

Esophageal stenosis and webs A congenital constriction of the esophagus with abnormal tissue forming webs that obstruct the passage of food.

Esophageal varices Varicose veins in the esophagus.

Esophagoscopy Endoscopic examination of the esophagus.

ESR (erythrocyte sedimentation rate) A test that measures the rate at which red blood cells fall to the bottom of a test tube, useful in diagnosing a number of conditions.

Estrogen A primarily female sex hormone produced by the ovaries, adrenal glands, and placenta. In women, it controls the development of secondary sex characteristics, menstruation, and pregnancy. A small amount of estrogen is produced in the testes and in fat tissue.

Eustacian tube The tube that connects the middle ear to the pharynx.

Evoked potentials A test to measure the rate at which impulses are conducted along the peripheral nerves in the spinal cord and brain.

Ewing's sarcoma A rapidly spreading tumor originating in the bone marrow cells. It is the second most common malignant bone tumor in children.

Exanthema subitum See **Roseola.**

Exchange transfusion A procedure in which a baby's total blood volume is gradually removed and replaced with donor blood. In a **partial exchange transfusion,** either packed red cells or plasma are exchanged with only part of the infant's blood volume to change the concentration of red cells in the infant's blood.

Exocrine glands Glands excreting substances directly to their target organs, such as mucous and sweat glands.

Exophthalmos Bulging eyeballs, which can be a symptom of a number of illnesses, including hyperthyroidism, tumors, and infection.

Exostoses Benign bone tumors that appear as outgrowths from bone surfaces.

Expectorant A medication believed to loosen mucus in the lower respiratory tract.

Expiration Breathing out.

Exstrophy A congenital malformation in which an organ, such as the bladder, is turned inside out or opens directly onto the skin.

Extracorporeal membrane oxygenation (ECMO) Oxygenation of the blood by means of a machine that does the job of the lungs. ECMO is an experimental treatment used when an infant suffers heart or lung failure.

Eyeglass aid A hearing aid similar to an aid worn behind the ear, with the battery and amplifier in the temple bar of eyeglasses.

Eyeteeth The pointed teeth between the incisors and molars. Also called canines.

Failure to thrive Absence of normal growth and weight gain in a child.

Fascia A sheet of fibrous tissue beneath the skin.

Febrile seizure A seizure associated with a high fever, usually seen in children between six months and three years of age.

Femur Thighbone.

Ferrous sulfate A form of iron taken orally to treat iron-deficiency anemia.

Fibula The long, thin bone found in the lower leg.

Fistula An abnormal connection between two body cavities.

Flaccid paralysis Paralysis in which muscle tone is lost and tendon reflexes are diminished or lost.

Floaters Spots in the visual field, often caused by debris in the vitreous humor.

Floppy infant syndrome See **Prader-Willi syndrome.**

Fluoride A chemical that in small amounts prevents tooth decay.

Focal infection A major infection arising from a smaller infection such as a dental abscess. May occur in the brain or spinal cord.

Focal segment sclerosis A severe, progressive form of glomerular (kidney) disease.

Focal seizure A type of epileptic seizure arising in only one part of the brain. Also called **partial seizure.** Types include: **single partial seizures,** involving only one limb without loss of consciousness; and **complex partial seizures,** involving changes in mental status such as hallucinations.

Follicle stimulating hormone A pituitary hormone that causes production of reproductive cells (eggs and sperm) in both sexes.

Fontan procedure A surgical procedure to correct tricuspid atresia. An opening is created between the right atrium of the heart and the pulmonary artery, and the accompanying hole in the atrial wall is repaired.

Fontanel A membrane-covered spot on a baby's head where the skull bones have not fused together.

Fracture A broken bone. Types include: **compound fracture,** or a broken bone that partially protrudes through the skin; **greenstick** or **incomplete fracture,** a partially broken bone; and **simple fracture,** a complete break.

Fructose intolerance An inborn metabolic error in which absence of an enzyme prevents metabolism of fructose, or fruit sugar.

Fulminating Developing quickly and with great severity.

Fundus The largest part or base of a large organ.

Fungus A low form of vegetable life including some that can cause infection.

Funnel chest A congenital depression of the sternum, the flat bone in the middle of the chest. Also called **pectus excavatrum.**

Furuncle See **Boil.**

Galactosemia An inborn metabolic error in which the body cannot convert galactose, a type of sugar, into glucose, the sugar utilized by the body.

Gallbladder A membranous sac that is situated below the liver and condenses and stores the bile drained from the liver.

Gamma globulin The type of blood protein that contains antibodies to fight infection. Gamma globulin can be separated from the other constituents of the blood and used to prevent or treat infections.

Ganglia A mass of nerve tissue outside the brain or spinal cord.

Gangrene Death of body tissue usually due to loss of blood supply. Affected area becomes shrunken and black.

Gastritis Inflammation of the stomach.

Gastroenteritis Inflammation of the mucous membranes of the stomach and intestines.

Gastroesophageal reflux Backward flow of stomach contents into the esophagus and mouth. The most common cause of spitting up in babies.

Gastroscopy Endoscopic examination of the stomach.

Gaucher's disease A congenital disorder of lipid metabolism associated with enlarged spleen, increased skin pigmentation, and bone lesions.

Gavage feeding Delivering nutrients such as formula or glucose directly to the digestive system via a tube inserted through the nose and down the esophagus to the stomach, or directly into the stomach through a surgical opening.

Gelastic seizure A type of epileptic seizure marked by uncontrolled, inappropriate laughter.

Gender identity disorder of childhood A child's concern over assigned gender, with preference for clothes and activities appropriate for the other gender.

Genetic short stature An inherited growth pattern of consistent, age-appropriate growth despite height in the lowest percentiles.

Gestational diabetes Diabetes mellitus appearing in the late second or early third trimester of pregnancy and caused by the human placental hormone lactogen.

Gingivostomatitis Primary herpes infection affecting the gums and the mucous membranes of the mouth and throat.

Gliadin A protein present in wheat gluten.

Globin The protein portion of the hemoglobin molecule.

Glomerulus A small tuft of capillaries in the kidney, responsible for filtering out waste products from the blood.

Glottis The vocal cords within the larynx.

Glucagon A hormone that increases glucose concentration in the blood.

Glucose The most common simple sugar and the main source of energy for humans. It is stored as glycogen in the liver and can quickly be converted back into glucose.

Glucose-6-phosphate dehydrogenase deficiency (G6PD) An inherited deficiency of an enzyme, the lack of which causes hemolytic anemia. The disorder is a sex-linked trait, which means that symptoms are present only in the sons of women who carry the defective gene.

Gluten enteropathy See **Celiac disease.**

Glycogen The form in which carbohydrate (mainly glucose) is stored in the body, to be converted into glucose, which is used to fuel muscular work or converted into heat.

Glycogen storage disease An inborn metabolic error marked by abnormal accumulation and storage of glycogen in various tissues.

Goiter Enlargement of the thyroid gland.

Gonadotropin A hormone that stimulates the ovaries or testicles.

Gonads Primary sex glands—overies in the female, testes in the male.

Gonococcal ophthalmia Eye infection in newborns of mothers with gonorrhea.

Gonorrhea A common sexually transmitted disease caused by the gonococcus bacterium and characterized by inflammation of the urethra, difficulty in urination (in males), and inflammation of the cervix (in females). Newborns may also contract the disease as they pass through the birth canal.

Grand mal seizure See **Tonic-clonic seizure.**

Granulocyte White blood cell containing granules. Granulocytes are manufactured in the bone marrow to digest and destroy bacteria.

Granuloma A tumor or growth containing granulation

tissue, which is the type of tissue that grows in a healing wound.

Graves' disease Hyperthyroidism in a newborn or older infant. Symptoms in newborns include rapid heart rate and respiratory distress; in older infants, goiter, weight loss, muscle weakness, and bulging eyes may be apparent.

Growth hormone (GH) A pituitary hormone that promotes body growth and fat mobilization and inhibits glucose utilization.

Growth plate A thin, flat structure within each bone that serves as the center of bone formation and controls the bone's length.

Guillain-Barré syndrome Acute polyneuritis. A disease of the peripheral nerves causing progressive muscular weakness and sometimes culminating in paralysis. Usually follows a viral infection.

Harlequin color change Harmless, transitory reddening of one side of an infant's body when it lies on that side.

Hashimoto's thyroiditis Enlarged thyroid gland thought to be caused by an autoimmune reaction.

Hayfever An allergic reaction to pollen in which mucous membranes of the eyes, nose, and throat become inflamed. Also called **allergic rhinitis** or **seasonal rhinitis.**

HBHR (home-based health record) A child's health record, including data base, growth and development measurements, immunization and screening test results, and a summary of illnesses.

Heat stroke An emergency condition in which the sweating mechanism of the body fails, resulting in an extremely high body temperature.

Hematemesis Vomiting blood.

Hematocrit (HCT) The percentage of total blood volume consisting of red blood cells.

Hematologic growth factors Hormones that stimulate the bone marrow to produce different types of blood cells. The types include: **erythropoietin,** which stimulates growth of red blood cells; and **granulocyte colony stimulating factor, granulote macrophage colony stimulating factor,** and **interleukin-3,** all of which stimulate production of leukocytes.

Hematoma A blood-filled swelling resulting from blood vessels injured or ruptured by a blow.

Hematopoiesis The manufacture of blood cells, which takes place in the bone marrow.

Hematuria Blood in the urine.

Heme The iron-containing portion of the hemoglobin molecule.

Hemoglobin The red pigment contained in red blood cells and combining the iron-containing heme with the protein-containing globin. Hemoglobin is responsible for transporting oxygen to body tissue and removing carbon dioxide from body tissue.

Hemolysis Breaking down of red blood cells.

Hemolytic anemia A disorder in which mature red blood cells break down at a faster rate than new cells can be manufactured.

Hemolytic uremic syndrome A group of symptoms, the hallmarks of which are kidney failure and anemia, occurring in infants and small children for unknown reasons following a respiratory or gastrointestinal infection.

Hemophilia An inherited blood disorder in which the blood is unable to clot causing severe bleeding even from minor wounds. The disease is sex-linked, meaning that it only affects males but is carried by females, who pass it along to their sons.

Hemophilus influenza type B (HiB) A highly contagious disease leading to meningitis, pneumonia, and epiglottitis.

Hemorrhage Abnormal bleeding due to rupture of a blood vessel.

Hemothorax Bleeding into the pleura.

Henoch-Schoenlein purpura A disease characterized by small red spots on the legs and buttocks, as well as abdominal discomfort, pain in the legs and knees, and blood in the urine and stool. The cause is unknown. Also called **anaphylactoid purpura.**

Hepatitis Inflammation of the liver, usually as a result of a viral infection. **Hepatitis B** is transmitted through blood (shared hypodermic needles or blood transfused from a hepatitis B carrier). **Hepatitis A** is transmitted through fecal contact, usually via contaminated food. A third type, **non-A, non-B,** is not as well understood as the other two.

Hereditary angioedema (HAE) An inherited form of hives caused by a disorder in a blood protein involved in the immune system.

Hereditary nephritis A severe, inherited glomerular defect, often associated with nerve deafness and eye abnormalities. Also called **Alport's syndrome.**

Hernia The abnormal protrusion of part or all of an organ (usually the intestines) through the surrounding tissues.

Herpes encephalitis Brain infection due to herpes virus Type 1 or 2.

Herpes simplex Recurring infection caused by herpes virus Type 1 or Type 2. **Herpes Type 1 (HSV-1)** involves blisterlike sores usually around the mouth and referred to as cold sores or fever blisters. **Herpes Type 2 (HSV-2)** usually affects the mucous membranes of the genitalia and can be spread by sexual contact. In unusual circumstances, either type can cause damage to other parts of the body, including the brain and eyes; infants born to mothers with active herpes infections at the time of birth are particularly susceptible to such severe, system-wide herpes infections.

Herpes zoster A painful viral infection resulting in inflammation and blisters following the path of a nerve. It may be caused by the same virus that causes chicken pox, which remains in the body in a latent form and may erupt many years later. Also called **shingles.**

Hiatus An opening.

High density lipoproteins (HDLs) A type of blood fat that is chemically bound to a protein. High levels of HDLs seem to protect against heart disease.

Hirschsprung's disease A congenital disorder in which missing nerve cells cause permanent contraction of part of the lower colon or rectum. Also called **aganglionic megacolon.**

Histamine A chemical found in body tissue and released to stimulate production of mucus by mucous membranes and gastric juices for digestion. In an allergic reaction, excessive amounts of histamine are produced and cause surrounding tissue to become inflamed. Antihistamines are thus prescribed for relief from allergic attacks.

Histogenic stage The period in fetal development during which the various body tissues form and differentiate.

Histoplasmosis A fungal respiratory disease caused by inhaling spores from animal droppings infected with the *Histoplasma capsulatum* fungus. Occurs in Tennessee, Kentucky, and parts of the Midwest.

HIV See **Human immunodeficiency virus.**

Hives Itchy red and white swellings that appear in the skin, usually in an allergic reaction. Also called **urticaria.**

HLA antigens See **Human lymphocyte antigens.**

Hodgkin's disease A cancer of the lymph-forming organs that is most common in young adults.

Homeostasis Maintenance of all body functions at normal levels, regulated by the endocrine and nervous systems.

Homocystinuria An inherited metabolic disease in which a byproduct of the amino acid cystine cannot be metabolized.

Hookworms Intestinal parasites that enter the system when the soles of the feet contact soil contaminated with infected feces. Immature, microscopic worms pass through the capillaries and bloodstream and eventually, at maturity, migrate to the small intestine. Although two types of hookworms exist, only the *Necator americanus* is common in the U.S., mainly in the South.

Hordeolum See **Sty.**

Hormone Secretion from an endocrine gland transported by the bloodstream to various organs in order to regulate vital functions and processes.

Horseshoe kidney A usually benign, inherited, congenital defect in which the kidneys are connected at their lower ends.

Human immunodeficiency virus The virus that causes AIDS. Also called **HIV.**

Human lymphocyte antigens (HLA antigens) Proteins present on most types of cells that determine whether a transplanted organ or bone marrow will be accepted or rejected by the host. Also called **human histocompatibility antigens.**

Hyaline membrane disease See **Respiratory distress syndrome (RDS).**

Hydrocele An abnormal accumulation of fluid, usually in the sac of the membrane that covers the testicle.

Hydrocephalus (or **hydrocephaly**) An accumulation of cerebrospinal fluid within the ventricles of the brain.

Hydrochloric acid An acid, composed of hydrogen and chlorine, secreted by the stomach in the process of digestion.

Hydromyelia Increased cerebrospinal fluid in the central spinal cord canal.

Hyperbilirubinism Excess bilirubin in the blood, leading to jaundice.

Hypercalcemia Excess calcium in the blood.

Hyperfunction Overactivity.

Hyperhidrosis Excessive perspiration.

Hyperlipidemia Increased concentration of fatty substances in the blood.

Hyperlordosis An abnormally exaggerated curve in the lower back.

Hypernatremia Excess sodium in the blood.

Hyperopia Farsightedness caused by inadequate length of the eyeball.

Hyperparathyroidism Overactivity of the parathyroid glands, leading to hypercalcemia. Usually caused by a primary disorder such as chronic kidney failure.

Hypertrophy Enlargement.

Hyphemia Blood in the front chamber of the eye.

Hypnagogic phenomena Vivid hallucinations that occur just before sleep.

Hypocalcemia Low calcium levels in the blood.

Hypofunction Underactivity.

Hypoglycemia Low blood sugar.

Hyponatremia Decreased concentration of sodium in the blood.

Hypoparathyroidism Underactivity of the parathyroid glands, leading to hypocalcemia.

Hypopituitarism Impairment of the pituitary gland, causing low levels of pituitary hormones, particularly growth hormone.

Hypoplasia Incomplete or underdevelopment of tissue.

Hypospadias Congenital malformation of the penis, with the urethral opening on the underside.

Hypothalamus The part of the brain just above the pituitary gland. It has a part in controlling basic functions such as appetite, procreation, sleep, and body temperature and may be affected by the emotions.

Hypothyroidism Underactivity of the thyroid gland, which may be caused by poor development of the gland, enzyme deficiency, iodine deficiency, or several other malfunctions.

Hypotonia Loss of muscle tone, with or without weakness.

Hypoxia Lack of oxygen.

Idiopathic Peculiar to an individual or originating from unknown causes.

Idiopathic thrombocytopenic purpura (ITP) A platelet disorder, usually triggered by a viral infection, in which platelets are destroyed in an autoimmune reaction, causing symptoms such as multiple small bruises (petechiae) and nosebleeds.

Ileum The lower portion of the small intestine.

Immunization The procedure by which specific antibodies are induced in body tissue. In **active immunization,** a disease-causing agent is administered to induce antibody production without actually causing the disease. In **passive immunization,** preformed antibodies are transferred into the body.

Immunoglobulins The five major types of antibodies

produced by the immune system. **IgE** is the immunoglobulin activated in allergic reactions. The others—**IgA, IgD, IgG,** and **IgM**—are active in fighting infection.

Immunotherapy Desensitization by frequent injections of increasing amounts of an allergen.

Impedance testing Testing of hearing using a probe that bounces sound waves off the eardrum.

Imperforate anus Congenital narrowing, closure, or absence of the anal opening.

Impetigo Highly contagious inflammatory pustular skin disease caused by staphylocci or streptococci.

Incarcerated hernia A hernia that has become trapped in the muscle wall.

Incisors The four upper and four lower front teeth.

Incus The middle bone in the triad of small bones that magnify vibrations in the middle ear. Also called the **anvil.**

Infantile spasm A type of epileptic seizure appearing mostly in babies and apparently aggravated by feeding, handling, and waking.

Influenza Flu. A contagious viral infection that occurs in epidemics, caused by two different viruses with numerous subtypes.

Inguinal Pertaining to the groin.

Inguinal canal An opening in the lower abdominal muscles through which the fetal testicles descend to the scrotum about two months before birth.

Inguinal hernia Protrusion of the intestines through muscles that separate them from the inguinal area.

Inspiration Inhalation.

Insulin The hormone produced and secreted by the beta cells of the pancreas. Insulin is needed for proper metabolism, particularly of carbohydrates, and the uptake of sugar (glucose) by certain body tissues. Types of insulin used to treat diabetes mellitus include: **regular,** or rapid acting; **NPH** or **lente,** which acts less rapidly; and **ultra-lente,** or very slow acting.

Intertrigo Chafing. Superficial inflammation of opposing skin surfaces that rub together.

Intra-aterial baffle See **venous switch.**

Intrathecal scan A test to observe the flow of cerebrospinal fluid, done by withdrawing some fluid and injecting radioactive substances, the movement of which can then be followed.

Intrauterine growth retardation (IUGR) Failure of a fetus to achieve a weight equal to that of 90 percent of others at the same stage of development.

Intravenous pyelogram (IVP) An X-ray study of the kidneys taken after contrast dye, administered intravenously, reaches the kidneys, ureters, and bladder.

Intraventricular hemorrhage (IVH) Mild to severe bleeding into the three cavities in the center of the brain, a condition that affects almost half of infants born before 34 weeks' gestation.

Intussusception A type of intestinal obstruction in which one part of an intestine slips into another part below it.

IPV Inactivated polio vaccine given by injection, an alternative to the standard oral polio vaccine.

Iris The round, colored portion of the eye that surrounds the pupil.

Ischemia Localized blood deficiency, usually as a result of a circulatory problem. For example, cardiac ischemia results when a coronary artery is so occluded that it cannot deliver sufficient blood to the heart muscle.

Islets of Langerhans The groups of cells (alpha and beta) in the pancreas that secrete endocrine hormones; the alpha cells produce glucagon and the beta cells produce insulin.

Isoimmunization Development of antibodies against the blood of another individual, as in Rh factor immunization between mother and fetus.

Isometric Having equal dimensions. Refers to a type of muscle contraction in which tension increases without a change in muscle length.

Isotope One of a series of chemical elements with similar chemical properties but different atomic weights and electric charges. Many isotopes are radioactive.

Jaundice Yellow discoloration of the skin and eyes caused by excessive amounts of bile pigments in the bloodstream. Common in newborns due to short-term inability of the liver to excrete adequate bilirubin.

Jejunum Part of the small intestine situated between the duodenum and the ileum.

Juvenile rheumatoid arthritis A children's disease characterized by joint pain and inflammation, usually accompanied by systemic symptoms including fever, swollen lymph nodes, and anemia. The disease is divided into three broad subgroups. In **polyarticular onset** disease, several joints, including the spine, may be involved. In **pauciarticular onset,** the knees, ankles, and elbows are most frequently affected. In **systemic** disease, symptoms affecting parts of the body other than the joints predominate. Also called **Still's disease.**

Kaposi's sarcoma A type of skin cancer associated with AIDS.

Kawasaki disease An acute disease of childhood, most common in Japan and among Asian children, marked by fever, conjunctivitis, reddening of the mouth and tongue, and swelling of the lymph nodes in the neck. In 20 percent of cases, the heart is involved. The cause is unknown. Also called **mucocutaneous lymph node syndrome.**

Kernig sign Pain occurring when a patient attempts to straighten a bent knee while lying down. Appears in meningitis.

Ketones Highly acidic substances produced by fat metabolism. Buildup of ketone bodies is often associated with diabetes and can lead to fatal coma.

Kidney failure Loss of 70–80 percent of kidney function, resulting in uremia. May be **chronic** (occurring gradually) or **acute** (developing suddenly, over a few days or hours).

Kidney pelvis The end of the ureter connected to the kidney. At the kidney pelvis, where urine is collected, the ureter widens. Also called **renal pelvis.**

Kidney stones Mineral deposits formed in the kidneys

from overly high urinary concentrations of phosphates, calcium, urates, or other substances.

Koplik spots Small, white and red spots on the mouth or on other mucous membranes appearing before the generalized rash of measles.

Labyrinth The fluid-filled structure in the inner ear, consisting of two chambers and three semicircular canals, that controls equilibrium.

Lacrimal sac A structure at the corner of the eye into which tears flow before draining through the nose.

Lactoalbumin A protein in cow's milk that seems to be responsible for milk allergies.

Lactose A sugar contained in milk.

Laryngeal edema Swelling of the larynx.

Laryngeal webs Fused portions of false vocal cords that may obstruct breathing.

Laryngitis Inflammation of the pharynx, which may temporarily impede speech.

Larynx The speech organ, located below the base of the tongue.

Laser *Light Amplification by Stimulated Emission of Radiation.* A laser beam is a beam of intense light that can be used surgically to sever, eliminate, or fuse body tissue.

Lens The transparent tissue of the eye that focuses rays of light in order to form an image on the retina.

Leukemia A group of cancers of the blood-forming organs in which a proliferation of bone marrow and lymphoid tissue produces an overabundance of white blood cells (leukocytes) and disrupts normal production of red blood cells. The two main types are **lymphocytic,** in which there is an overproduction of immature lymphocytes; and **myelogenous,** in which granulocytes or monocytes are overproduced in the bone marrow. **Acute lymphocytic leukemia (ALL)** is the most common form of leukemia in children, as well as the most treatable. **Acute myelogenous leukemia** is less common and less treatable.

Leukocytes White blood cells, instrumental in fighting infection.

LHRH (luteinizing hormone releasing hormone) A hormone produced in the hypothalamus that controls synthesis of luteinizing hormone.

LHRH analogs Drugs that lower the secretion of gonadotropin and that are used to treat precocious puberty.

Limb-girdle dystrophy A myopathy (muscle disorder) that affects different limbs successively and is rare in children.

Lipase A digestive enzyme found in saliva and other body fluids that breaks down fats.

Lipidosis A disorder of fat metabolism.

Lobar emphysema Overinflation of part of a lung, caused by abnormal narrowing of the lower airways.

Lobectomy Surgical removal of one lobe of a lung. The left lung has two lobes and the right lung, three.

Luteinizing hormone A pituitary hormone that causes the gonads to produce sex hormones.

Luxation Dislocation or displacement of a bone from its normal position in a joint. A **subluxation** is a partial dislocation in which the ends of the bones in a joint are out of alignment but still touching.

Lyme disease An infectious disease caused by bacteria carried by ticks of the species *Ixodes dammini* (deer ticks). Symptoms include blotchy skin rash at the site of the tick bite, malaise, fever, and joint pain. Untreated Lyme disease can cause neurological symptoms such as encephalitis and meningitis, as well as heart problems.

Lymph Transparent yellowish fluid containing lymphocytes and found in lymphatic vessels.

Lymph nodes Oval-shaped organs located throughout the body that manufacture lymphocytes and filter germs and foreign bodies from the lymph.

Lymphocytes A disease-fighting type of leukocyte manufactured in the lymph nodes and distributed in the lymphatic fluid and blood.

Lymphoma A cancer of lymph-forming tissues.

Magnetic resonance imaging (MRI) A new diagnostic technique that measures differences in magnetic energy in the body to produce cross-section images of organs.

Malabsorptive states Disorders in the absorption of nutrients through the small intestine. The causes may include missing enzymes or cell abnormalities. Celiac disease and cystic fibrosis are the most common types.

Malleus The small bone in the middle ear attached to the eardrum. Also called the hammer.

Maple syrup urine disease An inherited metabolic disorder in which certain amino acids cannot be metabolized.

Marfan syndrome An inherited disorder characterized by long limbs, loose joints, and abnormalities of the blood vessels. The syndrome is inherited in the dominant genetic pattern, which means that children of couples in which one member carries the gene have a 50 percent chance of having the disorder.

Marrow See **Bone marrow.**

Mast cells Cells coated with large amounts of IgE allergic antibodies, present in most body tissues. Mast cells release chemical mediators such as histamine following antigen-antibody interactions.

Measles An acute infectious disease characterized by fever, rash, and inflammation of mucous membranes. It is caused by a virus.

Meatal stenosis Narrowing of the opening of the urethra.

Meckel's diverticulum A congenital blind pouch near the end of the small intestine, where a fetal duct between the umbilicus and intestine fails to close before birth.

Meconium The greenish or blackish, sticky discharge from the bowels of a newborn baby.

Mediators Chemicals released from mast cells during an allergic reaction that are responsible for allergy symptoms.

Medullary cystic disease A rare hereditary disease in which cysts appear in the inner portions of the kidney. Also called **nephronophthisis.**

Medullary sponge kidney A generally benign, congenital abnormality in which the ends of the renal tubules are dilated slightly.

Medulloblastoma A fast-growing tumor of the cerebellum and fourth ventricle of the brain.

Megacephaly Abnormally large head.

Megakaryocyte A large bone-marrow cell from which platelets are formed.

Megalencephaly Abnormally large brain.

Megaureter A congenital malformation in which abnormal muscle fibers at the end of the ureter that joins the bladder cause the ureter to become dilated.

Melanin Dark pigment found in hair, skin, and choroid of the eye.

Melanocyte Pigment cell of the skin.

Melanoma Tumor composed of cells containing melanin. Mostly benign, but malignant melanoma is a rare and serious form of skin cancer, which is related to early and long-term exposure to excessive sunlight.

Meningitis Inflammation of the membranes of the spinal column and brain. Bacterial meningitis is caused by a variety of bacteria, but in infants most commonly by group B streptococci bacteria. See also **Aseptic meningitis.**

Mesangiocapillary glomerulonephritis A severe, progressive form of glomerular disease. Also called **membranoproliferative glomerulonephritis.**

Mesoblastic nephroma A kidney tumor arising from certain embryonic cells and most often occurring in infants.

Metabolism The combination of chemical and physical changes in the body essential for maintaining life processes.

Methacholine A drug that causes constriction of the bronchi.

Micrencephaly Abnormally small brain.

Microcephaly Abnormally small head.

Micropenis A penis under three centimeters long in a full-term infant.

Migraine Periodic severe headaches usually affecting only one side of the head and often accompanied by nausea or vomiting, inability to look at light, and fluid retention.

Milia A skin condition of infancy characterized by tiny white facial papules from excess oil-gland activity due to maternal hormones.

Miliaria Heat rash. A rash characterized by small red bumps and caused by excess heat, especially when perspiration is not allowed to evaporate.

MMR Measles, mumps, and rubella vaccination, generally given at 12 to 15 months of age.

Molars The grinding teeth at the back of both jaws.

Mold spores A type of fungus living on decaying matter. Spores, microscopic airborne parts of the fungus, are often found outdoors, in attics, and in basements.

Molluscum contagiosum A benign, indolent infectious skin disease caused by a virus and characterized by the appearance of several waxy bumps with central white cores.

Mongolian spots Dark blue or black spots on the lower back or buttocks of an infant. The spots usually disappear spontaneously.

Monoclonal antibodies Antibodies derived from cells grown in a laboratory using gene-splicing techniques, widely used in diagnosis and potentially valuable in cancer treatment.

Monocyte The largest type of white blood cell.

Mononucleosis A communicable disease, caused by the Epstein-Barr virus, in which the number of monocytes in the bloodstream increases. Symptoms include fever, swollen lymph nodes, and general malaise.

Monospot test A microscopic examination of white blood cells to detect antibodies to Epstein-Barr virus.

Mucocutaneous lymph node syndrome See **Kawasaki disease.**

Mucopolysaccharidosis A group of inherited diseases in which missing enzymes lead to neurological problems, facial deformities, and short stature.

Multicystic kidney A congenital malformation in which cysts fill one kidney.

Mumps A contagious disease affecting mostly children. Symptoms include painful swollen glands.

Muscular spinal atrophy A fatal inherited childhood disease in which the spinal cord degenerates. Also called **Werdnig-Hoffman** disease.

Mustard (or Senning) procedure See **venous switch.**

Myasthenia gravis (MG) A disease characterized by muscle weakness and fatigability caused by development of autoantibodies that attack the junction of nerve and muscle at a critical point. **Congenital myasthenia gravis** is a form of the disease that is present at birth.

Myclonic seizure A type of epileptic seizure marked by bilateral muscle twitching but no loss of consciousness.

Mycobacterium A group of organisms that includes the organism that causes tuberculosis.

Myelin A fatlike substance that covers nerve fibers.

Myelodysplasia Defective formation of the spinal cord.

Myelography A diagnostic technique in which an X ray is taken of the spinal cord after dye is injected between two vertebrae. The test measures electrical conductivity of a nerve.

Myocarditis Inflammation of the heart muscle.

Myoelectric Relating to the electric properties of muscle.

Myopathy A muscle disorder that is not caused by a disorder of the central nervous system.

Myopia Nearsightedness; blurring of all but very near vision.

Myotonia Temporary rigidity of a muscle after contraction.

Myotonic dystrophy A slowly progressing inherited myopathy usually beginning in adolescence and characterized by mental impairment, facial abnormalities, and muscle weakness.

Myringotomy Surgical opening of the eardrum.

Narcolepsy A chronic condition marked by sudden, recurrent episodes of sleep occurring without warning at any time of day.

Necrotizing enterocolitis (NEC) Severe intestinal inflammation caused by retention of undigested milk in the intestine of a patient who has recently begun feedings after serious illness.

Neonatal conjunctivitis Conjunctivitis in newborns,

caused either by silver nitrate drops (used to protect against gonorrheal damage) or microorganisms in the birth canal.

Neonatal herpes Severe infection with herpes virus Type 1 or 2 acquired by a newborn during passage through the birth canal of an infected mother.

Neonatal intensive care unit (NICU) A hospital nursery with advanced lifesaving and monitoring equipment and specially trained staff to provide round-the-clock care for ill or high-risk newborns.

Neonatal pneumonia Serious pneumonia in the neonate (infant from birth to one month of age), usually caused by streptococcal bacteria.

Neonatal sepsis Infection with group B streptococcus bacteria in the bloodstream of a newborn.

Nephrogenic diabetes insipidus A disease caused by failure of the renal tubules to respond to a hormone in the blood that conserves the body's fluid volume. Symptoms include unremitting thirst and, in infants, dehydration.

Nephrons The parts of the kidney in which waste is removed from the blood and urine is formed.

Nephrotic syndrome A condition in which the kidneys fail to excrete salt, leading to excessive edema (fluid retention and swelling). The cause is unknown. In **minimal change nephrotic syndrome**, which is the most common form of the syndrome in children under six, the kidneys are seldom permanently damaged. Also called **nephrosis**.

Nerve A bundle of fibers that carries impulses between the nerve center (brain and spinal cord) and other parts of the body.

Nervous system A system of delicate, interlaced nerve cells made up of the brain, cranial nerves, spinal cord, spinal nerves, and all nerve cells outside the spinal cord. The system receives and responds to stimuli via the sense organs (eyes, ears, organs of taste and smell, and receptors all over the body). It is separated into two divisions: the **central nervous system**, which consists of the brain and spinal cord; and the **peripheral nervous system**, which is the network of nerves extending to other parts of the body.

Neural tube The embryonic structure that eventually becomes the brain and spinal cord.

Neurogenic bladder Poorly developed nerves in the bladder, causing constant urine leakage.

Neuron A nerve cell.

Neuropathy A disorder affecting the nerves of nerve cells.

Neutropenia Deficiency of neutrophils (a subgroup of granulocytes) that is a frequent side effect of cancer chemotherapy. Neutropenia creates susceptibility to infections.

Neutrophil A type of granulocyte.

Nevus A congenital pigment or elevated portion of skin. A birthmark.

Nevus flammeus A red discoloration of the skin, usually on the face or at the base of the neck, appearing at birth and caused by overgrowth of capillaries in the skin.

Night terrors A type of sleep disorder causing children to wake screaming and remain frightened for some time after waking.

Nits Lice eggs.

Nonconvulsive seizure A mild form of epileptic seizure characterized by brief loss of awareness. Unconsciousness and convulsions do not occur. Also called **absence seizure** or **petit mal seizure.**

Non-Hodgkin's lymphoma The cancer of lymph-forming tissue most common in children.

Nummular dermatitis A rash similar to ringworm in appearance, with circular weals usually appearing on the buttocks, legs, backs of hands, or forearms.

Nursing caries Severe tooth decay in an infant who goes to sleep while sucking a bottle containing milk or juice. Also called **bottle mouth.**

Nystagmus Rolling or twitching eyes caused by a variety of eye abnormalities as well as certain drugs.

Occlusion The closure of ducts or blood vessels. In dentistry, it refers to the fitting together of upper and lower teeth.

Occult spina bifida Failure of part of the spinal cord to fuse during fetal development.

Olfactory bulb A structure in the roof of the nose that contains the ends of the olfactory nerves.

Olfactory nerve The nerve running from the roof of the nose to the brain that transmits orders to the brain.

Ophthalmoscope An instrument for examining the interior of the eye.

Optic nerve The fiber that transmits optic impulses from the retina to the brain.

OPV Oral polio vaccine, given at two, four, and sometimes six months of age and later as booster shots.

Orbit Eye socket.

Orbital cellulitis A serious infection of the connective tissue surrounding the eyeballs, often originating as a sinus or dental infection.

Orchitis Bacterial infection of the testes.

Organogenesis The period in fetal development during which the organs form.

Orthodontics The branch of dental science dealing with the correction and prevention of irregularities of the teeth.

Orthostatic proteinuria Protein in urine excreted while a child is standing but absent from urine excreted while he or she is lying down.

Ossicles Three connected bones (the malleus, incus, and stapes) in the middle ear that magnify sound vibrations from the eardrum.

Ossification The process of becoming bone or the change from cartilage to bone.

Osteoblasts Bone-forming cells.

Osteochondroma A benign bone tumor arising from cartilage cells, most frequent in persons between ages 10 and 25 and usually located near the ends of long bones.

Osteoclasts Large, multinucleated cells that absorb and remove old bone cells.

Osteogenesis imperfecta An inherited disorder characterized by abnormally fragile bones susceptible to frequent fractures. Also called **brittle bone disease.** In its most severe form, **osteogenesis imperfecta congenita,** it is apparent at birth and rarely survived by infants. The less severe form, **osteogenesis imperfecta tarda,** has two subtypes: the *gravis* form, in which frequent fractures occur in infancy, and the *levis* form, in which fractures occur later in childhood and are not as frequent.

Osteogenic sarcoma   A tumor arising from bone-forming cells and usually occurring at the ends of the long bones. This is the most common malignant tumor in children, with greatest incidence between the ages of 10 and 20.

Osteoid osteoma   Benign bone tumor usually appearing in a bone of the lower extremities and arising from the bone-forming cells. Most common in adolescents and young adults.

Osteomyelitis   Inflammation of the bone and marrow resulting from infection.

Otitis externa   Bacterial infection of the outer ear. Also called **swimmer's ear.**

Otitis media   Inflammation of the middle ear, which often occurs in small children following colds. Cloudy, pus-filled fluid may fill the area behind the eardrum, a condition known as **purulent otitis media.**

Oxygen hood   A clear plastic hood fitted over a newborn's head to provide oxygen.

Oxytocin   A pituitary hormone that causes uterine contractions.

Palpate   Examine by feeling with the hand.

Pancreas   The gland situated behind the stomach. It secretes pancreatic juice containing enzymes to aid in food digestion, and also contains groups of specialized cells (islets of Langerhans) that secrete insulin and glucagon to regulate blood sugar levels.

Pandemic   A disease outbreak that begins in one area and extends to all parts of the world.

Panhypopituitarism   Failure of the pituitary to produce hormones, caused by tumors in the pituitary, hypothalamus, or both.

Papilloma   A tumor, usually benign, of the skin or mucous membrane. **Juvenile papillomas** are growths on the larynx and pharynx, usually in prepubescent boys.

Parainfluenzaviruses   A group of common cold viruses particularly prevalent in children.

Paranasal sinuses   Pairs of air-filled spaces between the facial bones on either side of the nose. They include the **maxillary sinuses,** in the cheekbones; the **frontal sinuses,** under the eyebrows; and the **ethnoid** and **sphenoid sinuses,** beneath the temples.

Paraphimosis   Irreversible retraction of the foreskin of the penis, requiring circumcision or partial circumcision.

Parathyroid glands   Four small glands embedded in the thyroid gland. The hormones secreted by the parathyroid glands control the body's calcium and phosphorous levels.

Parathyroid hormone (PTH)   A hormone secreted by the parathyroid glands that helps maintain stable phosphorous and calcium levels in the blood.

Parenchyma   The parts of an organ that are directly related to the function of the organ (as opposed to supportive or connective tissues).

Parotid glands   The salivary glands in front of and below the ears.

Paroxysm   A sudden spasm or convulsion that is not epileptic in nature.

Paroxysmal torticollis   Episodic tilting of the head to one side at a peculiar angle, lasting from a few minutes to several weeks. Also called **wry neck.**

Partial seizure   See **Focal seizure.**

Patch test   Skin application of a suspected allergen that is left in place and covered for 48 hours to test for sensitivity.

Patent ductus arteriosus (PDA)   Failure of the ductus arteriosus (a blood vessel that bypasses the lungs in the fetus) to close in the first few days after birth, the most common cardiac problem in premature infants.

Patent urachus   Failure of the urachus (a tube that connects the fetal bladder to the umbilicus) to disappear before birth.

Pathological short stature   Growth deficiency caused by disease or poor nutrition.

Pavor nocturnus   See **Night terrors.**

Pectus excavatrum   See **Funnel chest.**

Pediculosis   Lice infestation. In children, **pediculosis capitis,** or lice infestation of the scalp hair, often occurs in outbreaks among family members.

Pelvic inflammatory disease   Infection and inflammation of a woman's upper reproductive organs, including the fallopian tubes, which usually results from sexually transmitted diseases and which may lead to scarring and infertility.

Peptic ulcer   Ulcer in the stomach, duodenum, or esophagus that is related to pepsin, a protein-digesting enzyme secreted by the stomach.

Percutaneous umbilical fetal blood sampling   An experimental diagnostic test in which a fetal blood sample is obtained via a needle inserted through the uterine wall into a blood vessel in the umbilical cord.

Pericarditis   Inflammation of the pericardium, a two-layer membrane covering the heart.

Periodic breathing   Cycles during which breathing slows and quickens, interspersed with short nonbreathing periods.

Periodic paralysis   Recurrent episodes of muscular weakness or flaccid paralysis, often triggered by anxiety or postexercise fatigue.

Peripheral neuropathy   A disease of the peripheral nerves, causing weakness and numbness.

Peristalsis   A wave of muscular contractions that pushes materials along the digestive tract.

Peritoneum   The serous membrane that lines the abdominal organs.

Peritonitis   Inflammation of the peritoneum.

Permanent teeth   The 32 adult teeth that begin to erupt at about 6 years of age and are usually all in place between ages 16 and 20.

Peroneal muscular atrophy   A neuropathy that becomes apparent in the teen years and is characterized by footdrop and awkward gait, with occasional involvement of the arms and hands.

Persistent fetal circulation A condition in which a newborn's blood continues to bypass the lungs, as it did before birth.

Pertussis An infectious disease caused by the *Bordetella pertussis* bacillus and characterized by a paroxysmal cough. Whooping cough.

Pervasive developmental disorder Impaired development of social interaction, communication, and imaginative activities. Cognitive skills and personal habits may also be impaired.

Petechiae Small hemorrhages under the skin.

Petit mal seizure See **Nonconvulsive seizure.**

Pharyngitis Inflammation of the pharynx. A sore throat.

Pharynx The throat.

Phenylketonuria (PKU) A hereditary metabolic disease caused by a defective enzyme in the body. Untreated, it causes severe brain damage. By law, the blood of all newborn babies is tested for the condition and other serious metabolic diseases.

Phimosis Constriction of the foreskin of the penis.

Phlegm Mucus.

Phobia An abnormally excessive and irrational fear.

Phoropter A masklike instrument into which different strengths of corrective lenses are inserted during an eye examination.

Phosphate A salt of phosphoric acid, important in maintaining the blood's acid-base balance.

Photosensitive seizure A type of generalized epileptic seizure brought on by rapidly flashing lights.

Phototherapy Treatment of jaundice in a newborn, by exposure to ultraviolet light.

Physiologic anemia The dramatic reduction in red blood cell production that occurs in the first few weeks of life.

Pica Repetitive eating of nonnutritive substances as well as food for at least one month.

Pierre-Robin anomaly A condition in which a newborn's jaw is unusually small, allowing the tongue to block the airway.

Pigmented nevus A mole.

Pineal gland A small gland, conical in structure, located on the back of the midbrain. Its function is not fully understood but it may be concerned with regulation of growth or of the sex glands.

Pinworms Easily transmitted intestinal parasites, also called *Enterobius vermicularis,* that lay eggs in the anal region that can then be rubbed off on bedding or become airborne in dust.

Pituitary gland The pea-size gland located at the base of the brain. It is controlled by the hypothalamus and it, in turn, controls the hormone production in many other endocrine glands.

Pityriasis rosea A skin rash of oval red patches usually on the trunk and upper extremities.

PKU See **Phenylketonuria.**

Placenta The structure developed on the uterine wall about the third month of pregnancy. Through the placenta, the fetus receives nourishment and oxygen and eliminates waste products. It is expelled from the mother after childbirth. The afterbirth.

Plaque Patch or film of organic substance on tissues, such as teeth or arterial walls.

Plasma The part of the blood composed mostly of water (over 90 percent). The other constituents include electrolytes, nutrients, wastes, clotting agents, antibodies, and hormones.

Platelets The colorless bodies in the blood instrumental to blood clotting. Also called **thrombocytes.**

Pleura The membrane lining the chest cavity and covering the lungs.

Pleural empyema Pus in the area surrounding the lung.

Pleurisy Inflammation of the pleura.

Pneumocystis carinii pneumonia A chronic lung infection caused by a single-celled organism, mainly seen in patients with immunodeficiency diseases.

Pneumoencephalography A method of examining structures within the brain, done by withdrawing cerebrospinal fluid and injecting air into the remaining spaces, then taking X rays.

Pneumonectomy Removal of one lung.

Pneumonia Infection of the lungs. May be bacterial, viral, chemical, or mycotic (fungal). Bacterial types include **pneumoccal** (most common), **staphylococcal, H. influenzae, Friedlander's bacillus, chlamydial,** and **mycoplasma.** Viral pneumonias have several causative agents, including rhinovirus, adenovirus, influenza respiratory syncytial virus, and parainfluenza. Chemical pneumonia is most commonly caused by inhalation of hydrocarbons such as kerosene or charcoal lighter fluid. Mycotic pneumonia is most common in immunosuppressed individuals.

Pneumothorax Lung collapse due to air or gas in the chest cavity.

Poliomyelitis An infectious disease marked by inflammation of the gray matter of the spinal column.

Pollen Microscopic grains of plant protein used for reproduction.

Polycystic kidney disease In infants, an inherited, congenital disorder in which numerous cysts on the kidneys cause enlargement and reduced kidney function. In adults the disease is also hereditary but develops later in life.

Polycythemia Excess red blood cells.

Polyp A nodular tumor, usually benign, that grows on a mucous membrane.

Pompholyx See **Dyshidrotic eczema.**

Postauricular hearing aid A behind-the-ear hearing aid containing a battery and amplifier that are attached to an earphone that fits inside the ear.

Posterior urethral valves A congenital urethral obstruction in males.

Post-traumatic stress disorder Fear persisting for more than a month after a traumatic event, along with repeated recall of the event and, in children, loss of established developmental skills.

Prader-Willi syndrome Muscular hypotonia and difficulty swallowing in infancy, followed by mental retardation and obesity later in childhood. Also called **floppy infant syndrome.**

Precocious puberty Puberty beginning before age eight in girls and age nine and a half in boys.

Preeclampsia A toxic condition of pregnancy characterized by high blood pressure, edema, and kidney malfunction.

Prematurity Birth between the 20th and 38th weeks of gestation.

Prickly heat See **Miliaria.**

Primary irritant dermatitis Skin inflammation caused by direct contact with an irritant.

Primary teeth A baby's first 20 teeth.

Processus vaginalis A saclike projection of the peritoneum.

Proctoscopy Endoscopic examination of the rectum.

Prodrome A symptom or group of symptoms indicating the approach of an illness.

Prophylactic Preventive.

Prostaglandins Hormonelike substances, secreted by a wide range of body tissues, that perform varying functions in the body. They are instrumental in stimulating uterine contractions during labor and birth and are also important in muscle function.

Prosthesis An artificial limb or other body part.

Proteinurea Protein in the urine.

Prothrombin A substance in the blood that forms thrombin, an enzyme essential to blood coagulation.

Pseudohypoparathyroidism A low level of calcium in the blood because of present but ineffective parathyroid hormone.

Pseudomembranous enterocolitis Inflammation of the intestines and colon accompanied by development of a pseudomembrane, or false membrane.

Psittacosis A disease similar to pneumonia and transmitted to humans by exposure to infected birds, such as pigeons.

Psoriasis A chronic skin condition characterized by the appearance of red skin lesions covered with silvery scales, arising from the overgrowth of certain skin cells.

PT Prothrombin time. A blood test that measures the function of blood coagulation factors.

PTT Partial prothrombin time. A blood test that measures the function of blood coagulation factors.

Ptosis Drooping of an eyelid or both eyelids.

Pulmonary Pertaining to the lungs.

Pulmonary atresia A congenital heart defect in which the valve between the right ventricle of the heart and the pulmonary artery is closed.

Pulmonary edema Buildup of fluid in the lungs. May be **hemodynamic,** or caused by elevated pressure in pulmonary blood vessels, or **permeability,** caused by infections that impair the permeability of the membrane covering the alveoli.

Pulmonary hemorrhage Bleeding in and around the alveoli.

Pulmonary stenosis Narrowing of the pathway between the right side of the heart and the lungs.

Pulmonary valve The valve between the right ventricle of the heart and the pulmonary artery.

Pupil The opening in the iris of the eye that allows the passage of light to the retina.

Pyloric canal The narrow region, or antrum, of the stomach leading to the duodenum.

Pyloric stenosis Congenital obstruction of the pyloric valve.

Rabies Hydrophobia. A deadly disease of the central nervous system caused by the rabies virus and spread by the bite of an infected animal.

Radioallergosorbent test (RAST) A blood test that determines whether an individual is allergic to a substance.

Rales Abnormal sounds from the lungs or bronchi.

Rapid maturer A child whose physical maturation is ahead of chronological age.

Recessive gene A gene that, when inherited from only one parent, does not produce a trait but can be transmitted to the next generation.

Rectal prolapse Protrusion of rectal mucous membrane through the anus.

Rectum The portion of the large intestine closest to the anal opening. It consists of the rectal canal and the anal canal.

Red blood cells (or red cells) See **Erythrocytes.**

Reduction Realignment of the pieces of a broken bone in their proper position. In **open reduction,** this realignment is performed after an incision is made at the fracture site.

Reflex seizure A type of epileptic seizure precipitated by a specific stimulus.

Refsum's syndrome An inherited disease of fat metabolism that causes visual disturbances and heart disease.

Regionalized neonatal care A system under which certain hospitals (usually major medical centers) maintain the most advanced equipment and best trained personnel for neonatal care. All high-risk patients from a defined geographic area may receive care at such hospitals, also known as Level III, or tertiary care, centers.

REM Rapid eye movement. The first stage of sleep, marked by movement of the eyes beneath the eyelids.

Renal Pertaining to the kidneys.

Renal artery The branch of the aorta through which blood enters the kidney.

Renal glycosuria Glucose in the urine caused by some abnormality in the renal tubules rather than diabetes.

Renal tubular acidosis A congenital disorder in which the renal tubules cannot reabsorb bicarbonate.

Renal tubules Small tubes within the kidneys in which waste chemicals are filtered out of the blood, while water, nutrients, and salts are retained.

Renal vein The vein through which cleansed blood leaves the kidney.

Renin An enzyme released by the glomeruli to regulate blood pressure.

Respiratory distress syndrome (RDS) A condition affecting newborn, especially preterm infants. The most common cause is **hyaline membrane disease,** in which the immature lungs cannot produce pulmonary surfactant, without which breathing is difficult, and hypoxia occurs.

Respiratory syncytial virus (RSV) A type of common

cold virus that gets its name from changes it causes in cell cultures. RSV infections are particularly common in children and may progress to bronchiolitis.

Reticulocyte An immature red blood cell containing a network of granules and filaments.

Retina The layered lining of the eye that contains light-sensitive receptors (the rods and cones) and conveys images to the brain.

Retinal detachment Separation of the retina from the blood vessels at the back of the eyeball, usually caused by injury.

Retinitis pigmentosa A hereditary condition in which the retina gradually degenerates. Symptoms usually progress from loss of night vision to loss of peripheral vision during childhood, with central vision usually preserved into adulthood. The condition is sex-linked, which means that women without symptoms who carry the gene have a 50 percent chance of transmitting it to their children. Any sons who inherit the gene will have the disease.

Retinoblastoma Malignant tumor of the retina, which is hereditary in 20 percent of cases.

Retinopathy An injury or disease of the retina, particularly common in insulin-dependent diabetes. **Retinopathy of prematurity (ROP)** occurs in premature infants whose retinal capillaries cease to develop because of oxygen therapy and other unknown factors, then resume development in an abnormal pattern.

Retractile testicles Testicles that can, at times, be seen in the scrotum but usually are not visible.

Retropharyngeal abscess An abscess in the lymph nodes at the back of the larynx, often arising from a sore throat, sinus infection, or ear infection.

Retrovirus A virus containing the enzyme reverse transcriptase. Examples include HIV (human immunodeficiency virus) and several tumor viruses.

Reye's syndrome An illness of unknown origin occurring in children under 18 after a viral infection such as flu or chicken pox. Symptoms, including severe vomiting and changes in mental status, begin during recovery from the initial illness. Reye's syndrome has a high mortality rate if it is not treated promptly.

Rheumatic fever An acute, generalized inflammatory disease that may occur after an upper respiratory or skin infection with the group A streptococcus organism. Rheumatic fever can cause permanent heart damage. This can be prevented by appropriate treatment, usually with antibiotics.

Rheumatoid factor Abnormal protein present in the blood of most people with rheumatoid arthritis or other autoimmune diseases.

Rh factor A group of antigens in the blood. Some people lack the Rh factor and are therefore designated as Rh negative.

Rh factor disease The anemic condition in infants due to Rh incompatibility between mother and child. The condition is seen in Rh positive babies born to Rh negative women. The mother builds antibodies against the baby's blood, destroying the red blood cells. It is seen only rarely in first babies because the mother is not exposed to the baby's blood until delivery. The condition can now be prevented by giving the mother a shot of Rh immune globulin shortly after the birth of an Rh incompatible baby. Some doctors also administer the shot to an Rh negative woman during the last trimester of pregnancy if there is a chance that the baby may be Rh positive—that is, if the father has Rh positive blood. The disease is also called **erythroblastalis fetalis.**

Rhinitis Inflammation of the nasal passages and the back of the nose.

Rhinoviruses A group of about 100 viruses that cause common colds.

Rickets A childhood disease caused by a deficiency of vitamin D. (Also called nutritional rickets.) Symptoms include improper development of bones and teeth because of a calcium/phosphorus imbalance. **Vitamin D-resistant rickets** is a form of the disease resulting from a metabolic disorder in which the body is unable to utilize vitamin D.

Rickettsial disease A disease caused by a microorganism of the genus *Rickettsia*, usually transmitted by ticks, fleas, lice, or mites. Example: Rocky Mountain spotted fever.

Ringworm See **Tinea.**

Rocky Mountain spotted fever A rickettsial disease spread by ticks. Early symptoms include fever, vomiting, headache, and muscle pain. May progress to paralysis and death without antibiotic treatment.

Rod cells Specialized light-sensitive cells in the retina.

Root canal A dental procedure involving the pulp at the core of the tooth and descending below the gum.

Roseola Appearance of red spots of varying sizes on the skin. Also refers to an acute, febrile illness in children between six months and two years of age, a hallmark of which is a rash appearing as the fever subsides.

Rotavirus A wheel-shaped virus that commonly causes gastrointestinal illnesses, especially diarrhea in children and infants.

Rubella German measles. A mild infectious disease characterized by fever, cough, malaise, and the appearance of red spots on the body. May cause abnormalities, especially cataracts, in babies born to mothers who had the illness during pregnancy.

Rubeola Measles.

Rumination disorder of infancy Regurgitation of food, followed by chewing and reswallowing or ejection from the mouth, beginning at three months to one year of age and persisting at least a month.

Sacrum The triangular bone just above the coccyx (tailbone) near the lower end of the spine. It is composed of five vertebrae that have fused together. With the bones of the pelvis, it forms the sacroiliac joint.

Salmonella A group of bacteria primarily responsible for the gastrointestinal symptoms of food poisoning.

Salmon patch A flat red or pink birthmark usually on the nape of the neck, the eyelids, or the forehead.

Scabies Contagious skin infestation by the *Sarcoptes*

scabiei mite, which burrows under the skin to lay its eggs, causing intense itching.

Scarlet fever   A contagious disease characterized by sore throat, red tongue, and rash consisting of tiny red points covering all the body except the face. Caused by group A streptococci bacteria.

Sclera   White of the eye.

Scleroderma   A disease characterized by thickening of the skin because of swelling of the underlying fibrous connective tissue. Early symptoms may be similar to those of arthritis.

Scoliosis   An abnormal sideways curvature of the spine that often appears during the preadolescent growth spurt.

Sebaceous gland   An oil-producing gland at the base of a hair follicle.

Sebaceous gland hyperplasia   Papular facial lesions in an infant, caused by overactivity of the sebaceous glands in response to maternal hormones.

Seborrheic dermatitis   A scaly, yellowish, crusted rash on the scalp, face, and ears, caused in infants by over-active oil glands stimulated by maternal hormones.

Seizure   A sudden attack of any type of symptoms. Usually refers to an epileptic convulsion.

Sensorineural hearing loss   Hearing loss due to failure of the inner ear to transmit sound to the brain. In children, it may be congenital (caused by rubella, birth injury, Rh factor disease, or other conditions) or acquired (as a result of meningitis, encephalitis, drug side effects, tumors, or hereditary conditions).

Separation anxiety   Anxiety experienced by small children when separated from a parent. It may be severe enough to be classified as **separation anxiety disorder,** when anxiety reaches panic level and symptoms persist for at least two weeks.

Sepsis   The state of being infected by germs in the blood or tissues.

Septicemia   Blood poisoning.

Septum   A dividing wall between two compartments or cavities.

Sequestered lung   A lung that is partially cut off from the bronchial system or that receives only systemic, rather than pulmonary, circulation.

Serum   The fluid formed in the clotting of blood. Contains antibodies and is injected in vaccines to build up antibodies to specific diseases.

Serum sickness   An allergic reaction characterized by fever, lymph node enlargement, and joint pain, occurring from several days to three weeks after an immunization or drug treatment.

Severe combined immunodeficiency disease (SCID)   An inherited absence of disease-fighting antibodies.

Sex-linked   A term that describes the pattern of inheritance of traits from genes on the X and Y chromosomes, which are the chromosomes that determine gender.

Shigellosis   Dysentery. Bloody diarrhea caused by the shigella bacterium.

Shingles   See **Herpes zoster.**

Shunt   An artificial passage to divert flow of a fluid from one route to another.

Sickle-cell anemia   An inherited blood disorder in which the body manufactures an abnormal type of globin that twists red blood cells into a sickle shape, caus-ing chronic hemolytic anemia. Most prevalent among blacks, not to be confused with sickle trait, a benign condition.

Sickle thalassemia   A blood disorder similar to sickle-cell anemia that may occur in children of couples in which one member has sickle-cell trait (one copy of the sickle-cell anemia gene) and the other has beta-thalassemia trait (one copy of the beta-thalassemia gene).

SIDS   See **Sudden infant death syndrome.**

Sigmoid   The S-shaped portion of the descending colon.

Sigmoidoscopy   Endoscopic examination of the begin-ning of the large intestine.

Silo-filler's disease   A type of chemical pneumonia caused by high levels of nitrogen dioxide in recently-filled silos.

Sinusitis   Infection of the sinus passages, often caused by pneumococci and *Hemophilus influenzae* bacteria.

Skin test   Introduction of a suspected allergen into the skin to see whether a local reaction, indicative of al-lergy, appears.

Sleep terror disorder   See **Night terrors.**

Small for date   Smaller than normal birthweight. Also called **small for gestational age,** or **SGA.**

Smallpox   A contagious disease caused by the variola virus, now considered to have been eradicated.

Soft palate   The back of the roof of the mouth.

Solitary bone cyst   A growth containing fluid and connec-tive tissue that usually affects the shaft of a long bone and appears in children between the ages of five and fifteen.

Solitary kidney   A congenital abnormality in which a child is born with only one kidney instead of two.

Somnambulism   Sleepwalking. A state in which a sleep-ing person unconsciously performs activities associated with wakefulness.

Spasmodic croup   Nighttime croup attacks caused by al-lergies.

Spasticity   Increased muscle tone or contraction causing stiff, poorly controlled movements.

Sphincter   A ring of muscle that opens and controls open-ing of an orifice.

Spina bifida   A congenital defect in which some of the vertebrae fail to close and therefore expose the contents of the spinal canal.

Spinal abscess   A localized buildup of pus or focal infec-tion in the spinal column, usually arising from a lung or kidney infection.

Spinal tap   A procedure in which a needle is placed in the spinal canal to withdraw spinal fluid for diagnostic pur-poses or administration of anesthesia. Also called **lum-bar puncture.**

Spleen   A large lymphoid organ behind the stomach on the lower left side of the rib cage. Its functions include cleansing the blood of parasites and manufacturing lymphocytes. It is, however, not an organ essential to life since these functions can be performed elsewhere in the body.

Split nose A congenital fissure that divides the nose.

Sprain Injury to the supportive structures around a joint, usually including a ligament tear.

Squamous cell A flat, scalelike cell of the epithelium.

Stapes The innermost of the three small, vibration-magnifying bones of the middle ear. Also called **stirrup.**

Staphylococcus Spherical bacteria occurring in clusters and responsible for boils, toxic shock syndrome, food poisoning, osteomyelitis, bacterial arthritis, endocarditis, and other illnesses.

Static neurological disorder A disorder arising from an injury to the central nervous system during gestation, birth, or the neonatal period. Also called static incephalopathy.

Status asthmaticus Severe, persistent asthma that does not respond to treatment.

Stem cells Immature blood cells.

Stenosis Narrowing of a body passage, tube, or opening.

Stereotypy/habit disorder Repetitive, voluntary behaviors such as head banging that cause injury or disrupt activities.

Steroids Natural hormones or synthetic drugs that have many different effects. Some steroids are antiinflammatory and are used to treat arthritis, asthma, and a number of other disorders. Because of undesirable side effects, including growth retardation, steroids are used in treating children only for very short periods or applied directly to the inflamed tissue when no other treatments are available. Also called **cortisone** or **corticosteroids.**

Stillbirth Birth of a dead fetus after 20 weeks of pregnancy.

Still's disease See **Juvenile rheumatoid arthritis.**

Strabismus An eye disorder in which both eyes are unable to focus simultaneously. Cross-eyedness, walleye, or squint.

Strain Minor injury caused by misuse or overuse of a muscle.

Stranger anxiety Anxiety in an infant or small child when approached by an unknown person; often part of normal development.

Strawberry hemangioma See **Capillary hemangioma.**

Strep throat A severe sore throat caused by group A streptococci.

Streptococcus Spherical bacterium that grows in chains, responsible for infections such as strep throat and scarlet fever.

Stridor A harsh, croaking sound during breathing, caused by obstructed airways.

String test A test to detect duodenal parasites. The patient swallows a gelatin capsule containing a string, one end of which is taped to the cheek. After three to four hours, the string is removed and the mucus adhering to it is examined.

Stupor A state of impaired but not complete loss of consciousness and responsiveness.

St. Vitus' dance Involuntary twitching that sometimes occurs in rheumatic fever. Also called **Sydenham's chorea.**

Sty A pimple in an eyelash follicle, usually caused by staphylococcus bacteria. Also called **hordeolum.**

Subconjunctival hemorrhages Bright red spots in the white of the eye, usually caused by coughing or an injury.

Subdural hemorrhage Bleeding beneath the hard tissue that encloses the brain.

Subependymal hemorrhage The least severe form of intraventricular hemorrhage in which bleeding occurs only in a small area of the central brain.

Subglottis stenosis Narrowing of the trachea from prolonged use of an endotracheal tube.

Sudden infant death syndrome (SIDS) Death of a child between one month and one year of age (usually at two to four months) for no apparent cause, often during sleep. Also called **crib death.**

Supple flat foot A condition usually related to laxity of foot ligaments, in which the foot is flat when bearing weight but arched when resting. Treatment is usually unnecessary.

Suprapubic tap Method of obtaining a clean urine sample by inserting a needle through the skin above the pubic bone into the bladder.

Surfactant A lubricant manufactured by the lungs, necessary for the alveoli to remain inflated.

Swimmer's ear See **Otitis externa.**

Sympathetic ophthalmia Unexplained total blindness occurring after an injury-blinded eye is left in place for longer than 12 days.

Synapse The point of communication between nerve endings.

Syncope Fainting.

Synovial fluid The viscid fluid that lubricates joints.

Syphilis A chronic, sexually transmitted disease that usually begins with skin manifestations then progresses to neurological and cardiac symptoms if untreated. Babies of women with syphilis can be born with **congenital syphilis** and exhibit a number of symptoms, including rashes, persistent runny nose, and bone lesions.

Syringomyelia Development of a fluid-filled sac in the spinal cord, usually in the neck or shoulder area. May be congenital, but usually develops later in life.

Systemic lupus erythematosus An inflammatory autoimmune disease involving deterioration of the body's connective tissues.

Systole The contraction of the heart muscle. Systolic blood pressure is the greater of the two blood pressure readings.

Tachycardia Abnormally rapid heart rate.

Tachypnea Rapid breathing.

Tapeworm An intestinal parasite acquired by eating undercooked beef or pork.

Target organs Organs that are responsive to a given hormone.

Tay-Sachs disease An inherited disease affecting the fat metabolism and the brain and characterized by progressive weakness, disability, and blindness, and finally death. Most common among Jews of Eastern European descent, it is inherited in the recessive pattern, which means that both parents must transmit the disease gene to the child for the child to develop the disease.

T cells Lymphocytes that attack foreign and virus-infected cells.

Telangiectasis Dilatation and breakdown of blood vessels.

Telogen Resting or shedding phase of hair-growth cycle.

Telogen effluvium Shedding of scalp hair often occurring in both infant and mother after birth. May be caused by hormone fluctuation.

Testicular feminization, complete Female genitalia in a genetic male caused by inability to utilize the hormone testosterone.

Testicular feminization, incomplete Abnormal female genitalia (enlarged clitoris and partially fused labia) in a genetic male.

Testicular torsion Twisting of the spermatic cord from which a testicle is suspended in the scrotum.

Tetanus An infectious disease caused by the toxin of the *Clostridium tetani* bacillus growing at the site of a wound.

Tetralogy of Fallot A congenital heart defect consisting of four different malformations: (1) a hole between the ventricles, (2) a narrowing of the opening between the pulmonary artery and the right ventricle, (3) enlargement of the right ventricle, and (4) misplacement of the aorta, so that it receives blood from both ventricles.

Thalamus The egg-shaped mass of gray matter at the base of the cerebrum that acts as a relay station for the body's major sensory pathways.

Thalassemia A group of hereditary blood diseases caused by defective production or synthesis of a certain component of hemoglobin. **Beta-thalassemia** (also called **Cooley's anemia** or **Mediterranean anemia**) occurs when the beta-globin component is missing. In **alpha-thalassemia,** alpha-globin production is deficient.

Thorax The chest.

Thrombocytopenia Decrease in the number of platelets in the blood.

Thromboplastin A blood coagulation factor found in both blood and tissues.

Thrombosis The formation of a blood clot that partially or completely blocks the blood vessel.

Thrush A fungal infection (candidiasis) of the mouth, often occurring in infancy but also in conditions of immunosuppression.

Thyroid gland The ductless gland located in the neck. The secretions of the thyroid gland control the rate of metabolism, among other functions.

Thyroid stimulating hormone (TSH) A pituitary hormone that causes the thyroid gland to secrete thyroid hormone.

Thyroxine A hormone produced by the thyroid gland.

Tibia The shinbone. The larger (inner) of the two bones of the lower leg.

Tic Involuntary spasmodic movements or twitching.

Tick paralysis A temporary neuropathy caused by a bite from a tick carrying Rocky Mountain spotted fever.

Tinea A contagious fungal infection of the hair, skin, or feet, commonly called **ringworm. Tinea capitis** is infection of the hair shafts, causing lesions on the scalp. Often appears as a reddish, elevated ring accompanied by broken hairs and localized hair loss. **Tinea corporis** is infection of the skin. **Tinea pedia,** or athlete's foot, is fungal infection of the foot characterized by itching, small sores, and cracks on the skin.

Tine test A skin test for tuberculosis in which a tuberculosis antigen derivative is pressed into the skin on four small prongs. The site of the impression is then checked after 48 and 72 hours for signs of a reaction.

Tinnitus Ringing or other persistent sounds in the ears.

Tonic-clonic seizure A generalized convulsion marked by unconsciousness and involvement of all limbs. Also called **grand mal seizure.**

Tonsillectomy Surgical removal of the tonsils.

Tonsillitis Inflammation of the tonsils.

Tonsils The two masses of lymphoid tissue covered by mucous membrane that are located on each side of the back of the throat.

TORCH *T*oxoplasmosis, *r*ubella, *c*ytomegalovirus, and *h*erpes. The most common intrauterine infections that can harm the fetus. A test for each of these infections, called a TORCH test, may be performed when a neonate shows signs of infection.

Torsion Twisting.

Total anomalous pulmonary venous connection A congenital heart defect in which an abnormal vein carries oxygenated blood from the lungs to the right atrium instead of the left, where it normally goes. This defect is generally accompanied by an atrial septal defect.

Tourette's disorder (or syndrome) A neurological disorder with a variety of symptoms including tics, purposeless movement, and inappropriate vocalizing. The syndrome is believed to stem from a metabolic disorder.

Toxemia Blood poisoning. A condition in which poisonous compounds are present in the bloodstream. **Toxemia of pregnancy** is another name for eclampsia.

Toxicara An intestinal parasite that usually infects dogs and cats but may be contracted by children who touch soil contaminated by animal feces. Also called **visceral larva migrans.**

Toxic shock syndrome An acute form of blood poisoning caused by *Staphylococcus aureus* bacteria. It is associated with the use of superabsorbent tampons during menstruation but has been reported in men and children as well.

Toxoplasmosis A parasitic disease caused by an organism called *Toxoplasma gondii*, often contracted from cat feces or undercooked meat. Symptoms may be mild, but infection can be passed to the fetus during pregnancy, often causing severe birth defects such as blindness and neurological damage.

Trachea The windpipe. The tube that extends from the larynx to the bronchi.

Tracheal stenosis Congenital narrowing of the tracheal opening.

Tracheitis Inflammation of the windpipe.

Tracheoesophageal fistula A congenital abnormality in which the esophagus does not connect with the stomach and a false passage exists between the stomach and trachea.

Tracheomalacia Softening of the cartilage of the trachea, leading to excessive narrowing.

Tracheostomy A surgically created opening in the neck to admit an endotracheal tube below the vocal cords.

Traction Continuous pulling of a body part using weights and pulleys. Used in treatment of dislocations, deformity, fracture, and severe muscle spasm.

Transcutaneous monitoring A noninvasive method of measuring blood gases using electrodes attached to the skin.

Transient tic disorder Motor and/or vocal tics occurring several times a day for at least two weeks but no longer than 12 months.

Transposition of the great arteries A congenital heart defect in which the aorta and pulmonary arteries are reversed so that unoxygenated blood flows out of the heart through the aorta and oxygenated blood flows through the pulmonary artery.

Transverse myelitis Inflammation of a portion of the spinal cord, frequently following a viral infection.

Triage Screening and classification of patients in emergency settings according to the severity of their conditions in order to set priorities for their treatment.

Trichotillomania A tendency to pull out one's own hair.

Tricuspid atresia A congenital heart defect in which the tricuspid valve is closed.

Tricuspid valve The valve between the right atrium and ventricle of the heart.

Triglycerides The most common lipid found in fatty tissue. A high level of triglyceride may increase the risk of blood vessel or heart disease.

True hermaphroditism Presence of both ovarian and testicular tissue, either combined in one organ or as separate organs.

Truncus arteriosus A congenital heart defect in which the aorta and pulmonary artery come from a single blood vessel and there is a hole between the ventricles.

Tuberculin skin test A skin test used to detect tuberculosis or tuberculosis sensitivity. An extract of tubercle bacilli is injected into the skin and a positive reaction indicates possible tuberculosis or a previous exposure to the disease.

Tuberculosis (TB) An infectious disease affecting the lungs most often but also other parts of the body. It is caused by the tubercle bacillus and symptoms include cough, chest pains, fatigue, sweating, and weight loss.

Turner's syndrome Absence of one X chromosome, causing short stature, infertility, and underdeveloped ovaries.

Tympanic membrane Eardrum. A thin, tough membrane that stretches across the ear canal.

Typhoid fever A bacterial infection caused by *Salmonella typhi* organisms and spread through contaminated milk, water, or food, especially shellfish. Symptoms include fever and diarrhea, and the disease may cause fatal dehydration.

Ultrasonography Use of high-frequency sound waves, which travel at different velocities through tissues of different densities, to create an image of organs and tissues.

Umbilical artery catheter A tube inserted into a newborn's aorta through an umbilical artery.

Underdeveloped left heart A congenital heart defect in which either or both the aortic or mitral valves are absent. Also called **hypoplastic left ventricle** or **hypoplastic left heart.**

Undescended testes Failure of one or both testicles to have passed down from the peritoneal cavity to the scrotum. Also called **cryptorchid testes.**

Unilateral seizure A type of epileptic seizure caused by damage to one cerebral hemisphere and affecting one side of the body.

Urachal cyst Abnormal opening in the central portion of the urachus that remains after the ends adjoining the umbilicus and bladder have closed.

Urachus A tube connecting the fetal bladder to the umbilicus.

Urate A salt of uric acid that sometimes leaves pink stains on the diapers of newborns.

Urea The nitrogen-containing waste product of protein breakdown that is excreted as the main component of urine.

Uremia A condition in which toxic substances remain in the blood due to the failure of the kidneys to filter out and excrete them.

Ureter One of the two tubes connecting the kidneys to the bladder and through which urine passes (by means of muscle contractions) into the bladder.

Ureteral bud The primitive ureter that forms at about five weeks' gestation.

Ureteral duplication A congenital malformation in which two ureters connect one kidney to the bladder.

Ureterocele A congenital malformation in which the muscles at the junction of the ureter and bladder are absent, causing the ureter to balloon.

Ureteropelvic junction obstruction (UPJ) A congenital malformation in which the junction of the ureter and renal pelvis is narrowed, obstructing the flow of urine from the kidney to the bladder.

Uretero vesical reflux Backward flow of urine from the bladder to the ureters, a frequent cause of urinary tract infections in children.

Urethra The tube through which urine passes from the bladder to the outside. In the female, it is about an inch and a half long; in the male, it is eight to nine inches long.

Uric acid An acid that is the waste product of metabolism. It is usually excreted in the urine.

Urinalysis Examination and analysis of the urine for diagnostic purposes.

Urticaria See **Hives.**

Urushiol The resin in poison ivy, poison oak, and poison sumac that causes contact dermatitis in susceptible individuals.

Uvula The small tag of tissue that hangs from the center of the soft palate at the back of the throat.

Vagus The cranial nerve that extends from the brain to serve the stomach, intestines, esophagus, larynx, lungs, and heart.

Van Bogaert's disease   A rare disorder of lipid metabolism.

Varicella-zoster immune globulin (VZIG)   Immune globulins or proteins that act an antibodies to the chicken pox virus and are administered to children with various types of cancer to prevent infection after exposure to chicken pox.

Vas deferens   The duct of the testes through which the spermatozoa must pass in ejaculation.

Vasopressin   A pituitary hormone that controls water output through the kidney.

VDRL (venereal disease research laboratory)   A blood test that detects an antibodylike substance that indicates infection with syphilis.

Velopharyngeal insufficiency   A congenital malformation of the palate and back of the throat, making speech and swallowing difficult.

Venous switch   A surgical procedure to correct transposition of the great arteries of the heart. The surgeon makes a tunnel inside the right atrium, allowing oxygenated blood to flow through the right ventricle to the aorta and nonoxygenated blood to flow through the left ventricle to the pulmonary artery. Also called **intra-atrial baffle** or a **Mustard** or **Sennig procedure.**

Ventricles   The lower two chambers of the heart, whose function is to pump blood.

Ventricular septal defect   A congenital heart defect in which there is an opening between the right and left ventricles.

Ventricular tachycardia   Rapid heart rate, usually between 150 and 200 beats per minute, arising from one of the ventricles.

Vermiform appendix   A narrow tube, commonly referred to as appendix, connected to the cecum. See **Cecum.**

Vernix caseosa   A fatty substance that covers the fetus, consisting of dead skin cells and oil. The substance serves to protect the fetus's skin.

Verrucae   Warts. Benign skin growths caused by a virus. **Verruca vulgaris** is the common wart, a skin-colored bump or cluster of bumps, usually occurring on the sides of the fingers. **Verruca plana** is the flat wart, a skin-colored or light brown lesion usually occurring on the face, backs of hands, or arms and legs. **Verruca plantaris** is a wart on the sole of the foot.

Vertebra   One of the 33 flat, roundish bones that make up the spinal column.

Vertigo   Dizziness; a spinning sensation.

Villus   A microscopic finger-shaped projection such as those found in the mucous lining of the stomach walls.

Visual cortex   The area of the brain that interprets the electrical impulses that are converted from the light signals perceived by the eyes.

Vitiligo   White patches on the skin due to loss of pigment.

Vitreous chamber   The round area behind the lens of the eye, containing the vitreous humor.

Vitreous humor   The jellylike substance that is found between the lens and the retina and that supports the interior parts of the eye.

Voiding cytourethrogram (VCU)   An X ray of the bladder and urethra taken after the patient is catheterized and fluid is infused into the bladder.

Von Willebrand's disease   An inherited clotting disorder that appears in both sexes and is usually mild.

Werdnig-Hoffman disease   See **Muscular spinal atrophy.**

White blood cells   See **Leukocytes.**

Wilms' tumor   A kidney tumor, the most common urinary tract malignancy in children.

Wry neck   See **Paroxysmal torticollis.**

Index